D1172175

Surgical Decision Making

Surgical Decision Making

FIFTH EDITION

Robert C. McIntyre, Jr., MD
Associate Professor, Division of GI, Tumor, and
Endocrine Surgery, University of Colorado
Health Sciences Center, Denver, Colorado

Gregory V. Stiegmann, MD
Professor of Surgery and Division Head,
Division of GI, Tumor, and Endocrine Surgery,
University of Colorado Health Sciences Center;
Vice President of Clinical Affairs, University of
Colorado Hospital, Denver, Colorado

Ben Eiseman, MD
Professor of Emeritus Surgery,
University of Colorado Health Sciences Center,
Denver, Colorado

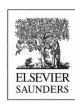

ELSEVIER
SAUNDERS

ELSEVIER
SAUNDERS

The Curtis Center
170 S Independence Mall W 300E
Philadelphia, Pennsylvania 19106

Notice

Surgery is an ever-changing field. Standard safety precautions must be followed, but as new research
and clinical experience broaden our knowledge, changes in treatment and drug therapy may become
necessary or appropriate. Readers are advised to check the most current product information
provided by the manufacturer of each drug to be administered to verify the recommended dose, the
method and duration of administration, and contraindications. It is the responsibility of the treating
physician, relying on experience and knowledge of the patient, to determine dosages and the best
treatment for each individual patient. Neither the publisher nor the authors assume any liability for
any injury and/or damage to persons or property arising from this publication.

Previous editions copyrighted 2000, 1993, 1986, 1978

Library of Congress Cataloging-in-Publication Data

Surgical decision making / [edited by] Robert C. McIntyre, Gregory V. Stiegmann, Ben
    Eiseman.–5th ed.
        p. ; cm.
    Includes bibliographical references and index.
    ISBN 0-7216-0290-8
        1. Surgery–Decision making. I. McIntyre, Robert C. II. Stiegmann, Gregory Van. III.
Eiseman, Ben, 1917-
    [DNLM: 1. Decision Making. 2. Surgical Procedures, Operative. 3. Decision Trees. WO
100 S9623 2004]
    RD31.5.S87 2004
    617–dc22

                                                                    2003066252

Printed in the United States of America

Last digit is the print number: 9   8   7   6   5   4   3   2   1

CONTRIBUTORS

Ruben J. Alvero, MD
Associate Professor of OB-GYN, University of
Colorado Health Sciences Center, Aurora, Colorado;
Attending Physician, University of Colorado, Denver,
Colorado; Adjunct Associate Professor, OB-GYN
Uniformed Services University of Health Sciences,
Bethesda, Maryland
  Endometriosis

Christopher D. Anderson, MD
Surgical Fellow, Department of Surgery,
Vanderbilt University Medical Center, Nashville,
Tennessee
  Liver Tumor

Erica D. Anderson, MD
Fellow, Division of Plastic Surgery, University of
Colorado Health Sciences Center, Denver,
Colorado
  Non-Melanoma Skin Cancer of the Face

Robert J. Anderson, MD
Meiklejohn Professor of Medicine, Professor and
Division Chief, University Medicine, University of
Colorado Health Sciences Center, Denver, Colorado
  Acute Renal Failure

Jyoti Arya, MD
Assistant Professor of Surgery, GI Tumor and
Endocrine Surgery, University of Colorado Health
Sciences Center, Denver, Colorado
  Occult Breast Lesions

Glenn T. Ault, MD, MSEd
Assistant Professor of Surgery, Department of
Colorectal Surgery, Keck School of Medicine,
University of Southern California, Los Angeles,
California
  Ulcerative Colitis

Thomas E. Bak, MD
Assistant Professor of Transplant Surgery, University
of Colorado Health Sciences Center, Denver,
Colorado
  Jaundice; Kidney Transplantation;
  Liver Transplantation

Carlton C. Barnett, Jr., MD
Assistant Professor, Department of Surgery,
University of Texas Southwestern Medical Center,
Dallas, Texas
  Cancer of Unknown Primary

Katherine A. Barsness, MD
Chief Resident, Department of Surgery, University of
Colorado Health Sciences Center, Denver,
Colorado
  Small Bowel Obstruction

Robert Bartlett, MD
Professor of Surgery, Director of Surgical
Critical Care, University of Michigan, Ann Arbor,
Michigan
  Acute Respiratory Failure

Robert W. Beart, Jr., MD
Professor and Chairman, Department of
Colorectal Surgery, University of Southern California
Keck School of Medicine, Los Angeles,
California
  Ulcerative Colitis

Kian Behbakht, MD
Assistant Professor of OB-GYN, Gynecologic,
Oncology, University of Colorado Health Sciences
Center; Attending Physician of OB-GYN,
Gynecologic Oncology, University of Colorado
Health Sciences Center, Denver, Colorado
  Ovarian Mass

Denis D. Bensard, MD
Associate Professor of Surgery/Pediatrics,
Department of Surgery, University of Colorado
Health Sciences Center; Director, Trauma, Surgery
Department, The Children's Hospital, Denver,
Colorado
  Infantile Hypertrophic Pyloric Stenosis;
  Neonatal Bowel Obstruction

Michael Bergen, MD
Fellow, Department of Oncology, Division of
Cutaneous Oncology, University of Colorado Health
Sciences Center, Denver, Colorado
  Melanoma

Ross S. Berkowitz, MD
William H. Baker Professor of Gynecologic
Oncology, Department of Obstetrics and
Gynecology, Harvard Medical School; Director of
Gynecology and Gynecologic Oncology, Brigham
and Women's Medical Hospital; Director of
Gynecology and Gynecologic Oncology, Dana
Farber Cancer Institute, Boston, Massachusetts
  Endometrial Carcinoma

Mark R. Bielefeld, MD
Assistant Professor, Department of Pediatrics, Texas
A&M University Health Science Center, College
Station, Texas; Attending Pediatric Cardiothoracic
Surgeon, Driscoll Children's Hospital, Corpus Christi,
Texas
  Neonatal Cyanosis; Cyanotic Congenital Heart Disease

Walter L. Biffl, MD
Chief, Division of Trauma and Surgical Critical Care,
Rhode Island Hospital, Associate Professor of
Surgery, Brown Medical School, Providence, Rhode
Island
  Blunt Abdominal Trauma

Michael Sean Boger, MD, PharmD
House Officer, Department of Internal Medicine, Wake Forest University Baptist Medical Center, Winston-Salem, North Carolina
Cushing's Syndrome

Robert E. Breeze, MD
Professor, Neurosurgery, University of Colorado Health Sciences Center, Denver, Colorado
Closed Head Injury; Cervical Spine Fractures

Murray F. Brennan, MD
Chairman, Department of Surgery, Memorial Sloan-Kettering Cancer Center, New York, New York
Retroperitoneal Mass

Laurence H. Brinckerhoff, MD
Chief Resident, Cardiothoracic Surgery, Division of Cardiothoracic Surgery, University of Colorado Health Sciences Center, Denver, Colorado
Pleural Effusion and Empyema; Carcinoma of the Lung

L.D. Britt, MD, MPH
Brickhouse Professor and Chairman, Eastern Virginia Medical School, Department of Surgery, Norfolk, Virginia
Penetrating Neck Injury

James M. Brown, MD
Associate Professor of Surgery, Department of Surgery/Division of Cardiac Surgery, University of Maryland—School of Medicine; Associate Professor of Surgery, Department of Surgery/Division of Cardiac Surgery, University of Maryland Medical System, Baltimore, Maryland
Perioperative Arrythmia

Tommy Brown, MD
Chief, Surgical Oncology, Madican Army Medical Center, Tacoma, Washington
Carcinoma of the Oral Cavity

Jon M. Burch, MD
Professor of Surgery, Department of Surgery, University of Colorado Health Sciences Center; Chief, General and Vascular Surgery, Denver Health Medical Center, Denver, Colorado
Shock; Thoracic Aorta Injury; Penetrating Injury of the Colon; Popliteal Artery Injury

Blake Cady, MD
Professor of Surgery, Brown University; Director of Breast Health Center, Women and Infants Hospital, Providence, Rhode Island
Recurrent Breast Carcinoma

Christopher A. Caldarone, MD
University of Iowa; University of Iowa Hospitals & Clinics, Cardiothoracic Surgery, Iowa City, Iowa
Patent Ductus Arteriosus

Mark P. Callery, MD
Associate Professor of Surgery, Harvard Medical School; Chief, Division of General Surgery, Beth Israel-Deaconess Medical Center, Boston, Massachusetts
Liver Tumor

John L. Cameron, MD
Alfred Blalock Distinguished Professor of Surgery, Department of Surgery, The Johns Hopkins University School of Medicine, Baltimore, Maryland
Periampullary Carcinoma

John P. Campana, MD
Assistant Professor, Department of Otolaryngology, University of Colorado Health Sciences Center, Denver, Colorado
Epistaxis

David N. Campbell, MD
Professor of Surgery, Division of Cardiothoracic Surgery, University of Colorado Health Sciences Center; Staff Surgeon, Pediatric Cardiothoracic Surgery, The Children's Hospital, Denver, Colorado
Congenital Obstructive Cardiac Anomalies; Congenital Septal Defects; Heart Transplantation

Soren N. Carlsen, MD
Urology Resident, Department of Surgery/Urology, University of Colorado Health Sciences Center, Denver, Colorado
Urinary Diversion

Peter R. Carroll, MD
Professor and Chair, Department of Urology, University of California, San Francisco, California
Bladder Tumor

Frank H. Chae, MD, CM
Assistant Professor of Surgery, Department of Surgery, University of Colorado Health Sciences Center; Attending Physician, Department of Surgery, University of Colorado Health Sciences Center, Denver, Colorado
Cholelithiasis (Gallstones); Choledocholithiasis (Common Bile Duct Stones)

Paul J. Chai, MD
Fellow, Cardiothoracic Surgery, Department of Surgery, Duke University Medical Center, Durham, North Carolina
Coarctation of the Aorta

Michael C. Chang, MD
Associate Professor of Surgery; Director, Trauma and Burn Services, Wake Forest University Health Sciences, Winston-Salem, North Carolina
Goal-Directed Resuscitation

Ravi S. Chari, MD
Associate Professor of Surgery and Cancer Biology, Department of Surgery, Vanderbilt University Medical Center, Nashville, Tennessee
Liver Tumor

W. Randolph Chitwood, Jr., MD
Senior Associate Vice Chancellor—Health Sciences, Professor of Surgery, Chief, Division of Cardiothoracic and Vascular Surgery, Brody School of Medicine, East Carolina University, Greenville, North Carolina
Pulmonary Embolism

Maureen Chung, MD, PhD

Assistant Professor, Department of Surgery, Brown University, Providence, Rhode Island

Recurrent Breast Carcinoma

David J. Ciesla, MD

Assistant Professor of Surgery, Department of Surgery, University of Colorado School of Medicine; Chief of Pediatric Trauma, Department of Surgery, Denver Health Medical Center, Denver, Colorado

Postoperative Fever

William G. Cioffi, Jr., MD

J. Murray Beardsley Professor and Chairman, Brown Medical School Department of Surgery; Surgeon-in-Chief, Rhode Island Hospital, Providence, Rhode Island

Burns

David R. Clarke, MD

Professor of Cardiothoracic Surgery, Department of Surgery, University of Colorado Health Sciences Center; Staff Surgeon, Children's Hospital, Denver, Colorado

Neonatal Cyanosis; Cyanotic Congenital Heart Disease

Joseph C. Cleveland, Jr., MD

Assistant Professor of Surgery, Division of Cardiothoracic Surgery, University of Colorado Health Sciences Center and Veterans Affairs Medical Center, Denver, Colorado

Preoperative Cardiac Evaluation

C. Clay Cothren, MD

Assistant Professor of Surgery, University of Colorado Health Sciences Center; Chief, Surgical Oncology, Department of Surgery, Denver Health Medical Center, Denver, Colorado

Acute Right Lower Quadrant Pain; Primary Hyperaldosteronism; Occult Breast Lesions

E. David Crawford, MD

Professor, Division of Urology, University of Colorado Health Sciences Center, Denver, Colorado

Testis Tumor

Anthony M. D'Alessandro, MD

Professor, Department of Surgery, University of Wisconsin Medical School; Executive Director, Organ Procurement Organization, University of Wisconsin Hospital and Clinics, Madison Wisconsin

Organ Donation

Thomas A. D'Amico, MD

Associate Professor, Department of Surgery, Duke University Medical Center, Durham, North Carolina

Mediastinal Tumor

Susan A. Davidson, MD

Associate Professor, Department of Obstetrics and Gynecology, Director of Gynecologic Oncology, University of Colorado Health Sciences Center; University of Colorado Hospital, Department of Obstetrics and Gynecology, Denver, Colorado

Carcinoma of the Cervix

Karlotta M. Davis, MD, MPH

Associate Professor of Obstetrics and Gynecology, University of Colorado Health Sciences Center, Denver, Colorado

Vaginal Bleeding in Reproductive Years; Postmenopausal Vaginal Bleeding; Adnexal Mass

Gerard M. Doherty, MD

Norman W. Thompson Professor of Surgery, General Surgery, University of Michigan; Second Head, University of Michigan, Department of General Surgery, Ann Arbor, Michigan

Insulinoma

Robert E. Donohue, MD

Professor of Surgery, Division of Urology, University of Colorado Health Sciences Center; Professor of Surgery, Department of Urology, University Hospital; Chief of Urology, Department of Urology, Veterans Administration Medical Center, Denver, Colorado

Scrotal Mass

Janette D. Durham, MD

Professor of Radiology, Department of Radiology, University of Colorado School of Medicine; University of Colorado Hospital, Department of Radiology, Denver, Colorado

Obstructive Jaundice: Interventional Options

Matthew J. Eagleton, MD

Department of Vascular Surgery, The Cleveland Clinic Foundation, Cleveland, Ohio

Peripheral Arterial Embolism

Matthew S. Edwards, MD

Vascular Surgery Fellow, Division of Surgical Sciences, Wake Forest University School of Medicine, Winston-Salem, North Carolina

Renovascular Disease

Fritz C. Eilber, MD

Fellow, Department of Surgery, Memorial Sloan-Kettering Cancer Center, New York, New York

Retroperitoneal Mass

E. Christopher Ellison, MD

Associate VP for Health Sciences and Vice Dean of Clinical Affairs, The Ohio State University Medical Center; Robert M. Zollinger Professor and Chair, Department of Surgery, The Ohio State University Medical Center, Columbus, Ohio

Zollinger-Ellison Syndrome

Abdusalam A. Elalem, MD

Chief Resident, Thoracic Surgery, Toronto General Hospital, University of Toronto, Toronto, Canada

Lung Abscess

Richard A. Falcone, Jr., MD

Fellow in Pediatric Surgery, Division of Pediatric Surgery, Cincinnati Children's Hospital Medical Center, University of Cincinnati College of Medicine, Cincinnati, Ohio

Hirschsprung's Disease

David R. Farley, MD

Consultant in Surgery, Division of Gastroenterologic and General Surgery, Mayo Clinic; Associate Professor of Surgery, Mayo Medical School, Rochester, Minnesota

Pheochromocytoma

David V. Feliciano, MD

Professor of Surgery, Emory University School of Medicine, Atlanta Georgia; Chief of Surgery, Grady Memorial Hospital, Atlanta, Georgia

Penetrating Abdominal Injury; Abdominal Vascular Injury

Adolfo Z. Fernandez, Jr., MD
Laparoscopy Fellow, Department of Surgery, Virginia Commonwealth University, Richmond, Virginia
                                        Morbid Obesity

Christina A. Finlayson, MD
Associate Professor of Surgery, Division of GI, Tumor, and Endocrine Surgery; Director of the Breast Center, University of Colorado Health Sciences Center, Denver, Colorado
                    Gastrointestinal Lymphoma; Gynecomastia;
                                Early Breast Carcinoma

Josef E. Fischer, MD
Mallinckrodt Professor of Surgery and Chair, Department of Surgery, Harvard Medical School and Beth Israel Deaconess Medical Center, Boston, Massachusetts
                              Enterocutaneous Fistula

Robert C. Flanigan, MD
Albert J. Jr. and Claire R. Speh Professor and Chairman, Department of Urology, Loyola University Medical Center, Maywood, Illinois
                                        Renal Mass

Brian J. Flynn, MD
Assistant Professor of Surgery/Urology, Department of Urology, University of Colorado Health Sciences Center; Director of Female Urology, Reconstructive Urology and Urodynamics, University of Colorado Health Sciences Center, Denver, Colorado
                                    Urinary Diversion

Reginald J. Franciose, MD
Assistant Professor of Surgery, University of Colorado Health Sciences Center; Attending Trauma Surgeon, Denver Health Medical Center, Denver, Colorado; Trauma Director, Vail Valley Medical Center, Vail, Colorado
        Postoperative Fever; Penetrating Injury of the Colon;
        Damage Control Laparotomy/Abdominal Compartment
                                        Syndrome

Julie Freischlag, MD
William Stewart Halsted Professor; Chair of the Department of Surgery; Surgeon-in-Chief, Johns Hopkins Medical Institutions, Baltimore, Maryland
                              Thoracic Outlet Syndrome

Charles F. Frey, MD, FACS
Professor of Surgery Emeritus, University of California Davis Medical Center, Sacramento, California
                              Chronic Pancreatitis

David A. Fullerton, MD
Professor of Surgery, Head of Cardiothoracic Surgery, University of Colorado; Head of Cardiothoracic Surgery, University of Colorado Hospital, Denver Colorado
                                    Mitral Stenosis

Aubrey C. Galloway, MD
Professor of Surgery, Director of Cardiac Surgical Research, Division of Cardiothoracic Surgery, New York University School of Medicine, New York, New York
                              Coronary Artery Disease

James S. Gammie, MD
Assistant Professor, Division of Cardiac Surgery, University of Maryland Medical Center, Baltimore, Maryland
                              Perioperative Arrhythmia

David A. Geller, MD
Associate Professor of Surgery, University of Pittsburgh; University of Pittsburgh Medical Center, UPMC Liver Cancer Center, Starzl Transplant Institute, Pittsburgh, Pennsylvania
                              Hepatocellular Carcinoma

C. Parker Gibbs, Jr., MD
Associate Professor, Department of Orthopaedic Surgery, Division of Musculoskeletal Oncology, University of Florida, Gainesville, Florida
                    Soft Tissue Masses of the Extremities

George K. Gittes, MD
Associate Professor of Surgery, UMKC School of Medicine; Holder and Ashcraft Professor of Surgical Research, Medical Research Department, Children's Mercy Hospital; Director, Laboratory for Surgical Organogenesis, Medical Research Department, Children's Mercy Hospital; Associate Professor Anatomy and Cell Biology, Kansas University School of Medicine, Kansas City, Missouri
                        Abdominal Mass in Childhood

Philip L. Glick, MD
Vice Chairman and Professor, Department of Surgery, State University of New York at Buffalo; Director of the Buffalo Institute of Fetal Therapy, Department of Pediatric Surgery, The Women & Children's Hospital of Buffalo; Executive Director of the Miniature Access Surgery Center, Department of Pediatric Surgery, The Women & Children's Hospital of Buffalo, Buffalo, New York
                        Congenital Diaphragmatic Hernia

Peter Gloviczki, MD
Professor of Surgery, Mayo Medical School; Chair, Division of Vascular Surgery; Director, Gonda Vascular Center, Mayo Clinic and Mayo Foundation, Rochester Minnesota
                              Venous Stasis Ulcer

Rene Gonzalez, MD
Associate Professor, Department of Medicine, Division of Medical Oncology, University of Colorado Health Sciences Center, Denver, Colorado
                                        Melanoma

Howard M. Goodman, MD
Assistant Clinical Professor, Obstetrics and Gynecology, Duke University Medical Center, Durham, North Carolina; Director of Gynecologic Oncology, Good Samaritan Hospital, West Palm Beach, Florida
                              Endometrial Carcinoma

Michael J.V. Gordon, MD
Director, The Hand Center, Department of Surgery, Division of Plastic and Hand Surgery, University of Colorado Hospital, Denver, Colorado
                              Hand and Wrist Fractures

Clive S. Grant, MD
Professor, Department of Surgery, Mayo Clinic, Rochester, Minnesota
                                    Thyroid Carcinoma

Gary D. Grossfeld, MD
Director, Genitourinary Oncology Program, Division of Urology, Mavin General Hospital, San Rafael, California
                                        Bladder Tumor

James M. Hammel, MD

Department of Surgery, Division of
Cardiothoracic Surgery, University of Iowa; Roy J.
and Lucille A. Carver College of Medicine, Iowa
City, Iowa

Patent Ductus Arteriosus

Kimberley J. Hansen, MD

Professor of Surgery, Division of Surgical Sciences,
Wake Forest University School of Medicine,
Winston-Salem, North Carolina

Renovascular Disease

Alden H. Harken, MD

Chairman, University of California, San Francisco
East Bay Surgery Program; Professor of Surgery,
Department of Surgery, University of California,
San Francisco, San Francisco, California; Chair,
Department of Surgery, Alameda County Medical
Center, Oakland, California

Aortic Valve Stenosis

David T. Harrington, MD

Assistant Professor of Surgery; Associate
Residency Program Director, Department of
Surgery, Brown Medical School, Providence,
Rhode Island

Burns

Bryan R. Haugen, MD

Associate Professor of Medicine and Pathology,
University of Colorado Health Sciences Center,
Denver, Colorado

Thyrotoxicosis; Thyroid Nodule

Julie K. Heimbach, MD

Transplant Center, Mayo Clinic, Rochester,
Minnesota

Acute Right Lower Quadrant Pain;
Primary Hyperaldosteronism

R. Phillip Heine, MD

Assistant Professor and Director, Division of
Maternal-Fetal Medicine; Vice Chair of
Administrative Affairs, Department of Obstetrics and
Gynecology, Duke University Medical Center,
Durham, North Carolina

Pelvic Inflammatory Disease

Scott W. Helton, MD

Professor of Surgery, Chief, Section of General Surgery,
University of Illinois at Chicago, Chicago, Illinois

Hepatic Abscess

Richard J. Hendrickson, MD

Instructor, Department of Surgery, University of
Colorado; Fellow, Pediatric Surgery, Children's
Hospital, Denver, Colorado

Tracheoesophageal Fistula/Esophageal Atresia; Infantile
Hypertrophic Pyloric Stenosis; Neonatal Bowel
Obstruction; Surgical Jaundice in Infancy

J. Laurance Hill, MD

Professor of Surgery, Chief of Pediatric Surgery,
Department of Surgery, University of Maryland,
Baltimore, Maryland

Imperforate Anus

Hung Ho, MD

Associate Professor of Surgery, University of California,
Davis School of Medicine, Davis, California

Chronic Pancreatitis

Mary A. Hooks, MD

Associate Professor, Department of Surgery, East
Tennessee State University, Johnson City, Tennessee

Dominant Breast Mass

Tracy L. Hull, MD

Staff Surgeon, Department of Colon and Rectal
Surgery, The Cleveland Clinic Foundation,
Cleveland, Ohio

Crohn's Disease of the Small Bowel

Matthew M. Hutter, MD

Instructor in Surgery, Harvard Medical School;
Assistant in Surgery, Division of General Surgery,
Massachusetts General Hospital, Boston,
Massachusetts

Pancreatic Pseudocysts

Bruce W. Jafek, MD

Professor and Former Chair (1976-1998),
Otolaryngology—Head and Neck Surgery,
University of Colorado Medical School; Active Staff,
Otolaryngology—Head and Neck Surgery,
University of Colorado Medical School; Active Staff,
Otolaryngology—Head and Neck Surgery,
Denver VA Hospital, Denver Colorado

Epistaxis

James Jaggers, MD

Associate Professor of Surgery, Duke University
Medical Center; Chief, Pediatric Cardiac Surgery,
Duke University Medical Center, Durham,
North Carolina

Coarctation of the Aorta

Herman A. Jenkins, MD

Professor and Chair, Department of Otolaryngology,
University of Colorado Health Sciences Center,
Denver, Colorado

Otorrhea

Jani R. Jensen, MD, MS

Resident Physician, Department of Obstetrics and
Gynecology, University of Colorado; Resident,
Obstetrics and Gynecology, University of Colorado
Hospital, Denver, Colorado

Endometriosis

Jeffrey L. Johnson, MD

Assistant Professor of Surgery, University of
Colorado Health Sciences Center; Director,
SICU, Denver Health Medical Center, Denver,
Colorado

Chest Injury

Steven C. Johnson, MD

Associate Professor of Medicine, Department of
Medicine, Division of Infectious Diseases, University
of Colorado Health Sciences Center; Director,
University of Colorado Hospital HIV/AIDS Clinical
Program, Denver, Colorado

HIV Disease in Surgical Patients

Michael R. Johnston, MD

Associate Professor of Surgery, University of
Toronto; Staff, Thoracic Surgery, University Health
Network—Toronto General Hospital; Associate
Scientist, Ontario Cancer Institute/Princess Margaret
Hospital, Toronto, Ontario, Canada

Lung Abscess

Gregory J. Jurkovich, MD

Professor of Surgery, University of Washington;
Chief of Trauma, Harborview Medical Center,
Seattle, Washington

Pancreatic Injury; Duodenal Injury

Manju Kalra, MBBS
Assistant Professor of Surgery, Mayo Medical School; Consultant, Division of Vascular Surgery, Gonda Vascular Center, Mayo Clinic and Mayo Foundation, Rochester, Minnesota
Venous Stasis Ulcer

Igal Kam, MD
Chief of Transplant Surgery, Professor of Surgery, University of Colorado Health Sciences Center, Denver, Colorado
Jaundice; Kidney Transplantation; Liver Transplantation

Frederick M. Karrer. MD
Associate Professor of Surgery, University of Colorado; Chairman & Program Director, Pediatric Surgery Department, Children's Hospital, Denver, Colorado
Tracheoesophageal Fistula/Esophageal Atresia; Surgical Jaundice in Infancy

George B. Kazantsev, MD, PhD
Assistant Professor of General Surgery, University of San Antonio, San Antonio, Texas; Attending Physician, Alta Bates Summit Medical Center, Oakland, California
Duodenal Ulcer

Lawrence L. Ketch, MD
Assistant Professor of Surgery, University of Colorado Health Sciences Center; Director, Division of Plastic Surgery, University of Colorado Hospital; Director, Plastic Surgery, Children's Hospital, Denver, Colorado
Non-Melanoma Skin Cancer of the Face; Flexor Tendon Injuries of the Hand

Robert E. H. Khoo, MD
Assistant Clinical Professor, Department of Surgery, University of Colorado School of Medicine, Denver Colorado; Attending Surgeon, Petaluma Valley Hospital, Petaluma, California
Anorectal Abscess/Fistula; Hemorrhoids; Pilonidal Disease

Fernando J. Kim, MD
Assistant Professor of Surgery/Urology, University of Colorado Health Sciences Center; Chief of Urology, Department of Surgery/Urology, Denver Health Medical Center, Denver Colorado
Traumatic Hematuria

Eric T. Kimchi, MD
Fellow, Surgical Oncology, Department of Surgery, University of Chicago Medical Center, Chicago, Illinois
Carcinoma of the Rectum or Anus

V. Suzanne Klimberg, MD
Professor of Surgery and Pathology; Director, Division of Breast Surgical Oncology, University of Arkansas for Medical Sciences; Staff Physician, Surgical Services, Central Arkansas Veterans Hospital Healthcare System, Little Rock Arkansas
Nipple Discharge

Badrinath R. Konety, MD, MBA
Assistant Professor of Urology and Epidemiology, Department of Urology, University of Iowa, Iowa City, Iowa
Staging and Management of Prostate Cancer

Gregory J. Landry, MD
Assistant Professor of Surgery, Division of Vascular Surgery, Oregon Health and Science University, Portland, Oregon
Chronic Limb-Threatening Ischemia

Anthony Laporta, MD
Chair, Department of Surgery, Rose Medical Center and Clinical Professor of Surgery, University of Colorado Health Sciences Center, Denver, Colorado
Diverticulitis

Michael Leo Lepore, MD
Professor of Otolaryngology—Head and Neck Surgery, University of Colorado School of Medicine; Director of Otolaryngology and Craniomaxillofacial Surgery, Denver Health Medical Center; Attending Otolaryngologist, Department of Surgery, Veterans Administration Medical Center, Denver, Colorado
Maxillary Fractures; Mandibular Fractures

Jonathan Lewis, RN, BSN, CPTC
Organ Procurement Coordinator, University of Wisconsin Hospitals and Clinics OPO, Madison, Wisconsin
Organ Donation

Mike Kuo Liang, MD
Chief Surgery Resident, Department of Surgery, University of Colorado Health Sciences Center, Denver, Colorado
Diverticulitis

Keith D. Lillemoe, MD
Professor and Vice Chairman, Department of Surgery, The Johns Hopkins Medical Institutions, Baltimore, Maryland
Periampullary Carcinoma

Charles M. Little, DO
Assistant Professor, Department of Surgery, Division of Emergency Medicine, University of Colorado Health Sciences Center, Denver, Colorado
Cardiopulmonary Resuscitation

James T. Maddux, MD
Interventional Cardiology Fellow, Cardiology/Medicine Department, University of Colorado Health Sciences Center; Interventional Cardiology Fellow, Veterans Affairs Medical Center, Denver, Colorado
Perioperative Myocardial Ischemia and Infarction

Sarah D. Majercik, MD
Department of Surgery, Brown University; Department of Surgery, Rhode Island Hospital, Providence, Rhode Island
Blunt Abdominal Trauma

Jack W. McAninch, MD
Professor of Urology, Department of Urology, University of California, San Francisco; Chief of Urology, San Francisco General Hospital, San Francisco, California
Ureteral Injuries

Martin D. McCarter, MD
Assistant Professor of Surgery, GI, Tumor, & Endocrine Surgery, University of Colorado Health Sciences Center, Denver, Colorado
Carcinoma of the Colon

Robert C. McIntyre, Jr., MD
Associate Professor, Division of GI, Tumor, and
Endocrine Surgery, University of Colorado Health
Sciences Center, Denver, Colorado
Preoperative Laboratory Evaluation;
Small Bowel Obstruction;
Volvulus; Thyrotoxicosis; Thyroid Nodule;
Primary Hyperaldosteronism

Margaret McQuiggan, MS, RD, CNSD
Clinical Dietician Specialist, Shock Trauma Intensive
Care, Herman Hospital, Houston, Texas
Nutritional Support

Randall B. Meacham, MD
Associate Professor and Head, Division of Urology,
Department of Surgery, The University of Colorado
School of Medicine, Denver, Colorado
Ureteral and Renal Calculi

Kristin L. Mekeel, MD
Chief Resident General Surgery, Department of
Surgery, University of Colorado Health Sciences
Center, Denver Colorado
Popliteal Artery Injury

David W. Mercer, MD
Associate Professor of Surgery, The University of
Texas Medical School—Houston; Chief of Surgery,
Department of Surgery, Lyndon B. Johnson General
Hospital; Vice Chairman, General Surgery,
The University of Texas Medical School – Houston,
Houston, Texas
Gastric Ulcer

Douglas E. Merkel, MD
Assistant Professor of Medicine, Department of
Medicine, Northwestern University Medical School,
Chicago; Senior Attending Physician, Department of
Medical Oncology, Evanston Northwestern
Healthcare, Evanston, Illinois
Advanced Breast Carcinoma

John C. Messenger, MD
Department of Medicine, University of Colorado
Health Sciences Center; Chief, Interventional
Cardiology, Cardiology Section, Denver VA Medical
Center; Attending Physician, Interventional Cardiology,
University of Colorado Hospital, Denver, Colorado
Perioperative Myocardial Ischemia and Infarction

Arlen D. Meyers, MD, MBA
Otolaryngology—Head and Neck Surgery,
University of Colorado School Medicine, Denver,
Colorado
Neck Mass

John D. Mitchell, MD
Assistant Professor of Surgery; Chief, Section of
General Thoracic Surgery, Division of Cardiothoracic
Surgery, University of Colorado Health Sciences
Center, Denver, Colorado
Pleural Effusion and Empyema;
Carcinoma of the Lung; Lung Transplantation

Max B. Mitchell, MD
Associate Professor of Surgery, Department of
Surgery, University of Colorado Health Sciences
Center; Pediatric Cardiothoracic Surgeon,
The Children's Hospital, Denver, Colorado
Congenital Obstructive Cardiac Anomalies

Kian A. Modanlou, MD
Surgery Resident, University of Colorado Health
Sciences Center, Denver, Colorado
Jaundice; Kidney Transplantation;
Liver Transplantation

Ernest Eugene Moore, MD
Professor and Vice Chairman of Surgery, University
of Colorado Health Sciences Center; Chief of
Surgery and Trauma Services, Denver Health
Medical Center, Denver, Colorado
Chest Injury; Thoracic Aorta Injury

Frederick A. Moore, MD
James H. "Red" Duke, Jr. Professor and
Vice Chairman, Department of Surgery,
University of Texas Houston Medical School;
Medical Director, Trauma Services, Trauma
Department, Memorial Hermann Hospital,
Houston, Texas
Nutrtional Support

Wesley S. Moore, MD
Professor of Surgery, Division of Vascular Surgery,
UCLA School of Medicine; Vascular Surgeon,
Division of Vascular Surgery, UCLA Center for the
Health Sciences
Extracranial Cerebrovascular Disease

J. Mark Morales, MD
Assistant Professor, Department of Pediatrics, Texas
A&M University Health Sciences Center, College
Station, Texas; Chief, Pediatric Cardiothoracic Surgery,
Driscoll Children's Hospital, Corpus Christi, Texas
Neonatal Cyanosis; Cyanotic Congenital Heart Disease

Steven J. Morgan, MD
Assistant Professor, Residency Program Director,
Department of Orthopedics, University of Colorado
Health Sciences Center; Associate Director,
Co-Director, Orthopedic Trauma, Department of
Orthopedics, Denver Health Medical Center, Denver,
Colorado
Pelvic Fractures; Mangled Extremity

Kenric M. Murayama, MD
Associate Professor of Surgery, Department of
Surgery, Northwestern University, Feinberg School
of Medicine; Associate Professor of Surgery,
Department of Surgery, Northwestern Memorial
Hospital, Chicago, Illinois
Hernia

Peter Muscarella, MD
Assistant Professor, Department of Surgery,
The Ohio State University Medical Center,
Columbus, Ohio
Zollinger-Ellison Syndrome

Alexander P. Nagle, MD
Advanced Laparoscopic Surgery Fellow, Department
of Surgery, Northwestern University Feinberg School
of Medicine; Advanced Laparoscopic Surgery
Fellow, Department of Surgery, Northwestern
Memorial Hospital, Chicago, Illinois
Hernia

Mark R. Nehler, MD
Associate Professor Vascular Section, Program
Director General Surgery, University of Colorado
Health Sciences Center, Denver, Colorado
Abdominal Aortic Aneurysm;
Varicose Veins

Christophe L. Nguyen, MD
Chief Resident in Surgery, Medical University of
South Carolina, Charleston, South Carolina
Cancer of Unknown Primary

Siam Oottamasathien, MD
Division of Urology, University of Colorado Health Sciences Center, Denver, Colorado
Testis Tumor

Daniel J. Ostlie, MD
Assistant Professor of Surgery, Department of Surgery, UMKC Medical School; Assistant Professor, Department of Surgery, Children's Mercy Hospital, Kansas City, Missouri
Abdominal Mass in Childhood

Kenneth Ouriel, MD
Professor of Surgery, Department of Surgery, Ohio State University, Columbus, Ohio; Chairman, Vascular Surgery, The Cleveland Clinic Foundation, Cleveland, Ohio
Peripheral Arterial Embolism

Jonathan M. Owens, MD
Resident, Department of Otolaryngology, University of Colorado Health Sciences Center, Denver, Colorado
Neck Mass

Norman A. Paradis, MD
Associate Professor, Surgery and Medicine, University of Colorado Health Sciences Center; Sr. Medical Director, Emergency Services, University of Colorado Hospital, Denver, Colorado
Cardiopulmonary Resuscitation

Bruce C. Paton, MD
Emeritus Clinical Professor of Surgery, Department of Surgery, University of Colorado Health Sciences Center, Denver, Colorado; Director, The Given Institute, Aspen, Colorado
Hypothermia

David A. Partrick, MD
Director of Surgical Endoscopy in Infants and Children, Department of Pediatric Surgery, The Children's Hospital; Assistant Professor of Surgery, Department of Surgery, University of Colorado Health Sciences Center, Denver, Colorado
Inguinal and Scrotal Conditions in Children

William H. Pearce, MD
Violet R. and Charles A. Baldwin Professor of Vascular Surgery, Department of Surgery, Northwestern University Feinberg School of Medicine; Chief, Division of Vascular Surgery, Department of Surgery, Northwestern Memorial Hospital, Chicago, Illinois
Acute Mesenteric Vascular Occlusion

Nathan W. Pearlman, MD
Professor of Surgery, Division of GI, Tumor, and Endocrine Surgery, University of Colorado Health Sciences Center, Denver, Colorado
Carcinoma of the Esophagus

Nancy Dugal Perrier, MD
Assistant Professor of Surgery, Wake Forest University School of Medicine, Winston-Salem, North Carolina
Cushing's Syndrome

DuyKhanh T. Pham, MD
Surgical Resident, Department of Surgery, Duke University Medical Center, Durham, North Carolina
Mediastinal Tumor

Mitchell C. Posner, MD
Professor of Surgery, Chief, Surgical Oncology, Department of Surgery, University of Chicago, Chicago, Illinois
Carcinoma of the Rectum or Anus

Christopher D. Raeburn, MD
Instructor, Department of Surgery, University of Colorado Health Sciences Center, Denver, Colorado
Preoperative Laboratory Evaluation; Aortic Valve Stenosis

Chitra Rajagopalan, MD
Associate Professor, Department of Pathology, University of Colorado Health Sciences Center, and Chief, Pathology; Laboratory Medicine Service, Eastern Colorado Healthcare System, Denver, Colorado
Bleeding Disorders in Surgical Patients

Sonia Ramamoorthy, MD
Assistant Professor of Surgery, Section of Colon and Rectal Surgery, UC San Francisco Medical Center, San Francisco, California
Lower Gastrointestinal Bleeding

David W. Rattner, MD
Associate Professor of Surgery, Harvard Medical School; Chief, Division of General Surgery, Massachusetts General Hospital, Boston, Massachusetts
Pancreatic Pseudocysts

John Ridge, MD, PhD
Chief, Head and Neck Surgery Section, Department of Surgical Oncology, Fox Chase Cancer Center, Philadelphia, Pennsylvania
Carcinoma of the Oral Cavity

David Rigberg, MD
Gonda (Goldschmied) Vascular Center, UCLA Medical Center, Los Angeles, California
Thoracic Outlet Syndrome

Emily K. Robinson, MD
Assistant Professor, Department of Surgery, The University of Texas—Houston; Attending Surgeon, The Department of General Surgery, LBJ Hospital, Houston, Texas
Gastric Ulcer

Thomas N. Robinson, MD
Assistant Professor of Surgery, Division of GI, Tumor, and Endocrine Surgery, University of Colorado Health Sciences Center, Denver, Colorado
Gastroesophageal Reflux Disease; Lower Gastrointestinal Bleeding

Alexander S. Rosemurgy, MD
Professor of Surgery, Professor of Medicine, Director of Sugical Digestive Disorders, The Reeves/Culverhouse Endowed Chair in Surgery, University of South Florida, Tampa, Florida
Acute Pancreatitis

Daniel Rosenstein, MD
Clinical Instructor, Stanford University, Department of Urology, Palo Alto, California; Associate Chief, Division of Urology, Santa Clara Valley Medical Center, San Jose, California
Ureteral Injuries

Sharona B. Ross, MD
Resident in Surgery, University of South Florida, Tampa, Florida
Acute Pancreatitis

Lisa A. Rutstein, MD
Surgical Oncology Fellow, Department of Surgery, University of Pittsburgh; University of Pittsburgh Medical Center, UPMC Cancer Center, Pittsburgh, Pennsylvania
Hepatocellular Carcinoma

Clare Savage, MD
Research Fellow, Department of Surgery, The University of Texas Medical Branch, Galveston, Texas
Esophageal Perforation; Caustic Ingestion

Mark T. Scarborough, MD
Associate Professor, University of Florida, Department of Orthopaedic Surgery, Division of Musculoskeletal Oncology, Gainesville, Florida
Soft Tissue Masses of the Extremities

Nancy Schindler, MD
Assistant Professor of Surgery, Northwestern University Feinberg School of Medicine, Chicago, Illinois; Attending Surgeon, Department of Surgery, Evanston Northwestern Hospital, Evanston, Illinois
Acute Mesenteric Vascular Occlusion

David P. Schnur, MD
Assistant Professor, Division of Plastic Surgery, University of Colorado Health Sciences Center, Denver Colorado
Flexor Tendon Injuries of the Hand

Charles F. Schwartz, MD
Assistant Professor of Surgery, Division of Cardiothoracic Surgery, New York University School of Medicine, New York, New York
Coronary Artery Disease

Wayne H. Schwesinger, MD
Professor of Surgery, Director of Surgical Endoscopy and Minimally Invasive Surgery, Department of Surgery, University of Texas Health Science Center at San Antonio, San Antonio, Texas
Duodenal Ulcer

Stephen M. Scott, MD
Assistant Professor, OB-GYN, University of Colorado Health Sciences Center; Associate Chair and Director of Pediatric Gynecology, The Children's Hospital of Denver, Denver, Colorado
Prepubertal Vaginal Bleeding

Walter W. Scott, Jr. MD
Assistant Professor of Surgery, Department of Surgery, East Carolina University, Greenville, North Carolina
Pulmonary Embolism

Peter A. Seirafi, MD
Cardiothoracic Surgeon, Baptist Medical Center Walker, Jasper, Alabama
Heart Transplantation

Craig H. Selzman, MD
Assistant Professor of Surgery, Division of Cardiothoracic Surgery, University of North Carolina, School of Medicine, Chapel Hill, North Carolina
Preoperative Cardiac Evaluation

Ashok R. Shaha, MD
Professor of Surgery, Memorial Sloan Kettering Cancer Center, New York, New York
Cancer of the Larynx

Brian D. Shames, MD
Surgical Transplant Fellow, Department of Surgery, University of Wisconsin, Madison, Madison, Wisconsin
Organ Donation

Irving Shen, MD
Assistant Professor, Department of Surgery, Oregon Health & Science University, Portland, Oregon
Congenital Septal Defects

Stephen Shorofsky, MD
Associate Professor, Department of Medicine, University of Maryland, Baltimore, Maryland
Perioperative Arrhythmia

Wade R. Smith, MD
Director of Orthopedic Surgery and Co-Director of Orthopedic Trauma Service, Department of Orthopedic Surgery, Denver Health Medical Center, University of Colorado Health Sciences Center, Denver, Colorado
Pelvic Fractures; Mangled Extremity

John I. Song, MD
Assistant Professor; Director of Head & Neck Oncology, Department of Otolaryngology, University of Colorado School of Medicine, Denver, Colorado
Salivary Gland Tumor

Christopher J. Sonnenday, MD
Fellow in Surgical Oncology, The Johns Hopkins University School of Medicine, Baltimore, Maryland
Adrenal Incidentaloma

Jennifer St. Croix, MD
Surgical Resident, Department of Surgery, University of Colorado Health Sciences Center, Denver, Colorado
Abdominal Aortic Aneurysm; Varicose Veins

Mark D. Stegall, MD
Professor of Surgery; Director, Kidney and Pancreas Transplant Surgery, Mayo Clinic College of Medicine, Rochester, Minnesota
Pancreas Transplantation

Gregory V. Stiegmann, MD
Professor of Surgery and Head, Division of GI, Tumor, and Endocrine Surgery, University of Colorado Health Sciences Center; Vice President for Clinical Affairs, University of Colorado Hospital, Denver, Colorado
Bleeding Esophageal Varices

Eric D. Strauch, MD
Assistant Professor of Surgery, Department of Surgery, University of Maryland, Baltimore, Maryland
Imperforate Anus

Choichi Sugawa, MD, PhD
Professor and Director of Surgical Endoscopy, Department of Surgery, Wayne State University School of Medicine; Professor of Surgery, Detroit Receiving Hospital; Professor of Surgery, Harper University Hospital, Detroit, Michigan
Upper Gastrointestinal Bleeding

Harvey T. Sugerman, MD
David M. Hume Professor of Surgery, Department of Surgery, Virginia Commonwealth University; Medical College of Virginia Hospitals, Richmond, Virginia
Morbid Obesity

Jon S. Thompson, MD
Professor & Vice Chair, Department of Surgery, University of Nebraska Medical Center; Attending Physician, General Surgery, University of Nebraska Hospital; Attending Physician, General Sugary, VAMC of Omaha, Omaha, Nebraska
Short Bowel Syndrome

Norman W. Thompson, MD, PhD
Professor Emeritus of Surgery, University of Michigan, Ann Arbor, Michigan
Hypercalcemia and Hyperparathyroidism

David S. Tichansky, MD
Laparoscopic Surgery Fellow, Department of Surgery, Medical College of Virginia/Virginia Commonwealth University, Richmond, Virginia
Morbid Obesity

Thadeus L. Trus, MD
Associate Professor of Surgery, Division of Minimally Invasive Surgery, Dartmouth-Hitchcock Medical Center, Lebanon, New Hampshire
Achalasia

Ryan L. Van De Graaf, MD
Ear, Nose and Throat Specialties, P.C., Lincoln, Nebraska
Otorrhea

Jon A. van Heerden, MD
Fred C. Anderden Professor of Surgery, Mayo Medical School; Consultant in Surgery, Division of Gastroenterologic and General Surgery, Mayo Clinic and Mayo Foundation, Rochester, Minnesota
Pheochromocytoma

Alex J. Vanni, MD
Resident in Urology, Lahey Clinic, Burlington, Massachusetts
Ureteral and Renal Calculi

Michael E. Wachs, MD
Associate Professor, Division of Transplant Surgery, University of Colorado Health Sciences Center, Denver, Colorado
Jaundice; Kidney Transplantation; Liver Transplantation

Jeffrey Wallace, MD, MPH
Associate Professor and Director of Clinical Geriatrics, Department of Medicine, University of Colorado Health Sciences Center, Denver, Colorado
Geriatric Surgery

Mark D. Walsh Jr., MD
Surgical Resident, Department of Surgery, University of Colorado Health Sciences Center, Denver, Colorado
Volvulus

Marjorie C. Wang, MD
Assistant Professor, Department of Neurosurgery, University of Washington and Harborview Medical Center, Seattle, Washington
Closed Head Injury; Cervical Spine Fractures

Brad W. Warner, MD
Professor of Surgery, University of Cincinnati College of Medicine; Attending Surgeon, Division of Pediatric Surgery, Cincinnati Children's Hospital Medical Center, Cincinnati, Ohio
Hirschsprung's Disease

Kelly J. White, MD
Assistant Professor of Medicine, University of Colorado Health Sciences Center; Chief of Surgery, Denver Veterans Administration Medical Center, Eastern Colorado Health Care System, Denver, Colorado
Acute Renal Failure

Thomas A. Whitehill, MD
Associate Professor of Surgery, Department of Surgery, University of Colorado, Denver, Colorado
Intermittent Claudication; Deep Vein Thrombosis

John A. Whitesel, MD
Past Chief, Division of Urology, Clinical Professor of Surgery, Department of Surgery/Urology, University of Colorado Health Sciences Center, University Hospital, and Denver Health Medical Center, Denver, Colorado
Prostatism

Harold C. Weisenfeld, MD, CM
Assistant Professor, Department of Obstetrics, Gynecology, and Reproductive Services, University of Pittsburgh School of Medicine, Pittsburgh, Pennsylvania
Pelvic Inflammatory Disease

Richard D. Williams, MD
Professor and Rubin Flocks Chair, Department of Urology, University of Iowa, Iowa City, Iowa
Staging and Management of Prostate Cancer

David P. Winchester, MD
Professor and Chair, Deptartment of Surgery, Evanston Northwestern Healthcare, Northwestern University Feinberg School of Medicine, Chicago, Illinois
Advanced Breast Carcinoma

Richard E. Wolfe, MD
Assistant Professor of Medicine, Harvard Medical School; Chief of Emergency Medicine, Department of Emergency Medicine, Beth Israel Deaconess Medical Center, Boston, Massachusetts
Airway Management

Tonia M. Young-Fadok, MD, MS
Associate Professor of Surgery, Mayo Medical School, Rochester, Minnesota; Consultant Surgeon, Division of Colon and Rectal Surgery, Mayo Clinic, Scottsdale, Arizona
Anal Fissure

Garret Zallen, MD
Pediatric Surgery Fellow Department of Pediatric Surgery, The Women's & Children's Hospital of Buffalo, Buffalo, New York
Congenital Diaphragmatic Hernia

Martha A. Zeiger, MD
Associate Professor of Endocrine and Oncologic Surgery, The Johns Hopkins University School of Medicine, Baltimore, Maryland
Adrenal Incidentaloma

Bernard E. Zeligman, MD
Associate Professor, Department of Radiology, University of Colorado School of Medicine; Radiologist, Department of Radiology, University of Colorado Hospital, Denver Colorado
Obstructive Jaundice: Interventional Options

Joseph B. Zwischenberger, MD
Professor of Surgery, Medicine and Radiology, Director of General Thoracic Surgery, ECMO/Critical Care Program; Co-Director of Multiple Disciplinary Thoracic Oncology Program, Division of Cardiothoracic Surgery, Department of Surgery, The University of Texas Medical Branch, Galveston, Texas
Esophageal Perforation; Caustic Ingestion

CONTENTS

PREFACE

Only those of us struggling to stay afloat in the fast-moving current of clinical surgery can fully appreciate the revolutionary changes that have occurred in our specialty during the past five to ten years. Students, residents, and young clinical surgeons blissfully unaware of the tranquility of the past surgical mainstream lack an appreciation of the magnitude of recent changes.

Editors who are responsible for producing a new edition of a textbook face special challenges—they must choose the right moment to launch their craft, as well as design and provision it so it stays on an even keel and remains a leader in the swift-moving current. Dr. Robert C. McIntyre, Jr., who is both an academic endocrine surgeon and a skilled "white water man," has done most of the heavy lifting in launching the fifth edition of this text and has managed to achieve our objective at a time of revolutionary change in clinical surgery.

Since the publication of the previous edition five years ago, the primary force for change has been the improved technology of minimally invasive surgical and endoscopic techniques. Other forces include the merging of operative surgery with endoscopy and invasive radiology, new techniques in solid organ and bone marrow transplantation, and major changes in chemotherapy and other medications supporting operative surgery.

We introduced our first edition of this book three decades ago and were rebuked by those who suggested that by using algorithms we were attempting to turn clinical surgery into a cookbook technology. It is with a good deal of satisfaction that our original emphasis on evidence-based medicine, outcome expectancy, and the importance of quality of life in decision analysis as illustrated in the form of algorithms is now an accepted form of teaching clinical practice.

We are continuing to use our original graphic and editorial format because it seems to be the most effective way to summarize the complex system of thought processes that constitutes clinical surgical practice. However, the subject matter of this edition has been radically changed to illustrate modern practice. Thirty three new chapters have been added with 105 new authors in this edition, and the focus of 10 chapters has been entirely revised. A major emphasis has been placed on the competing role of minimally invasive techniques and recent advances in monitoring and management in the pre- and postoperative period.

Thirty years of experience over four previous editions has demonstrated the success of this editorial format in helping students and residents to prepare for certifying and qualifying examinations. We have also found the format to be useful reassurance for practicing surgeons in areas where their day-to-day practice is limited. From my own experience as an examiner, I even found it occasionally reassuring before quizzing a series of bright candidates to take a surreptitious look at a chapter or two in areas in which I needed a little "refreshing" exposure.

We hope this new edition will serve all students of surgery, beginning with their second year in medical school, through residency and their practice years—and even into their retirement. Surgery continues to be an exciting and intellectually stimulating specialty. This edition is intended to improve current patient care and to give evidence of this dynamism.

Ben Eiseman, MD

Denver, Colorado

GENERAL

Chapter 1 *Preoperative Laboratory Evaluation*

CHRISTOPHER D. RAEBURN, MD • ROBERT C. MCINTYRE, JR., MD

(A) More than 3 billion dollars are spent each year on preoperative laboratory evaluation; however, approximately 60% of these tests are unnecessary and increase the cost of care without reducing perioperative morbidity or mortality. Additional testing to evaluate borderline or falsely abnormal results can lead to iatrogenic injury. Specific preoperative laboratory evaluation should be performed to confirm or to rule out medical conditions that are likely to impact a patient's perioperative course. A thorough history and physical alone is 96% accurate in predicting a patient's fitness for surgery.

(B) The magnitude and risk of the operative procedure should be considered when determining the extent of preoperative evaluation. Intracranial, thoracic, and abdominal operations carry higher risk than do operations that do not involve entering these cavities.

(C) Asymptomatic patients without any comorbid disease undergoing elective procedures need no preoperative laboratory evaluation regardless of age. Abnormal preoperative laboratory values in healthy, asymptomatic patients do not predict postoperative adverse outcomes.

(D) A basic metabolic panel (BMP) including electrolytes, glucose, blood urea nitrogen, and creatinine is useful in patients with seizure disorders because electrolyte abnormalities may lower the seizure threshold during the perioperative period and complicate antiseizure therapy. A complete blood count (CBC) and electrocardiogram (ECG) should be done for patients with a history of stroke that may indicate a cardiac condition such as atrial fibrillation or simply be a marker of systemic atherosclerotic disease, either of which may increase the risk of an adverse perioperative cardiac event and require preoperative evaluation.

(E) Perioperative adverse cardiac events are the most common cause of serious morbidity and mortality in patients undergoing elective surgery. Thus patients with a known history of coronary artery disease (CAD), as well as those with signs/symptoms or risk factors indicative of CAD, require further preoperative cardiac evaluation (see Chapter 2). Patients with evidence of peripheral vascular disease should be presumed to have CAD until proven otherwise.

(F) In patients with pulmonary disease and a recent change in symptoms, preoperative chest x-ray is indicated to assess for the presence of acute or progressive disease. Patients with stable disease need not undergo chest x-ray. Pulmonary function tests (PFTs) and arterial blood gases (ABGs) may be warranted in patients with significant obstructive/reactive airway disease undergoing thoracic or upper abdominal surgery but should not be done in all patients. Optimal use of preoperative spirometry is in patients who are to undergo thoracic or upper abdominal surgery and who have symptoms of significant respiratory tract disease on a careful history and physical examination. In addition, spirometry may be helpful in a patient with chronic obstructive pulmonary disease or asthma if, after clinical assessment, it is uncertain whether the degree of airflow obstruction has been optimally reduced. A partial pressure of arterial carbon dioxide ($PaCO_2$) greater than 45 mmHg is a risk factor for pulmonary complications. Risk reduction can include cessation of smoking for 8 weeks before operation, airflow reduction with bronchodilators or steroids, elimination of infection, and instruction on lung expansion maneuvers.

(G) Liver function tests (LFTs), prothrombin time (PT), international normalized ratio (INR), and a partial thromboplastin time (PTT) are indicated in patients with a history of advanced liver disease because these patients are at increased risk for perioperative infections, hemorrhage, and wound complications. It remains controversial whether diabetes mellitus is an independent risk factor for perioperative complications; however, it is a significant risk factor for other comorbidities such as coronary artery disease and chronic renal insufficiency. Serum albumin concentration is a better predictor of surgical outcomes than many other preoperative patient characteristics. Whereas mild to moderate malnutrition does not impact perioperative complications, patients with severe malnutrition may have significant anemia, electrolyte disturbances, and coagulation defects. Severely malnourished patients undergoing elective surgery may benefit from preoperative nutritional support. Serum albumin level is a very reliable indicator of increased operative risk.

(H) Renal dysfunction predisposes to electrolyte disturbances, which increase the risk of anesthetic complications and perioperative arrhythmias. Thus assessment and normalization of preoperative electrolyte abnormalities and anemia is indicated.

(I) A history of hematologic disorders such as anemia, thrombocytopenia, or bleeding tendency should be investigated. Malignancy affects perioperative morbidity and warrants a search for anemia, thrombocytopenia, and coagulation abnormalities.

(J) A social history is important in identifying patients with a significant history of alcohol or tobacco abuse. Identification of liver disease in patients with a significant history of alcohol abuse may permit medical optimization before elective surgery. Cessation of smoking 8 weeks before surgery significantly reduces perioperative pulmonary complications; however, some benefit may occur when patients stop smoking for even a few days preceding surgery. A preoperative chest x-ray, PFTs, and ABGs may be indicated as discussed above (see F).

(K) A careful review of medications is important because certain medications such as anticoagulants and diuretics may increase the risk of perioperative morbidity.

REFERENCES
Alsumait BM, Alhumood SA, Ivanova T et al: A prospective evaluation of preoperative screening laboratory tests in general surgery patients. Med Princ Pract 11:42–45, 2002.

Arozullah AM, Daley J, Henderson WG et al: Multifactorial risk index for predicting postoperative respiratory failure in men after major noncardiac surgery. The National Veterans Administration Surgical Quality Improvement Program. Ann Surg 232:242–253, 2000.

Dzankic S, Pastor D, Gonzalez C et al: The prevalence and predictive value of abnormal preoperative laboratory tests in elderly surgical patients. Anesth Analg 93:301–308, 2001.

Gibbs J, Cull W, Henderson W et al: Preoperative serum albumin level as a predictor of operative mortality and morbidity: Results from the National VA Surgical Risk Study. Arch Surg 134:36–42, 1999.

Johnson RK, Mortimer AJ: Routine pre-operative blood testing: Is it necessary? Anaesthesia 57(9):914–917, 2002.

Litaker D: Preoperative screening. Med Clin North Am 83:1565–1581, 1999.

Narr BJ, Warner ME, Schroeder DR et al: Outcomes of patients with no laboratory assessment before anesthesia and a surgical procedure. Mayo Clin Proc 72:505–509, 1997.

Parker BM, Tetzlaff JE, Litaker DL et al: Redefining the preoperative evaluation process and the role of the anesthesiologist. J Clin Anesth 12:350–356, 2000.

Roizen MF: More preoperative assessment by physicians and less by laboratory tests. N Engl J Med 342:204–205, 2000.

Smetana GW: Preoperative pulmonary evaluation. N Engl J Med 340:937–944, 1999.

Velanovich V: Preoperative laboratory evaluation. J Am Coll Surg 183:79–87, 1996.

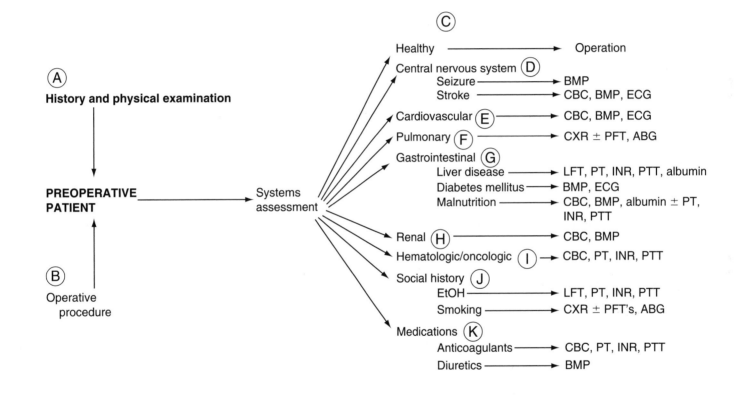

Chapter 2 **Preoperative Cardiac Evaluation**

CRAIG H. SELZMAN, MD • JOSEPH C. CLEVELAND, JR., MD

(A) A careful history and physical examination, as well as prudent evaluation of electrocardiograms and selected laboratory tests, should be able to screen the majority of patients at risk for noncardiac surgery. Independent risk factors are previous or existing coronary artery disease, cerebrovascular disease, congestive heart failure, insulin-requiring diabetes, and renal insufficiency (i.e., creatinine greater than 2 mg/dl).

(B) Numerous studies have attempted to identify risk factors for patients at high risk for cardiac morbidity and mortality following noncardiac surgery. The Goldman and Eagle criteria have been validated in several large studies. In addition, a consensus statement addressing preoperative evaluation for noncardiac surgery has recently been updated. The following recommendations depend heavily upon these recommendations as well as on the Lee revised cardiac risk index. Several caveats to the following algorithm exist: Patients with active major clinical predictors should be stabilized before surgery (e.g., unstable coronary syndromes, decompensated congestive heart failure, significant arrhythmias, and severe valvular disease). In the majority of cases, preoperative cardiac evaluation should not delay or change plans for the primary presenting problem. Finally, "cleared by cardiology" should not substitute for good judgment and communication between surgeon, anesthesiologist, and other treating physicians.

(C) Specific procedure-related risks are important. High-risk procedures carry a cardiac risk of greater than 5% and include emergent operations (especially in the elderly), aortic and infra-inguinal vascular surgery, or long operations associated with large fluid shifts and blood loss. Intermediate risk procedures generally carry a cardiac risk of less than 5% and include carotid endarterectomy, head and neck surgery, intraperitoneal or intrathoracic procedures, orthopedic surgery, and prostate surgery. Low-risk procedures carry a cardiac risk of less than 1% and include endoscopic procedures, superficial procedures, cataract surgery, and breast surgery. High-risk procedures score a 1 on the revised cardiac risk index (as high as a previous stroke).

(D) Whereas the risk of cardiac events in this group is generally less than 1% to 2%, one may still consider adding β-blockers before surgery. Patients with 2 or more minor criteria (e.g., age greater than 65 years, hypertension, current smoker, hypercholesterolemia, or noninsulin-dependent diabetes) should receive β-blockade.

(E) The intermediate group generally carries a cardiac risk of 2% to 4%; β-blocker therapy can decrease this risk to less than 1%. In a group of 1351 patients undergoing major vascular surgery, more than 80% had less than 3 risk factors, and those on β-blockers had a less than 1% cardiac event rate. However, if the patient carries a strong history of coronary artery disease, has a poor functional status (i.e., less than 4 METs, or metabolic equivalents as defined by the American Heart Association), and will be undergoing a high-risk procedure, it would be reasonable to suggest noninvasive testing in this intermediate group.

(F) A variety of noninvasive tests are now available. Stress testing can be from exercise, usually on a treadmill with continuous ECG monitoring; or pharmacologic, as seen with dobutamine, dipyridamole, and adenosine. Imaging studies, including echo and radionucleotide studies (e.g., thallium and sesta-MIBI), reveal not only exercise capacity but the presence of previous myocardial infarction and the extent of reversible ischemia. The choice of stressor and imaging techniques should be determined by the degree of institutional experience.

(G) Both echo and nuclear imaging techniques are able to segmentally quantify areas of wall motion abnormalities induced by stress. These results can be helpful in identifying patients requiring further invasive testing.

(H) Although most would consider any abnormality on stress imaging an indication for invasive testing, the aforementioned study would suggest that patients with less than 4 segmental wall abnormalities, treated with β-blockers, would carry a cardiac event rate of less than 3%. However, this is only one retrospective study. Traditionally, any patient with a positive noninvasive study should proceed to coronary angiography.

(I) In a study of 1000 patients undergoing vascular surgery, 25% had severe correctable coronary artery disease. The issue of prophylactic revascularization remains unclear. While awaiting results from randomized trials, revascularization strategies should be based on standard indications as outlined by the American College of Cardiology/ American Heart Association practice guidelines.

(J) Significant controversy exists as to the role of percutaneous coronary interventions (PCI) for asymptomatic single- or double-vessel coronary disease. If the area of blockage correlates to segments of ischemia by noninvasive testing, one may wish to revascularize this region. Importantly, any PCI with stent placement necessitates treatment with antiplatelet agents, which will require a 4- to 6-week delay before surgery.

(K) Coronary artery bypass grafting (CABG) in asymptomatic patients should be reserved for patients with classic indications such as severe 3-vessel disease with reduced left ventricular function and left main stenosis. The anticipated morbidity and mortality from CABG must be weighed against the risk reduction afforded with β-blockade or the urgency/indications for the noncardiac surgical problem.

(L) Several large, randomized studies have reported significant reduction in cardiac events associated with perioperative β-blockade. Patients should be given cardioselective agents (e.g., atenolol, metoprolol, or esmolol) with a goal to lower the heart rate to less than 65 bpm both preoperatively (best if more than 1 to 2 weeks before surgery) and postoperatively (both immediately and upon discharge). Few absolute contraindications

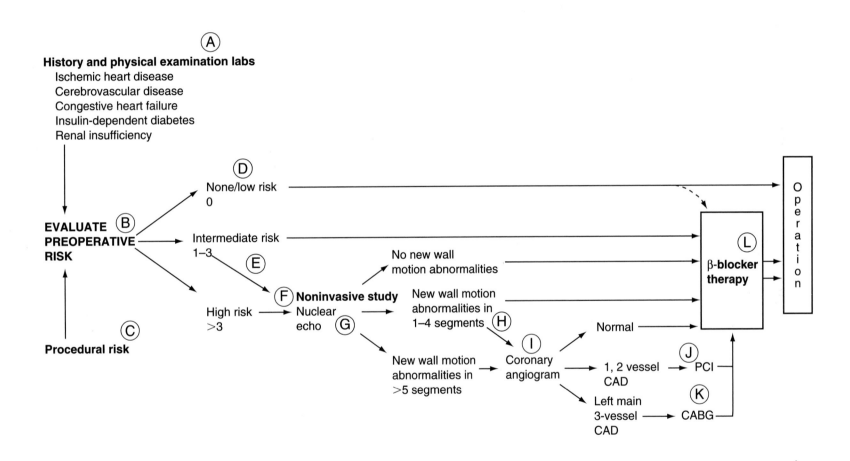

Ⓐ
History and physical examination labs
  Ischemic heart disease
  Cerebrovascular disease
  Congestive heart failure
  Insulin-dependent diabetes
  Renal insufficiency

EVALUATE Ⓑ
PREOPERATIVE
RISK

Ⓒ
Procedural risk

Ⓓ
None/low risk
0

Intermediate risk
1–3

Ⓔ

High risk → Nuclear
>3   echo Ⓖ

Ⓕ **Noninvasive study**

No new wall
motion abnormalities

New wall motion
abnormalities in
1–4 segments Ⓗ

New wall motion
abnormalities in
>5 segments

Ⓘ Coronary
angiogram

Normal

1, 2 vessel Ⓙ
CAD → PCI

Left main
3-vessel → CABG
CAD Ⓚ

Ⓛ
β-blocker
therapy

Operation

to β-blocker therapy exist; these include severe bronchospasm, decompensated CHF, and high-degree heart block. As such, β-blocker therapy is an essential component to most patients at risk for cardiac events following noncardiac surgery.

REFERENCES

Auerbach AD, Goldman L: β-Blockers and reduction of cardiac events in noncardiac surgery. JAMA 287:1435–1442, 2002.

Boersma E, Poldermans D, Bax JJ et al: Predictors of cardiac events after major vascular surgery. JAMA 285:1865–1873, 2001.

Eagle KA, Berger PB, Calkins H et al: ACC/AHA Guideline update for perioperative cardiovascular evaluation for noncardiac surgery: Executive summary. Circulation 105:1257–1267, 2002.

Hertzer NR, Beven EG, Young JR et al: Coronary artery disease in peripheral vascular patients: A classification of 1000 coronary angiograms and results of surgical management. Ann Surg 199:223–233, 1984.

Lee TH, Marcantonio ER, Mangione CM et al: Derivation and prospective validation of a simple index for prediction of cardiac risk of major noncardiac surgery. Circulation 100:1043–1049, 1999.

Mangano DT, Goldman L: Preoperative assessment of patients with known or suspected coronary disease. N Engl J Med 333:1749–1756, 1995.

Poldermans D, Boersma E, Bax JJ et al: The effect of bisoprolol on perioperative mortality and myocardial infarction in high-risk patients undergoing vascular surgery. N Engl J Med 341:1789–1794, 1999.

Poldermans D, Boersma E, Bax JJ et al: Bisoprolol reduces cardiac death and myocardial infarction in high-risk patients as long as 2 years after successful major vascular surgery. Eur Heart J 22:1353–1358, 2001.

Selzman CH, Miller SA, Zimmerman MA et al: The case for β-adrenergic blockade as prophylaxis against perioperative cardiovascular morbidity and mortality. Arch Surg 136:286–290, 2001.

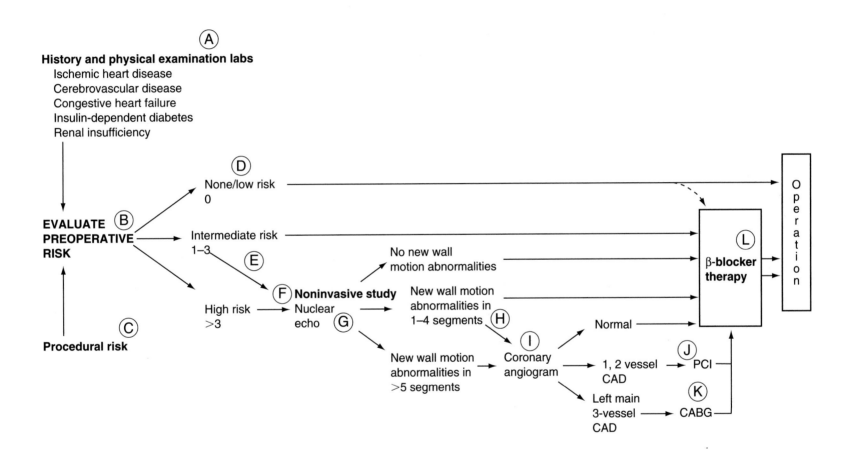

Ⓐ
History and physical examination labs
   Ischemic heart disease
   Cerebrovascular disease
   Congestive heart failure
   Insulin-dependent diabetes
   Renal insufficiency

Ⓑ **EVALUATE PREOPERATIVE RISK**

Ⓒ **Procedural risk**

Ⓓ None/low risk
0

Intermediate risk
1–3

High risk
>3

Ⓔ

Ⓕ **Noninvasive study**
Nuclear echo

Ⓖ

No new wall motion abnormalities

New wall motion abnormalities in 1–4 segments Ⓗ

New wall motion abnormalities in >5 segments

Ⓘ Coronary angiogram

Normal

1, 2 vessel CAD

Left main 3-vessel CAD

Ⓙ PCI

Ⓚ CABG

Ⓛ β-blocker therapy

Operation

Chapter 3 *Perioperative Arrhythmia*

JAMES M. BROWN, MD • JAMES S. GAMMIE, MD • STEPHEN SHOROFSKY, MD

(A) In the preoperative phase, a complete history and physical should be used to assess perioperative risk. A history of heart failure should prompt further investigation as to its cause and to determine whether it is compensated or uncompensated. A history of angina, ischemic heart disease, myocardial infarction, or a murmur of any kind should prompt further investigation. A history of perioperative arrhythmias of course is significant; however, it is significant as a marker for potential morbidity and mortality based on underlying cardiac abnormalities.

(B) Laboratory data will help identify remediable medical problems and abnormalities, especially in patients on diuretic therapy. PVCs on a preoperative ECG are significant as a marker of underlying heart disease. PVCs in the presence of a normal heart confer minimal added risk to operative intervention; however, PVCs in the presence of an abnormal heart indicate increased risk of cardiovascular morbidity and mortality. Elderly patients and patients with reduced ventricular function are at an increased risk of new perioperative arrhythmias. Based on preoperative evaluation, patients can be grouped as low-risk patients (e.g., patients with normal hearts or with mild stable symptoms). High-risk patients include the elderly, those with a history of heart failure, or those with unstable symptoms. Uncompensated or decompensated heart failure is an extremely high-risk situation and needs attention before operative intervention.

(C) Patients at high risk should undergo further testing and intervention. This might include determination of ventricular function, stress testing to determine reversible myocardial ischemia, or coronary angiography. Any evidence of active metabolic electrolyte or pulmonary system problem should be corrected, especially in elderly patients. High-risk patients who are candidates for β-blocker therapy will have reduced perioperative and long-term risk from institution of β-blocker therapy

before intervention. In addition, patients with heart failure that is uncompensated need to be treated with low-dose β-blocker therapy and angiotensin-converting enzyme inhibitors or receptor blockers in addition to diuretic therapy and stabilized over a period of days to weeks if time allows.

(D) During and after operative interventions, rhythm and conduction system abnormalities can generally be grouped as to whether they are tachyarrhythmias or bradyarrhythmias. The tachyarrhythmias are dominated by new-onset superventricular tachycardia or atrial fibrillation. Patients with preoperative atrial or ventricular arrhythmias will almost always manifest the same arrhythmia perioperatively.

(E) The bradyarrhythmias can be divided into AV conduction disturbances or frank asystole. Asystole should prompt cardiopulmonary resuscitation per ACLS protocol, which will include temporary pacing by external leads or transvenous pacemaker. Asystole leading to ventricular fibrillation should be treated by standard ACLS protocol involving immediate cardioversion. AV conduction disturbances can be divided into first-degree heart block; or PR interval prolongation on ECG, management of which is observation. Second-degree heart block can be either of the Mobitz I or Mobitz II variety. Mobitz I or Wenckebach is a progressive lengthening of the PR interval until an atrial impulse fails to conduct. This cycle then repeats itself. This is benign and requires no therapy. It may occur after an inferior myocardial infarction and is self-limiting; no pacemaker is required. Mobitz II involves either repetitive or paroxysmal loss of atrial impulse conduction without progressive lengthening of the PR interval. It can progress to complete heart block; placement of a temporary pacemaker is warranted. Third-degree AV block involves no atrial impulse conduction to the ventricle. A ventricular escape rhythm often fixes the heart rate at approximately 40 bpm. Acute onset usually follows acute myocardial infarction involving

the blood supply to the atrioventricular node. Treatment is immediate insertion of a pacemaker.

(F) Stable tachyarrhythmias need not be treated precipitously before careful consideration as to their nature and cause. Causes may include ischemia, hypoxia, pulmonary embolism, catecholamine excess or administration, pain, nebulizer treatments, electrolyte abnormalities, hypothermia, mechanical irritation (e.g., a Swann-Ganz catheter in the right ventricle), and hyperthyroidism. All of these factors should be corrected before operative intervention. Elderly patients with pulmonary surgery, a pulmonary process, or volume overload are also at risk for superventricular tachyarrhythmias.

(G) Patients who suffer tachyarrhythmias and are unstable (e.g., systolic blood pressure less than 90) require more immediate intervention. Ventricular tachycardia should be treated by immediate cardioversion and administration of lidocaine or amiodarone. Ventricular fibrillation, of course, requires immediate cardioversion per ACLS protocol. Atrial fibrillation associated with hypotension requires synchronized cardioversion, correction of all underlying remediable problems, and administration of amiodarone. In unstable patients, amiodarone must be given slowly. Its purpose is to prevent regression to atrial fibrillation after cardioversion.

(H) In a patient with atrial fibrillation and a blood pressure greater than 90, the primary initial goal is rate control and stabilization. In this set of patients, it is important to identify from the preoperative evaluation the presence of an abnormal heart. With severe ventricular dysfunction, institution of progressive doses of intravenous β-blocker therapy may result in morbidity from low cardiac output or bradycardia. Therefore, in patients with severe underlying heart disease who suffer atrial fibrillation postoperatively, recommended therapy is correction of all extra cardiac medical problems followed by loading with amiodarone (150 mg IV over 15 minutes followed by PO amiodarone dosing) and early cardioversion for any decompensation.

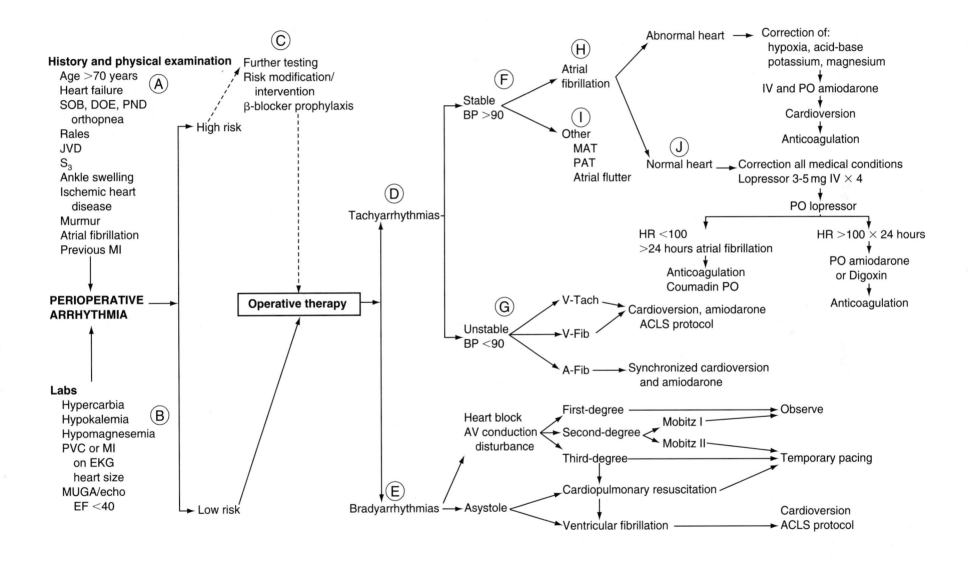

History and physical examination
Age >70 years
Heart failure
SOB, DOE, PND
  orthopnea
Rales
JVD
S_3
Ankle swelling
Ischemic heart
  disease
Murmur
Atrial fibrillation
Previous MI

**PERIOPERATIVE
ARRHYTHMIA**

Labs
Hypercarbia
Hypokalemia
Hypomagnesemia
PVC or MI
  on EKG
  heart size
MUGA/echo
  EF <40

Ⓐ

Ⓒ Further testing
Risk modification/
  intervention
β-blocker prophylaxis

High risk

Ⓑ

Low risk

Operative therapy

Ⓓ Tachyarrhythmias

Ⓔ Bradyarrhythmias

Ⓕ Stable
BP >90

Ⓗ Atrial
fibrillation

Abnormal heart → Correction of:
hypoxia, acid-base
potassium, magnesium
↓
IV and PO amiodarone
↓
Cardioversion
↓
Anticoagulation

Ⓘ Other
MAT
PAT
Atrial flutter

Ⓙ Normal heart → Correction all medical conditions
Lopressor 3-5 mg IV × 4
↓
PO lopressor

HR <100
>24 hours atrial fibrillation
↓
Anticoagulation
Coumadin PO

HR >100 × 24 hours
↓
PO amiodarone
or Digoxin
↓
Anticoagulation

Ⓖ Unstable
BP <90

V-Tach
V-Fib → Cardioversion, amiodarone
ACLS protocol

A-Fib → Synchronized cardioversion
and amiodarone

Heart block
AV conduction
  disturbance

First-degree —————————→ Observe
Second-degree
  Mobitz I
  Mobitz II —————→ Temporary pacing
Third-degree ——————————→ Temporary pacing

Cardiopulmonary resuscitation

Asystole

Ventricular fibrillation ——————→ Cardioversion
ACLS protocol

(I) There are other types of superventricular tachycardia that include multifocal atrial tachycardia or MAT. This is a rapid atrial arrhythmia that responds poorly to conventional therapy because it is usually caused by underlying severe cardiopulmonary disease (e.g., cor pulmonale and congestive heart failure). Treatment should include magnesium replenishment in addition to correcting the underlying disease process and treatment of heart failure. Atrial flutter involves a rapid and regular atrial rate of approximately 300 bpm, although this rate can vary. AV node conduction is usually at a ratio of 2 for 1, giving a ventricular rate of approximately 150. Vagal stimulation or medically induced AV nodal blockade may change the 2-to-1 block to one of higher degree. In the perioperative setting, control of atrial flutter with medical therapy is disappointing and primary efforts should be directed at correcting underlying metabolic and electrolyte abnormalities followed by conversion either by DC countershock or rapid atrial pacing. Paroxysmal atrial tachycardia or PAT results from either an ectopic automatic focus stemming from the atrium at one point or several points. It usually begins abruptly and lasts from minutes to hours. Atrial rates can be from 160 to 250 bpm and are often conducted at a ratio of 1 to 1. Management should include rate control using β-blockers, amiodarone, and digitalis. Of note, although amiodarone has surfaced as a dominant anti-arrhythmic for both superventricular tachycardias and ventricular tachycardias, it is not without cost and risk of complication. Pulmonary toxicity has received the most notoriety; however, amiodarone in combination with other AV nodal blocking agents can cause bradycardia and, in rare instances, may precipitate thyrotoxicosis. Amiodarone, like any medication, must be used appropriately and with caution.

(J) For the patient with a normal heart, correction of all remediable medical problems should be accomplished. These patients should be treated initially with intravenous β-blocker therapy followed by oral dosing. If heart rate is controlled at less than 100 bpm, but the patient persists in atrial fibrillation after 24 hours, PO anticoagulation is started. If heart rate control is not achieved after 24 hours of β-blocker therapy, PO amiodarone, 400 mg three times per day for 5 days, followed by 200 mg a day or digitalis and PO anticoagulation is added. Amiodarone is a very useful medication. It is, however, associated with a risk of pulmonary toxicity, thyrotoxicosis, and bradycardia. Intravenous heparin administration should be used cautiously in the early perioperative period, and its risk must be balanced against the risk of thromboembolism and stroke, which is approximately three times baseline in the perioperative population in the presence of atrial fibrillation.

REFERENCES

Amar D: Postoperative atrial fibrillation. Heart Dis 4: 117–123, 2002.

Ashrafian H, Davey P: Is amiodarone an underrecognized cause of acute respiratory failure in the ICU? Chest 120: 275–282, 2001.

Braunwald E, Zipes DP, Libby P (eds): Heart Disease: A Textbook of Cardiovascular Medicine, 6th ed. Braunwald, E, Zipes, DP, Libby, P (eds). Philadelphia: WB Saunders, 2000, pp 2084–2087.

Carlson MD: How to manage atrial fibrillation: An update on recent clinical trials. Cardiol Rev 9:60–69, 2001.

Lee JK, Klein GJ, Krahn AD et al: Rate-control versus conversion strategy in postoperative atrial fibrillation: a prospective, randomized pilot study. Am Heart J 140:871–877, 2000.

Leung PM, Quinn ND, Belchetz PE: Amiodarone-induced thyrotoxicosis: Not a benign condition. Int J Clin Pract 56: 44–46 2002.

Mahla E, Rotman B, Rehak P et al: Perioperative ventricular dysrhythmias in patients with structural heart disease undergoing noncardiac surgery. Anesth Analg 86:16–21, 1998.

Maisel WH, Rawn JD, Stevenson WG: Atrial fibrillation after cardiac surgery. Ann Intern Med 135:1061–1073, 2001.

Rho RW, Bridges CR, Kocovic D: Management of postoperative arrhythmias. Semin Thorac Cardiovasc Surg 12:349–361, 2000.

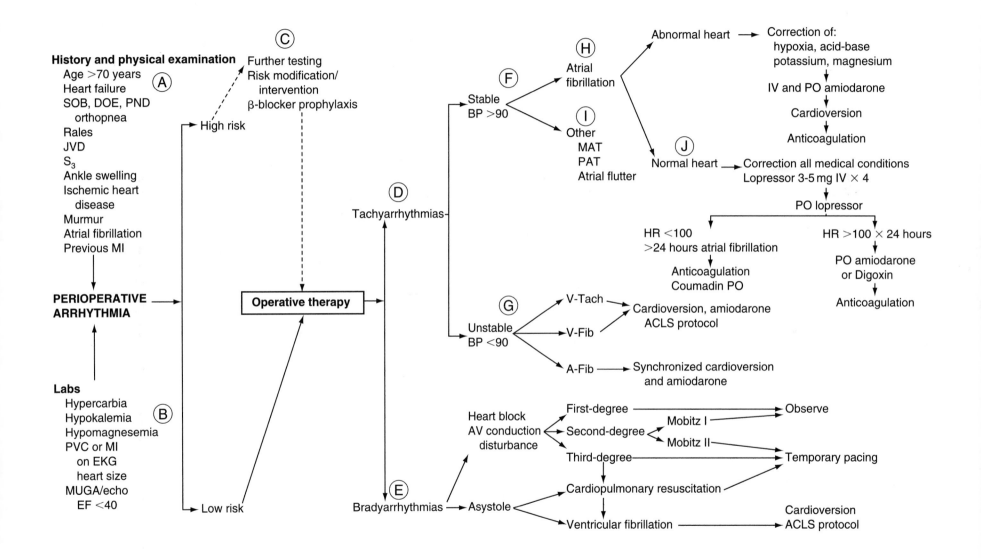

History and physical examination
Age >70 years   ⒶHeart failure
SOB, DOE, PND
  orthopnea
Rales
JVD
S_3
Ankle swelling
Ischemic heart
  disease
Murmur
Atrial fibrillation
Previous MI

**PERIOPERATIVE
ARRHYTHMIA**

Labs
Hypercarbia   ⒷHypokalemia
Hypomagnesemia
PVC or MI
  on EKG
  heart size
MUGA/echo
  EF <40

Ⓒ Further testing
Risk modification/
  intervention
β-blocker prophylaxis

→ High risk

→ Low risk

Operative therapy

Ⓓ Tachyarrhythmias

Ⓔ Bradyarrhythmias

Ⓕ Stable
BP >90

Ⓗ Atrial
fibrillation

Ⓘ Other
MAT
PAT
Atrial flutter

Abnormal heart → Correction of:
hypoxia, acid-base
potassium, magnesium
↓
IV and PO amiodarone
↓
Cardioversion
↓
Anticoagulation

Ⓙ Normal heart → Correction all medical conditions
Lopressor 3-5 mg IV × 4
↓
PO lopressor

HR <100
>24 hours atrial fibrillation
↓
Anticoagulation
Coumadin PO

HR >100 × 24 hours
↓
PO amiodarone
or Digoxin
↓
Anticoagulation

Ⓖ Unstable
BP <90

V-Tach
V-Fib
→ Cardioversion, amiodarone
ACLS protocol

A-Fib → Synchronized cardioversion
and amiodarone

Heart block
AV conduction
disturbance

First-degree —————→ Observe
Second-degree
  Mobitz I → Observe
  Mobitz II → Temporary pacing
Third-degree —————→ Temporary pacing
↓
Cardiopulmonary resuscitation

Asystole

Ventricular fibrillation —————→ Cardioversion
ACLS protocol

Chapter 4 *Cardiopulmonary Resuscitation*

CHARLES M. LITTLE, DO • NORMAN A. PARADIS, MD

(A) Verify unresponsiveness by stimulating patient.

(B) In witnessed arrest caused by ventricular fibrillation (VF) or pulseless ventricular tachycardia (VT) on ECG monitor, defibrillate immediately. Pads or quick-look paddles should be applied at once. VF or pulseless VT should be identified and defibrillation performed without delay. Cardiopulmonary resuscitation (CPR) using external chest compression provides less than 25% of pre-arrest cerebral and myocardial bloodflow. Rapid conversion of a treatable rhythm disturbance, therefore, is the first priority if neurologic injury is to be prevented. VF and VT are treatable rhythms, but successful defibrillation falls steadily with delays. In patients with unwitnessed arrest or in arrest more than 5 minutes, consider 1 to 2 minutes of chest compressions before countershock.

(C) Determine if you are using a monophasic or biphasic defibrillator: Biphasic defibrillators are more effective. An initial defibrillation dose of 200 joules (J) in monophasic defibrillators maximizes successful defibrillation and minimizes myocardial damage and the development of postcountershock pulseless bradyarrhythmias. Subsequent defibrillations are done at 300 J, then 360 J. With biphasic defibrillators, use approximately half as many joules. Employ the proper pad (or paddle) position with one just beneath the left nipple and the other beneath the clavicle to the right of the sternum (with paddles, use firm pressure and a conducting paste). Deliver the shock in the expiratory phase of ventilation (to minimize air resistance in the lungs); and deliver three consecutive countershock pulses (successive defibrillations lower skin resistance). Between countershocks, pause only long enough to check for a return of a spontaneous rhythm. Consider anterior-to-posterior paddle/pad position in patients who fail to defibrillate at maximal output.

(D) Start chest compressions if the patient is pulseless. Place the heel of one hand on top of the other on the lower half of the sternum. Compress forcefully at a rate of 80 to 100 compressions per minute. Each thrust should depress the sternum 1.5 to 2 inches in adults. Change providers frequently because of fatigue. There is no perfusion during interruptions in CPR; keep these to a minimum.

Open the airway; to relieve obstruction, displace the mandible (and the attached tongue and epiglottis) anteriorly using head tilt and chin lift. Care should be taken in patients who may have suffered a cervical injury. Suction the oropharynx, use a finger sweep to remove vomitus and debris, and insert a plastic oral airway. Assist ventilation with bag-valve-mask. If airway adjuncts are unavailable, administer mouth-to-mouth or mouth-to-pocket mask ventilation in patients suffering respiratory arrest.

Although the correct use of the bag-valve-mask can provide ventilation, endotracheal intubation protects the airway from aspiration and is the most effective means of ventilation and oxygen delivery. Emergent cricothyrotomy may be necessary in the context of severe craniofacial trauma, foreign body aspiration, anaphylaxis, or epiglottitis.

End-tidal CO_2 may be used as a crude indicator of CPR perfusion. ET-CO_2 levels above 15 appear predictive of the return of spontaneous circulation. Blood gas analysis may be useful to delineate hypoventilation.

Venous access is critical. Peripheral access is fastest, but central venous cannulation may optimize drug delivery. Do not delay pharmacotherapy by waiting for a central line. In the absence of venous access, the endotracheal tube provides a route for administering epinephrine, atropine, or lidocaine. In children, fluids and drugs can be administered via the intraosseous route.

(E) Reversible causes of respiratory arrest in a patient who is not breathing but has a pulse include CNS depression and primary asphyxia (e.g., respiratory failure, foreign body aspiration, epiglottitis, or cervicofacial trauma).

(F) Vasopressin (40 units) and epinephrine (1 mg) augment aortic diastolic blood pressure and increase the coronary perfusion pressure. The standard dose of epinephrine, 1 mg, can be repeated every 3 to 5 minutes. Higher doses (e.g., 0.2 mg/kg every 3 to 5 min) may be needed to maximize coronary perfusion pressure. After the administration of vasopressin or epinephrine, countershocks at 360 J should be repeated.

(G) Bradyasystole can result from a vagal response in MI or to drugs or metabolic processes. IV epinephrine (1 mg or 0.2 mg/kg every 3 to 5 minutes during arrest) should be used in asystole. Atropine is given (1 mg IV, repeated to 0.3 mg/kg every 3 to 5 minutes). Asystole artifact must be ruled out by checking cable connections and monitor leads. The monitor leads can be rotated to exclude fine VF.

Asystole that is unresponsive to initial ventilation, chest compression, and atropine has a grim prognosis. Success rates of electrical pacing in asystolic patients are negligible except in those who develop asystole immediately after cardioversion and in selected patients with heart block or bradyarrhythmias in the setting of acute MI or conduction system disease.

Pulseless electrical activity (PEA) is characterized by ECG evidence of electrical activity (QRS complexes) in the absence of effective myocardial contractions. If possible, confirm PEA with arterial monitoring or ultrasonography. Severe shock can be confused with PEA.

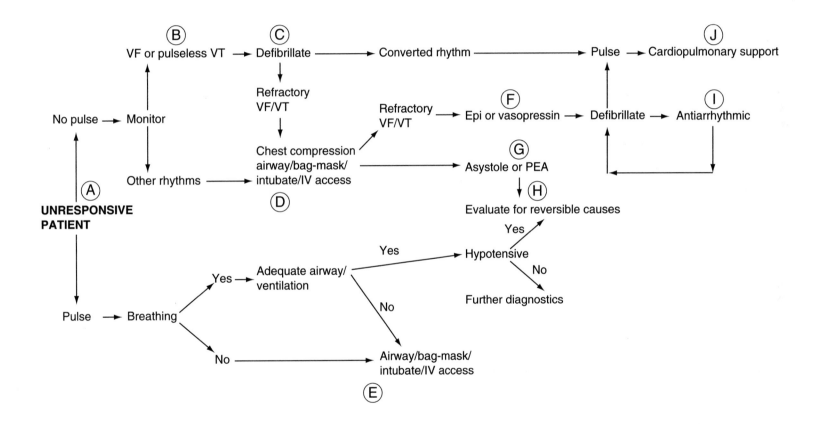

(H) The principal determinants of outcome in PEA are identification of reversible causes and the quality of CPR. Reversible causes (and treatments) of PEA include hypovolemia (crystalloid infusion), severe acidemia (ventilation and bicarbonate administration), hyperkalemia (calcium chloride and sodium bicarbonate), pneumothorax (decompression), and cardiac tamponade (pericardiocentesis).

(I) After failure of pressor drugs, consider antidysrhythmic therapy. Amiodarone (300 mg) is considered the first-line drug for incessant VF or VT. Lidocaine (1-1.5 mg/kg) and procainamide (17 mg/kg slow) have been used for many years. Magnesium (2 g) should be administered for VT with the appearance of torsades de pointes in a patient who may have a prolonged QT.

Calcium is generally ineffective for patients without cardiac mechanical activity. Intracellular calcium concentrations may reach toxic levels during arrest and reperfusion and contribute to cellular injury. Calcium may be beneficial, however, to some patients with PEA or severe shock (e.g., those with a wide QRS complex, a prolonged resuscitation effort, hypocalcemia,

hyperkalemia, or calcium channel blocker toxicity).

Sodium bicarbonate is generally not needed in the first 10 to 15 minutes of cardiac arrest if adequate ventilation is maintained. If severe metabolic acidosis (pH less than 7.2) develops, sodium bicarbonate (1 mEq/kg IV) may be considered. In general, the acidemia of cardiopulmonary arrest is better managed by aggressive alveolar ventilation than by bicarbonate administration.

(J) It is important in patients with restoration of circulation that secondary ischemic events be prevented through close monitoring of cardiopulmonary status post-arrest.

The neurologic outcome of patients in coma after cardiac arrest may be improved by induction of mild hypothermia (34°C).

REFERENCES

Becker LB, Weisfeldt ML, Weil MH et al: The PULSE initiative: Scientific priorities and strategic planning for resuscitation research and lifesaving therapies. Circulation 105(21): 2562–2570, 2002.

Bernard SA, Gray TW, Buist MD et al: Treatment of comatose survivors of out-of-hospital cardiac arrest with induced hypothermia. N Engl J Med 346:557–563, 2002.

Brown CG, Martin DR, Pepe PE et al: A comparison of standard-dose and high-dose epinephrine in cardiac arrest outside the hospital. The Multicenter High-Dose Epinephrine Study Group. N Engl J Med 327:1051–1055, 1992.

Caffrey SL, Willoughby PJ, Pepe PE et al: Public use of automated external defibrillators. N Engl J Med 347:1242–1247, 2002.

Gueugniaud PY, Mols P, Goldstein P et al: A comparison of repeated high doses and repeated standard doses of epinephrine for cardiac arrest outside the hospital. European Epinephrine Study Group. N Engl J Med 339:1595–1601, 1998.

Guidelines 2000 for cardiopulmonary resuscitation and emergency cardiovascular care. Circulation 102(8 Suppl):I1–I403, 2000.

Lindner KH, Dirks B, Strohmenger HU et al: Randomised comparison of epinephrine and vasopressin in patients with out-of-hospital ventricular fibrillation. Lancet 349:535–537, 1997.

Niemann JT, Cairns CB, Sharma J et al: Treatment of prolonged ventricular fibrillation: Immediate countershock versus high-dose epinephrine and CPR preceding countershock. Circulation 85:281–287, 1992.

Paradis NA, Martin GB, Rosenberg J et al: The effect of standard- and high-dose epinephrine on coronary perfusion pressure during prolonged cardiopulmonary resuscitation. JAMA 265:1139–1144, 1991.

Weil MH, Tang W: Cardiopulmonary resuscitation: A promise as yet largely unfulfilled. Dis Mon 43:429–501, 1997.

Wik L, Hansen TB, Fylling F et al: Delaying defibrillation to give basic cardiopulmonary resuscitation to patients with out-of-hospital ventricular fibrillation: A randomized trial. JAMA 289:1389–1395, 2003.

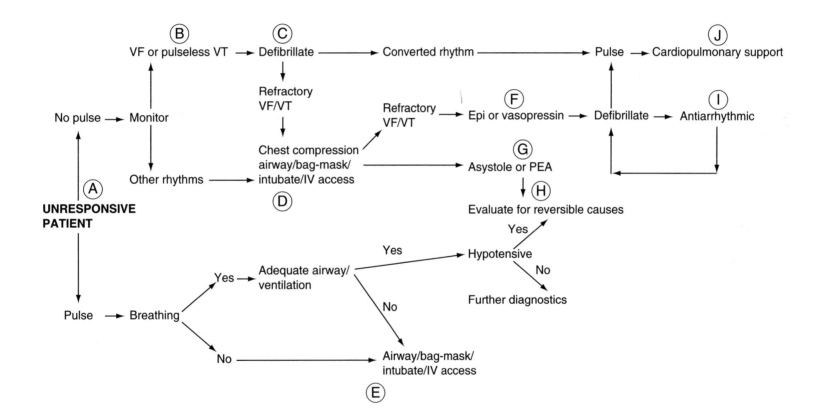

Chapter 5 Shock

JON M. BURCH, MD • ERNEST E. MOORE, MD

(A) Pneumothorax must be suspected and treated early in the course of resuscitation.

(B) Given flat neck veins; low central venous pressure (CVP); and a history of fluid loss, blood loss, trauma, or surgery, resuscitation begins with fluid challenge. The volume given should be based on an estimate of the patient's weight. Ringer's lactate (30 ml/kg) should be infused rapidly.

(C) If neck veins are distended, CVP is increased, or arrhythmia is present, a cardiac cause must be considered.

(D) If shock persists, a pulmonary artery line (Swan-Ganz catheter) should be inserted.

(E) Treatment of arrhythmia is followed by consideration of a pacemaker and long-term pharmacologic support.

(F) Causes of low or normal filling pressures include severe hypovolemia, sepsis, severe trauma, and neurogenic shock.

(G) High filling pressures and poor cardiac function suggest several compressive causes. Mechanical causes should be considered and treated early. This may require pericardiocentesis for treatment of cardiac tamponade and pericarditis, ventilation for support of patients with pulmonary embolism, and surgery for some cardiac problems. Therapy for the failing heart is directed at offloading the intravascular space by diuresis. Subsequent therapy is more specific to the pattern of cardiac failure. During resuscitation, constant monitoring of the level of oxygenation and of acid-base balance is necessary. The use of nitrates for vasodilation is based on the combined cardiac assessment.

(H) Cardiac tamponade occurs in a variety of clinical scenarios including trauma, postoperative states, tuberculosis, tumors, aortic dissection, uremia, and anticoagulation. The hallmark of cardiac tamponade is equalization of cardiac pressure in all four chambers. Although tamponade can be confused with left ventricular failure, noninvasive cardiac testing is diagnostic.

(I) If the systemic vascular resistance (SVR) is high and the cardiac output (CO) is low, the patient is hypovolemic and needs volume expansion with attention to acidosis. Be prepared for continued fluid needs if third-space losses are ongoing. Treat the cause of blood or fluid loss.

(J) With low SVR, the diagnostic possibilities are as follows: (1) sepsis and (2) neurogenic shock. Primary treatment aims to remove the cause of shock, provide fluids (balanced crystalloids), and optimize electrolytes and acid-base balance. Renal dose dopamine may help to preserve renal function. If CO is very low, use dobutamine, 5 µg/kg/min. α–adrenergic agents should be used to provide vasoconstriction only after other therapy fails. Start vasoconstrictive therapy using phenylephrine, 100 µg, to increase resistance; or use norepinephrine starting at 0.01 µg/kg/min. Monitor organ function and peripheral circulation closely.

(K) Diuresis can begin with furosemide, 40 mg, and increase as the patient improves. CO and pulmonary wedge pressure (PWP) should be monitored. An inotrope can be added.

(L) If shock persists, SVR should be reduced. If the heart rate is slow, it should be increased by using isoproterenol 0.2 µg/kg/min. If filling pressures are high, nitroglycerin, 25 µg/min, can be used.

(M) If filling pressures (CVP and PWP) are normal or low, use an afterload-reducing agent such as sodium nitroprusside, 0.5 µg/kg/min. If filling pressures are high, nitroglycerin, 25 µg/min, can be used.

REFERENCES

Gattinoni L, Brazzi L, Pelosi P et al: A trial of goal-oriented hemodynamic therapy in critically ill patients. N Engl J Med 333:1025–1032, 1995.

Miller PR, Meredith JW, Chang MC: Randomized, prospective comparison of increased preload versus inotropes in the resuscitation of trauma patients: Effects on cardiopulmonary function and visceral perfusion. J Trauma 44:107–113, 1998.

Velmahos GC, Demetraides D, Shoemaker WC et al: Endpoints of resuscitation of critically injured patients: Normal or supranormal? A prospective randomized trial. Ann Surg 232:409–418, 2000.

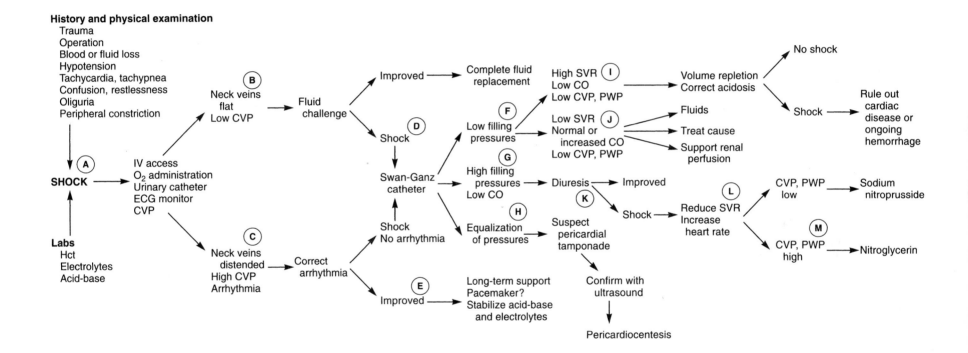

History and physical examination
Trauma
Operation
Blood or fluid loss
Hypotension
Tachycardia, tachypnea
Confusion, restlessness
Oliguria
Peripheral constriction

SHOCK

Labs
Hct
Electrolytes
Acid-base

Ⓐ IV access
O_2 administration
Urinary catheter
ECG monitor
CVP

Ⓑ Neck veins flat
Low CVP

Ⓒ Neck veins distended
High CVP
Arrhythmia

Fluid challenge

Correct arrhythmia

Improved → Complete fluid replacement

Ⓓ Shock

Swan-Ganz catheter

Shock
No arrhythmia

Ⓔ Improved → Long-term support
Pacemaker?
Stabilize acid-base and electrolytes

Ⓕ Low filling pressures

Ⓖ High filling pressures
Low CO

Ⓗ Equalization of pressures

High SVR Ⓘ
Low CO
Low CVP, PWP

Low SVR Ⓙ
Normal or increased CO
Low CVP, PWP

Diuresis → Improved

Ⓚ Shock

Suspect pericardial tamponade

Confirm with ultrasound

Pericardiocentesis

Volume repletion
Correct acidosis

Fluids
Treat cause
Support renal perfusion

No shock

Shock → Rule out cardiac disease or ongoing hemorrhage

Ⓛ Reduce SVR
Increase heart rate

CVP, PWP low → Sodium nitroprusside

Ⓜ CVP, PWP high → Nitroglycerin

Chapter 6 *Goal-Directed Resuscitation*

MICHAEL C. CHANG, MD

(A) Patients can be in shock for any of several reasons (e.g., hemorrhagic, cardiogenic, spinal, or septic shock). Untreated dead or injured tissue can also cause systemic shock because of deranged inflammatory status. Shock can be assessed by physical examination or by measuring markers of metabolic acidosis including the arterial base deficit and the serum lactate.

(B) Resuscitation from shock should always start with assessment of the airway, pulmonary status, and circulation. Intravenous access for rapid fluid administration should be obtained, a urinary catheter should be placed to monitor hourly urine output, and an ECG monitor should be placed to monitor cardiac rhythm.

(C) Oxygen transport is assessed by calculating oxygen delivery (DO_2) and oxygen consumption (VO_2). Oxygen delivery is calculated as the product of arterial oxygen content (CaO_2) and cardiac index ($DO_2 = Hg \times SaO_2 \times 1.39 \times CI$). Oxygen consumption is calculated as the arterial-venous oxygen content difference and cardiac index ($VO_2 = [CaO_2 - CvO_2] \times CI$). Mixed venous oxygen saturation (SvO_2) provides a continuous real time indicator of the balance between oxygen delivery and consumption and oxygen demand. Thus the major determinants of the SvO_2 are hemoglobin, SaO_2, CI, and VO_2. Inadequate oxygen delivery, excessive oxygen demand, or inadequate oxygen consumption can all contribute to shock status.

(D) Adequate oxygen delivery is defined at the level of oxygen delivery that provides optimal oxygen consumption. This is usually greater than $600\,ml/min/m^2$. The determinants of oxygen delivery are arterial oxygen saturation (SaO_2), hemoglobin concentration, and cardiac index.

(E) Adequate cardiac index and blood pressure are defined according to oxygen delivery and clinical tissue perfusion. Generally, a cardiac index greater than $3.5\,L/min/m^2$ is desired, and a mean arterial pressure greater than 80 to 85 mm Hg

is desirable. Hemoglobin or hematocrit should be titrated to optimize oxygen delivery for any given cardiac index. Arterial saturations should be maintained at greater than 0.90.

(F) Excessive oxygen demand in the face of the normal or supranormal oxygen delivery can lead to ongoing tissue acidosis and shock.

(G) Oxygen demand can be lowered primarily by eradicating the source of systemic inflammation (e.g., dead or injured tissue, infection, or abscess). Sedation and pharmacologic paralysis, when necessary, can lower oxygen demand. Ensuring normal heat status by warming hypothermic patients will also lower oxygen demand.

(H) Rate, rhythm, preload, afterload, and myocardial contractility are the independent determinants of cardiac function. These should be assessed individually, and abnormalities should be corrected to optimize cardiac index and mean arterial pressure.

(I) The first step in optimizing the independent determinants of cardiovascular function is to measure and optimize preload status. Intravascular volume status can be estimated at the bedside with a pulmonary artery catheter, measuring right ventricular end diastolic volume index (RVEDVI) and pulmonary artery occlusion pressure (PAOP). If pulmonary artery catheterization is not possible, response to a fluid challenge is an excellent way to assess the presence of a volume deficit. Echocardiography can also give an estimate of volume status and cardiac contractility.

(J) If preload is inadequate, fluid administration should be begun to optimize preload before moving on to assessing or improving contractility and/or afterload. Fluid administration should be according to the patient's needs, either isotonic crystalloid or blood products as necessary.

(K) If preload is adequate, and cardiac index and mean arterial pressure are still low, then myocardial contractility and afterload should

be assessed. Myocardial contractility can be difficult to assess at the bedside but can be inferred as the underlying deficit by the process of elimination if preload and afterload are deemed adequate. Another way to assess myocardial contractility is to calculate ventricular end systolic elastance (i.e., the slope of the ventricular end systolic pressure volume relationship). Afterload can be assessed by calculating systemic vascular resistance index (SVRI) from mean arterial pressure (MAP), the central venous pressure (CVP) and cardiac index ($SVRI = [(MAP - CVP) \times 80]/CI$) or by measuring the slope of the aortic input impedance relationship.

(L) If the hemoglobin concentration is decreased, packed red blood cells should be administered. This improves oxygen transport, oxygen carrying capacity, and preload. If the PT and PTT are abnormal, fresh frozen plasma can be administered. This corrects the underlying coagulopathy as well as provides a colloid fluid bolus.

(M) If no indications exist for administration of packed red blood cells or fresh frozen plasma, and preload is not adequate, isotonic fluid, usually either lactated Ringer's solution or normal saline, should be administered in a stepwise fashion to obtain adequate preload.

(N) If afterload is adequate and decreased myocardial contractility is present, then administration of positive inotropic agents with relatively pure inotropic effects should be undertaken. This would include dobutamine at clinical doses (2 to 20 µg/kg/min) and dopamine (5 to 10 µg/kg/min) at alpha/beta-range doses.

(O) If both contractility and afterload are noted to be inadequate, then administration of agents with both positive inotropic and vasopressor activities should be undertaken. This includes dopamine 10 µg/kg/min and epinephrine at any dose greater than 0.15 to 0.25 µg/kg/min. Doses should be titrated to achieve the appropriate clinical response.

REFERENCES

Chang MC, Mondy JS III, Meredith JW et al: Clinical application of ventricular end-systolic elastance and the ventricular pressure-volume diagram. Shock 7:6:413–419, 1997.

Chang MC, Blinman TA, Rutherford EJ et al: Preload assessment in trauma patients during large-volume shock resuscitation. Arch Surg 131:728–731, 1996.

Chang MC: Monitoring of the critically injured patient. New Horizons 7:35–45, 1999.

Kincaid EH, Miller PR, Meredith JW et al: Elevated arterial base deficit in trauma patients: A marker of impaired oxygen utilization. J Am Coll Surg 187:384–392, 1998.

Nelson LD: Continuous venous oximetry in surgical patients. Ann Surg 203:329–333, 1986.

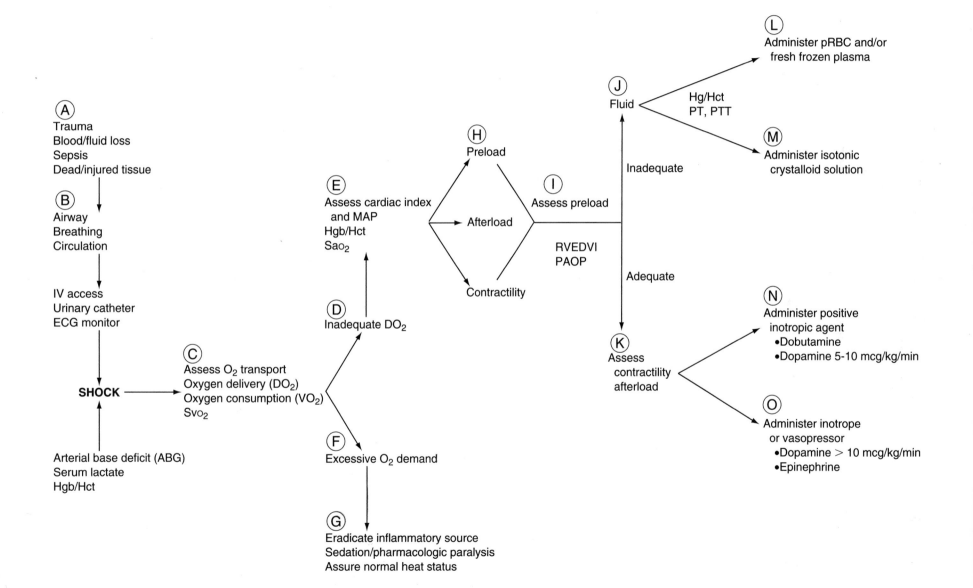

Chapter 7 **Bleeding Disorders in Surgical Patients**

CHITRA RAJAGOPALAN, MD

(A) The best screening test for a potential hemostatic disorder is a history of excessive bleeding during surgery, dental extraction, or minor trauma; easy bruising; heavy menstrual flow; and prior history of transfusions. Medical illnesses associated with bleeding tendencies include chronic liver disease, collagen vascular disease, hematological disease, and chronic renal disease. The presence of petechiae, hematomas, ecchymoses, hematuria, melena, or hemarthrosis suggests a problem. Medication history (specifically, aspirin, nonsteroidal anti-inflammatory drugs, and broad-spectrum antibiotics) and information on anticoagulant therapy and heparin flushes of IV lines must be obtained.

(B) Surgical bleeding may be caused by problems with vascular integrity or an acquired platelet dysfunction. Localized bleed typically indicates surgical (technical) bleed and diffuse bleed, a defect in hemostasis.

(C) Significant morbidity is noted with preoperative hemoglobin less than 9 g/dl. Examination of the peripheral smear provides clues to the presence of significant anemia (macrocytosis or microcytosis), splenic hypofunction (target cells), hemolytic anemia (schistocytes or spherocytes), increased reticulocyte count, or the presence of cold agglutinins (rouleaux formation).

(D) Qualitative and quantitative defects in platelets are seen in uremia and liver disease, or as direct effect of certain medications. Evaluation thrombocytopenia includes the platelet count; platelet morphology; and, possibly, bone marrow examination. In the absence of thrombocytopenia, platelet aggregation studies and platelet function assays may identify a qualitative defect.

(E) The prothrombin time (PT), INR, and activated partial thromboplastin time (aPTT) are assayed for the diagnosis of vitamin K deficiency, presence of a lupus anticoagulant, coagulation factor inhibitors, congenital and acquired clotting factor deficiencies, disseminated intravascular coagulation, and to monitor warfarin and heparin therapy.

(F) Measurement of fibrinogen levels is helpful in the diagnosis of congenital or acquired hypofibrinogenemia, which may be seen in liver disease, DIC, and thrombolytic therapy. Fibrinogen levels greater than 100 mg/dl are associated with a greater bleeding tendency.

(G) The bleeding time is sometimes used as a screening test for the diagnosis of acquired and congenital platelet disorders, qualitative platelet disorders, and von Willebrand's disease. In most patients, a normal bleeding time (2 to 9 min) indicates normal platelet function. A prolonged preoperative bleeding time does not always correlate with the risk of surgical bleeding and has little value in patients whose platelet counts are lower than 100,000/mm^3. A prolonged bleeding time caused by uremia may be corrected by administering 1-desamino (8-D-arginine) vasopressin (DDAVP) if not contraindicated. Additionally, cryoprecipitate or platelet transfusions may be necessary to maintain hemostasis.

(H) Activated clotting time: This test is used to monitor the effectiveness of heparin therapy. The test is affected by hemodilution, hypothermia, and protamine sulfate administration.

(I) Thromboelastogram: This test measures initiation of clot formation, strength, and the eventual clot lysis or retraction of clot.

(J) Replacement of more than one blood volume may cause dilutional coagulopathy and hypothermia. To achieve surgical hemostasis, platelets and fresh frozen plasma may be necessary. If hypothermia is anticipated, blood warmers are used.

(K) Platelet dysfunction with prolonged bleeding is seen with aspirin and with antiplatelet medications (e.g., ticlopidine hydrochloride [Ticlid], and clopidogrel [Plavix]). Additionally, eptifibatide (Integrelin), abciximab (Reo Pro), and tirofiban hydrochloride (Aggrastat) may increase postoperative bleeding. Heparin-induced thrombocytopenia (HIT) is usually seen within 2 to 12 days of initiation of heparin therapy and is followed by an abrupt 50% drop from the baseline platelet count. Discontinuing heparin often reverses the thrombocytopenia. When the diagnosis of HIT is confirmed, alternatives such as recombinant hirudin (Refludan) or argatroban (Acova) may be considered.

(L) Excess coumadin is identified by a prolonged PT and INR and, if possible, should be discontinued 24 hours before the surgical procedure. For quick correction of the PT, FFP and/or low-dose vitamin K may be considered. Usually 2 to 4 units of FFP will correct prolongation of PT/aPTT.

(M) Patients with significant liver disease have deficiencies of clotting factors and platelet abnormalities. All screening tests may be abnormal. Treatment with FFP, platelets, and cryoprecipitate may be necessary.

(N) DIC or consumption coagulopathy can occur in the presence of sepsis, excessive bleeding, or thrombosis. In addition to the labile factors V and VIII being consumed, platelets and fibrinogen levels are rapidly decreased. PT and aPTT are prolonged and platelet count and fibrinogen level are decreased. The d-dimer test to detect in vivo clot lysis is positive. Management of DIC is directed at treating the cause. Treatment may also include FFP; cryoprecipitate; platelet transfusions (if thrombocytopenia is life threatening); and, in some instances, infusion of heparin.

(O) Patients receiving streptokinase, urokinase, or recombinant tPAs (Activase and Retavase) may have excess unneutralized plasmin, resulting in systemic bleeding. Management is by transfusion therapy and/or the judicious use of e-aminocaproic acid (EACA, Amicar), aprotinin (Trasylol), or tranexamic acid (Cyklokapron). Postprostatectomy hemorrhage may be caused by urokinase; it results in local surgical bleed. Laboratory evaluation of hyperfibrinolysis should include PT, aPTT, fibrinogen

History and physical examination (A)
    Previous surgical bleed
    Bruising
    Family history
    Medications
    Chronic liver disease
    Chronic renal disease
    Hematological disease
    Collagen vascular disease

(B)
BLEEDING DISORDERS

Labs
    Hemogram (C)
    Platelet count (D)
    Protime/INR/activated partial thromboplastin time (E)
    Fibrinogen (F)
    Bleeding time (G)
    Activated clotting time (H)
    Thromboelastogram (I)

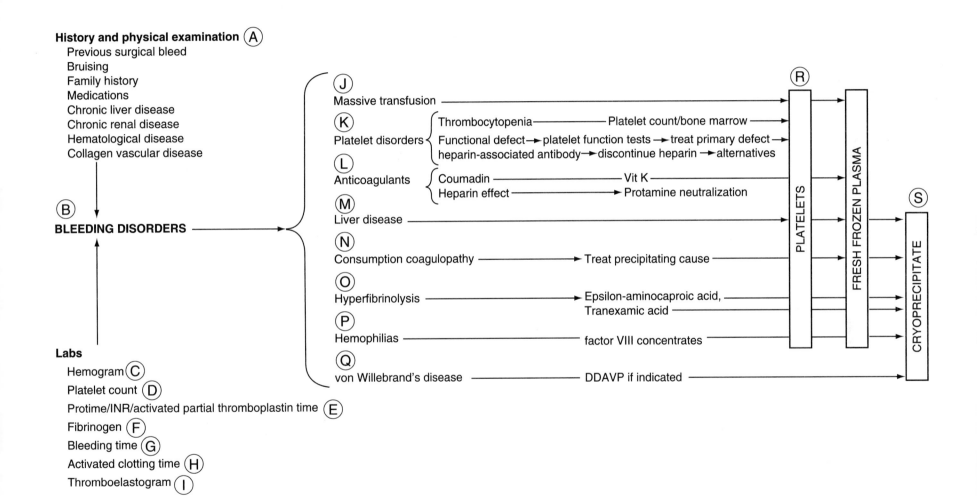

(J) Massive transfusion

(K) Platelet disorders
    Thrombocytopenia —— Platelet count/bone marrow
    Functional defect → platelet function tests → treat primary defect
    heparin-associated antibody → discontinue heparin → alternatives

(L) Anticoagulants
    Coumadin —— Vit K
    Heparin effect —— Protamine neutralization

(M) Liver disease

(N) Consumption coagulopathy —— Treat precipitating cause

(O) Hyperfibrinolysis —— Epsilon-aminocaproic acid, Tranexamic acid

(P) Hemophilias —— factor VIII concentrates

(Q) von Willebrand's disease —— DDAVP if indicated

(R) PLATELETS

FRESH FROZEN PLASMA

(S) CRYOPRECIPITATE

level, plasminogen level, fibrin degradation product (FDP), d-dimer, and alpha 2-antiplasmin levels. Intraoperative assessment of hyperfibrinolysis may be done using a thromboelastograph or whole blood viscoelastic clot detection. Management of this type of bleeding should take into account the underlying clinical condition.

(P) Hemophilia A is an inherited X-linked disorder caused by deficiency of factor VIII procoagulant activity. Severity of the hemorrhage depends on the factor VIII levels. Management depends on factor VIII levels, presence of inhibitors, and site of surgical procedure. DDAVP for mild hemophilia, factor VIII concentrates, or cryoprecipitate may be used to control bleeding. Hemophilia B is a sex-linked recessive disorder caused by factor IX deficiency. Severity correlates with factor IX levels and presence of inhibitors. Typically, bleeding after surgery is delayed.

Treatment with factor IX-containing concentrates may be required for severe deficiencies.

(Q) Von Willebrand's disease is the most common inherited congenital bleeding disorder. Mild cases may be treated with DDAVP except in type IIb, in which it is contraindicated. In severe cases, cryoprecipitate and FFP may be required.

(R) Apheresis or single-donor platelets are the equivalent of 6 to 8 random platelet units. Platelet transfusions for patients whose platelet count is 50,000 to 100,000/mm^3 must be evaluated on a case-by-case basis.

(S) Cryoprecipitate is typically issued as a pooled product. The amount of cryoprecipitate required depends on the severity of the bleed. Cryoprecipitate contains vWF, FVIII, fibrinogen, and FXIII and can also be used topically as fibrin glue or as fibrin sealant.

REFERENCES

Armas-Loughran B, Kalra R, Carson JL: Evaluation and management of anemia and bleeding disorders in surgical patients. Med Clin N Am 87:229–242 2003.

Bergqvist D, Agnelli G, Cohen AT et al: Duration of prophylaxis against venous thromboembolism with Enoxaparin after surgery for cancer. N Engl J Med 346:975–980, 2002.

Eckman MH, Erban JK, Singh SK et al: Screening for the risk for bleeding or thrombosis. Ann Intern Med 138:W15–W24, 2003.

Hender U: Recombinant factor VIIa (NovoSeven) as a hemostatic agent. Dis Mon 49:39–48, 2003.

Kearon C, Hirsh J: Management of anticoagulation before and after elective surgery. N Engl J Med 336:1506–1511, 1997.

Moiniche S, Romsing J, Dahl JB et al: Nonsteroidal anti-inflammatory drugs and the risk of operative site bleeding after tonsillectomy: A quantitative systematic review. Anesth Analg 96:68–77, 2003.

Winkelmayer WC, Levin R, Avorn J: Chronic kidney disease as a risk factor for bleeding complications after coronary artery bypass surgery. Am J Kidney Dis 41:84–89, 2003.

History and physical examination (A)
    Previous surgical bleed
    Bruising
    Family history
    Medications
    Chronic liver disease
    Chronic renal disease
    Hematological disease
    Collagen vascular disease

(B)

BLEEDING DISORDERS

Labs
    Hemogram (C)
    Platelet count (D)
    Protime/INR/activated partial thromboplastin time (E)
    Fibrinogen (F)
    Bleeding time (G)
    Activated clotting time (H)
    Thromboelastogram (I)

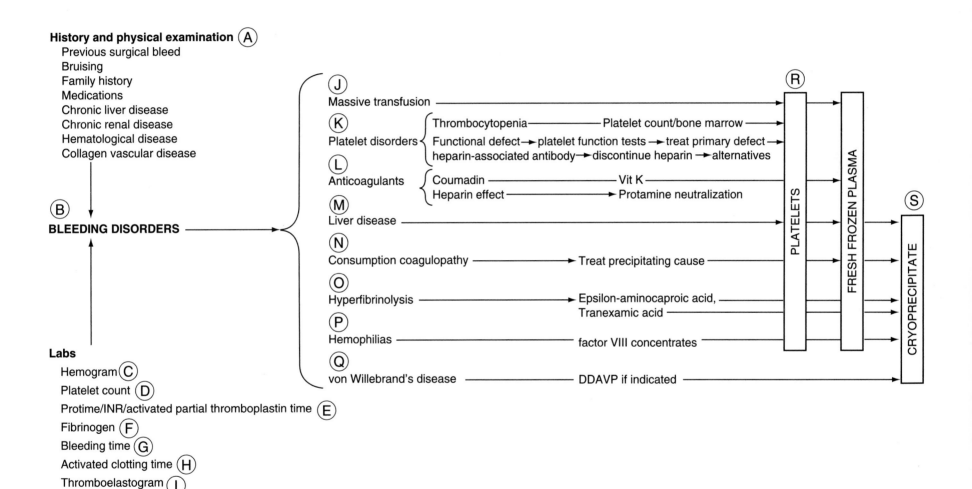

(J)
Massive transfusion

(K)
Platelet disorders
- Thrombocytopenia —————— Platelet count/bone marrow ——→
- Functional defect —→ platelet function tests —→ treat primary defect —→
- heparin-associated antibody —→ discontinue heparin —→ alternatives

(L)
Anticoagulants
- Coumadin —————— Vit K ——————
- Heparin effect —————→ Protamine neutralization

(M)
Liver disease

(N)
Consumption coagulopathy —————→ Treat precipitating cause ——→

(O)
Hyperfibrinolysis —————→ Epsilon-aminocaproic acid, ——
Tranexamic acid ——————

(P)
Hemophilias —————— factor VIII concentrates ——→

(Q)
von Willebrand's disease —————— DDAVP if indicated ——————

(R) PLATELETS

FRESH FROZEN PLASMA

(S) CRYOPRECIPITATE

Chapter 8 *Postoperative Fever*

DAVID J. CIESLA, MD • REGINALD J. FRANCIOSE, MD

(A) A postoperative fever is a common event and occurs in 15% to 47% of patients. Two temperature elevations to greater than 38.5°C within a 24-hour period constitute a postoperative fever. A thorough history (Hx) and physical examination (PE) will elucidate the cause of postoperative fever in the majority of patients. Comorbidities including malignancy, immunosupression, and renal failure may contribute to postoperative fever. Diabetes does not increase the incidence of postoperative wound infection but may increase its severity. Physical examination requires special attention to the operative site; extremities; vascular access sites; indwelling urinary catheter; and the lungs, especially in the early postoperative period.

(B) Laboratory tests are more likely to be significant when ordered specifically in response to physical examination findings. There is no routine battery of tests or studies that is appropriate for all patients.

(C) The majority of early postoperative fevers are the result of noninfectious causes and are self-limited. Early postoperative fever with T greater than 39°C demands immediate examination of the operative site to rule out necrotizing wound infection.

(D) Fever in the late postoperative period prompts a thorough Hx and PE with significant findings dictating further evaluation and treatment with a minimum number of additional tests.

(E) The incidence of positive blood cultures in the postoperative febrile patient is extremely low (0% to 3%) but postoperative mortality can be as high as 35% in bacteremic patients and 40% to 60% in the critically ill. Blood cultures are most likely to be positive and impact therapy when drawn more than 72 hours after surgery from patients at high risk for postoperative infection. Blood cultures are not warranted in the presence of a known infection confirmed by other culture evidence unless the pathogen has a propensity to seed other tissue spaces. Repeat blood cultures after a known bacteremia have little diagnostic utility.

(F) The critically ill differ from other postoperative patients in that numerous confounding variables are often present, making the clear identification of a febrile source difficult. Hx and PE can be unreliable, which often leads to an extensive work-up to identify occult infection. Risk factors include malnutrition, indwelling intravenous catheters, and broad-spectrum antibiotics.

(G) Serosanguinous drainage from an abdominal wound 3 to 5 days after surgery suggests a wound dehiscence, which is best explored in the operating room under sterile conditions where control of evisceration and secondary wound closure can be managed. Drainage of purulent fluid from the wound mandates opening the wound to allow for healing by secondary intention. Antibiotics are not necessary for most routine wound infection but may be indicated for cellulitis.

(H) Computed tomography (CT) has a 90% sensitivity and specificity for diagnosing intra-abdominal sepsis and is most useful 5 to 7 days following surgery when routine postsurgical fluid collections have largely resolved. CT-guided catheter drainage can also effectively treat the majority of intra-abdominal abscesses.

(I) In addition to physical examination, the detection of occult sepsis in the critically ill includes evaluation for acalculous cholecystitis (ultrasound/HIDA scan), intra-abdominal abscess (ultrasound/CT scan), and sinusitis (CT scan) that may require operative or image-guided drainage.

(J) Onset of a new heart murmur and presence of fever suggests subacute bacterial endocarditis (SBE) and should prompt ECG/echocardiogram and blood culture.

REFERENCES

Badillo AT, Sarani A, Evans SR: Optimizing the use of blood cultures in the febrile postoperative patient. J Am Coll Surg 194:477–487, 2002.

Bearcroft PW, Miles KA: Leukocyte scintigraphy or computed tomography for the febrile post-operative patient? Eur J Radiol 23:126–129, 1996.

Bohen JM, Solomkin JS, Dellinger EP: Guidelines for clinical care: Anti-infective agents for intra-abdominal infection. A Surgical Infection Society policy statement. Arch Surg 127:83–89, 1992.

Christou NV, Barie PS, Dellinger EP: Surgical Infection Society intra-abdominal infection study: Prospective evaluation of management techniques and outcome. Arch Surg 128:193–198, 1993.

Clarke DE, Kimelman J, Raffin TA: The evaluation of fever in the intensive care unit. Chest 100:213–220, 1991.

Cunha BA: The clinical significance of fever patterns. Infect Dis Clin North Am 10:33–44, 1996.

Freischlag J, Busittil RW: The value of postoperative fever evaluation. Surgery 94:358–363, 1983.

Garibaldi RA, Cushing D, Lerer T: Risk factors for postoperative infection. Am J Med 91:158S–163S, 1991.

Haley RW, Culver DH, Morgan DH: Identifying patients at high risk of surgical wound infection: A simple multivariate index of patient susceptibility and wound contamination. Am J Epidemiol 121:206–215, 1985.

Jarvis WR, Edwards JR, Culver DH: Nosocomial infection rates in adult and pediatric intensive care units in the United States. National Nosocomial Infections Surveillance System. Am J Med 91:185S–191S, 1991.

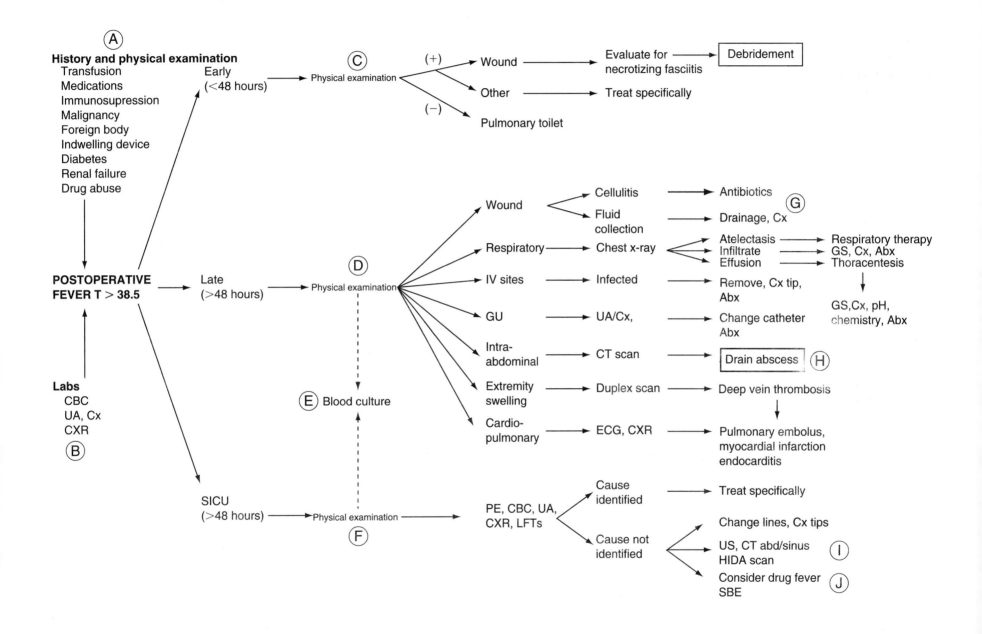

Ⓐ
History and physical examination
Transfusion
Medications
Immunosupression
Malignancy
Foreign body
Indwelling device
Diabetes
Renal failure
Drug abuse

POSTOPERATIVE FEVER T > 38.5

Labs
CBC
UA, Cx
CXR
Ⓑ

Early
(<48 hours)

Late
(>48 hours)

SICU
(>48 hours)

Ⓒ Physical examination

(+)
→ Wound → Evaluate for necrotizing fasciitis → Debridement
→ Other → Treat specifically
(−)
Pulmonary toilet

Ⓓ Physical examination

Ⓔ Blood culture

Ⓕ Physical examination

Wound
→ Cellulitis → Antibiotics Ⓖ
→ Fluid collection → Drainage, Cx

Respiratory → Chest x-ray
→ Atelectasis → Respiratory therapy
→ Infiltrate → GS, Cx, Abx
→ Effusion → Thoracentesis
→ GS,Cx, pH, chemistry, Abx

IV sites → Infected → Remove, Cx tip, Abx

GU → UA/Cx, → Change catheter Abx

Intra-abdominal → CT scan → Drain abscess Ⓗ

Extremity swelling → Duplex scan → Deep vein thrombosis

Cardio-pulmonary → ECG, CXR → Pulmonary embolus, myocardial infarction endocarditis

PE, CBC, UA, CXR, LFTs
→ Cause identified → Treat specifically
→ Cause not identified
→ Change lines, Cx tips
→ US, CT abd/sinus HIDA scan Ⓘ
→ Consider drug fever SBE Ⓙ

Chapter 9 *Nutritional Support*

MARGARET MCQUIGGAN, MS, RD, CNSD • FREDERICK A. MOORE, MD

(A) Patients are screened for nutritional risk in a timely manner. Assessment includes a medical history, nutritional history, and physical examination to assess muscle mass and energy reserves. Stress level and current level of organ function is determined.

(B) Laboratory measurements include serum protein markers and timed urinary nitrogen (TUN) for nitrogen balance calculations. C-reactive protein (CRP) is a sensitive acute phase response protein that peaks 3 to 4 days after injury. Only when this begins to decline will albumin, prealbumin, and transferrin be produced. The degree of stress and/or malnutrition can be classified by the following measurements:

(C) Preoperative nutritional repletion of surgical patients improves outcome in patients with severe deficits. Well-nourished to moderately malnourished patients should begin early enteral nutrition support (within 48 hours) once postoperative resuscitation is complete.

(D) Oral nutrition requires that one be able to meet more than 2/3 of nutritional needs by mouth. Interruptions in intake because of repeated procedures, operations, sedation, and NPO status should be considered.

(E) When the oral route is unavailable for nutritional support, enteral nutrition is preferred because it is more cost-effective and is associated with less risk than parenteral nutrition. Enteral nutrition offers better substrate utilization and maintains gut mucosal integrity and immunocompetence. Recent literature supports its use in pancreatitis. Concurrent parenteral and enteral nutrition is an option in patients with extraordinary demands (e.g., burns) or mild GI intolerance.

(F) Parenteral nutrition is useful when the GI tract is totally nonfunctional. It may also be employed when decreased splanchnic perfusion is suspected (e.g., when high-dose α-agonists or pressors are utilized).

(G) The stomach is accessed by blind nasal or oral intubation. Gastric feedings are suited for stable, nonventilated patients with normal gastric motility who are at low risk for aspiration. Risk of pulmonary aspiration decreases from stomach to duodenum to jejunum. Gastric residuals and abdominal distention should be checked initially every 4 hours, then every 8 hours. An acceptable residual volume is less than 200 cc. Continuous feedings are preferred in the critical care setting.

(H) Nasoduodenal tubes are placed by blind intubation with radiologic verification of placement. Tubes may be easily displaced by coughing, vomiting, patient agitation, or tube migration back into the stomach.

(I) Nasojejunal feeding tube placement can also be achieved by the "push" technique, either endoscopically, at bedside, or fluoroscopically. Jejunal feeding tubes are not as easily displaced as are nasoduodenal tubes. Although gastric ileus persists 1 to 2 days after surgery, and colon peristalsis is impaired for 3 to 5 days, small bowel motility is preserved. Full enteral support is possible in 85% of patients.

(J) Percutaneous endoscopic gastrostomy (PEG) is a safe, cost-effective alternative to the traditional operative gastrostomy when prolonged enteral support is anticipated. A concurrent percutaneous jejunostomy may be placed to facilitate feeding while the PEG is used for gastric drainage and/or medication administration (PEG/PEJ).

(K) A feeding jejunostomy can be placed at the time of exploratory laparotomy and feedings begun shortly thereafter.

(L) Patients requiring parenteral support for greater than 7 days should receive central TPN through a dedicated subclavian port.

(M) Although rare, peripheral parenteral nutrition (PPN) is employed when a central venous catheter is contraindicated or as a short-term therapy (i.e., 7 to 10 days) pending either oral or enteral feeding.

(N) Isotonic, polymeric formulas are those with long-chain proteins, carbohydrates, and a normal fat load. They are designed for patients with intact digestive and absorptive ability and can be used in the majority of patients.

(O) Fiber-containing formulas are polymeric formulas with added insoluble and, sometimes, soluble fiber. They may be of use in promoting a more-formed stool in patients with diarrhea. They are most useful in stable, long-term care patients because they reduce laxative usage and simulate a normal diet.

(P) Specialized immune-enhancing formulas are supplemented with glutamine, arginine, omega-3 fatty acids, and nucleotides. Glutamine helps maintain gut mucosal integrity and is thought to be conditionally essential during stress. The other nutrients are directed at wound healing and modulating monocyte and lymphocyte function to reverse postoperative inflammation and immunosuppression. These formulas are expensive and usage

Laboratory Monitoring of Nutritional Status				
Test	**Normal**	**Mild**	**Moderate**	**Severe**
Albumin (gm/dl)	>3.5	2.8–3.2	2.5–2.8	<2.5
Transferrin (mg/dl)	>200	180–200	150–180	<150
Prealbumin (mg/dl)	>18	15–18	10–15	<10
TUN (gm/day)	0.1 gm/kg body weight	8–10 g/day	10–12 g/day	>12 g/day
CRP (mg/dl)	0.0–0.8	<15	15–25	>25

History and
physical examination
  History of weight loss
  Anorexia
  Dysphagia
  Substance abuse
  Chronic disease
  Previous GI surgery   (A)
  Muscle mass
  Adipose reserves
  Trauma
  Sepsis
  Organ function

NUTRITIONAL
SUPPORT

Labs
  Albumin
  Prealbumin   (B)
  Transferrin
  Total urinary nitrogen
  C-reactive protein
  Serum glucose

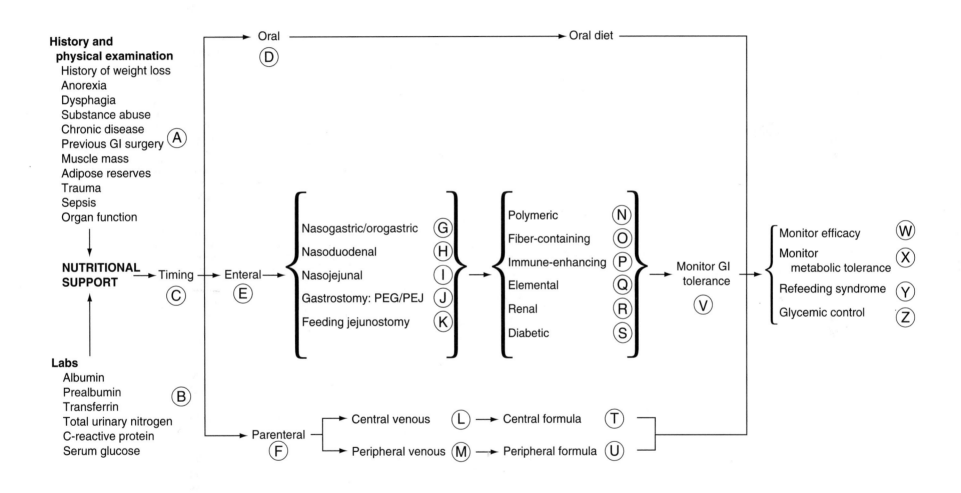

should be limited to patient populations in whom enhanced outcome has been proven (i.e., patients undergoing surgery for upper gastrointestinal cancer, ICU patients, or multiple trauma patients).

(Q) Elemental formulas contain amino acids, short-chain peptides, glucose, and a limited quantity of fat to prevent essential fatty acid deficiency. These are easily absorbed and minimize pancreatic and bile secretion, and are often used in short gut, in pancreatitis, or as initial feedings after prolonged gut disuse.

(R) Renal formulas are concentrated (2 kcal/cc) products that are low in potassium, phosphorus, and vitamins A and D. They are targeted for the patient with acute renal failure with or without hemodialysis. Continuous dialysis permits usage of standard formulas.

(S) Diabetic formulas are high-fat, fiber-containing products. They have been tested in ambulatory Type 1 diabetics and long-term care Type 2 diabetics. Usage in acute care has been shown to effect a modest reduction in blood glucose but no demonstrable effect on outcome. Current glycemic control recommendations favor the usage of insulin for glycemic control.

(T) Central TPN solutions are highly concentrated formulas that meet the need for protein, carbohydrate, fat, electrolytes, multivitamins, and most minerals.

(U) Peripheral parenteral solutions should have a final osmolarity of less than 800 mOsm/liter to avoid thrombophlebitis; thus only a moderate amount of kilocalories are provided in a large volume of solution. Additional lipids increase kilocalories and reduce osmolarity.

(V) Enteral tolerance should be monitored routinely. Vomiting, distention, diarrhea, increased NG output, or gastric residuals merit assessment and intervention.

(W) Serial measurements of body weight, body cell mass, wound healing, and serum proteins demonstrate the efficacy of the support provided.

(X) Serial analysis of electrolytes, LFTs, glucose, and pCO_2 provide impetus for tailoring the feeding regimen.

(Y) Nutritionally deplete patients may experience refeeding syndrome. This may result from alcoholism, cancer, anorexia nervosa, or prolonged NPO status/clear liquid diet. Precipitous declines in serum potassium, magnesium, phosphorus, and calcium occur while hyperglycemia appears. It is essential to gradually increase feedings to target goals, monitor blood glucose, and include ample electrolytes.

(Z) Maintaining glycemic control at less than 110 mg/dl has been shown to promote significant decreases in morbidity and mortality in surgical patients.

REFERENCES

A.S.P.E.N. Board of Directors and the Clinical Guidelines Task Force: Guidelines for the use of enteral and parenteral nutrition in adult and pediatric patients. JPEN 26(suppl 1):1SA–138SA, 2002.

Beyers P, Silver H, Restler C: Hyperglycemia: Is a disease-specific enteral formula indicated? Presented at the A.S.P.E.N. 19th Clinical Congress, Miami Beach, 1996.

Havala T, Shronts E: Managing the complications associated with refeeding. Nutrition in Clinical Practice 5:23–29, 1990.

Homann HH, Kemen M, Fussenich C: Reduction in diarrhea incidence by soluble fiber in patients receiving total or supplemental enteral nutrition. JPEN 18:486–490, 1994.

Kozar R, McQuiggan M, Moore F: Trauma. In Shikora S, Martindale RG, Schwaitzburg S (eds): Nutritional Considerations in the Intensive Care Unit. Silver Spring, MD: A.S.P.E.N. Publishers, 2002.

McClave SA, Spain DA, Snider HL: Nutritional management in acute and chronic pancreatitis. Gastroenterol Clin North Am 27:421–434, 1998.

McQuiggan MM, Marvin RG, McKinley BA et al: Enteral feeding following major torso trauma: From theory to practice. New Horizons 7:131–146, 1999.

Moore FA, Feliciano DV, Andrassy RJ et al: Early enteral feeding compared with parenteral reduces postoperative septic complications: The results of a meta-analysis. Ann Surg 216:172–183, 1992.

Moore FA, Moore EE, Kudsk KA et al: Clinical benefits of an immune-enhancing diet for early postinjury enteral feeding. J Trauma 37:607–615, 1994.

Reed RL, Eachempati SR, Russell MK et al: Endoscopic placement of jejunal feeding catheters in critically ill patients by a "push" technique. J Trauma 45:388–393, 1998.

Van den Berghe G, Wouters P, Weekers F et al: Intensive insulin therapy in critically ill patients. N Engl J Med 345:1359–1367, 2001.

Veterans Administration: Cooperative trial of perioperative total parenteral nutrition in malnourished surgical patients: Background, rationale, and study protocol. Am J Clin Nutrition 47(2 Suppl):351–391, 1988.

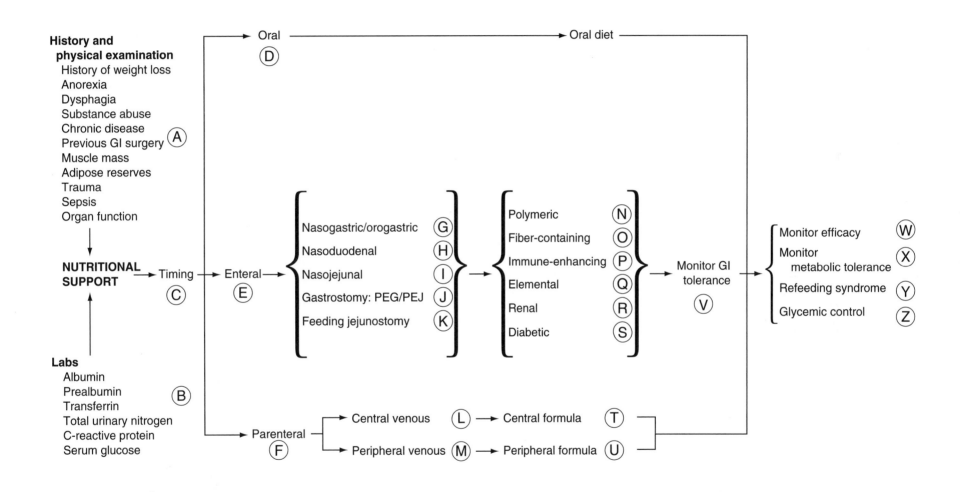

**History and
  physical examination**
  History of weight loss
  Anorexia
  Dysphagia
  Substance abuse
  Chronic disease
  Previous GI surgery Ⓐ
  Muscle mass
  Adipose reserves
  Trauma
  Sepsis
  Organ function

**NUTRITIONAL
SUPPORT**

Timing
Ⓒ

Labs
  Albumin
  Prealbumin Ⓑ
  Transferrin
  Total urinary nitrogen
  C-reactive protein
  Serum glucose

Oral
Ⓓ

Enteral →
Ⓔ

Nasogastric/orogastric Ⓖ
Nasoduodenal Ⓗ
Nasojejunal Ⓘ
Gastrostomy: PEG/PEJ Ⓙ
Feeding jejunostomy Ⓚ

Polymeric Ⓝ
Fiber-containing Ⓞ
Immune-enhancing Ⓟ
Elemental Ⓠ
Renal Ⓡ
Diabetic Ⓢ

Monitor GI
tolerance
Ⓥ

Oral diet

Monitor efficacy Ⓦ
Monitor
  metabolic tolerance Ⓧ
Refeeding syndrome Ⓨ
Glycemic control Ⓩ

Parenteral
Ⓕ

Central venous Ⓛ → Central formula Ⓣ
Peripheral venous Ⓜ → Peripheral formula Ⓤ

Chapter 10 **Hypothermia**

BRUCE C. PATON, MD

(A) History includes circumstances of exposure (e.g., obvious accidental exposure, old age, or living conditions). It also notes associated diseases (i.e., neurologic, cardiovascular, or endocrine); drug or alcohol intoxication; and psychiatric disorders.

(B) Hypothermia produces bradycardia, hypotension, and unconsciousness. Peripheral pulses are often impalpable. Inability to feel a pulse, measure blood pressure, or hear a heartbeat does not mean a cold patient is dead. Unconsciousness with a core temperature of greater than 32°C may be caused by associated drugs or head injury and not by hypothermia. Bradycardia and atrial fibrillation are common arrhythmias when temperature falls to less than 30°C. Ventricular fibrillation or asystole can occur with a temperature less than 25°C.

(C) Any core temperature (e.g., esophageal, high rectal, bladder, or tympanic membrane) less than 35°C constitutes hypothermia. Accepted classifications include mild, 35 to 32°C; moderate, 32 to 28°C; deep, 28 to 25°C; and profound, less than 25°C.

(D) Abnormalities of serum K+, Na+, and glucose are common. Blood urea nitrogen and creatinine are elevated if there is renal shutdown. Acidosis is common, especially during rewarming. Measurements of pH should not be corrected for temperature. A toxicant screen is essential to exclude drugs or alcohol as the cause of hypothermia.

(E) Barring head injury or drug overdose, unconsciousness in a cold patient is considered to be caused by hypothermia (temperature usually less than 32°C). Those who arrive in the emergency room conscious should survive.

(F) Unconscious cold patients must be admitted to the ICU or operating room (if extracorporeal circulation is to be used), and treatment of both hypothermia and associated condition must be started.

(G) Arrhythmias with ineffective cardiac output may occur during rewarming. Most arrhythmias disappear with normothermia. Active rewarming is commonly necessary before ventricular defibrillation is possible. Rewarming may cause relative hypovolemia, which should be treated with volume replacement as indicated by standard criteria.

(H) Passive rewarming consists of removing wet clothing, covering the patient with warm blankets, monitoring the ECG and temperature, and allowing endogenous metabolism to rewarm the body. This can be done in the emergency room, the ICU, or a hospital room.

(I) Determination of heartbeat can be difficult. Shivering interferes with ECG monitoring, and pulse blood pressure may not be palpable. Arterial cutdown may be necessary to measure blood pressure.

(J) If the heart is beating, the patient should be treated with full intensive care monitoring. Treatment must be carefully controlled and cautious rather than overzealous. The patient is handled gently. Endotracheal intubation and the insertion of Swan-Ganz catheters must be done gently, but these measures should not be withheld for fear of inducing ventricular fibrillation. Acidosis and electrolyte abnormalities are corrected slowly as is the hypotension caused by vasodilation during rewarming.

(K) Cardiopulmonary resuscitation is started as soon as the absence of a heartbeat is confirmed. Cardiopulmonary resuscitation started in the field must be continued until cardiac action can be definitively determined and treated.

(L) Active rewarming may be external or internal. External methods are less traumatic than internal ones and are more readily available but less efficient. The chosen method should be appropriate to the situation and, if possible, should allow resuscitation during rewarming. External rewarming may include hot water bottles, piped suits or blankets, radiant heat, warmed circulating air, or warm water tub (45°C). Immersion in warm water is the most efficient external method. Internal rewarming always begins with the administration of warm, humidified oxygen. This prevents further heat loss and provides additional heat. Body cavity lavage (peritoneum, pleura) is efficient and requires minimal equipment. Femorofemoral or total cardiopulmonary bypass with a heat exchanger is the most efficient method of rewarming but requires special equipment in a cardiac center. It is the optimal treatment for profound hypothermia with cardiac arrest.

(M) Survival depends more on associated diseases and injuries than on the degree of hypothermia. Mild hypothermia should not cause death. Deep hypothermia with cardiac arrest treated by cardiopulmonary bypass has a 50% mortality. Elevated blood urea nitrogen or K+ and the need for resuscitation outside a hospital are associated with a poor prognosis. Serum K+ greater than 10 mEq/1 signifies inability to resuscitate. Hypothermia incidental to severe trauma adds significantly to mortality.

REFERENCES

Danzl DF: Accidental Hypothermia. In Auerbach PS (ed.): Wilderness Medicine, 4th ed. St. Louis: Mosby, 2001.

Giesbrecht CG: Emergency treatment of hypothermia. Emerg Med 13:9–16, 2001.

Walpoth BH, Walpoth-Aslan BN, Mattle HP, et al: Outcome of survivors of accidental deep hypothermia and circulatory arrest treated with extracorporeal blood warming. New Eng J Med 337:1500–1505, 1997.

Wittmers LE, Jr.: Pathophysiology of cold exposure. Minn Med 84:30–36, 2001.

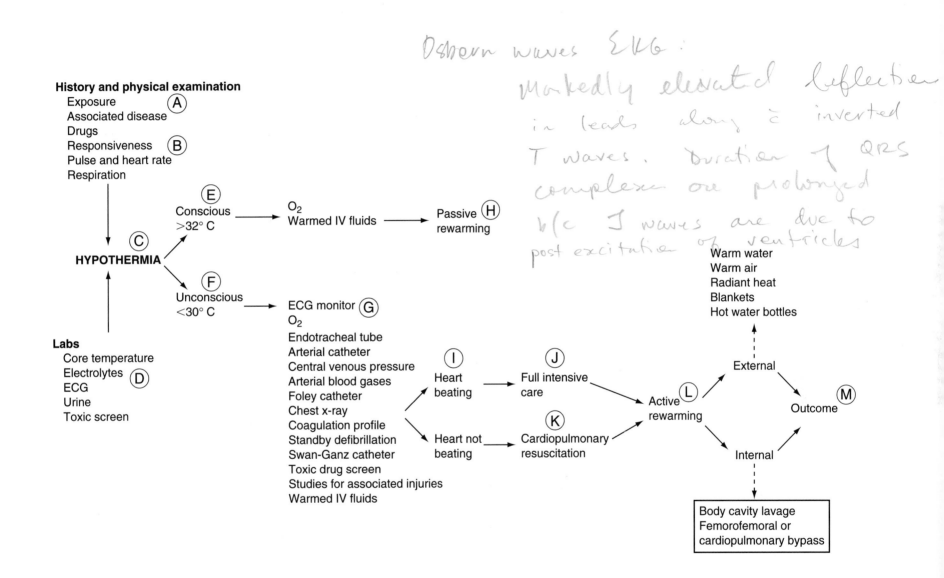

History and physical examination
Exposure (A)
Associated disease
Drugs
Responsiveness (B)
Pulse and heart rate
Respiration

→ **HYPOTHERMIA** (C)

Labs
Core temperature
Electrolytes (D)
ECG
Urine
Toxic screen

(E) Conscious >32° C → O₂ / Warmed IV fluids → Passive rewarming (H)

(F) Unconscious <30° C → ECG monitor (G)
O₂
Endotracheal tube
Arterial catheter
Central venous pressure
Arterial blood gases
Foley catheter
Chest x-ray
Coagulation profile
Standby defibrillation
Swan-Ganz catheter
Toxic drug screen
Studies for associated injuries
Warmed IV fluids

(I) Heart beating → Full intensive care (J)

(K) Heart not beating → Cardiopulmonary resuscitation

→ Active rewarming (L)

External → Warm water / Warm air / Radiant heat / Blankets / Hot water bottles

Internal

→ Outcome (M)

Body cavity lavage
Femorofemoral or
cardiopulmonary bypass

Handwritten note:
Osborn waves EKG:
Markedly elevated deflection in leads along c inverted T waves. Duration of QRS complexes are prolonged b/c J waves are due to post excitation of ventricles

Chapter 11 *Acute Respiratory Failure*

ROBERT BARTLETT, MD

Acute respiratory failure in surgical patients is usually mild to moderate and very responsive to treatment. This condition is identified as "mild respiratory failure" in the diagram. **Initial management** includes ventilation and systemic monitoring and treatment. If the goals of initial management are met, proceed to weaning from ventilation.

Patients who fail to respond to initial management have **severe respiratory failure. Advanced management** of severe respiratory failure includes pressure controlled inverse ratio ventilation, diuresis to dry weight, prone positioning, normal hematocrit, and normal serum albumin. Patients who fail despite advanced treatment have a very high mortality risk and are candidates for extracorporeal support.

(A) Mortality risk in acute respiratory failure. In a recent study of mechanical ventilation by the NIH-ARDS Net the mortality for 7000 patients who met the definition of acute lung injury or ARDS was 44%, and the mortality for the 902 patients entered into the ventilation study was 35%.

(B) Plateau pressure (Pplat: the airway pressure after a brief inspiratory hold on a mechanical ventilator) is the best indication of alveolar inflation or over inflation. Over inflation causes stretch injury to alveoli. The level of plateau pressure which invariably causes alveolar injury has not been determined, but any plateau pressure greater than 35 cm of water should be avoided, even in severe respiratory failure.

(C) Optimizing end expiratory pressure (PEEP). PEEP is used to maintain inflation of alveoli which would deflate at lower pressure. Positive end expiratory pressure should be set just above the critical closing pressure of dependent alveolar units. Optimal PEEP is determined as the point of maximal O_2 delivery (highest SVO_2) or the point of maximal effective compliance (volume/pressure).

(D) Oxygen delivery (DO_2) is normally 600 cc/m^2/min. DO_2 is cardiac output times the arterial oxygen content (Hb gm/dl × % sat × 1.36 = CO_2/dl).

PEEP can increase O_2 content by increasing saturation, but can decrease cardiac output. The ideal level of positive end expiratory pressure is that which prevents small airway collapse in vulnerable lung units, but is not high enough to inhibit venous return into the chest. The optimal level of PEEP will vary with the tidal volume, inspiratory pressure, blood volume, cardiac function, and respiratory rate. Therefore, optimal PEEP may change hour to hour. This combination of factors is best identified by the maximal venous blood saturation if a pulmonary artery catheter is in place. In the absence of a pulmonary artery catheter these variables can be estimated by the maximal effective compliance or by identifying the inflection point on the inspiratory side of the volume pressure curve. Optimizing PEEP will help to optimize the cardiac output. Systemic oxygen delivery is further optimized by assuring a normal amount of hemoglobin (15 grams %) in the blood.

(E) Dilution of plasma proteins with associated decrease in plasma colloid osmotic pressure (COP) commonly occurs in patients with acute respiratory failure. One goal of treatment (which will facilitate normalizing extracellular fluid volume) is to be sure that plasma albumin levels are in the normal range (>3 grams/dl).

(F) When oxygen delivery is limited by respiratory failure, attention should be paid to measuring oxygen consumption (VO_2) and reducing oxygen consumption and hypermetabolism to normal levels by treating sepsis or other underlying conditions.

(G) The combination of normalizing oxygen consumption when possible and optimizing systemic oxygen delivery (DO_2) will result in the normal ratio of oxygen delivery to oxygen consumption at 4 or 5 to 1. The relationship between oxygen delivery and consumption is conveniently measured continuously by continuous monitoring of mixed venous blood oxyhemoglobin saturation.

(H) Extracellular fluid overload is common in patients who have acute respiratory failure,

partly from high venous pressures induced by mechanical ventilation, but primarily due to fluid given as resuscitation or treatment. Fluid overload plays a major role in respiratory failure, pathogenesis, and outcome. Normal extracellular fluid volume (normal body weight) is a goal of treatment in ventilator patients.

(I) When patients have apparently recovered from acute respiratory failure and appear to be ready for extubation, the weaning criteria are measured (Table 11.1). These criteria measure the strength of the patient's effort (inspiratory force, tidal volume, and vital capacity), the patient's ability to understand and cooperate (vital capacity), the ability to sustain a period of spontaneous breathing (respiratory rate) and some measure of the ability to excrete metabolically produced carbon dioxide (minute ventilation). Acceptable weaning criteria are: inspiratory force > −20 cm H_2O, tidal volume >5 cc/kg, vital capacity >2× tidal volume, respiratory rate <20, minute ventilation >100 cc/kg/min. If the patient meets these criteria it is generally safe to extubate the patient.

(J) Patients who fail to respond to the management discussed in initial management are typically characterized by alveolar arterial gradient

TABLE 11.1
Weaning Criteria

Parameter	Value
Pao$_2$ on Fio$_2$	>80 torr on <0.6
PaCo$_2$	<45 torr
Respiratory rate (RR)	<35/min
Tidal Volume (Vt)	>5 ml/kg
Vital Capacity	>10 ml/kg
Minute Ventilation	<10 L/min
Negative Inspiratory Force	<−20 cm H_2O
Rapid Shallow Breathing Index	<104

(RR/Vt in L)

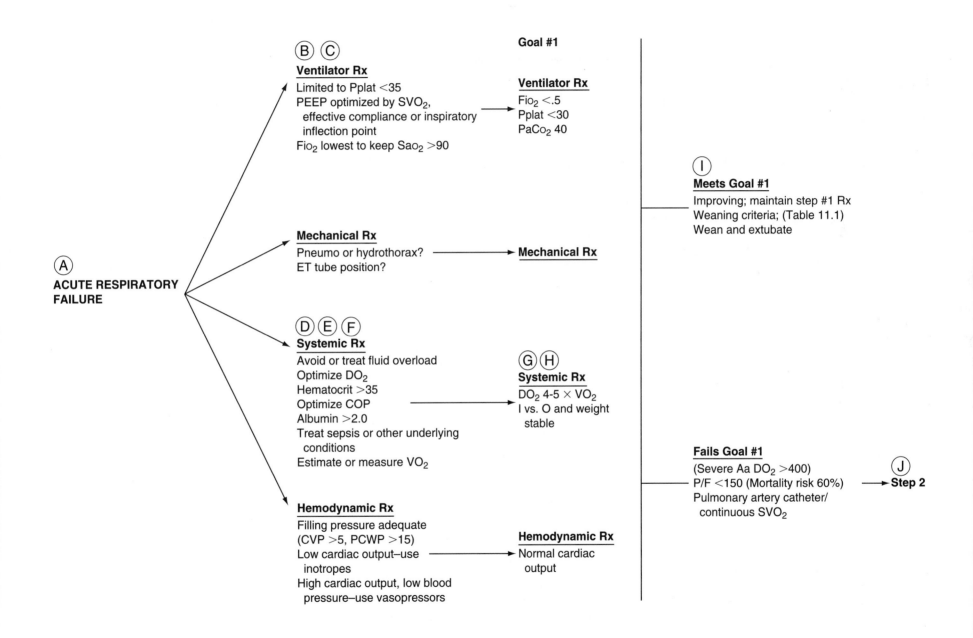

Ⓑ Ⓒ

Ventilator Rx

Limited to Pplat <35
PEEP optimized by SVO_2,
  effective compliance or inspiratory
  inflection point
Fio_2 lowest to keep Sao_2 >90

Goal #1

Ventilator Rx

Fio_2 <.5
Pplat <30
$PaCo_2$ 40

Ⓘ

Meets Goal #1

Improving; maintain step #1 Rx
Weaning criteria; (Table 11.1)
Wean and extubate

Mechanical Rx

Pneumo or hydrothorax?
ET tube position?

Mechanical Rx

Ⓐ

**ACUTE RESPIRATORY
FAILURE**

Ⓓ Ⓔ Ⓕ

Systemic Rx

Avoid or treat fluid overload
Optimize DO_2
Hematocrit >35
Optimize COP
Albumin >2.0
Treat sepsis or other underlying
  conditions
Estimate or measure VO_2

Ⓖ Ⓗ

Systemic Rx

DO_2 4-5 × VO_2
I vs. O and weight
  stable

Fails Goal #1

(Severe Aa DO_2 >400)
P/F <150 (Mortality risk 60%)
Pulmonary artery catheter/
  continuous SVO_2

Ⓙ

→ **Step 2**

Hemodynamic Rx

Filling pressure adequate
(CVP >5, PCWP >15)
Low cardiac output–use
  inotropes
High cardiac output, low blood
  pressure–use vasopressors

Hemodynamic Rx

Normal cardiac
  output

>400 or PaO_2/FiO_2 <150. These patients have a mortality risk which is greater than 60% and the treatment outline in advanced management should be followed.

(K) Pressure controlled ventilation (PCV). Pressure controlled ventilation is the preferred mode in severe respiratory failure because each breath has the possibility of recruiting more alveolar units (unlike volume-controlled ventilation). Since the goal is achievement and maintenance of alveolar inflation more time is spent during inspiration than exhalation, resulting in "inverse ratio" (PCIRV).

(L) Accept hypoxia and hypercarbia rather than overdistend alveoli. Using high pressure and rapid rate to achieve CO_2 clearance causes more harm than good if stretch injury results. Similarly using FiO_2 levels greater than 80% depletes alveolar nitrogen and leads to alveolar collapse. For these reasons it is safer to accept hypoxemia and hypercarbia than to cause further lung injury with high plateau pressures and high inspired oxygen.

(M) Inhaled nitric oxide is an excellent pulmonary vasodilator which is very effective in cases of pulmonary arterial spasm. This occurs in newborn respiratory failure and post-lung transplant. Inhaled nitric oxide (NO) has been attempted for other forms of respiratory failure in children and adults, but vasospasm is not a major component of the pathophysiology so NO is not effective as treatment. High frequently oscillation is a mode of mechanical ventilation which has been used in newborn infants with success. In adults with respiratory failure high frequency ventilation is still under investigation.

(N) The simple weight of interstitial fluid in severe respiratory failure presses down on dependent alveoli causing alveolar collapse and transpulmonary shunting of the blood which is perfusing those collapsed alveoli. Because patients are often managed in the supine position, these compressed alveoli are found in the posterior aspects of the lung.

By turning the patient prone the effects of the weight of water are reversed; the posterior alveolar units open up and the shunt is decreased.

Prone positioning has become an essential step in management of severe respiratory failure. Alveolar inflation, and VQ matching improves dramatically thereby improving oxygenation. Typically patients are turned prone for 6 hours, then supine, then prone, etc until FiO_2 requirement is less than 50%. It is important to treat the fluid overload in the patient during this stage of management, otherwise the benefit of prone positioning will not be realized.

(O) Intubation for more than 3 days leads to nosocomial pneumonia and requires sedation and may cause vocal cord damage. Tracheostomy eliminates these problems but has some inherent risks. If tracheostomy can routinely and easily be performed without complications, it should be carried out for patients with severe respiratory failure. Ventilator weaning is also facilitated by tracheostomy.

(P) Meduri has presented convincing evidence that high-dose steroids are effective in weaning patients from mechanical ventilation in the late stages of ARDS (after 7 days). Meduri dosage schedule is Solu-Medrol 2 mg/kg per day for 1 week, then 1 mg/kg per day until the patient is off the ventilator.

(Q) Patients who have an Aa gradient greater than 600 despite all the treatment outlined in advanced management have a very high risk of dying. Extracorporeal circulation and gas exchange (often called extracorporeal membrane oxygenation, ECMO) is indicated in this situation. The survival rate for children with severe respiratory failure and treated with ECMO is approximately 70% and for adults is approximately 60%. An alternative to full extracorporeal gas exchange support is the use of extracorporeal circulation to remove CO_2 as the primary goal. This allows decrease in the ventilator pressure and rate to very low levels while achieving oxygenation across the native lung.

REFERENCES

Amato MB, Barbas CSV, Mederos DM, et al: Effect of a protective ventilator strategy on mortality in the acute respiratory distress syndrome. N Engl J Med 338:347–354, 1998.

The Acute Respiratory Distress Syndrome Network. Ventilation with lower tidal volumes as compared with traditional tidal volumes for acute lung injury and the acute respiratory distress syndrome. N Eng J Med 342:1301–1308, 2000.

Bartlett RH: Extracorporeal life support in the management of severe respiratory failure. Clinics in Chest Medicine 21:555–561, September 2000.

Bartlett RH: Use of the Mechanical Ventilator. Chapter 92 in ACS Surgery, Principles and Practice, Web MD. New York, NY, 2003.

Bartlett RH, Dechert RE, Mault J, Ferguson S, Kaiser AM, Erlandson EE: Measurement of metabolism in multiple organ failure. Surgery 92:771–779, 1982.

Bartlett RH, Rich P: Pulmonary Insufficiency. Chapter 71 in ACS Surgery, Principles and Practice, Web MD. New York, NY, 2003.

Dreyfuss D, Saumon G: Ventilator-induced lung injury: lessons from experimental studies. Am J. Critical Care Med. 157:1–30, 1998.

Gattinoni L, Tognoni G, Pesenti A, et al: Effect of prone positioning on the survival of patients with acute respiratory failure. N Engl J Med 345:568–573, 2001.

Hickling K, Walsh J, Henderson S, et al: Low mortality in adult respiratory distress syndrome using low-volume, pressure-limited ventilation with permissive hypercapnia: a prospective study. Crit Care Med 22:1568–1578, 1994.

Mangialardi RJ, Martin GS, Bernard GR, et al: For the Ibuprofen in Sepsis Study Group: Hypoproteinemia predicts acute respiratory distress syndrome development, weight gain, and death in patients with sepsis. Critical Care Med 28, 3137–3145, 2000.

Meduri GU, Headley AS, Golden E, et al: Effect of prolonged methyl prednisolone therapy in un-resolving acute respiratory distress syndrome: a randomized controlled study. JAMA 280:159–165, 1998.

Mitchell JP, Schuller D, Calandrino FS, Schuster DP: Improved outcome based on fluid management in critically ill patients requiring pulmonary artery catheterization. American Review of Respiratory Disease 145(5), 990–998, 1992.

Squara P, Dhainaut J-FA, Artigas A, Carlet J: Hemodynamic profile in severe ARDS: results of the European Collaborative ARDS Study. Intensive Care Med 24:1018–1028, 1988.

Vasilyev S, Schaap R, Mortenson JD: Hospital survival rate of patients with acute respiratory failure in modern intensive care units: an international multi-center, prospective study. Chest 107:1083–1088, 1995.

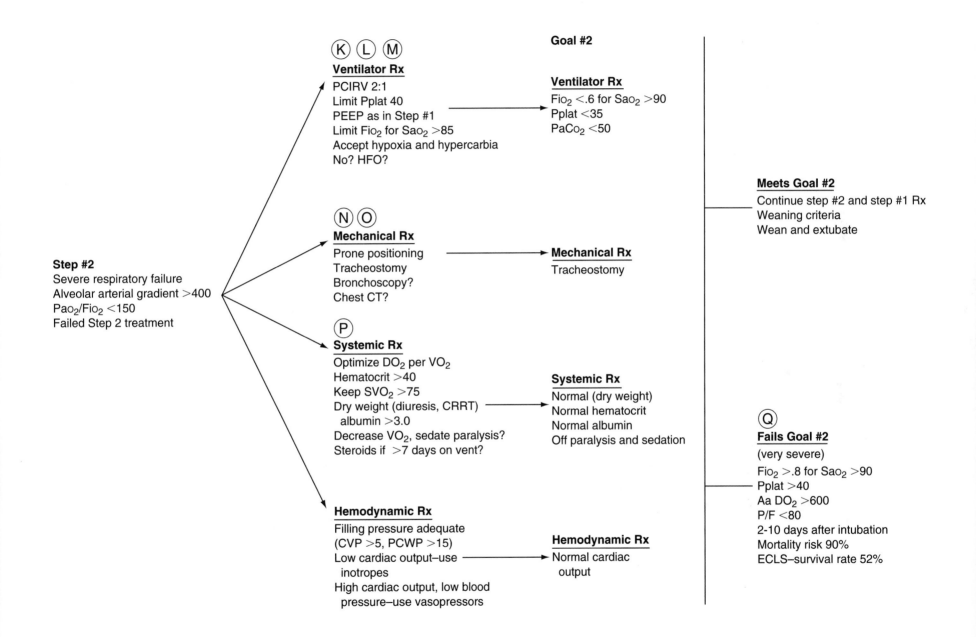

Ⓚ Ⓛ Ⓜ

Goal #2

Ventilator Rx
PCIRV 2:1
Limit Pplat 40
PEEP as in Step #1
Limit Fio_2 for Sao_2 >85
Accept hypoxia and hypercarbia
No? HFO?

Ventilator Rx
Fio_2 <.6 for Sao_2 >90
Pplat <35
$PaCo_2$ <50

Meets Goal #2
Continue step #2 and step #1 Rx
Weaning criteria
Wean and extubate

Ⓝ Ⓞ

Mechanical Rx
Prone positioning
Tracheostomy
Bronchoscopy?
Chest CT?

Mechanical Rx
Tracheostomy

Step #2
Severe respiratory failure
Alveolar arterial gradient >400
Pao_2/Fio_2 <150
Failed Step 2 treatment

Ⓟ

Systemic Rx
Optimize DO_2 per VO_2
Hematocrit >40
Keep SVO_2 >75
Dry weight (diuresis, CRRT)
   albumin >3.0
Decrease VO_2, sedate paralysis?
Steroids if >7 days on vent?

Systemic Rx
Normal (dry weight)
Normal hematocrit
Normal albumin
Off paralysis and sedation

Ⓠ

Fails Goal #2
(very severe)
Fio_2 >.8 for Sao_2 >90
Pplat >40
Aa DO_2 >600
P/F <80
2-10 days after intubation
Mortality risk 90%
ECLS–survival rate 52%

Hemodynamic Rx
Filling pressure adequate
(CVP >5, PCWP >15)
Low cardiac output–use
   inotropes
High cardiac output, low blood
   pressure–use vasopressors

Hemodynamic Rx
Normal cardiac
   output

Chapter 12 *Acute Renal Failure*

KELLY J. WHITE, MD • ROBERT J. ANDERSON, MD

———

(A) The diagnosis of acute renal failure (ARF) is based on an acute (hours to days) rise in creatinine and blood urea nitrogen (BUN) levels. This may or may not be accompanied by oliguria (urine output of less than 400 ml/day). A rise in creatinine of 0.5 to 1.5 mg/dl, an increase of creatinine of 50% from baseline, or a 25% decrease in glomerulalar filtration rate (GFR) are all indicators of ARF. Early recognition of ARF is critical.

(B) A thorough review of the patient's history is essential. A focus on exposures to potential nephrotoxins such as contrast agents, pigments (e.g., myoglobin or hemoglobin), or drugs (e.g., angiotension converting enzymes (ACE) inhibitors, nonsteroidal anti-inflammatory drugs (NSAIDs), or aminoglycosides) is especially important in the hospitalized patient. The physical examination should focus on the patient's volume status (i.e., blood pressure, pulse, orthostatics, mucous membranes, axillary sweat, and edema).

(C) Additional laboratory data may be helpful. Hyperkalemia should be ruled out and treated when indicated. Abnormal hepatic function tests may indicate primary liver disease. An elevated creatinine kinase may indicate myoglobinuria. A decreased hematocrit may indicate hemorrhage or hemolysis.

(D) Certain findings should prompt assessment of need for emergent renal replacement therapy. Refractory hyperkalemia, volume overload, or acidosis can be indications for emergent intervention. Mental status changes or seizures secondary to uremia may also indicate a need for emergent intervention.

(E) Acute anuria (urine output of less than 50 ml/day) should prompt an emergent evaluation of possible causes. A urinary catheter should be placed or flushed if already in place. An emergent ultrasound should be obtained to rule out obstruction. Less common causes of anuria include cessation of renal blood flow and rapidly progressive glomerulonephritis.

(F) Urinalysis and urine electrolytes are essential in delineating the cause of renal failure. The urine and serum electrolytes should be obtained simultaneously for calculation of FENa (urine Na × serum creatinine/serum Na × urine creatinine × 100). A low FENa (less than 1%) generally indicates intact tubular function. An elevated FENa (greater than 2%) may indicate damaged tubules or reflect a history of renal insufficiency, recent administration of diuretics, or osmotic diuresis.

(G) A low FENa suggests a prerenal cause. Supportive findings include compatible history and physical examination, BUN/creatinine ratio of greater than 20, urinary specific gravity greater than 1.020, urine Na less than 20, and a normal urinary sediment with or without hyaline casts.

The volume status of the patient, along with pertinent history and lab findings, should help delineate the cause. Prerenal azotemia is often reversible if recognized and treated promptly, but it may lead to acute tubular necrosis if untreated.

(H) When postrenal causes are suspected, urinary catheterization and renal ultrasound should be obtained expeditiously. An elevated postvoid residual (PVR) (greater than 100 cc) or hydronephrosis on ultrasound confirm obstructive uropathy. An evaluation for the cause of obstruction should include prostatic enlargement; pelvic masses and malignancies; bladder masses; and intratubular obstruction secondary to crystals, proteins, or stones. Relief of obstruction or diversion is indicated.

(I) An active urine sediment and FENa greater than 1 indicate a renal etiology. Specific urine abnormalities are often suggestive of an underlying cause. Management is directed appropriately and should include renal consultation.

REFERENCES

Agrawal M, Swartz R: Acute renal failure. Am Fam Phys 61: 2077–2088, 2000.

Albright R: Acute renal failure: A practical update. Mayo Clin Proc 76:67–74, 2001.

Nolan C, Anderson R: Hospital acquired acute renal failure. J Am Soc Nephrol 710–718, 1998.

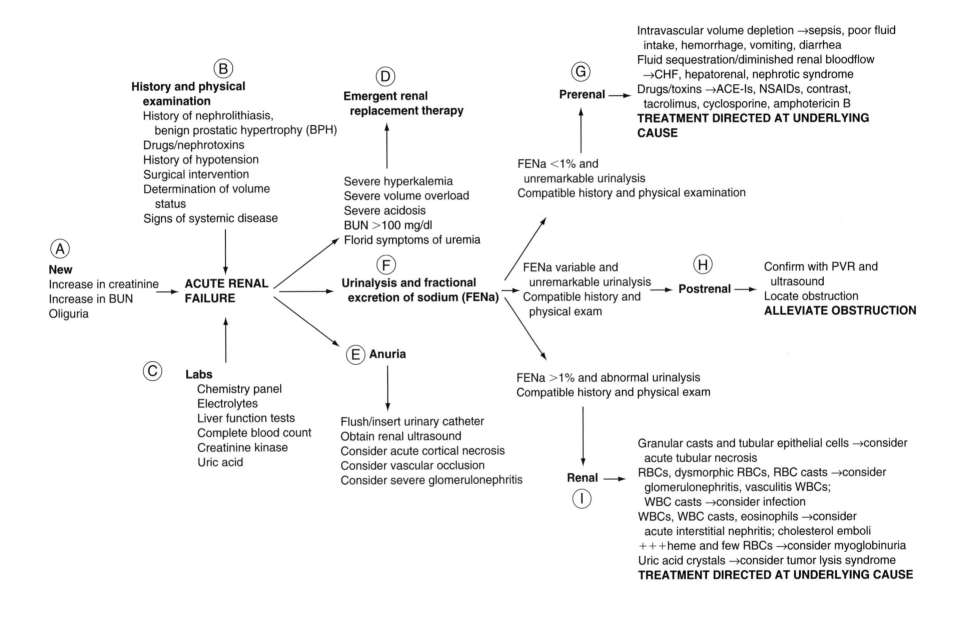

(B) **History and physical examination**
History of nephrolithiasis,
   benign prostatic hypertrophy (BPH)
Drugs/nephrotoxins
History of hypotension
Surgical intervention
Determination of volume
   status
Signs of systemic disease

(D) **Emergent renal replacement therapy**

Severe hyperkalemia
Severe volume overload
Severe acidosis
BUN >100 mg/dl
Florid symptoms of uremia

(G) **Prerenal** →
Intravascular volume depletion →sepsis, poor fluid
   intake, hemorrhage, vomiting, diarrhea
Fluid sequestration/diminished renal bloodflow
   →CHF, hepatorenal, nephrotic syndrome
Drugs/toxins →ACE-Is, NSAIDs, contrast,
   tacrolimus, cyclosporine, amphotericin B
TREATMENT DIRECTED AT UNDERLYING CAUSE

FENa <1% and
unremarkable urinalysis
Compatible history and physical examination

(A) **New**
Increase in creatinine
Increase in BUN
Oliguria

ACUTE RENAL FAILURE

(F) **Urinalysis and fractional excretion of sodium (FENa)**

FENa variable and
unremarkable urinalysis
Compatible history and
physical exam

(H) **Postrenal** →
Confirm with PVR and
ultrasound
Locate obstruction
ALLEVIATE OBSTRUCTION

(C) **Labs**
   Chemistry panel
   Electrolytes
   Liver function tests
   Complete blood count
   Creatinine kinase
   Uric acid

(E) **Anuria**

Flush/insert urinary catheter
Obtain renal ultrasound
Consider acute cortical necrosis
Consider vascular occlusion
Consider severe glomerulonephritis

FENa >1% and abnormal urinalysis
Compatible history and physical exam

Renal →
(I)
Granular casts and tubular epithelial cells →consider
   acute tubular necrosis
RBCs, dysmorphic RBCs, RBC casts →consider
   glomerulonephritis, vasculitis WBCs;
   WBC casts →consider infection
WBCs, WBC casts, eosinophils →consider
   acute interstitial nephritis; cholesterol emboli
+++heme and few RBCs →consider myoglobinuria
Uric acid crystals →consider tumor lysis syndrome
TREATMENT DIRECTED AT UNDERLYING CAUSE

Chapter 13 *Geriatric Surgery*

JEFFREY WALLACE, MD, MPH

(A) Patients aged 65 years and older now represent over half of the average general surgical practice. This population presents with different diseases, greater risks, more challenging decisions, and a more demanding level of perioperative care. Initial assessment must include careful review of medical conditions, assessment of cardiopulmonary stability (if concerns exist, preoperative medical consultation is appropriate), review of all medications (both prescription and nonprescription), and clarification of usual functional and cognitive abilities (this often requires input from family and other care providers). Although most older surgical patients have significant comorbidities (one-third have three or more pre-existing medical conditions), chronological age per se should not preclude surgery because acceptable outcomes have been reported for both elective and emergent operations even among patients 100 years of age and older.

(B) Although even extreme age is not a contraindication to surgery, decision making regarding the risks and benefits of surgical procedures should take into account factors such as expected survival based on current age and health status (Table 13-1). Further, physiologic changes of aging do place older surgical patients at greater risk for perioperative complications, and an improved understanding of these physiologic changes (Table 13-2) can help surgeons minimize morbidity and mortality risks in their older patients. When polypharmacy is present, the risk of delirium and other adverse drug effects increases substantially and consideration should be given to obtaining geriatric medicine consultation. Nutritional status is an important predictor of hospitalization outcomes, and because there is evidence to suggest that simple interventions such as oral protein and energy supplements can improve outcomes, assessment of nutritional status should be a routine part of surgical perioperative care.

TABLE 13–1
Life Expectancy at Selected Ages by Gender and Health Status

Men

At Age	70	75	80	85	90	95
Healthy	18.0	14.2	10.8	7.9	5.8	4.3
Average	12.4	9.3	6.7	4.7	3.2	2.3
Frail	6.7	4.9	3.3	2.2	1.5	1.0

Women

At Age	70	75	80	85	90	95
Healthy	21.3	17.0	13.0	9.6	6.8	4.8
Average	15.7	11.9	8.6	5.9	3.9	2.7
Frail	9.5	6.8	4.6	2.9	1.8	1.7

Adapted from Walter LC, Covinsky KE: Cancer screening in elderly patients: A framework for individualized decision making. JAMA 285(21):2750–2756, 2001.

(C) Common and at least partially preventable events that occur among hospitalized and postoperative older adults include the following: acute renal insufficiency, adverse drug events (10% to 15%), dehydration (7%), delirium (10% to 50%), depression (20%), electrolyte disturbances, functional decline (32%), infection, malnutrition (prevalence as high as 60%), pressure ulcers (5%), thromboembolism (20% to 30% deep vein thrombosis; 1% to 5% pulmonary embolism), and untreated/undertreated pain.

(D) The risk of adverse drug events (ADEs) rises with the number of medications used; therefore every effort should be made to limit medications in older adults to only those that are absolutely indicated and necessary. Sedative-hypnotics and drugs with anticholinergic activity are among the most common offending agents. For sleep complaints, nonpharmacologic approaches

TABLE 13–2
Selected Physiologic Changes with Aging and Potential Perioperative Problems

Organ System	Age-related change	Clinical Effects
Body composition	↓ lean body mass, ↑ total and visceral body fat	↓ metabolic rate, ↑ effects fat soluble drugs
Cardiovascular	↑ left ventricle and arterial stiffness, ↓ β-adrenergic responsiveness, ↓ max heart rate and cardiac output	↑ risk CHF, ↓ tolerance atrial fibrillation ↑ risk postural hypotension
Pulmonary	↓ chest wall compliance, ↓ lung elasticity at rest, mucociliary clearance, ↓ diaphragmatic strength	↑ risk infection, ↑ A-a gradient and ↓ PO_2* ↑ atelectasis at rest, ↑ risk post-op hypoxia
Renal/Volume regulation	↓ GFR (variable but averages 10 ml ↓/decade) ↓ ADH/renal response to hypovolemia ↓ sodium excretion response to hypervolemia	↓ renal excretion of drugs, ↓ ability to compensate for volume depletion or volume overload
Gastrointestinal	↓ swallow coordination, ↓ esophageal secondary contractions, ↓ colon motility, ↓ lactase levels	↑ risk aspiration, ↑ lactose intolerance, predisposed to constipation
Immunity	Skin and mucous membrane changes, ↓ efficacy of barrier functions, altered cytokine and humoral antibody responses to infection	Increased susceptibility to skin, urinary, and pulmonary infections, ↓ febrile response to infections (up to 25% septic elders afebrile)

*Age-adjusted normal for A-a gradient estimated by formula (age/4) + 4; age-adjusted PO_2 estimated by 110–(0.4 × age).

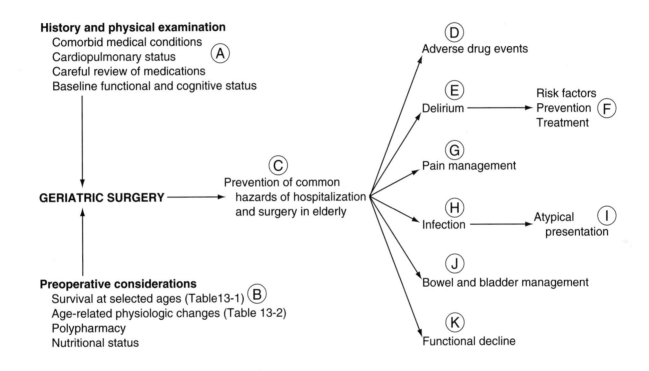

History and physical examination
Comorbid medical conditions
Cardiopulmonary status (A)
Careful review of medications
Baseline functional and cognitive status

GERIATRIC SURGERY ⟶ (C) Prevention of common hazards of hospitalization and surgery in elderly

Preoperative considerations
Survival at selected ages (Table13-1) (B)
Age-related physiologic changes (Table 13-2)
Polypharmacy
Nutritional status

(D) Adverse drug events

(E) Delirium ⟶ Risk factors
Prevention (F)
Treatment

(G) Pain management

(H) Infection ⟶ Atypical (I) presentation

(J) Bowel and bladder management

(K) Functional decline

(e.g., increased activity, avoidance of daytime naps, and quiet environment) should be undertaken first, and diphenhydramine (Benadryl) in particular should be avoided as a sleeping pill. Medication doses must be adjusted for reduced renal function, and because serum creatinine often does not accurately reflect renal function in older adults, glomerular filtration rate should be calculated using standard formulas.

(E) Postoperative delirium or cognitive decline affects 5% to 50% of older surgical patients; it should be routinely looked for because it is often a sign of an underlying new acute process (e.g., ADE, infection, or hypoxia) as well as a predictor of adverse outcomes that might be averted with early detection and intervention. The onset of delirium typically occurs on the first to third postoperative day and is characterized by acute onset, fluctuating course, inattention or difficulty focusing, and either disorganized thinking and/or altered level of consciousness (e.g., hyperalert or lethargic).

(F) Age (especially older than 80 years), preexisting cognitive impairment, severity of acute illness, and extent of surgical procedure are risk factors for delirium that are not readily modifiable. Medications are the single most common (and modifiable) cause of delirium, followed by infection and metabolic abnormalities. Interventions that have focused on minimizing the number of medications, monitoring for hypoxia and metabolic abnormalities, appropriately managing pain, early mobilization, enhancing nutrition, and maintaining normal bowel and bladder function have been shown to substantially reduce the incidence of delirium.

(G) Because of ischemic heart disease, diminished pulmonary function, and increased drug sensitivity, older patients are more vulnerable to the physiologic consequences of inadequate analgesia as well as to the side effects of analgesia use. Undertreated pain appears to increase the risk for delirium as well as impede rehabilitation and adversely affect functional status at discharge. Conversely, analgesics are the class of drug associated with the highest number of ADEs. One study among hip fracture patients successfully used scheduled Tylenol with low dose morphine as needed for early stage pain and oxycodone for later stage pain. Avoid meperidine, methadone, and propoxyphene.

(H) Risk for pneumonia and urinary tract infections can be decreased by early mobilization, incentive spirometry/deep breathing exercises, and early removal of bladder catheters. Evaluation of postoperative fever is addressed elsewhere; however, it is important to note that older adults with postoperative infections may present atypically, without fever or leukocytosis.

(I) Afebrile infection is common in elderly persons. Older adults may also have lower peak temperatures with acute infectious illness. Serious infection may thus present atypically, with little or no fever, but instead as new confusion, incontinence, or falling.

(J) Urinary catheters should be removed as early as possible, ideally by postoperative day 2, with patients subsequently monitored for retention or incontinence problems (the former will be minimized by early mobilization, avoidance of drugs with anticholinergic activity, and judicious use of narcotics). Patients should be monitored for constipation with the goal of a bowel movement by postoperative day 2 and every 48 hours thereafter (assuming oral feeding has resumed). Narcotic use should automatically prompt an accompanying bowel program.

(K) Early mobilization is a key to avoiding functional decline (and other complications) that commonly accompanies acute illness and hospitalization in older adults. Because of age-related lung changes, by age 65 years full lung expansion does not occur while a person is sitting, and hence chair rest does not optimally prevent atelectasis or reduce pneumonia risk. Nursing staff and/or physical therapy should help mobilize patients on postoperative day 1, advancing from chair sitting to standing and walking as rapidly as possible. Immobilization for 2 days or more increases the risk of pulmonary complications, muscle weakness, anorexia, and deep-vein-thrombosis, and almost guarantees a decline in functional status at the time of hospital discharge.

REFERENCES

Cullen DJ, Sweitzer BJ, Bates DW et al: Preventable adverse drug events in hospitalized patients. Crit Care Med 25:1289–1297, 1997.

Katz PR, Grossberg GT, Potter JF et al: Geriatrics Syllabus for Specialists, 2002. New York: American Geriatrics Society, 2002.

Marcantonio ER, Flacker JM, Wright RJ et al: Reducing delirium after hip fracture: A randomized trial. J Am Geriatr Soc 49:516–522, 2001.

Milne AC, Potter J, Avenell A: Protein and energy supplementation in elderly people at risk from malnutrition. Cochrane Database Syst Rev (3):CD003288, 2002.

Morrison RS, Magaziner J, Gilbert M et al: Relationship between pain and opioid analgesics on the development of delirium following hip fracture. J Gerontol A Biol Sci Med Sci 58:76–81, 2003.

Warner MA, Saletel RA, Schroeder DR et al: Outcomes of anesthesia and surgery in people 100 years of age and older. J Am Geriatr Soc 46:988–993, 1998.

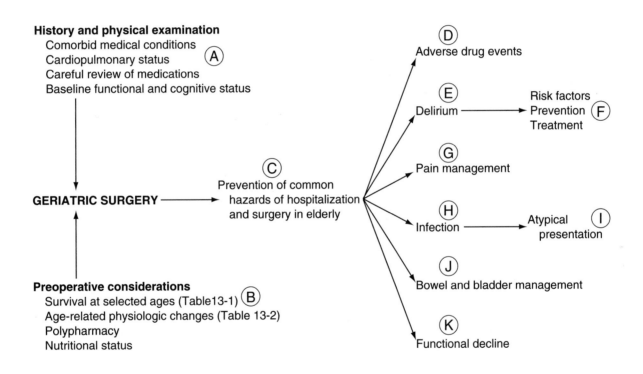

History and physical examination
   Comorbid medical conditions
   Cardiopulmonary status   (A)
   Careful review of medications
   Baseline functional and cognitive status

(D)
Adverse drug events

(E)
Delirium ──────────► Risk factors
                      Prevention (F)
                      Treatment

(G)
Pain management

(C)
Prevention of common
hazards of hospitalization
and surgery in elderly

GERIATRIC SURGERY ──────►

(H)
Infection ──────────► Atypical (I)
                       presentation

(J)
Bowel and bladder management

Preoperative considerations
   Survival at selected ages (Table13-1) (B)
   Age-related physiologic changes (Table 13-2)
   Polypharmacy
   Nutritional status

(K)
Functional decline

Chapter 14 HIV Disease in Surgical Patients

STEVEN C. JOHNSON, MD

(A) Human immunodeficiency virus (HIV) infection is common, currently affecting approximately 1 million persons in the United States. HIV targets the CD4+ T-lymphocyte, a white blood cell critical for immune function, leading to a progressive immunodeficiency allowing opportunistic infections or malignancies to occur. Without treatment, these illnesses commonly result in the patient's death. The development of antiviral agents that inhibit HIV (termed antiretroviral agents) has greatly improved the outcome of HIV infection. For example, the annual mortality rate at the University of Colorado HIV/AIDS program has declined from 13% in 1995 to less than 2% in 2003. In addition, *Pneumocystis carinii* pneumonia (PCP), the most common opportunistic infection, occurred in less than 1% of the program's HIV+ patients in 2003. Consequently, the impact of HIV infection on the diagnosis and management of surgical diseases will vary widely from patient to patient based on individual factors such as the state of the immune system and the presence or absence of HIV-related complications.

Most HIV-infected patients will now present with the typical signs and symptoms of surgical diseases and will have similar indications for surgical intervention as patients without HIV infection. Some patients with HIV infection, especially those with advanced HIV disease (AIDS), may present with atypical manifestations of surgical diseases. This may reduce the ability of the patient to manifest focal infection (e.g., an abscess). In addition, intra-abdominal opportunistic infections (e.g., disseminated *Mycobacterium avium* complex disease, AIDS cholangiopathy, and cytomegalovirus colitis) may simulate surgical diseases such as cholecystitis, cholangitis, and appendicitis. These clinical situations have become much less common in recent years with the marked decline in opportunistic infections. Infectious complications of HIV are typically not subtle, often presenting with specific syndromes such as pneumonia, meningitis, focal neurologic symptoms, diarrhea, or fever. Patients with advanced HIV disease may also have wasting, malnutrition, chronic pain, chronic diarrhea, or peripheral neuropathy. The preoperative history and physical examination should usually uncover these complications without difficulty. Elective operations should be postponed until acute infections have been adequately treated.

Patients with HIV infection often have other significant illnesses. Approximately 15% to 20% of HIV+ patients are co-infected with hepatitis B or hepatitis C. These illnesses may cause substantial morbidity or mortality even if the HIV infection is under good control. Mental illness (e.g., depression or bipolar disease) and substance abuse are also relatively common. A consequence of the improved prognosis with HIV is that many patients are now living much longer. As this population ages, heart and lung diseases common to the general population will also occur in this patient population.

(B) Patients with AIDS often have leukopenia and may only mount a relative leukocytosis in response to infection. This may reduce the ability of the patient to manifest focal infections such as an abscess. The normal range for the CD4+ T-lymphocyte count is generally between 500 and 1200 cells/mm^3. The viral load is the level of plasma HIV mRNA. In interpreting the CD4 lymphocyte count, measurements should be relatively recent, preferably within the last 3 months.

(C) HIV+ patients with a CD4 lymphocyte count in the normal range will have a similar prognosis to patients without HIV infection and will likely handle most surgical procedures without additional risk of complications. HIV+ patients with a CD4 lymphocyte count between 200 and 500 cells/mm^3 are likely to be immunosuppressed to a moderate degree but remain at a relatively low risk for an AIDS-related opportunistic infection. HIV+ patients with a CD4 lymphocyte count of less than 200 cells/mm^3 (which is one of the CDC's definitions for AIDS) are at a substantially higher risk for infection and may have impaired wound healing. In this group, the prognosis of HIV may impact substantially on surgical decision-making. The primary care physician or infectious disease consultant may be helpful in formulating a prognosis for this patient group.

History and physical examination
    Acute signs and symptoms
    HIV complications
        Pneumonia
        CNS symptoms
        Diarrhea
        Malnutrition
    Hepatitis
    Substance abuse

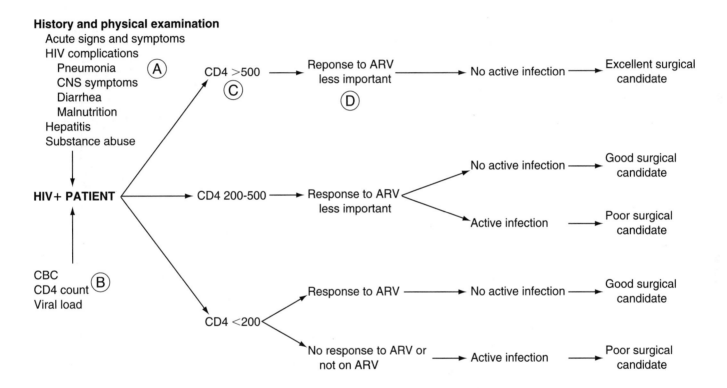

TABLE 14–1
Currently Available Antiretroviral Agents

Agent, Initials	Trade Name	Drug Class*	Usual Dose†
Zidovudine, AZT, ZDV	Retrovir	Nucleoside RTI	300 mg PO bid
Didanosine, ddI	Videx	Nucleoside RTI	200 mg PO bid
Zalcitabine, ddc	HIVID	Nucleoside RTI	0.75 mg PO tid
Stavudine, d4T	Zerit	Nucleoside RTI	40 mg PO bid
Lamivudine, 3TC	Epivir	Nucleoside RTI	150 mg PO bid
Abacavir, ABC	Ziagen	Nucleoside RTI	300 mg PO bid
Fixed dose Zidovudine and Lamivudine	Combivir	Two nucleoside RTIs in a single tablet	One 300 mg/150 mg tablet PO bid
Fixed dose Zidovudine, lamivudine, and abacavir	Trizivir	Three nucleoside RTIs in a single tablet	One 300 mg/150 mg/300 mg tablet PO bid
Tenofovir	Viread	Nucleotide RTI	300 mg PO qd
Nevirapine	Viramune	Non-nucleoside RTI	200 mg PO bid
Delavirdine	Rescriptor	Non-nucleoside RTI	400 mg PO tid
Efavirenz	Sustiva	Non-nucleoside RTI	600 mg PO qhs
Saquinavir (hard gel capsule)	Invirase	Protease inhibitor	600 mg PO tid
Saquinavir (soft gel capsule)	Fortovase	Protease inhibitor	1200 mg PO tid
Ritonavir	Norvir	Protease inhibitor	600 mg PO bid
Indinavir	Crixivan	Protease inhibitor	800 mg PO tid
Nelfinavir	Viracept	Protease inhibitor	750 mg PO tid
Amprenavir	Agenerase	Protease inhibitor	1200 mg PO bid
Lopinavir with ritonavir	Kaletra	Protease inhibitor	400 mg/100 mg PO bid
Atazanavir	Reyataz	Protease inhibitor	400 mg PO qd
Enfuvirtide (T-20)	Fuzeon	Fusion inhibitor	90 mg SC bid

*RTI: reverse transcriptase inhibitor.
†Usual doses are provided. Doses may vary based on weight, the presence of renal or hepatic failure, or when using combinations which have pharmacokinetic interactions.
NOTE: Most patients with HIV infection will be on combination antiretroviral therapy. Some patients with more advanced disease may also be on prophylactic antibiotics or treatments for opportunistic infections. Every attempt should be made to continue these medications in the peri-operative period and to minimize the number of missed doses. However, these medications can have important drug interactions with medications used in the surgical patient. Certain benzodiazepines (e.g., triazolam and midazolam) and lipid-lowering agents (e.g., simvastatin and lovastaitin) are actually contraindicated in patients taking protease inhibitors. Two of the non-nucleoside reverse transcriptase inhibitors (i.e., efavirenz and nevirapine) induce the cytochrome p450 enzymes and may lower the levels of coadministered drugs. The pharmacist or infectious disease consultant may be useful in evaluating for potentially dangerous drug interactions. In addition, drug interaction tables are available at: Centers for Disease Control and Prevention: Updated U.S. Public Health Service guidelines for the management of occupational exposures to HBV, HCV, and HIV and recommendations for postexposure prophylaxis. MMWR 50(RR11):1–42, 2001.

(D) Treatment for HIV infection typically involves a combination of 3 or 4 antiretroviral drugs (Table 14-1). Response to therapy is measured both in terms of a rise in the CD4 lymphocyte count and a fall in the plasma HIV RNA level (also called the viral load). Patients responding optimally to therapy will often have a normal CD4 lymphocyte count and an undetectable plasma viral load. However, many patients have a substantial benefit from therapy without reaching a normal CD4 count or an undetectable viral load.

REFERENCES

Barlett JG, Gallant JE: 2003 Medical Management of HIV Infection. Johns Hopkins University, Division of Infectious Diseases and AIDS, 2003.
Centers for Disease Control and Prevention: Updated U.S. Public Health Service guidelines for the management of occupational exposures to HBV, HCV, and HIV and recommendations for postexposure prophylaxis. MMWR 50(RR11):1–42, 2001.
Centers for Disease Control and Prevention: Revised guidelines for HIV counseling, testing, and referral. MMWR 50(RR19): 1–58, 2001.
Department of Health and Human Services and the Henry J. Kaiser Family Foundation: Guidelines for the Use of Antiretroviral Agents in HIV-infected Adults and Adolescents. Revised November 10, 2003. Available at www.aidsinfo.nih.gov.
2001 USPHS/IDSA Guidelines for the Prevention of Opportunistic Infections in Persons Infected with Human Immunodeficiency Virus. U.S. Public Health Service (USPHS) and Infectious Diseases Society of America (IDSA), November 28, 2001. Available at www.aidsinfo.nih.gov.

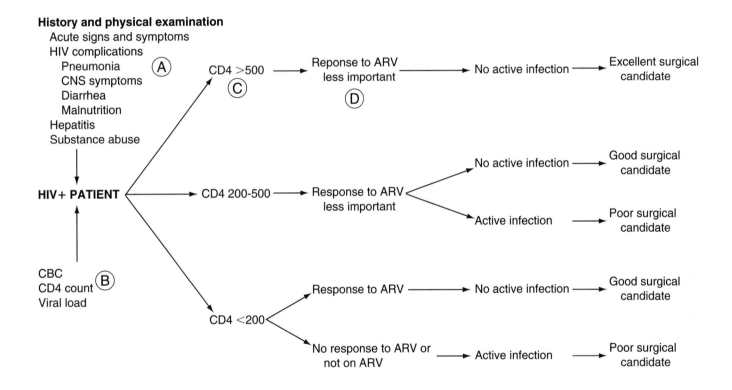

History and physical examination
　　Acute signs and symptoms
　　HIV complications
　　　　Pneumonia
　　　　CNS symptoms
　　　　Diarrhea
　　　　Malnutrition
　　Hepatitis
　　Substance abuse

Ⓐ

HIV+ PATIENT

CBC
CD4 count Ⓑ
Viral load

CD4 >500
Ⓒ

Reponse to ARV
less important
Ⓓ

No active infection

Excellent surgical
candidate

CD4 200-500

Response to ARV
less important

No active infection

Good surgical
candidate

Active infection

Poor surgical
candidate

CD4 <200

Response to ARV

No active infection

Good surgical
candidate

No response to ARV or
not on ARV

Active infection

Poor surgical
candidate

HEAD AND NECK

Chapter 15 *Otorrhea*

RYAN L. VAN DE GRAAF, MD • HERMAN A. JENKINS, MD

(A) Otorrhea is drainage from the ear. This symptom can be the only finding present or can be accompanied by other symptoms including pain, fever, otalgia (ear pain), hearing loss, vertigo, or pruritus. This can occur acutely secondary to infection, trauma, or an iatrogenic etiology. It can also be a chronic symptom caused by chronic infection, cholesteatoma, systemic diseases, or carcinoma. The type of otorrhea can also vary. Purulent or malodorous otorrhea is usually indicative of acute bacterial otitis, whereas clear otorrhea is seen more often in CSF otorrhea and chronic otitis media with perforation of the tympanic membrane. The source of the otorrhea can be the external ear; the middle ear; or, possibly, CSF. Hearing loss may accompany otorrhea. Conductive hearing loss suggests a middle ear lesion; sensorineural hearing loss and vertigo indicate involvement of the inner ear. Pruritus is common, especially in eczematous conditions and otomycosis, but may be secondary to drainage from middle ear lesions.

(B) The first step, after a thorough history, in the evaluation of otorrhea involves examining the ear canal; tympanic membrane (TM); and middle ear, if possible. The use of a handheld otoscope is often sufficient, but in some cases the diagnosis cannot be made without examining the ear under an operating microscope. If necessary, the ear should be suctioned of fluid and debris in order to provide better visualization. In cases refractory to antibiotic therapy or in immunocompromised patients, cultures should be obtained to drive appropriate antibiotic therapy.

(C) If edema of the external canal prevents TM visualization, a Merocel wick is placed in the canal and antibiotic otic drops are instilled or "wicked" into the canal several times a day. This allows the drops to penetrate deeper into the canal than they otherwise would. Periodic suctioning and replacement of the wick are performed until the canal is patent and the TM visualized. Not only does this aid in diagnosis, it is also therapeutic.

(D) Bacterial otitis externa, or swimmer's ear, is an infection of the external ear canal skin. It begins with breakdown of the ear canal epithelium, caused by either trauma (e.g., Q-tip use) or maceration of the skin from excessive moisture. This results in a bacterial infection, usually pseudomonas. Symptoms include severe otalgia; otorrhea; and, occasionally, cellulitis extending onto the pinna or cheek and upper neck. Treatment includes manual suctioning of the ear canal, placing a wick if necessary, and the use of topical antibiotic drops. If the cellulitis extends onto the pinna or cheek, oral antibiotics are also recommended. Using a 50%/50% solution of isopropyl alcohol and white vinegar after water exposure can prevent recurrent otitis externa.

(E) Fungal otitis externa or otomycosis is usually caused by aspergillus or other saprophytic fungi. Itching is prominent and discharge usually scant and serous. Gray, black, or white velvety debris typically covers an erythematous canal. Mycelia and spores are seen under the microscope. Treatment is through cleaning the canal under the operating microscope and the application of antifungal agents such as cresylate, 4% acetic acid (Domeboro solution), Merthiolate, or Lotrimin cream.

(F) Eczematous external otitis may be associated with similar scalp conditions. Treatment involves the use of topical steroid drops or creams. Occasionally, patients can develop an allergic reaction to neomycin otic drops resulting in striking erythema of the ear canal.

(G) Acute otitis media is most common in children with poor eustachian tube function during an upper respiratory infection. A purulent effusion may develop and, if enough pressure exists, the tympanic membrane may spontaneously rupture leading to otorrhea. This is classically described as severe pain followed by immediate resolution of the pain with voluminous otorrhea. The most common pathogens include pneumococcus,

Haemophilus influenzae, and *Moraxella catarrhalis*. Treatment can generally be limited to topical antibiotic drops because local concentrations reach supratherapeutic levels. In the presence of a perforation, the use of ototoxic drugs (e.g., neomycin) should be discouraged because there is a potential risk of permanent hearing loss. Fluorquinolone otic preparations (e.g., ciprofloxacin and ofloxacin) are not ototoxic and are acceptable for use when the middle ear is exposed. Only in complicated or resistant cases should systemic antibiotics be used. Complications of acute otitis media include serous labyrinthitis, meningitis, facial paralysis, coalescent mastoiditis, and intracranial abscess. Treatment is IV antibiotics and, generally, mastoidectomy.

(H) Chronic otitis media is recurrent or persistent purulent otorrhea associated with TM perforation and conductive hearing loss. Contamination of the middle ear with water exacerbates the problem. Chronic eustachian tube dysfunction prevents healing of the perforation. The mucosa may become edematous, and granulation tissue may occur. Therapy includes water precautions, frequent suctioning, and topical antibiotic drops. Patients who respond and remain without otorrhea for more than 3 months may be candidates for a myringoplasty or tympanoplasty to repair the perforation. Continued otorrhea despite vigorous medical management implies irreversible disease that requires tympanomastoidectomy. A CT scan may be beneficial in determining the extent of diseased tissue. Drilling out the mastoid not only removes diseased mucosal tissue but also improves ventilation of the middle ear, which increases the success of the tympanoplasty.

(I) Cholesteatoma is the presence of squamous epithelium in the middle ear or mastoid space. It generally results as a complication of chronic poor eustachian tube dysfunction. This leads to negative pressure in the middle ear space, which can cause retraction of the TM, most often in the posterior, superior quadrant (the pars flaccida).

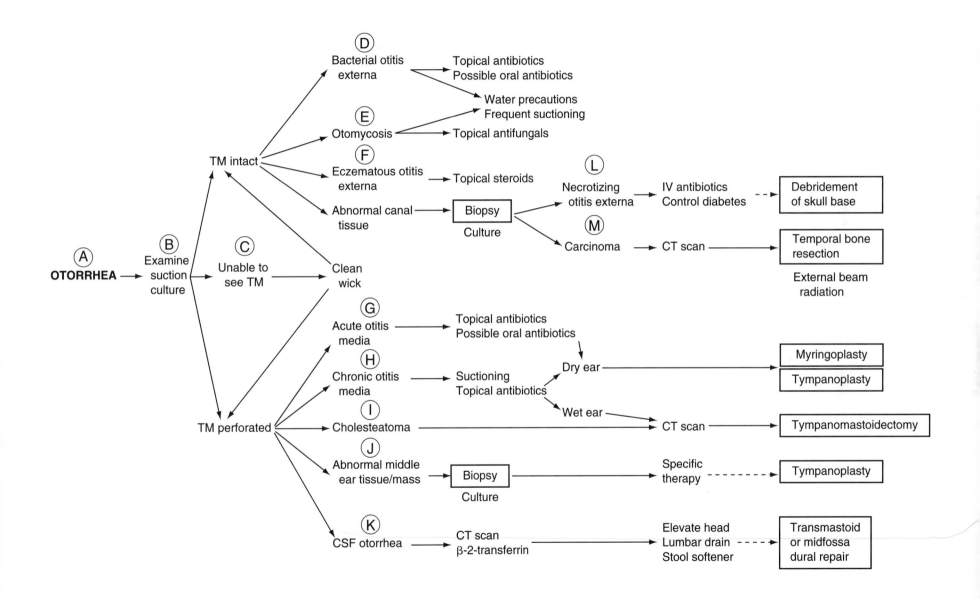

Such a retraction pocket can bottleneck, leading to retained squamous epithelium, which invades into the middle ear and mastoid. Chronic perforations, especially if located marginally on the TM, can allow for migration of squamous epithelium into the middle ear, thus creating a cholesteatoma. Rarely, congenital cholesteatomas can occur. Cholesteatomas can locally destroy structures through enzymatic resorption of bone. This can lead to ossicular destruction; or, less commonly, vertigo, sensorineural hearing loss, and intracranial complications. Treatment includes surgical removal of the cholesteatoma through various forms of tympanomastoidectomy.

Ⓙ   Abnormal tissue in the middle ear can be chronic granulation tissue, cholesteatoma, neoplasm, or granuloma. Biopsy and culture usually determine the diagnosis. Granulomas such as tuberculosis or Wegener granulomatosis are treated systemically. Tympanoplasty for correction of persistent perforation is delayed until the underlying disease process is eradicated.

Ⓚ   CSF otorrhea usually occurs iatrogenically or secondary to a temporal bone fracture. Less often, advanced temporal bone malignancy causes CSF otorrhea. Aural CSF placed on filter paper shows a clear halo around a serosanguineous center (target sign) because CSF diffuses distally from blood and serum. A positive β-2-transferrin indicates the presence of CSF. Leakage of CSF from the ear can occur through the ear canal, down the back of the throat or out the nose via the eustachian tube, or out a postauricular incision. In the presence of a fracture or malignancy, a CT of the temporal bone should be obtained to determine the site of the leak. If not treated, meningitis may occur. There is controversy over the use of prophylactic antibiotics. Initial treatment includes elevating the head of bed, placing a pressure dressing over the ear and mastoid, and the use of stool softeners. If this does not work, a lumbar drain may be placed to reduce CSF pressure. Finally, transmastoid or cranial repair of the injured dura may be necessary to stop the leak.

Ⓛ   Necrotizing ("malignant") otitis externa (NOE) is usually seen in diabetic patients. It is an osteomyelitis usually caused by *Pseudomonas aeruginosa* and is characterized by deep, severe otalgia with granulation tissue at the bony-cartilaginous junction of the ear canal. A markedly elevated ESR and a temporal bone CT scan demonstrating osteomyelitis are indicative of this disease. A technetium 99m pyrophosphate bone scan can also be utilized. NOE can lead to generalized skull base osteomyelitis and rapid death. Involvement of cranial nerves usually indicates a poor prognosis. Early and aggressive treatment is necessary and involves local debridement, the use of topical antibiotic drops, long-term antipseudomonal intravenous antibiotics, and control of the diabetes. Aggressive debridement of the skull base may also be necessary. Intravenous antibiotics should continue for at least 4 to 6 weeks. A gallium scan may be checked at the onset of the disease and on intervals to assess response to treatment. Alternatively, a normalized ESR can be used to determine when to discontinue antibiotics.

Ⓜ   Malignancies of the ear canal include squamous cell carcinoma (most common), basal cell carcinoma, and adenocarcinoma of adenexal glands. Foul-smelling otorrhea may be present. Persistent pain is a clue to diagnosis because otalgia is uncommon in uncomplicated chronic otitis. Advanced tumors can invade the middle ear and cranial cavity, giving rise to hearing loss, facial paralysis, or other cranial neuropathies. The threshold for biopsy should be low because what may look like chronic granulation tissue could be carcinoma. Realize that the facial nerve may be exposed or even involved by the process. Treatment usually involves temporal bone resection followed by radiation therapy. Some tumors (e.g., rhabdomyosarcoma) present more commonly in younger patients, may be sensitive to chemoradiation, and may not require resection. Prognosis of carcinoma of the ear canal is poor and distant metastases are common, often despite adequate local control.

REFERENCES

Bailey BJ, Calhoun KH, Healy GB et al (eds): Head and Neck Surgery–Otolaryngology. Philadelphia: Lippincott Williams & Wilkins, 2001.

Coker NJ, Jenkins HA: Atlas of Otologic Surgery. Philadelphia: WB Saunders, 2001. Cummings CW, Fredrickson JM, Harker LA et al (eds): Otolaryngology–Head and Neck Surgery. St. Louis: CV Mosby, 1998.

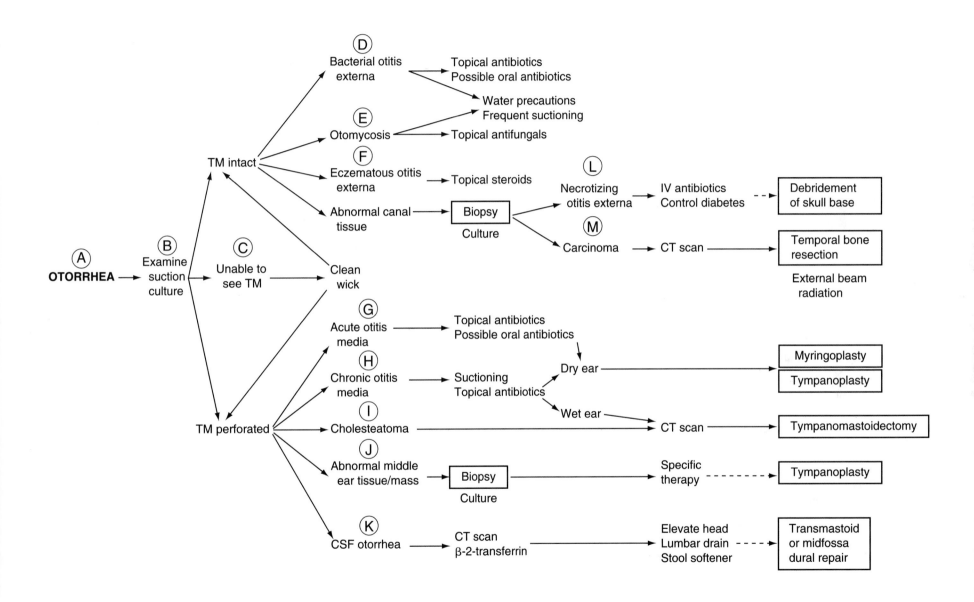

Chapter 16 *Epistaxis*

JOHN P. CAMPANA, MD ● BRUCE W. JAFEK, MD

(A) The causes of epistaxis are multiple and differ depending on the patient's age. Common causes include trauma (a lack of supporting stroma and thin mucosal lining makes vessels inherently vulnerable—this is the most common cause of epistaxis in children); decreased humidity and subsequent drying of the mucosa (epistaxis is more common in drier climates and during winter); inflammation (e.g., upper respiratory infections, allergic rhinitis); blood dyscrasias (e.g., leukemia, hemophilia, and idiopathic thrombocytopenic purpura); tumors and foreign bodies (e.g., neoplasia, juvenile nasopharyngeal angiofibroma—the classic cause of severe epistaxis in the adolescent male); vascular anomalies (e.g., hereditary hemorrhagic telangiectasia, capillary ectasia); and pharmacologic (e.g., prescription drugs such as coumadin or heparin or OTC drugs such as ASA, ibuprofen, vitamin E, vitamin C, St. John's wort, ginko, or a combination of these).

(B) Other evidence of hemorrhage or of mucosal or vascular anomalies should be sought and the source of the bleeding identified. This requires equipment such as a suction device, nasal speculum, good lighting, local anesthesia, and proper protection for the physician. Most bleeding (90%) is anteroinferior along the septum (Kiesselbach's plexus, Little's area). The younger the patient, the more likely the bleeding site is to be anterior and of traumatic origin.

(C) Ambulatory treatment begins with application of gentle, constant pressure. The patient pinches the nose just distal to the bony cartilaginous junction for 15 to 20 minutes, sitting up to decrease the blood pressure in the nose. This measure may have failed at home, prompting the visit to the emergency room.

(D) Application of Gelfoam or Surgicel to the site is recommended for patients with blood dyscrasias because these topical, hemostatic, absorbable agents need not be removed later.

(E) If a bleeding site is found, silver nitrate ($AgNO_3$) is applied to cauterize the area. The area is dried with suction before attempting to identify additional bleeding sites. Alternatively, or in addition, hot electrocautery may be used.

(F) If these measures fail, the nose is packed anteriorly with Surgicel placed directly onto the bleeding point, followed by a 1- to 2-inch impregnated gauze. Apply the gauze in layers from the nasal floor to the nasal roof. This stops bleeding in 90% of patients. If the packing has been placed properly but the bleeding persists, then posterior packing is required. This treatment is unpleasant for the patient. It requires intravenous antibiotics. For elderly patients, admission to the ICU is prudent because the posterior packing significantly lowers alveolar oxygenation and can cause hypercapnia. Those with marginal cardiopulmonary function may be pushed toward decompensation. Early embolization, ligation, or endoscopic cautery may be more appropriate.

(G) The patient may be sent home with antibiotics to return in 2 to 3 days for removal of the packing. If there is crusting and dryness of the nasal mucosa, saline rinses (1 pint of water with 1 teaspoon of salt and a pinch of baking soda) and application of an antibiotic ointment (e.g., Bactroban, Neosporin) on an outpatient basis are helpful.

(H) When ambulatory treatment fails, the patient is hospitalized. Any coagulopathy is corrected. Anterior bleeding is cauterized. An important rule is to cauterize only one side of the septum, to prevent septal perforation. Only the bleeding point is cauterized, to avoid mucosal scarring with subsequent atrophic rhinitis. Electric cautery may be used for more vigorous bleeders.

(I) Posterior packing should be done by an otolaryngologist or other experienced clinician.

(J) If packing fails, arterial ligation or embolization may be necessary. Because both the internal and the external carotid artery systems supply the nose, arteriographic study may be warranted before such therapy is initiated. Embolization may, of course, be done at the time of arteriography. Endoscopic clipping of the sphenopalatine artery is a promising new method of control of refractory posterior epistaxis.

REFERENCES

Barlow DW, Deleyiannis F, Pinczower EF: Effectiveness of surgical management of epistaxis at a tertiary care center. Laryngoscope 107:21–23, 1997.

Chopra R: Epistaxis: A review. J Royal Soc Health 120:31–33, 2000.

Cullen MM, Tami TA: Comparison of internal maxillary artery ligation versus embolization for refractory posterior epistaxis. Otol–HN Surg 118:636–642, 1998.

O'Flynn PE, Shadaba A: Management of posterior epistaxis by endoscopic clipping of the sphenopalatine artery. Otol Clin NA 25:374–377, 2000.

Peyvandi F, Mannucci PM: Rare coagulation disorders. Thrombosis & Haemostasis 82:1207–1214, 1999.

Pond F, Sizeland A: Epistaxis: Strategies for management. Australian Family Physician 29:933–938, 2000.

Tan LK, Calhoun KH: Epistaxis. Med Clin NA 83:43–56, 1999.

Valavanis A, Christoforidis G: Applications of interventional neuroradiology in the head and neck. Sem Roentgenol 35:72–83, 2000.

Walshe P: The use of fibrin glue to arrest epistaxis in the presence of a coagulopathy. Laryngoscope 112:1126–1128, 2002.

History and physical examination
Trauma
Decreased humidity
Inflammation
Blood dyscrasias
Tumors, foreign bodies
Vascular anomalies
Medications
Nasal examination

Labs
Hematocrit
Coagulation studies
Liver function tests
BUN

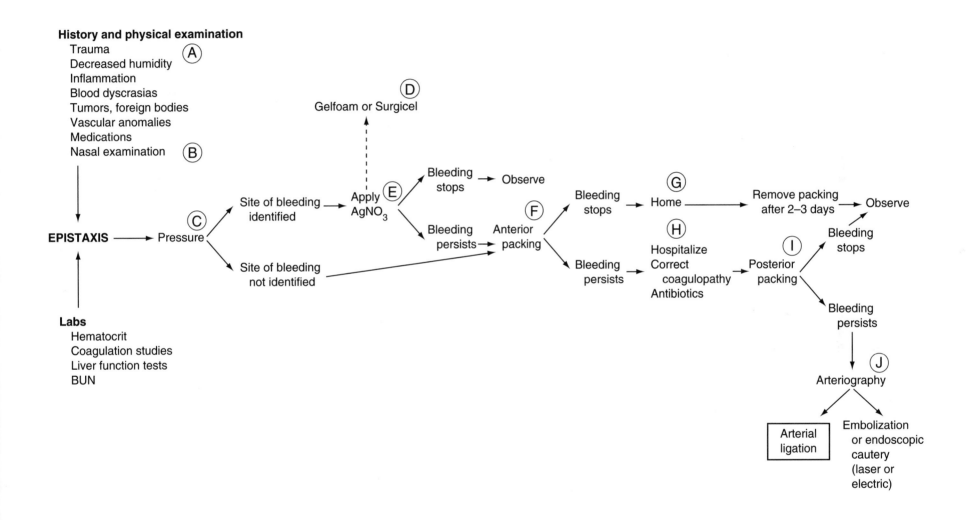

Chapter 17 *Non-Melanoma Skin Cancer of the Face*

ERICA D. ANDERSON, MD • LAWRENCE L. KETCH, MD

(A) The key to preventing skin cancer is reducing sun exposure. This can be achieved by avoiding sunlight during the middle of the day, by using sunscreens with an SPF greater than 15, and by wearing protective clothing.

(B) Risks for increased incidence of skin cancer include fair complexion, light hair, blue or green eyes, inability to tan, propensity to sunburn, history of multiple or severe sunburns, age, and Celtic ancestry. Other factors such as occupation, habits (tanning booths), and residential geography are considered indirect causes of increased sun exposure.

(C) Genetic syndromes (e.g., xeroderma pigmentosum and basal cell nevus syndrome) predispose to the development of multiple basal cell carcinomas, often at an early age.

(D) Actinic keratosis, Bowen's disease, and keratoacanthoma are premalignant.

(E) Skin cancer is the most common malignancy, with the majority of these tumors arising on the sun-exposed regions of the head and neck. The incidence of skin cancer has been rising rapidly since the 1960s, with over 1 million cases of non-melanoma skin cancer (NMSC) in the United States each year. The mortality caused by NMSC is low, with an estimated 95% 5-year survival rate. NMSC can, however, be locally aggressive and result in considerable disfigurement, loss of function, and health care costs.

(F) A histological diagnosis is needed to ensure proper identification and adequate treatment. The microscopic features of each lesion are predictive of clinical behavior, recurrence, and metastasis. A full-thickness skin biopsy consisting of the epidermis, dermis, and a portion of the subcutaneous tissue including the margin of uninvolved skin is indicated.

Punch, shave, incisional, and excisional biopsies are easily performed in an office setting. The choice of a particular technique depends on the size, location, and suspected nature of the lesion, as well as the cosmetic result desired.

(G) Actinic keratoses (AK) are scaly, circumscribed, rough, erythematous, sun-induced premalignant lesions that histologically may mimic squamous cell cancer. They are typically found on the head and neck of middle-aged and elderly individuals. Malignant conversion to SCC is estimated at 0.1% per year.

(H) Basal cell cancer (BCC) is the most common cutaneous malignancy and represents 75% of all NMSCs. Over half a million BCCs are diagnosed annually in the United States. The lifetime risk for the development of BCC in whites is approximately 33%, and men are slightly more at risk than women. The incidence of BCC peaks around age 70 years.

Eighty percent of BCCs arise on the sun-exposed areas of the head and neck, and 30% alone are found on the nose, making it the most common site for BCC.

BCCs spread primarily by local growth and invasion. Metastatic disease is rare (less than 0.1%).

BCCs can be divided into several subtypes based on clinical and histologic patterns (e.g., nodular, superficial, micronodular, infiltrative, morpheaform, and basosquamous carcinoma). Nodular BCC (75%) clinically presents as a well-defined, pearly, translucent nodule with a rolled border. Telangiectasias are commonly seen on the surface of the nodule. Central ulceration or bleeding may be present.

Superficial BCCs (10%) are erythematous, scaly, discrete macules or slightly elevated papules that can resemble an eczematous dermatitis.

Micronodular, infiltrative, and morpheaform BCCs (10%) have a more aggressive histologic appearance and clinical course. They appear as flat, white or yellow plaques with ill-defined margins.

Basosquamous carcinomas are rare, showing histologic evidence of both basal cell and squamous cell differentiation with increased rates of growth and metastasis compared with BCC.

Location of the tumor also can influence the chance of incomplete excision and recurrence. Significantly more BCCs recur in the midface or around the ears. Recurrence rates also increase with tumor size, duration, and with neglected or inadequately excised tumors.

(I) Squamous cell cancer (SCC) (20%) is a flesh-colored or erythematous nodule with elevated and ill-defined borders but may present with hyperkeratotic centers or cutaneous horns.

The cumulative rate of metastasis for SCC of the skin is estimated to be between 2% and 6%, and the 5-year survival rate for metastatic SCC is approximately 34%. SCC can metastasize to regional lymph nodes or to distant sites, primarily the lungs and the liver. SCCs located on the ear and the lip have higher rates of recurrence and metastasis, approaching 10% and 14% respectively, as do those found in the nasolabial creases, periorbital, and preauricular regions.

Tumors that arise in scars or in chronic wounds are more aggressive, with a metastatic rate between 18% and 38%. SCCs arising in immunocompromised patients may be multiple, grow rapidly, and have aggressive clinical courses.

(J) Merkel cell carcinoma is a highly malignant tumor derived from neuroendocrine cells that are believed to function as touch receptors. It is commonly associated with high recurrence and metastatic rates (40%). A poor prognosis can be related to the presence of lymph node metastases at the time of presentation.

(K) Superficial destructive measures including topical 5-fluorouracil cream, cryosurgery, electrodessication and curettage, CO_2 laser,

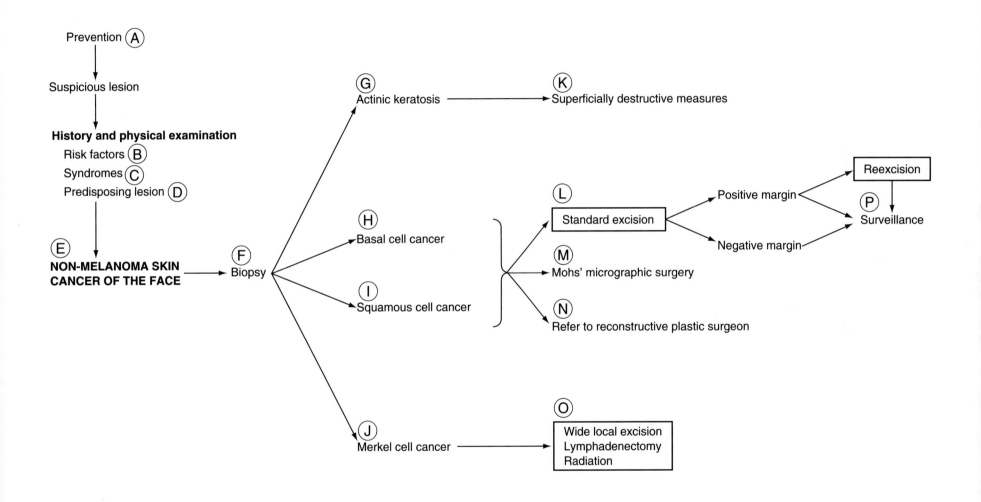

Prevention (A)

↓

Suspicious lesion

↓

History and physical examination

Risk factors (B)

Syndromes (C)

Predisposing lesion (D)

(E)

NON-MELANOMA SKIN CANCER OF THE FACE → (F) Biopsy

(G) Actinic keratosis → (K) Superficially destructive measures

(H) Basal cell cancer

(I) Squamous cell cancer

(L) Standard excision → Positive margin → Reexcision → Surveillance (P)

Standard excision → Negative margin → Surveillance (P)

(M) Mohs' micrographic surgery

(N) Refer to reconstructive plastic surgeon

(J) Merkel cell cancer → (O) Wide local excision / Lymphadenectomy / Radiation

dermabrasion, and chemical peels all provide adequate treatment for AKs. If the AK is raised and hyperkeratotic, shave or punch biopsy may be more appropriate.

(L) Excision is the treatment of choice for most BCCs and SCCs. Although there is no uniform recommendation about the size of the margin, many surgeons use margins of 2 to 4 mm with a depth of mid to deep subcutaneous tissue for small (less than 2 cm) primary basal or squamous cell carcinomas with well-defined borders and nonaggressive histology. For larger or more aggressive subtypes, many recommend greater than 7 mm margins to a depth that includes all of the subcutaneous tissue. All specimens are evaluated by frozen or permanent section to determine if the margins are free of tumor.

(M) Mohs' micrographic excision uses horizontal frozen sections and intraoperative tumor mapping to provide a higher cure rate for SCCs and BCCs while leaving a smaller wound. It can be considered in cases of recurrent tumor, aggressive histology, perineural invasion, or ill-defined margins. Disadvantages include expertise, time, and expense.

(N) If the tumor is located where maximal conservation of normal tissue is important (e.g., eyelid, nose, ear, or lip), a referral to a plastic and reconstructive surgeon should be considered. Periorbital lesions can be particularly difficult to manage. Ectropion, or eversion of the lid margin away from the globe, can occur after surgical reconstruction of facial defects that encroach on the lower eyelid. Chronically this can lead to exposure keratitis of the cornea and loss of vision. When closing a defect in the periorbital region, the flap should be constructed so that any tension on the lower lid is horizontal. Permanent anchoring sutures from the undersurface of the flap to the periosteum of the orbital rim and lateral canthus aid flap support. Finally, tightening of the lower lid may be required by canthopexy or canthoplasty.

(O) Wide local excision with lymphadenectomy as clinically indicated is standard treatment. Sentinel lymph node mapping may be useful. Postoperative radiation is recommended for all patients.

(P) Continued follow-up of patients with NMSC facilitates the early detection of new tumors and recurrences. Yearly skin examinations are appropriate for those who have had skin cancer or who are at high risk for skin cancer in order to decrease functional, psychological, and financial effects of these potentially morbid tumors.

REFERENCES

Goldberg DP: Assessment and surgical treatment of basal cell skin cancer. Clin Plast Surg 24:673–686, 1997.

Padgett JK, Hendrix JD: Cutaneous malignancies and their management. Otolaryng Clin N Am 34:523–553, 2001.

Preston DS, Stern RS: Nonmelanoma cancers of the skin. N Engl J Med 327:1649–1662, 1992.

The National Comprehensive Cancer Network (NCCN): Guidelines of care for nonmelanoma skin cancers. Dermatol Surg 26:289–292, 2000.

Zbar RI, Cottel WI: Skin tumors I: Nonmelanoma skin tumors. Selected Readings in Plastic Surgery 9:1–34, 2000.

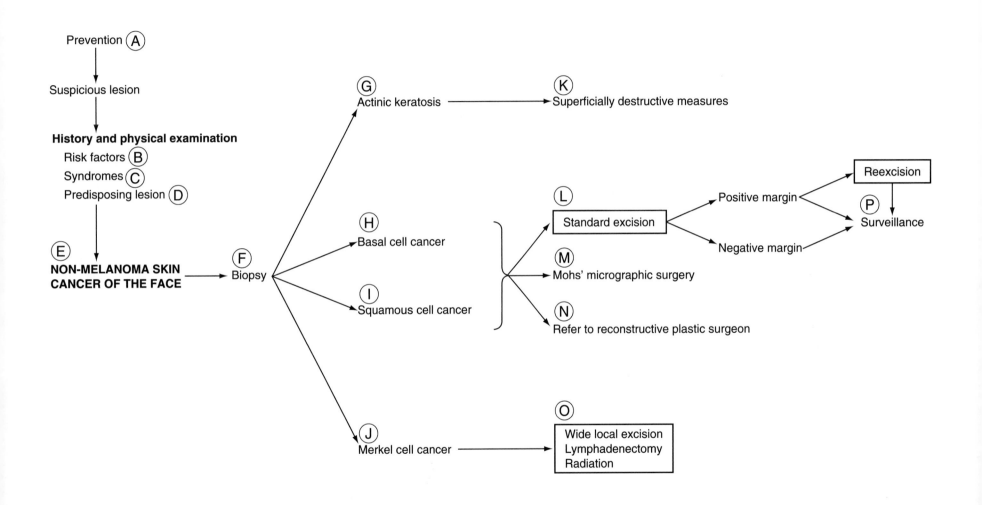

Chapter 18 *Carcinoma of the Oral Cavity*

TOMMY BROWN, MD ● JOHN RIDGE, MD, PHD

(A) Exposure to alcohol and tobacco is the chief cause of carcinoma of the oral cavity. The risk for those abusing both alcohol and tobacco is 38 times that of those who abstain from both. Chronic exposure to these agents creates a "field effect," leaving the entire upper aerodigestive mucosa at risk. This results in a high incidence of second primary cancers even after successful treatment of the index lesion. The oral cavity includes the lip, anterior two-thirds of the tongue, floor of the mouth, gingiva, retromolar trigone, buccal mucosa, and hard palate. The tongue is the most common site of cancer in the oral cavity, representing 43% of cases; this is followed by the floor of the mouth, representing 14%; and the remaining sites, representing less than 10% each. Symptoms of oral carcinoma include mass, ulceration, pain, symptoms related to cranial nerve involvement, bleeding, and change in speech. Initial evaluation should include site and duration of symptoms, a thorough history of etiologic risk factors, and the patient's overall physical and emotional health. The patient's social history and compliance also play significant roles in selection of treatment and the patient's ability to tolerate rehabilitation. A comprehensive head and neck examination should be performed documenting appearance, size, thickness, and mobility of the lesion as well as relationship to surrounding structures. Cranial nerve evaluation should include sensation over the chin, tongue mobility, facial nerve function, gag reflex, and trapezius function. Careful examination for second malignancies is mandatory. Erythroplakia and suspicious areas of leukoplakia should be biopsied. Erythroplakia has the highest risk of associated carcinoma, and any red lesions should be biopsied. Masses in the neck should be characterized by size, mobility, and involvement of the overlying skin.

(B) Oral cancer is the sixth leading cause of cancer worldwide. In the United States, more than 20,300 cases are diagnosed and 5300 people die each year of oral cancer. Ninety percent of oral cancers are squamous cell cancer. Surgical resection remains the mainstay of treatment.

(C) Preoperative evaluation also includes chest x-ray to screen for metastatic disease or synchronous lung cancer. CT scan of the head and neck to evaluate the extent of nodal disease is worthwhile if no "staging" supraomohyoid neck dissection is planned (see F).

(D) A biopsy of the suspicious lesion should be obtained in the office or during examination under anesthesia. A simple punch biopsy or incisional biopsy is usually adequate. The lesion should not be removed entirely during biopsy except by the surgeon who will render the cancer care.

(E) Enlarged neck nodes are evaluated using FNA if no primary lesion is identified. Excisional biopsy of suspected nodal metastasis should be avoided because this almost invariably complicates definitive management of the neck disease.

(F) Examination under anesthesia (EUA) with endoscopy (direct laryngoscopy with esophagoscopy and/or bronchoscopy) should be performed on patients with enlarged neck nodes whose primary lesion is not found with imaging studies and complete head and neck examination. The role of PET scan is uncertain. EUA may also be used as an adjunct to evaluate the extent, staging, and resectability of known oral cancers before definitive resection. If the location and extent of disease is apparent on physical examination and imaging studies, this may obviate the need for EUA.

(G) In stage I oral carcinoma (T1M0), lesions are smaller than 2 cm and the neck is clinically negative. Stage I oral cancer is usually treated by primary surgical resection, but definitive radiotherapy may be employed. Both treatment modalities offer equivalent survival of 75% to 85%. Surgery includes the attendant risks of anesthesia and resection as well as potential functional deficits. The overall treatment period is short and surgery can be repeated as necessary. Margins of 1.5 to 2 cm are appropriate. Primary radiotherapy avoids the physical loss of tissue; however, the course involves treatment 5 days per week for 6 to 7 weeks. Additionally, mucositis and long-term dry mouth are universal complications that have a devastating impact on quality of life. A "staging" supraomohyoid neck dissection is recommended if the likelihood of nodal metastasis runs greater than 20% based on the characteristics of the primary lesion. The incidence of nodal metastasis is related to T stage and depth of invasion. For any oral cancers greater than 2 mm thick, a staging neck dissection warrants serious consideration. If radiation therapy is employed as the primary modality, the neck should usually be treated.

(H) Stage II (T2N0M0) includes patients with a primary lesion between 2 and 4 cm with the neck negative. Again, surgery or radiotherapy have equivalent cure rates of 60% to 70%. Neck dissection and radiotherapy are based on the tumor size and thickness as described for stage I disease. Most patients will experience lower morbidity from resection.

(I) Stage III patients have a primary tumor larger than 4 cm (T3N0M0) or a single ipsilateral node larger than 3 cm (T1-3N1M0). Treatment typically involves both radiation and surgery. For resectable disease, surgery is often followed by adjuvant radiation within 6 weeks of the operation. Postoperative radiotherapy is recommended when the estimated risk of locoregional recurrence is greater than 20%. Indications may include positive or close (less than 5 mm) margins, high grade histology, perineural/vascular invasion, and T3 or T4 lesions. The indications for cervical radiation include multiple metastatic nodes, extracapsular extension, and lymph node size greater than 3 cm. Neck treatment should be included in surgical planning for virtually all stage III patients. Survival ranges from 35% to 50%.

(J) Stage IV (T4N0-3M0, T1-3N2-3M0, and AnyTAnyNM1) represents a diverse group of lesions. Patients who are resectable should undergo surgery to include complete extirpation of the primary lesion with neck dissection, followed by radiotherapy. Those not resectable should receive radiotherapy or chemotherapy. Cure rate ranges from 15% to 35% for resectable cancers.

REFERENCES

Adelstein DJ: Induction chemotherapy in head and neck cancer. Hematol Oncol Clin North Am 13:689–698, 1999.

American Joint Committee on Cancer: Manual for Staging of Cancer, 6th ed. Philadelphia: Lippincott Williams & Wilkins, 2002.

Boyle JO, Strong EW: Oral Cavity Cancer. In Shah JP (ed): Cancer of the Head and Neck. Hamilton, Ontario: BC Decker Inc; 2001.

Franceschi D, Gupta R, Spiro RH et al: Improved survival in the treatment of squamous carcinoma of the oral tongue. Am J Surg 166:360–365, 1993.

Fukano H, Matsuura H, Hasegawa Y et al: Depth of invasion as a predictive factor for cervical lymph node metastasis in tongue carcinoma. Head Neck 19:205–210, 1997.

Jemal A, Thomas A, Murray T et al: Cancer statistics, 1999. CA Cancer J Clin 52:23–47, 2002.

Kramer S, Gelber RB, Snow JB et al: Combined radiation therapy and surgery in the management of advanced head and neck cancer: Final report of study 73-03 of the Radiation Therapy Oncology Group. Head Neck Surg 10:19–30, 1987.

Wijers OB, Levendag PC, Braaksma MMJ et al: Patients with head and neck cancer cured by radiation therapy: A survey of the dry mouth syndrome in long-term survivors. Head Neck 24:737–747:2002.

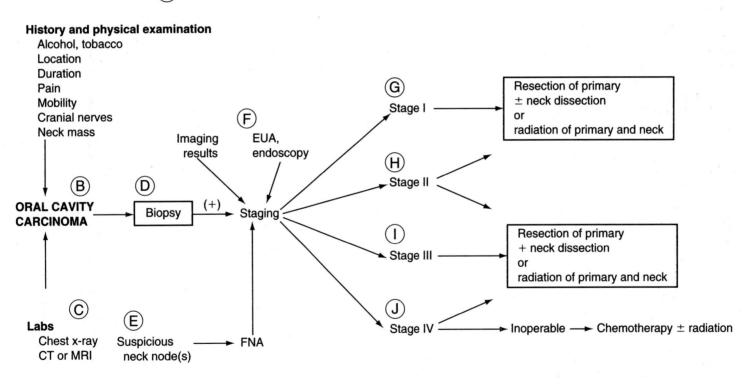

Chapter 19 Salivary Gland Tumor

JOHN I. SONG, MD

(A) Salivary gland neoplasms can present as slow-growing, painless masses or as recurrent swellings. A history of tobacco and/or alcohol abuse should be elicited to rule out metastasis from the upper aerodigestive tract. A complete head and neck examination should be performed to assess the extent of disease. Deep-lobe parotid masses can mimic oropharyngeal masses, whereas submandibular masses may simulate neck masses. In parotid masses, symptoms of sicca syndrome (e.g., keratoconjunctivitis or xerostomia) can suggest underlying Sjögren's syndrome.

(B) Facial nerve paralysis (in parotid masses) or other cranial nerve deficits, fixation of the mass, involvement of the overlying skin, and trismus are all suggestive of malignancy.

(C) Sjögren's syndrome can cause diffuse unilateral or bilateral parotid swelling, most commonly in middle-aged women. If Sjögren's syndrome is suspected, lab studies including rheumatoid factor (RF), sedimentary rate (ESR), antinuclear antibody (ANA), and antibodies to Sjögren's syndrome antigens (SS-A; SS-B) should be obtained. Definitive diagnosis of Sjögren's syndrome may require a minor salivary gland biopsy from the lower lip. CT, MRI, or both are recommended to assess extent of disease. MRI can also assess perineural invasion. Sialograms may be useful in detecting salivary gland stones. Diffuse parotid enlargement in a young person should raise the suspicion for HIV infection. These intraparotid lymphoepithelial cysts may be unilateral or bilateral.

(D) Fine-needle aspiration (FNA) can help differentiate between salivary neoplasms, metastatic disease, inflammatory processes, or lymphoma. FNA has a greater than 90% sensitivity and specificity rate and most studies to date have not demonstrated tumor seeding with this technique.

(E) Approximately 25% of parotid gland tumors are malignant, whereas 75% of submandibular, sublingual, and minor salivary gland tumors are malignant. In general, the smaller the salivary gland, the more likely a mass is malignant.

(F) Most parotid neoplasms (greater than 75%) are benign. In contrast, only 25% of submandibular gland neoplasms are benign. Benign salivary gland neoplasms include pleomorphic adenomas, monomorphic adenomas, Warthin's tumors, and oncocytomas. Some 75% of parotid tumors are found within the superficial lobe, and a superficial lobectomy with facial nerve preservation is curative. Benign deep lobe parotid tumors are treated by limited total parotidectomy with facial nerve preservation. Submandibular gland resection with preservation of the marginal mandibular and lingual nerves is curative for benign submandibular gland tumors. Simple enucleation of tumor, especially within the parotid gland, can result in violation of the capsule, tumor spillage, and a high rate of local recurrence and should be avoided.

(G) Patients with Sjögren's syndrome have a greater than 40 times relative risk of developing lymphoma in the parotid gland. Non-Hodgkin's lymphoma is the most common type to arise in major salivary glands. Primary resection is rarely indicated in lymphoma, but additional core biopsy or incisional biopsy may be needed to obtain tissue for flow cytometry or to assess cytoarchitecture.

(H) Primary squamous cell carcinoma (SCC) of salivary gland origin must be differentiated from metastasis to adjacent cervical lymph nodes. In order to diagnose primary SCC, the tumor must originate from the parenchymal epithelial cells within the gland itself. High-grade mucoepidermoid carcinoma can also mimic SCC.

(I) Low-grade malignant tumors include acinic cell carcinomas and low- and intermediate-grade mucoepidermoid carcinomas. Treatment of low-grade malignancies is similar to benign tumors. A superficial or total parotidectomy with facial nerve sparing or submandibular gland resection is indicated. Neither regional lymph node dissection nor postoperative radiotherapy or chemotherapy is indicated.

(J) High-grade malignancies include undifferentiated carcinoma, SCC, high-grade mucoepidermoid carcinoma, adenocarcinoma, adenoid cystic carcinoma, and malignant mixed tumor.

(K) If a diagnosis of SCC or undifferentiated carcinoma is decided upon, a thorough search for an upper aerodigestive tract primary tumor should be made. This may include an examination under anesthesia and a panendoscopy. In addition, primary cancers of the skin, lung, breast, and kidney can also metastasize to salivary glands and adjacent lymph nodes and must be ruled out.

(L) Treatment of high-grade salivary gland malignancies includes an en-bloc resection of the primary tumor. This may include: (1) total parotidectomy; (2) wide local resection of the submandibular triangle including floor of mouth, tongue, and mandible if involved with tumor; and (3) palatectomy (near total or total) for minor salivary gland carcinomas. Regional lymph node dissection is also indicated in high-grade malignancies. Clinically N_0 nodes are addressed by selective or functional neck dissection sparing surrounding muscles, vessels, and nerves. Clinically palpable N+ nodes are addressed by modified radical or radical neck dissections. The facial nerve can usually be spared unless there is pre-existing nerve paralysis or gross tumor invasion at the time of surgery. Adenoid cystic carcinomas have a high incidence of perineural invasion. Frozen-section biopsy of the facial nerve or submandibular ganglion is indicated until negative margins are obtained. Additional resection of the facial nerve may require a mastoidectomy to access the temporal bone. Whenever possible, the facial nerve should be reconstructed with a nerve graft in addition to facial reanimation procedures for maximal ocular protection and cosmesis.

(M) In patients with high-grade carcinomas, postoperative radiation therapy can improve locoregional control and long-term survival in some tumor types. In general, perineural or angiolymphatic invasion, facial nerve paralysis, cervical metastases,

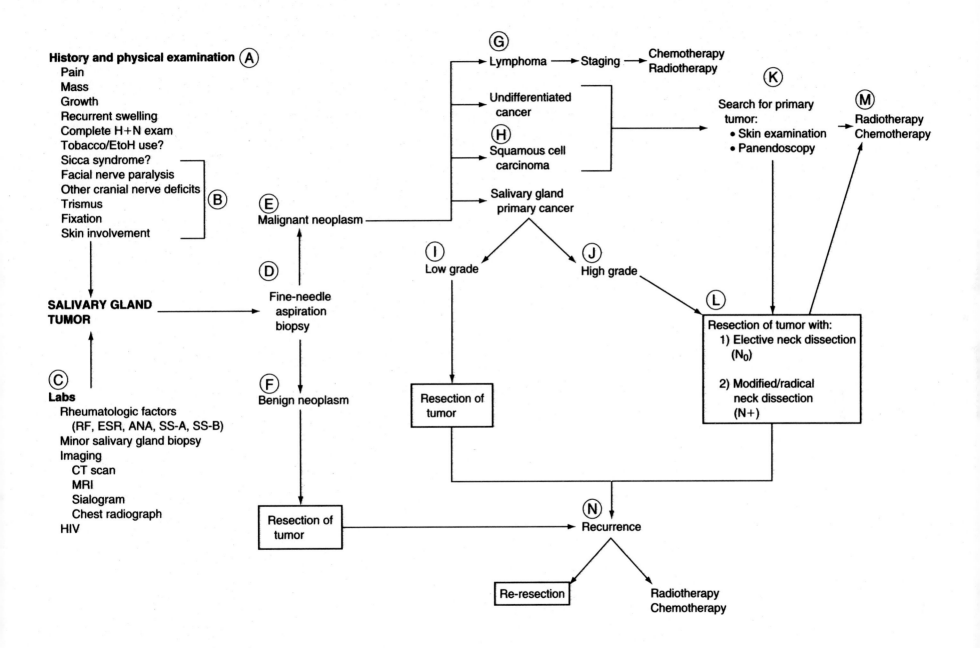

History and physical examination Ⓐ
Pain
Mass
Growth
Recurrent swelling
Complete H+N exam
Tobacco/EtOH use?
Sicca syndrome?
Facial nerve paralysis
Other cranial nerve deficits
Trismus
Fixation
Skin involvement

Ⓑ

SALIVARY GLAND TUMOR

Ⓒ
Labs
Rheumatologic factors
    (RF, ESR, ANA, SS-A, SS-B)
Minor salivary gland biopsy
Imaging
    CT scan
    MRI
    Sialogram
    Chest radiograph
HIV

Ⓓ
Fine-needle
aspiration
biopsy

Ⓔ
Malignant neoplasm

Ⓕ
Benign neoplasm

Resection of
tumor

Ⓖ
Lymphoma → Staging → Chemotherapy
                                Radiotherapy

Undifferentiated
cancer
Ⓗ
Squamous cell
carcinoma

Salivary gland
primary cancer

Ⓚ
Search for primary
tumor:
• Skin examination
• Panendoscopy

Ⓜ
Radiotherapy
Chemotherapy

Ⓘ
Low grade

Ⓙ
High grade

Ⓛ
Resection of tumor with:
1) Elective neck dissection
   (N$_0$)

2) Modified/radical
   neck dissection
   (N+)

Resection of
tumor

Ⓝ
Recurrence

Re-resection

Radiotherapy
Chemotherapy

and positive surgical margins are indications for postoperative radiation therapy. In cases of metastatic disease to the salivary gland, radiation and chemotherapy may be indicated as part of the treatment for the primary tumor. Salivary gland tumors with overexpression of Her-2/neu may benefit from chemotherapy.

Ⓝ Local recurrence of benign salivary gland tumors should be re-resected. In rare cases, pleomorphic adenomas can degenerate into malignant carcinomas. Careful pathologic evaluation is indicated in these cases, especially if the mass recurs after a prolonged period from initial surgery. Whenever possible, re-resection and radiation therapy is indicated in high-grade carcinoma recurrences. Radiation alone may be used for palliation but is less likely to achieve local control.

REFERENCES

Aijaz A, Myers EN, Carrau R: Malignant Tumors of the Salivary Glands. In Myers EN, Suen JY (eds): Cancer of the Head and Neck. Philadelphia: WB Saunders, 1996.

Batsakis JH: Tumors of the Head and Neck: Clinical and Pathological Consideration, 2nd ed. Baltimore: Williams & Wilkins, 1979.

Eisele DW, Johns ME: Salivary Gland Neoplasms. In Bailey BJ, Calhoun KH, Deskin RW et al (eds): Head and Neck Surgery—Otolaryngology, 3rd ed. Philadelphia: WB Saunders, 1993.

Gallia LJ, Johnson JT: The incidence of neoplastic versus inflammatory disease in major salivary gland masses diagnosed by surgery. Laryngoscope 91:512–516, 1981.

Hanna EY, Suen JY: Neoplasms of the Salivary Glands. In Cummings CW, Fredrickson JM, Harker LA et al (eds): Otolaryngology—Head and Neck Surgery, 3rd ed. St. Louis: Mosby, 1998.

Spiro RH, Armstrong J, Harrison L et al: Carcinoma of the major salivary glands: Recent trends. Arch Otolaryngol Head Neck Surg 115:316–321, 1989.

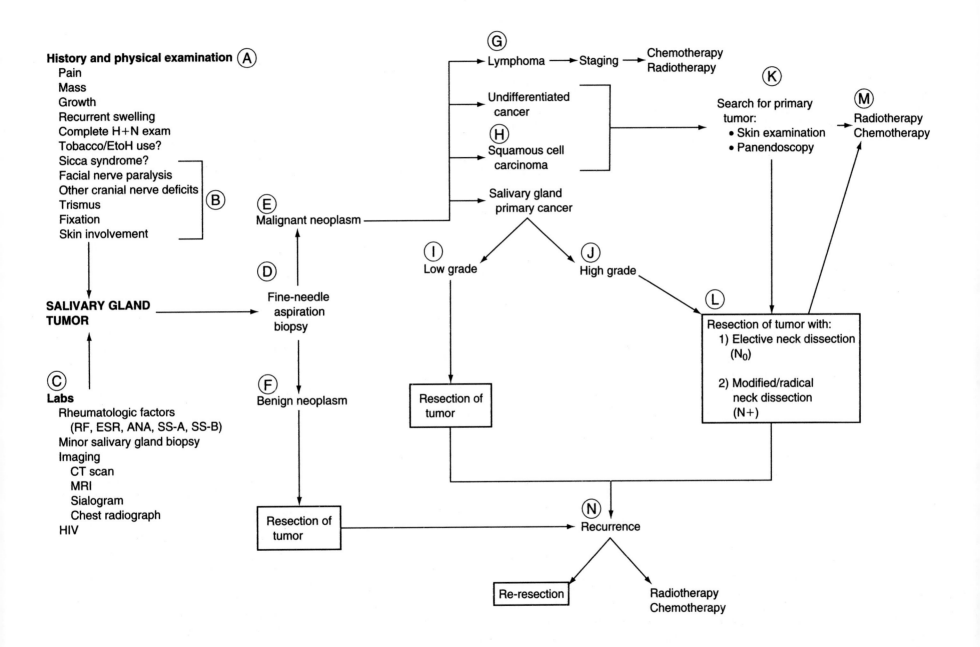

History and physical examination Ⓐ
Pain
Mass
Growth
Recurrent swelling
Complete H+N exam
Tobacco/EtOH use?
Sicca syndrome?
Facial nerve paralysis
Other cranial nerve deficits
Trismus
Fixation
Skin involvement
Ⓑ

SALIVARY GLAND TUMOR

Ⓒ
Labs
Rheumatologic factors
(RF, ESR, ANA, SS-A, SS-B)
Minor salivary gland biopsy
Imaging
CT scan
MRI
Sialogram
Chest radiograph
HIV

Ⓓ
Fine-needle
aspiration
biopsy

Ⓔ
Malignant neoplasm

Ⓕ
Benign neoplasm

Resection of
tumor

Ⓖ
Lymphoma → Staging → Chemotherapy
Radiotherapy

Undifferentiated
cancer

Ⓗ
Squamous cell
carcinoma

Salivary gland
primary cancer

Ⓘ
Low grade

Ⓙ
High grade

Resection of
tumor

Ⓚ
Search for primary
tumor:
• Skin examination
• Panendoscopy

Ⓛ
Resection of tumor with:
1) Elective neck dissection
(N$_0$)

2) Modified/radical
neck dissection
(N+)

Ⓜ
Radiotherapy
Chemotherapy

Ⓝ
Recurrence

Re-resection

Radiotherapy
Chemotherapy

Chapter 20 **Neck Mass**

JONATHAN M. OWENS, MD • ARLEN D. MEYERS, MD, MBA

(A) Age is an important consideration in neck mass evaluation. Neck masses in children and young adults are benign in 90% of cases, whereas the "rule of 80" can be applied after age 40 years. This states that 80% of nonthyroid neck masses are neoplastic and that 80% of the neoplastic masses are malignant. Although 80% of neck malignancies in adults are epidermoid (squamous cell) carcinomas, 90% of cervical cancers in children are of mesenchymal origin.

(B) A persistent lump in the neck of an adult is usually metastatic cancer and originates from a primary tumor above the clavicle. At least 70% of patients seen with a neck mass diagnosed as cancer by a node biopsy will be found to have an obvious primary lesion of the head or neck at initial examination.

(C) CT scan of the neck is the radiologic study of choice for neck mass evaluation. The greatest utility of CT is in evaluation of masses that are difficult to assess by physical examination, such as those in a deep lobe of the parotid gland or in the parapharyngeal space. CT may also be helpful in identifying a primary tumor of the head and neck that is not readily apparent on initial physical examination. CT and MRI are not reliable in predicting the presence or absence of malignancy in enlarged cervical nodes. The role of PET scan in staging head and neck cancer is controversial; currently, its greatest role is evaluating primary and nodal sites following radiation.

(D) All mucosal surfaces of the pharynx, oral cavity, and larynx should be examined before performing an open node biopsy in a patient with a neck mass. Furthermore, at the time of the biopsy, careful endoscopic evaluation of these areas should be performed. Biopsy of suspicious lesions should be performed. If biopsy reveals cancer, the neck mass should be considered to be metastatic disease and biopsy of the neck mass is not necessary.

(E) Cervical lymphadenopathy in HIV-positive patients is a common finding; this most often represents lymph node hyperplasia rather than a neoplastic process. The most common malignant neck mass in HIV patients is lymphoma. These lymphomas are generally high-grade, or B-cell origin, and often involve extranodal sites such as the parotid gland or soft tissue of the neck. Kaposi's sarcoma is the most common neoplastic process in HIV patients. It generally presents as a cutaneous or mucosal lesion; associated neck masses are rare. Atypical infections (e.g., mycobacteria, actinomyces, and nocardia) should also be considered when evaluating a neck mass in an HIV patient.

(F) A tender neck mass strongly suggests infection. The presence of fluctuance suggests a neck abscess. Needle aspiration may be performed to confirm the presence of purulent material. A neck abscess should be treated with incision and drainage; cultures should also be obtained. CT scan may be helpful in differentiating an abscess from other infectious responses (e.g., phlegmon or reactive adenopathy). If no abscess is present and infection is suspected, antibiotics should be administered. If the mass persists for 4 weeks despite adequate antibiotic therapy, biopsy should be performed.

(G) Differential diagnosis of a midline neck mass includes:

Thyroglossal duct cyst
Dermoid cyst
Pyramidal lobe of thyroid
Sebaceous cyst

Most midline neck masses in children are congenital and benign. Thyroglossal duct cyst is the most common midline neck mass in children. It most commonly arises just inferior to the hyoid bone. In thyroid hypoplasia, a small area of aberrant ectopic thyroid tissue may be mistaken for a thyroglossal duct cyst. The incidence of such aberrant tissue is low (1% to 2% of all thyroglossal abnormalities). The use of preoperative ultrasound for patients with thyroglossal duct cysts has been advocated to avoid excising the only functioning thyroid tissue present.

(H) Branchial cleft cysts or sinuses are commonly associated with a small pit in the skin along the anterior border of the sternocleidomastoid muscle. The patient may report recurrent swelling or infection of the mass. Other lateral neck masses may represent inflammatory lymph nodes from infections, enlargement of salivary glands, carotid body tumors, or metastatic cancer from the head and neck.

(I) Supraclavicular nodes are usually either lymphoma or metastases from cancer of the breast, lung, pancreas, or stomach (Virchow's node). Biopsy is indicated if the primary is not evident.

(J) Fine-needle aspiration (FNA) biopsy for cytologic diagnosis is the single most important test in the work-up of a neck mass. FNA should be performed on all persistent neck masses unless an obvious primary tumor is located. The use of ultrasound to guide FNA is often helpful. If cells are examined by an experienced pathologist, the sensitivity for the presence of neoplasm is 92% and the specificity for the absence of tumor is 98%. Various molecular studies may augment routine analysis of FNA specimens when the diagnosis is uncertain. Flow cytometry is useful in detecting non-Hodgkin's lymphoma on FNA specimens; the sensitivity is 77% to 100% and specificity 100%. Epstein-Barr virus (EBV) is associated with nasopharyngeal carcinoma, and the detection of EBV DNA by polymerase chain reaction (PCR) in a cervical metastatic lymph node FNA is predictive of this diagnosis. The cost of an FNA sample and analysis is about $500.

(K) Panendoscopy of the upper aerodigestive tract includes direct laryngoscopy, rigid esophagoscopy, and rigid bronchoscopy. The purposes of panendoscopy are to stage and biopsy a known primary tumor; identify an unknown primary tumor; and to screen for a second primary cancer

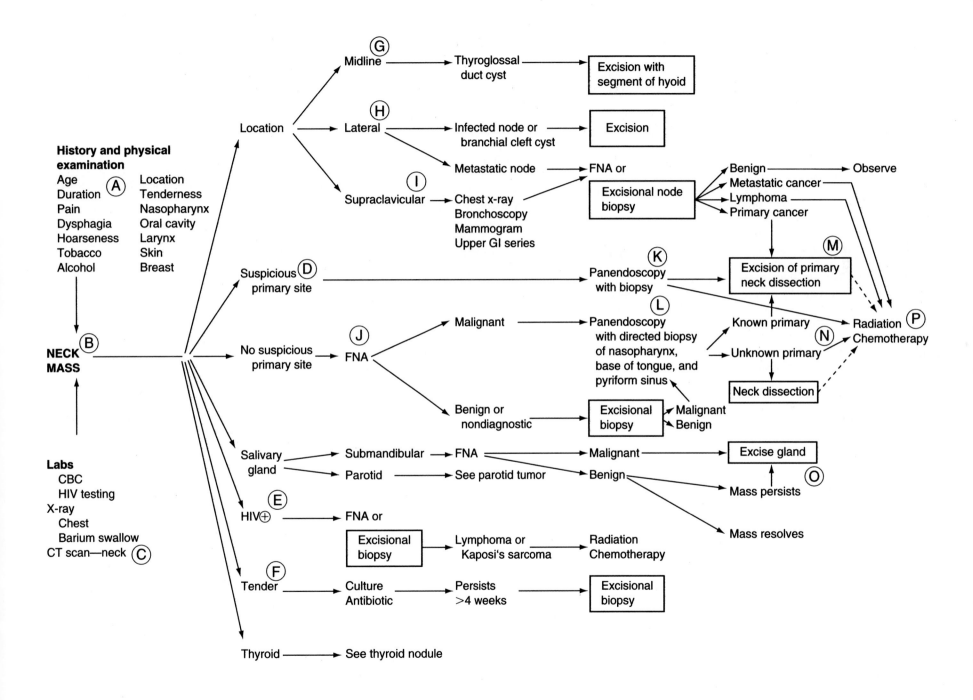

History and physical examination

Age   (A) Location
Duration   Tenderness
Pain   Nasopharynx
Dysphagia   Oral cavity
Hoarseness   Larynx
Tobacco   Skin
Alcohol   Breast

NECK MASS (B)

Labs
 CBC
 HIV testing
X-ray
 Chest
 Barium swallow
CT scan—neck (C)

Location

Midline (G) → Thyroglossal duct cyst → Excision with segment of hyoid

Lateral (H) → Infected node or branchial cleft cyst → Excision

→ Metastatic node → FNA or

Supraclavicular (I) → Chest x-ray / Bronchoscopy / Mammogram / Upper GI series → Excisional node biopsy → Benign → Observe
 Metastatic cancer
 Lymphoma
 Primary cancer

Suspicious primary site (D) → Panendoscopy with biopsy (K) → Excision of primary neck dissection (M)

No suspicious primary site → FNA (J) → Malignant → Panendoscopy with directed biopsy of nasopharynx, base of tongue, and pyriform sinus (L) → Known primary / Unknown primary → Neck dissection → Radiation (P) / Chemotherapy (N)

→ Benign or nondiagnostic → Excisional biopsy → Malignant / Benign

Salivary gland → Submandibular → FNA → Malignant → Excise gland (O)
 Parotid → See parotid tumor → Benign → Mass persists / Mass resolves

HIV⊕ (E) → FNA or

Excisional biopsy → Lymphoma or Kaposi's sarcoma → Radiation Chemotherapy

Tender (F) → Culture Antibiotic → Persists >4 weeks → Excisional biopsy

Thyroid → See thyroid nodule

at a separate site, such as the esophagus. The incidence of a synchronous second primary tumor is approximately 3%.

(L) The nasopharynx, base of tongue, tonsil, and pyriform sinus are notorious sites for squamous cell carcinoma in the neck with no obvious primary. Bilateral tonsillectomy and directed biopsy of these sites should be performed on the patient with a cancerous neck mass and no known primary, even if the mucosa at these sites is normal in appearance. As many as 25% of unknown primary lesions may be identified in this manner. Up to 35% of primary lesions may be identified with PET scan when evaluating an unknown primary lesion.

(M) When the primary cancer is in the neck and the mass is a local metastasis, excision of the primary tumor with en bloc resection of the regional nodes can be curative. Preoperative studies should include liver function tests and a chest x-ray or CT scan to evaluate for metastatic disease. Postoperative radiation is usually advisable, especially with multiple involved nodes or extracapsular extension from lymph nodes.

(N) In 5% to 8% of patients with squamous cell carcinoma in a neck node, no primary tumor site is found. Neck dissection is often adequate therapy for a single, small lymph node. The treatment of a large, single node or multifocal disease is controversial and may involve neck dissection alone, radiation alone, or both.

(O) Excision of parotid and submandibular salivary gland masses is often warranted regardless of preoperative cytologic determination of malignancy. A salivary gland mass yielding nonneoplastic diagnosis by FNA may be observed rather than excised because these masses often resolve over time. A persistent salivary gland mass should be excised regardless of FNA findings. When FNA is performed by experienced pathologists for the evaluation of salivary gland masses, the sensitivity for neoplasm is 93% and specificity is 99%.

(P) Unresectable metastatic squamous cell carcinoma commonly responds to radiation and chemotherapy for palliation. Lymphoma also often responds to radiation, chemotherapy, or a combination of the two.

REFERENCES

Carbone A, Vaccher E, Barzan L et al: Head and neck lymphomas associated with human immunodeficiency virus infection. Arch Otolaryngol Head Neck Surg 121:210–218, 1995.

Frable MA, Frable WJ: Fine-needle aspiration biopsy of salivary glands. Laryngoscope 101:245–249, 1991.

Gupta P, Maddalozzo J: Preoperative sonography in presumed thyroglossal duct cysts. Arch Otolaryngol Head Neck Surg 127:200–202, 2001.

Iganej S, Kagan R, Anderson P et al: Metastatic squamous cell carcinoma of the neck from an unknown primary: Management options and patterns of relapse. Head Neck 24:236–246, 2002.

Knappe M, Louw M, Gregor RT: Ultrasonography-guided fine-needle aspiration for the assessment of cervical metastases. Arch Otolaryngol Head Neck Surg 126:1091–1096, 2000.

Macdonald MR, Freeman JL, Hui MF et al: Role of Epstein-Barr virus in fine-needle aspirates of metastatic neck nodes in the diagnosis of nasopharyngeal carcinoma. Head Neck 17:487–493, 1995.

McGuirt WF: Differential diagnosis of neck masses. In Cummings CW, Fredrickson JM et al (eds): Otolaryngology-Head and Neck Surgery, 3rd ed. St. Louis: Mosby, 1998.

McGuirt WF, Greven K, Williams D III et al: PET scanning in head and neck oncology: A review. Head Neck 20:208–215, 1998.

Park YW: Evaluation of neck masses in children. Am Family Physician 51:1904–1912, 1995.

Young NA, Al-Saleem TI, Ehya H et al: Utilization of fine-needle aspiration cytology and flow cytometry in the diagnosis and subclassification of primary and recurrent lymphoma. Cancer 84:252–261, 1998.

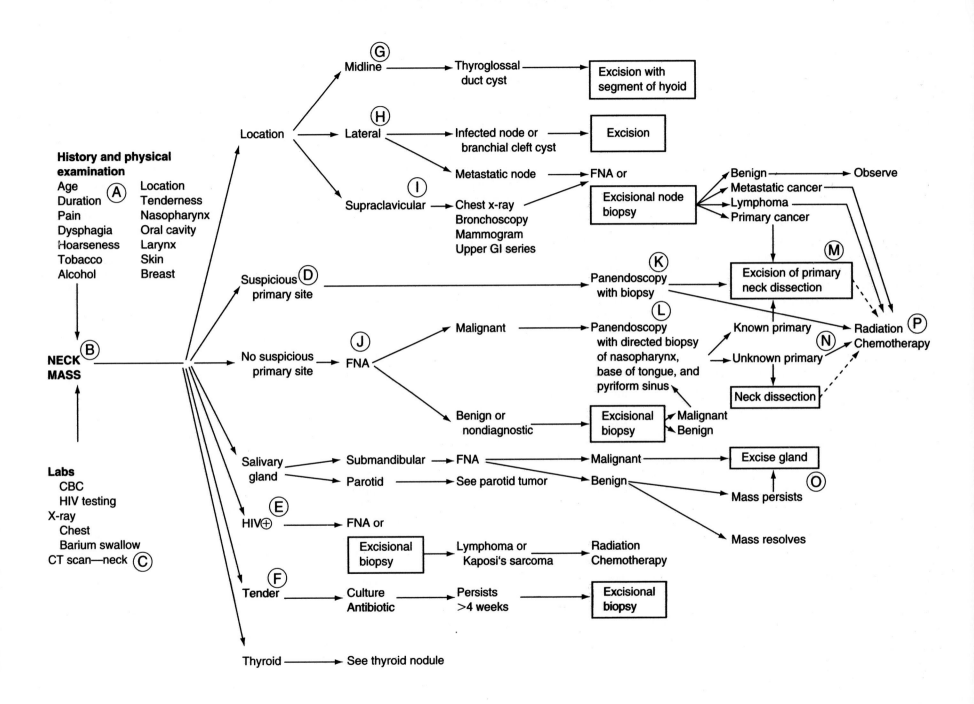

Chapter 21 *Cancer of the Larynx*

ASHOK R. SHAHA, MD

(A) The most common initial symptom of cancer of the larynx is hoarseness of the voice, because the majority of these patients have a lesion on the vocal cord. Hoarseness in any elderly individual should not be neglected, and a full evaluation is necessary to rule out laryngeal cancer. Vague sore throat, hemoptysis, ear pain, and neck node metastasis are also symptoms. Ear pain may be a presenting symptom of supraglottic cancer.

(B) The most common risk factor is smoking. The treating physician should appreciate the high incidence of field cancerization, which will require appropriate endoscopy to evaluate the extent of the primary disease and rule out second primary in the lung, the esophagus, or other regions of the upper aerodigestive tract. Fortunately, the majority of the patients with glottic cancer present in early stage because early onset of hoarseness occurs whenever there is a tiny lesion on the free border of the vocal cord.

(C) Appropriate initial evaluation includes a good history and physical examination; indirect laryngoscopy; and fiberoptic laryngoscopy to evaluate the extent of the disease, the status of the endolaryngeal and vocal cord mucosa, and mobility of the true vocal cord. The examination should determine the extent of the primary tumor and status of regional nodes. Lesions of the supraglottic larynx need detailed evaluation of the extent of the disease, including the proximity of the lesion to the anterior commissure. The tumors of the subglottic larynx, though rare, need to be evaluated carefully because they could be easily missed. Appropriate photodocumentation should be considered, as should video documentation, if available. The appreciation of the vocal cord mobility is critical in appropriate clinical staging of the extent of the disease and therapeutic modalities. The examination should also determine the adequacy of the airway and include a search for a second primary in the upper aerodigestive tract.

(D) Approximately 40,000 new patients with head and neck cancer (4% of all cancers) are seen in the United States each year. The incidence of cancer of the larynx includes approximately 10,000 new patients every year. Management of cancer of the larynx revolves around the major vital function of speech; in advanced cases, laryngectomy has a major impact on quality of life. Approximately 50% of larynx cancer patients present in early stage (stage I and II). The remainder of patients present in advanced stage (stage III and IV) with either advanced primary tumor or lymph node metastasis. Survival drops by approximately 50% in patients with advanced laryngeal cancer. The incidence of nodal metastasis is high in patients with supraglottic laryngeal cancer, whereas the nodal metastasis in vocal cord cancer is quite rare unless the patient presents in advanced stage primary tumor. There is considerable paucity of lymphatics in the free border of the vocal cord.

The definitive treatment of laryngeal cancer depends on factors such as the location of the tumor, the extent of the disease, proximity of the lesion to the vocal cord, vocal cord mobility, pre-epiglottic or paraglottic extension of the disease, and extension of the tumor into pyriform sinus or base of the tongue. Treatment requires careful planning and consultation with other services such as medical oncology and radiation therapy, and also input from the patient. The treatment decisions generally revolve around quality of life and voice function.

(E) Imaging studies such as computed tomography (CT) or magnetic resonance imaging (MRI) are quite helpful to evaluate the extent of the disease; however, in early stage lesions the imaging studies are of limited benefit. In advanced stage disease or in nodal metastasis, the imaging is helpful to evaluate the extent of the nodal disease and the paraglottic or pre-epiglottic extension of the tumor. CT and MRI are extremely helpful to evaluate the status of the soft tissue extension of the disease, cartilage destruction, involvement of the anterior commissure, and paraglottic region. Chest x-ray evaluates for a synchronous lung tumor. CT scan of the chest may be considered if any abnormality is noted on chest x-ray.

(F) Direct laryngoscopy is performed to evaluate the extent of the disease and to perform biopsy for diagnosis. The direct laryngoscopy should include microlaryngoscopy, whenever necessary, with the use of a video telescope (e.g., 0-degree, 30-degree, 90-degree, and 120-degree). Video telescopes will evaluate the exact extent of the disease (especially the involvement of the anterior commissure and subglottic region). It is also very important to evaluate the location of the supraglottic laryngeal cancer and its proximity to the vocal cord. The trachea and bronchus, as well as the esophagus, can be inspected via endoscopy.

(G) The larynx is divided into supraglottic, glottic, and subglottic regions, with respective distributions of malignancy at 44%, 55%, and 1%. If the lesion appears very superficial, vocal cord stripping should be considered as an initial diagnostic evaluation. This will be both diagnostic and therapeutic in many instances. The white lesions of the vocal cord may represent hyperkeratosis, parakeratosis, dysplasia, severe dysplasia with atypia, in situ carcinoma, or infiltrating squamous cell carcinoma. The most common histopathologic variety is squamous cell carcinoma, found in more than 95% of these lesions. Other tumors (e.g., minor salivary gland tumors) are quite rare.

(H) Early stage supraglottic laryngeal cancers can be treated with radiation therapy or with surgery. The surgery will require supraglottic laryngectomy; however, in most circumstances, the majority of patients with supraglottic laryngeal cancer are treated with an organ preservation protocol. There is a very high incidence of nodal metastasis (commonly bilateral) in supraglottic laryngeal cancer, and due consideration must be given to the management of the neck along with management of the primary.

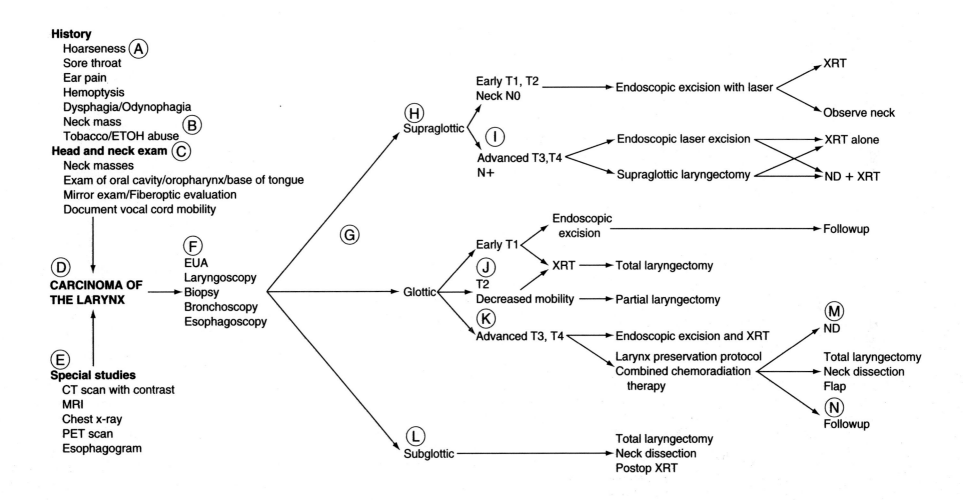

History
   Hoarseness Ⓐ
   Sore throat
   Ear pain
   Hemoptysis
   Dysphagia/Odynophagia
   Neck mass Ⓑ
   Tobacco/ETOH abuse
Head and neck exam Ⓒ
   Neck masses
   Exam of oral cavity/oropharynx/base of tongue
   Mirror exam/Fiberoptic evaluation
   Document vocal cord mobility

Ⓓ
CARCINOMA OF THE LARYNX

Ⓔ
Special studies
   CT scan with contrast
   MRI
   Chest x-ray
   PET scan
   Esophagogram

Ⓕ
EUA
Laryngoscopy
Biopsy
Bronchoscopy
Esophagoscopy

Ⓖ

Ⓗ Supraglottic
  Early T1, T2 Neck N0 → Endoscopic excision with laser → XRT / Observe neck
  Ⓘ Advanced T3, T4 N+ → Endoscopic laser excision → XRT alone / ND + XRT
   Supraglottic laryngectomy → XRT alone / ND + XRT

Glottic
  Early T1 → Endoscopic excision → Followup
  Early T1 → XRT → Total laryngectomy
  Ⓙ T2 → XRT
   Decreased mobility → Partial laryngectomy
  Ⓚ Advanced T3, T4 → Endoscopic excision and XRT
   Larynx preservation protocol / Combined chemoradiation therapy → Ⓜ ND / Total laryngectomy, Neck dissection, Flap / Ⓝ Followup

Ⓛ Subglottic → Total laryngectomy, Neck dissection, Postop XRT

(I) The supraglottic laryngectomy, a popular operation in the past, has considerable issues related to the need of tracheostomy; occasional difficulty in weaning from the tracheostomy is seen, especially in radiated patients and voice dysfunction. The supracricoid laryngectomy, a common surgical procedure in Europe, has not become very popular yet in the United States; however, it should be included in the surgical armamentarium.

(J) Early stage glottic (vocal cord) cancers can be treated effectively with endoscopic laser excision and close follow-up; or, if there is an infiltrating tumor, with radiation therapy. Partial laryngectomy is generally reserved for T2 tumors or tumors with diminished vocal cord mobility. Radiation therapy probably offers better voice function compared with partial laryngectomy; however, patients who fail radiation therapy may require a total laryngectomy as a salvage surgical procedure.

(K) A majority of patients with advanced laryngeal cancer are treated with an organ preservation protocol. The primary total laryngectomy is rarely considered today in view of the relatively effective alternate treatment approaches such as larynx preservation protocol. Endoscopic laser excision may be considered in select circumstances depending upon the experience and the expertise of the treating physician. However, experience with this approach appears to be limited at this stage in the United States.

ORGAN PRESERVATION PROTOCOL

Since the classic Veterans' Administration study on treatment of larynx cancer was published, there appears to be enormous interest in treating advanced stage laryngeal cancer (requiring total laryngectomy) with a combination of chemotherapy and radiation therapy as an organ preservation protocol. The overall success of this treatment appears to parallel that of primary surgery with postoperative radiation therapy; however, the functioning larynx could be preserved in 66% of the surviving patients. Obviously this requires a careful evaluation of the extent of the disease, patient participation in decision making, and appropriate involvement of multi-modality approaches. Imaging studies are quite important to evaluate the extent of the disease. Generally, the treatment regimen includes a concurrent chemoradiation therapy with cis-platinum and 5FU as major chemotherapeutic drugs, along with radiation therapy and hyperfractionation towards the end of the treatment. The post-treatment follow-up is critical to evaluate the status of the larynx and to rule out recurrent cancer. This may require further imaging studies; appropriate endoscopy and biopsy, if necessary; and PET scanning in select individuals. The overall results of organ preservation protocol appear to be quite promising and rewarding in view of voice preservation. At the same time, long-term complications related to mucositis and esophageal stricture need further analysis. The diagnosis of persistent or recurrent cancer may be delayed because of difficulty in evaluating the endolarynx, which may delay the salvage surgical procedure. The incidence of complications related to wound necrosis and pharyngeal fistula appears to be quite high in salvage surgical procedures. A planned neck dissection may be necessary in patients with persistent neck disease or in patients presenting initially with N2 or N3 neck disease.

(L) The subglottic tumors are quite rare and form only 1% of the overall incidence. The majority of the patients with subglottic tumors are truly glottic cancers with extension into subglottic region. These patients are best treated with surgical intervention and postoperative radiation therapy. The surgery may invariably require total laryngectomy.

(M) Even though larynx preservation protocol appears to be the current approach in management of advanced laryngeal cancer, it is very important to appreciate the high cost of this treatment modality and the necessity of close follow-up with clinical examination and appropriate imaging studies. Patients who present with extensive primary tumor (e.g., T4 lesions with extension into the soft tissue of the neck; cartilage destruction; or extensive pre-epiglottic, paraglottic, or massive subglottic tumors) may benefit from primary laryngectomy and tracheoesophageal puncture, with postoperative radiation therapy in select circumstances.

(N) In early stage laryngeal cancer (stage I), the 5-year survival is 90% to 95%, whereas in advanced stage supraglottic laryngeal cancer the survival is 55% to 60%. In glottic laryngeal cancer, the 5-year survival in early stage is 95% to 98%, whereas in advanced stage it is 60% to 65%.

REFERENCES

The Department of Veterans Affairs Laryngeal Cancer Study Group: Introduction chemotherapy plus radiation compared with surgery plus radiation in patients with advanced laryngeal cancer. N Engl J Med 324:1685–1690, 1991.

Kraus DH, Pfister DG, Harrison LB et al: Salvage laryngectomy for unsuccessful larynx preservation therapy. Ann Otol Rhinol Laryngol 104:936–941, 1995.

Laccourreye O, Brasnu D, Perie S et al: Supracricoid partial laryngectomies in the elderly: Mortality, complications, and functional outcome. Laryngoscope 108:237–242, 1998.

Lefebvre J-L, Chevalier D, Luboinsk B et al: Larynx preservation in pyriform sinus cancer: Preliminary results of a European Organization for Research and Treatment of Cancer phase III trial. J Natl Cancer Inst 88:890–899, 1996.

Lima RA, Freitas EQ, Kligerman J et al: Supracricoid laryngectomy with CHEP: Functional results and outcome. Otolaryngol Head Neck Surg 124:258–260, 2001.

Mendenhall WM, Parsons JT, Mancuso AA et al: Radiotherapy for squamous cell carcinoma of the supraglottic larynx: An alternative to surgery. Head Neck 18:24–35, 1996.

Myers EN, Wagner RL, Johnson JT: Microlaryngoscopic surgery for T1 glottic lesions: A cost-effective option. Ann Otol Rhinol Laryngol 103:28–30, 1994.

Pfister DG, Harrison LB, Strong EW, Borl GJ: Current status of larynx preservation with multimodality therapy. Oncology 6:33–35, 1992.

Pfister DG, Shaha AR, Harrison LB: The role of chemotherapy in the curative treatment of head and neck cancer. Surg Oncol Clin N Am 6:749–768, 1997.

Pignon JP, Bourhis J, Komenge C et al, on behalf on the MACH-NC Collaborative Group: Chemotherapy added to locoregional treatment for head and neck squamous-cell carcinoma: Three meta-analyses of updated individual data. Lancet 355:949–955, 2000.

Pradhan SA, D'Cruz AK, Pai PS et al: Near-total laryngectomy in advanced laryngeal and pyriform cancers. Laryngoscope 112:375–380, 2002.

Shaha AR, Hoover EL, Marti JR et al: Synchronicity, multicentricity, and metachronicity of the head and neck cancer. Head Neck 10:225–228, 1988.

Zeitels SM: Surgical management of early supraglottic cancer. Otolaryngol Clin North Am 30:59–78, 1997.

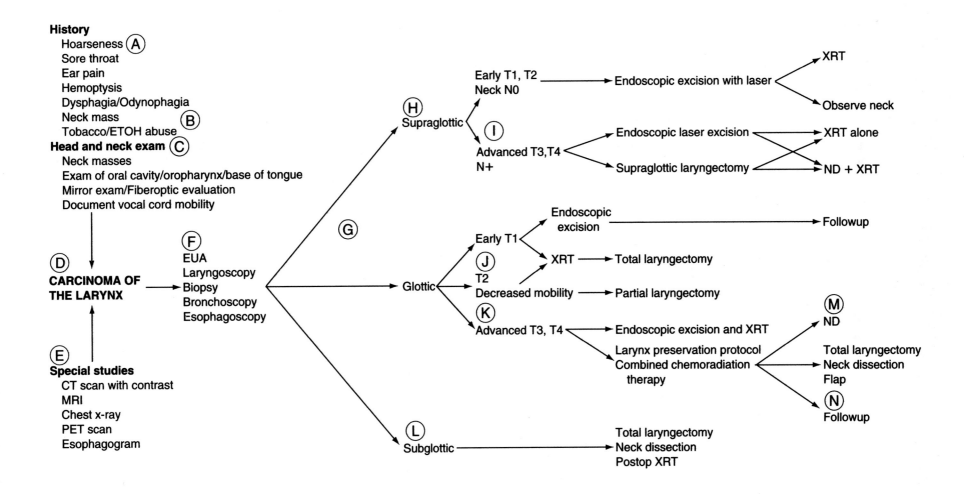

History
Hoarseness Ⓐ
Sore throat
Ear pain
Hemoptysis
Dysphagia/Odynophagia
Neck mass Ⓑ
Tobacco/ETOH abuse
Head and neck exam Ⓒ
Neck masses
Exam of oral cavity/oropharynx/base of tongue
Mirror exam/Fiberoptic evaluation
Document vocal cord mobility

Ⓓ
CARCINOMA OF THE LARYNX

Ⓔ
Special studies
CT scan with contrast
MRI
Chest x-ray
PET scan
Esophagogram

Ⓕ
EUA
Laryngoscopy
Biopsy
Bronchoscopy
Esophagoscopy

Ⓖ

Ⓗ
Supraglottic

Early T1, T2
Neck N0 ——→ Endoscopic excision with laser ⟨ XRT / Observe neck

Ⓘ
Advanced T3,T4
N+ → Endoscopic laser excision → XRT alone / ND + XRT
→ Supraglottic laryngectomy → XRT alone / ND + XRT

Glottic

Early T1 ⟨ Endoscopic excision ——————→ Followup
XRT → Total laryngectomy

Ⓙ
T2
Decreased mobility ——→ Partial laryngectomy

Ⓚ
Advanced T3, T4 → Endoscopic excision and XRT
→ Larynx preservation protocol
Combined chemoradiation therapy

Ⓜ
ND
Total laryngectomy
Neck dissection
Flap

Ⓝ
Followup

Ⓛ
Subglottic ——————→ Total laryngectomy
Neck dissection
Postop XRT

CARDIOPULMONARY

Chapter 22 **Pulmonary Embolism**

WALTER W. SCOTT, JR., MD ● W. RANDOLPH CHITWOOD, JR., MD

(A) Most clinically significant pulmonary emboli (PE) originate from iliac or femoral deep venous thrombosis. Many tests are available to diagnose deep venous thrombosis, including duplex ultrasonography, impedance plethysmography, magnetic resonance imaging, and the plasma D-dimer assay. Although contrast venography has been the gold standard, duplex ultrasonography is becoming the test of choice because it is noninvasive and highly accurate. Major predisposing factors for deep venous thrombosis and pulmonary emboli include congestive heart failure (CHF), malignancy, prolonged bedrest, trauma, oral contraceptives, advanced age, previous pelvic or lower extremity surgery, previous thrombophlebitis or pulmonary embolism, pregnancy, and obesity.

(B) The most common presenting symptoms include dyspnea (77%), chest pain (63%), hemoptysis (26%), and altered mental status (23%). Common physical findings include tachycardia (59%), fever (43%), rales (42%), and tachypnea (38%).

(C) PE occurs commonly after surgery. Both operative mortality and hospital costs are increased significantly by this complication. The expense of hospitalization may be more than doubled by a major thromboembolic event. Effective prophylaxis, rapid diagnosis, and precise treatment are important for both patient and cost benefits.

(D) The chest x-ray ($65)* is often normal, but it may demonstrate diminished pulmonary vascularity (Westermark's sign). The ECG ($70) may show rhythm disturbances, T wave and ST segment changes, and P wave enlargement. Arterial blood gases ($90) may be more helpful. Approximately 75% of patients with an acute PE have a $PaCO_2$ of less than 36 mm Hg and/or a PaO_2 of less than

80 mm Hg. Plasma D-dimers, which are specific cross-linked fibrin derivatives, are sensitive markers for venous thromboembolism but lack specificity. However, patients with a low probability of PE and a negative D-dimer do not require any further diagnostic testing.

(E) Unstable hemodynamics (i.e., elevated CVP, pulmonary artery pressure diastolic greater than 25 mmHg, and systolic blood pressure [SBP] less than 80 mmHg) indicate cardiovascular collapse.

(F) Helical CT scanning ($750) has come into broad usage as a first test for pulmonary embolus. It is a highly accurate test for large pulmonary emboli but lacks adequate sensitivity for emboli in subsegmental or smaller pulmonary arteries. Likewise, echocardiography (echo) is helpful in the diagnosis of large pulmonary emboli but lacks sensitivity for smaller emboli. Transthoracic echo offers the advantage of being a rapid, noninvasive, bedside examination with the ability to diagnose multiple types of pathology in the critically ill patient. Cardiomyopathy, aortic dissection, acute myocardial infarction, pericardial effusion, and valve disease all are detectable on echo. Echo signs suggestive of pulmonary embolus include right heart volume overload, a patent foramen ovale (with or without a significant shunt), and right ventricular thrombus. Massive embolus in the main pulmonary artery is also visible on echo. Transesophageal echo improves resolution in multiple areas including the pulmonary arteries.

(G) A ventilation-perfusion (VQ) lung scan ($900) performed within 48 hours of onset of symptoms, combined with a high level of clinical suspicion, is a powerful predictor of PE. VQ scan results are reported as low probability (5% to 10%), intermediate probability, or high probability (greater than 90%) for PE. A low-probability scan combined with low clinical suspicion essentially rules out the diagnosis of pulmonary embolism; however, 40% of patients with a low-probability scan

but a very high clinical index of suspicion have a PE. These patients and those with intermediate-probability scans should undergo pulmonary arteriography. Segmental or lobar parenchymal disease on CXR caused by pneumonia, cancer, or other infiltrates precludes the need for VQ scanning.

(H) Precise pulmonary arterial pressure monitoring is necessary to resuscitate patients who are hemodynamically unstable after a large embolus. Swan-Ganz pulmonary arterial monitoring ($165) is essential. β-agonists (e.g., dopamine, dobutamine, and epinephrine) often are required. The need for vasoactive α-adrenergic agents suggests profound hemodynamic collapse. Pulmonary arterial vasodilators usually are ineffective.

(I) Persistent and refractory hypotension, despite maximal pharmacologic and respiratory support, in the presence of documented pulmonary emboli, is an indication for thrombolytic therapy. In the presence of a specific contraindication to thrombolysis, percutaneous or surgical embolectomy should be performed. The evolution of radiographic techniques for thrombectomy and catheter-directed thrombolysis have made surgical embolectomy less common. The mortality of patients requiring embolectomy remains high (20% to 60%).

(J) Pulmonary angiography ($760) is still considered the definitive test (greater than 95% accuracy) for diagnosing pulmonary emboli. It should be done within 24 to 72 hours of onset of symptoms. Resolution of emboli begins early because of natural thrombolysis and extends to 21 days after the event. Elevation in mean pulmonary artery pressure and levels of hypoxemia correlate linearly with the degree of acute pulmonary embolic vascular obstruction.

(K) Patients with a demonstrable pulmonary embolus should be anticoagulated immediately with heparin (80 IU/kg bolus followed by continuous drip therapy at a rate of 18 IU/kg/hr using actual patient weight). Activated partial

---

*Cost estimates represent the sum of the hospital charge at our institution (a tertiary-care, university-affiliated hospital) and the Medicare physician reimbursement for performing and/or interpreting that study.

History and physical examination
　Predisposing factors Ⓐ
　Dyspnea
　Chest pain
　Hemoptysis Ⓑ
　Altered mental status

PULMONARY EMBOLISM Ⓒ

Labs Ⓓ
　Chest x-ray
　ECG
　Arterial blood gases
　D-dimer

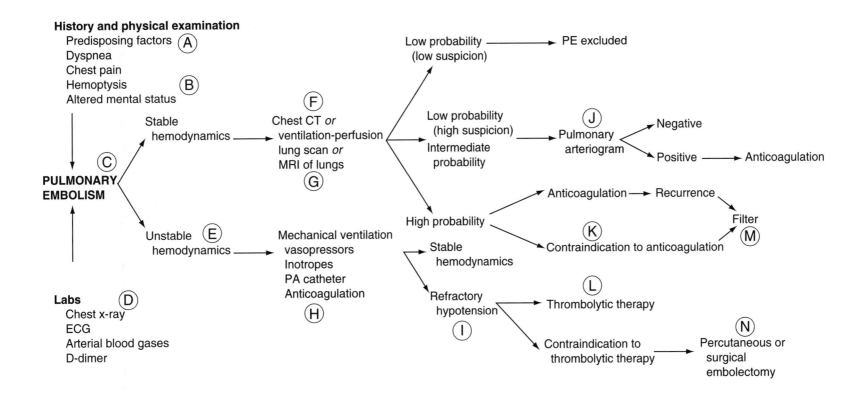

thromboplastin times are used to regulate heparin. A therapeutic level is 2 to 2.5 times the control level. Platelet counts are followed daily. IV heparin therapy is continued until the international normalized ratio (INR) is elevated to 2.5 to 3.5 after starting warfarin therapy. Warfarin is continued for a minimum of 12 weeks. There is no evidence that bedrest prevents clot propagation. Currently, a 2-day ICU stay and the remaining care in a monitored hospital bed (7 days) adds approximately $8100 to hospital charges.

(L) Streptokinase ($1400), urokinase ($9000), and recombinant tissue plasminogen activator (r-TPA) ($3500) have all been approved by the FDA to treat pulmonary embolism. Several studies have demonstrated accelerated clot lysis with these agents as compared with heparin alone. These agents may be administered peripherally or directly into the pulmonary artery (i.e., catheter-directed thrombolysis). Bleeding complications pose the greatest risk; approximately 1% of patients with PE treated with thrombolytic agents experience intracranial bleeding. Absolute contraindications for thrombolytic therapy include previous hemorrhagic stroke, intracranial neoplasm, recent cranial surgery or trauma, and active or recent internal bleeding. Relative contraindications include bleeding diathesis, uncontrolled severe hypertension, cardiopulmonary resuscitation, nonhemorrhagic stroke, and surgery within the previous 10 days.

(M) A vena cava filter ($2840) may be required to prevent recurrent emboli; however, such filters are not uniformly successful because smaller emboli can pass through them or emboli can propagate around the devices through collateral venous channels. Specific indications for a filter include recurrent emboli despite adequate anticoagulation, heparin-induced thrombocytopenia or sensitivity, active peptic ulcer or other bleeding problems, septic emboli, pulmonary hypertension from recurrent chronic emboli, a recent neurosurgical procedure, and recent pulmonary embolectomy.

(N) Indications for pulmonary embolectomy include a contraindication to thrombolytic therapy and failed thrombolysis (with ongoing hemodynamic compromise). Bilateral pulmonary embolectomy requires cardiopulmonary bypass. Unilateral pulmonary arterial embolectomy can be done when extracorporeal circulation is not available. Survival after acute embolectomy is 40% to 70%. The charge for this procedure is approximately $11,300.

REFERENCES

Burke B, Sostman HD, Carroll BA et al: The diagnostic approach to deep venous thrombosis. Clin Chest Med 16:253–268, 1995.

Gray HH, Morgan JM, Paneth M et al: Pulmonary embolectomy for acute massive pulmonary embolism: An analysis of 71 cases. Br Heart J 6:196–200, 1988.

Goldhaber SZ: Echocardiography in the management of pulmonary embolism. Ann Int Med May:691–700, 2002.

Kelly J, Rudd A, Lewis RR et al: Plasma D-dimers in the diagnosis of venous thromboembolism. Arch Intern Med 162:747–756, 2002.

Lassen MR, Borris LC, Nakov RL: Use of the low-molecular weight heparin reviparin to prevent deep venous thrombosis after leg injury requiring immobilization. N Engl J Med 347:726–730, 2002.

Lee RW: Pulmonary embolism. Chest Surg Clin N Am 12:417–437, 2002.

Marino PL: The ICU Book. Philadelphia: Lippincott, 1998.

Nazario R, Delorenzo LJ, Maguire AG: Treatment of venous thromboembolism. Cardiol Rev 10:249–259, 2002.

PIOPED Investigators: Value of the ventilation/perfusion scan in acute pulmonary embolism: Results of the Prospective Investigation of Pulmonary Embolism Diagnosis (PIOPED). JAMA 263:2753–2759, 1990.

History and physical examination
Predisposing factors (A)
Dyspnea
Chest pain
Hemoptysis (B)
Altered mental status

PULMONARY EMBOLISM (C)

Labs (D)
Chest x-ray
ECG
Arterial blood gases
D-dimer

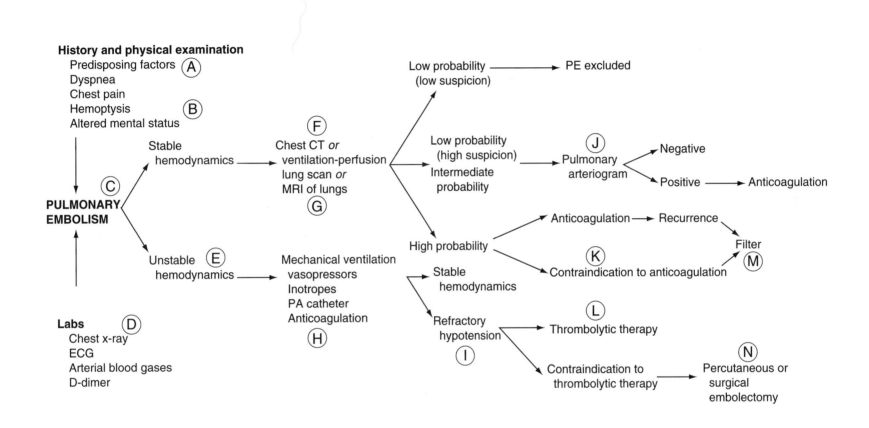

Chapter 23 *Pleural Effusion and Empyema*

LAURENCE H. BRINCKERHOFF, MD • JOHN D. MITCHELL, MD

(A) Patients with pleural effusion most commonly present with symptoms of shortness of breath, chest pain, and fever; however, symptoms may include localized purulent drainage and even hemoptysis. History may include recent infections such as pneumonia. Patients should be asked about tobacco use, exposure history, cancer, and causes of depressed immune function such as HIV or immunosuppressive therapy. They should also be queried about recurrent effusions that required thoracentesis.

(B) A chest x-ray is used as the initial step in evaluation. Characteristics of the effusion, such as the size and whether it is free-flowing or loculated, may be discerned. The presence of other thoracic pathology ranging from pneumonia to evidence of neoplastic disease may also be seen. If these issues cannot be fully addressed by chest x-ray, a CT scan may be useful.

(C) Once diagnosed, the patient with pleural effusion should undergo thoracentesis or chest tube placement. These procedures should attempt to completely evacuate the effusion if possible. Fluid obtained from thoracentesis or tube thoracostomy is allocated for cultures (i.e., aerobic, anaerobic, fungal, and acid-fast bacilli); and for cytologic and laboratory analysis (e.g., cell count, pH, lactic dehydrogenase, glucose, and amylase). Bronchoscopy is considered for patients with persistent unexpanded lung fields after drainage of the effusion to rule out endobronchial obstruction.

(D) An air-fluid level on chest x-ray before any drainage may reflect a bronchopleural fistula. Such fistulas may resolve with chest tube drainage or may require open thoracotomy.

(E) If postdrainage chest x-ray/CT scan demonstrates complete evacuation of the fluid collection, further efforts at drainage may be deferred. Treatment is directed by the laboratory results of the removed fluid and the underlying disease state.

(F) If postdrainage chest x-ray/CT scan demonstrates loculations or incompletely drained fluid, an attempt at percutaneous treatment with installation of streptokinase or tissue plasminogen activator (tPA) may be considered. This approach is most effective with early (less than 7 to 10 days old) empyemas. CT evaluation is particularly helpful in characterizing the extent of the loculations and the response to therapy.

(G) Recurrent effusions are usually treated with talc pleurodesis if neither malignancy nor evidence of infection exists. The efficacy of talc pleurodesis is maximized utilizing a thoracoscopic approach, with bedside pleurodesis using talc slurry reserved for those judged too infirm to withstand a general anesthetic.

(H) There are four principles of empyema management: (1) complete drainage of purulent collection; (2) obliteration of empyema space; (3) investigation and treatment of underlying infection; and (4) management of associated conditions.

(I) If the fluid is sterile, a second drainage procedure may be attempted, usually guided by CT or ultrasound to locate fluid. If loculations persist after the second procedure, and it is more than 14 days since the diagnosis of loculated sterile pleural effusion, the patient should undergo video-assisted thoracoscopic surgery (VATS) decortication.

(J) The natural history of empyema is one of progressive fibrous deposits (the "rind" or "peel") encasing the lung and the empyema cavity. The longer an empyema is left untreated, the more likely it is to have a well-developed capsule/rind and to trap the lung. In this situation, percutaneous approaches to treatment are rarely effective. If findings after the initial drainage procedure indicate loculations and infection or trapped lung syndrome, the patient is evaluated for decortication.

(K) "Early" empyemas diagnosed within the first week or two of onset are usually amenable to effective decortication through a video-assisted approach. The surgeon must be careful not to compromise the operative goals merely to avoid thoracotomy.

(L) The presence of an empyema beyond 14 days usually indicates the need for decortication via thoracotomy, although exceptions exist. Careful removal of the fibrous peel from the visceral pleural surface is essential to allow complete lung expansion.

(M) Age, clinical condition, and comorbidities identify some patients as being at high risk from aggressive management. These patients often have malignant processes and limited life expectancy. Under these circumstances, the patient should undergo rib resection and/or placement of an empyema tube in the most dependent site of the loculated fluid collection.

REFERENCES

Alrawi SJ, Raju R, Acinapura AJ et al: Primary thoracoscopic evaluation of pleural effusion with local anesthesia: An alternative approach. J Soc Laparoendoscopic Surg 6:143–147, 2002.

Bouros D, Antoniou KM, Chalkiadakis G et al: The role of video-assisted thoracoscopic surgery in the treatment of parapneumonic empyema after the failure of fibrinolytics. Surg Endoscop 16:151–154, 2002.

Cameron RJ: Management of complicated parapneumonic effusions and thoracic empyema. Intern Med J 32:408–414, 2002.

Collins J: CT signs and patterns of lung disease. Radiol Clin N Am 39:1115–1135, 2001.

De Hoyos A, Sundaresan S: Thoracic empyema. Surg Clin N Am 82:643–671, 2002.

Hanna JW, Reed JC, Choplin RH: Pleural infections: A clinical-radiologic review. J Thorac Imaging 6:68–79, 1991.

Heffner JE: Infection of the pleural space. Clin Chest Med 20:607–622, 1999.

Heffner JE, Brown LK, Barbieri C et al: Pleural fluid chemical analysis in parapneumonic effusions: A meta-analysis. Am J Respir Crit Care Med 151:1700–1708, 1995.

Meyer DM, Jessen ME, Wait MA et al: Early evacuation of traumatic retained hemothoraces using thoracoscopy:

A prospective, randomized trial. Ann Thorac Surg 64: 1396–1401, 1997.

Miller JI (ed): Empyema, spaces, and fistula. Chest Surg Clin N Am 6:403–626, 1996.

Richardson JD, Carrillo E: Thoracic infection after trauma. Chest Surg Clin N Am 7:401–427, 1997.

Smith JA, Mullerworth MJ, Westlake GW et al: Empyema thoracis: 14-year experience in a teaching center. Ann Thorac Surg 51:39–42, 1991.

Wait MA, Sharma S, Hohn J et al: A randomized trial of empyema therapy. Chest 111:1548–1551, 1997.

Wallenhaupt SL: Surgical management of thoracic empyema. J Thorac Imaging 6:80–88, 1991.

Waller DA. Thoracoscopy in management of postpneumonic pleural infections. Current Opinion in Pulmonary Medicine. 8:323-6, 2002.

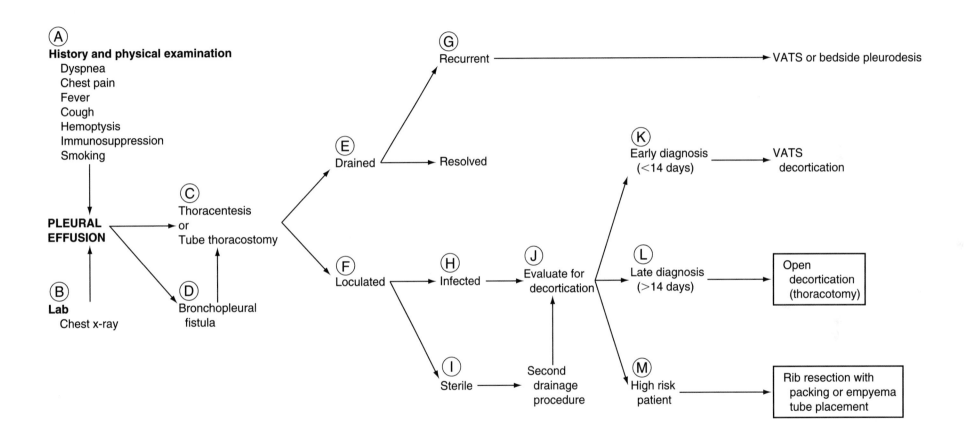

Chapter 24 **Lung Abscess**

ABDUSALAM A. ELALEM, MD • MICHAEL R. JOHNSTON, MD

(A) Lung abscess can affect anyone at any age. The most vulnerable are patients with diabetes, malnourishment, chronic disease, history of substance abuse, epilepsy, poor dental hygiene, stroke, and those with recent operation or blunt trauma. Lung abscess is associated with cancer in about 30% of patients over 45 years of age. Recently, immuno-suppression and AIDS have become significant risk factors. In children immune incompetence and malnutrition are the most important risk factors.

(B) Aspiration is responsible for 50% of all lung abscesses; it is most likely to occur in patients who are unconscious or in an altered state of consciousness because of drug abuse, anesthesia, alcohol, or seizures. Bronchial obstruction by foreign body, tumor, or extrinsic compression may also lead to a lung abscess. About 20% of necrotizing pneu-monias will develop into lung abscesses. An unusual cause is the transdiaphragmatic extension of a liver or subphrenic abscess. Multiple lung abscesses may be of hematogenous origin from thrombophlebitis, endocarditis, or vasculitis; or from primary pul-monary infections (i.e., *Staphylococcus aureus* and *Pneumocystis carinii)*.

(C) Adult patients usually have fever, chills, and chest pain. Children may or may not have chest pain, but they usually fail to thrive, suffer weight loss, and have high fever. Typically, symptoms appear 2 to 3 weeks after an inadequately treated pneumonia or aspiration. As the abscess progresses, about 75% of patients will cough up foul-smelling sputum. Hemoptysis, which can be massive and life threatening, is also common. Physical examination may reveal fever, altered sensorium, poor dental hygiene, and clubbing.

(D) Lung abscess is an acute or chronic infection of the lung marked by a localized collection of pus, inflammation, and destruction of lung tissue. It is the end result of different disease processes rang-ing from bacterial or fungal infection to cancer. Incidence of lung abscess has declined with the widespread availability of antibiotics.

Differential Diagnosis
1. Infected bullae
2. Cysts
3. Sequestration
4. Cavitating tumor
5. Tuberculous and fungal infection
6. Loculated empyema

(E) The chest radiograph typically shows a solitary cavitary lesion with an air-fluid level; multiple cavities are more common in immunocompromised individuals. Patients without a strong history of aspi-ration and with indolent symptoms should be thor-oughly investigated for carcinoma. A history of an abnormal chest x-ray in the past may suggest an infected bulla or cyst.

(F) Chest CT scan will define the anatomic location of the abscess (the posterior segment of the upper lobe and superior segment of the lower lobe on the right side are most common); the size, extent, and content of the abscess; and the thickness of the abscess wall. It can also suggest bronchial obstruction by foreign body or tumor. Rare cases of sequestration with abnormal systemic blood supply can be defined by a contrast-enhanced CT scan.

(G) Bronchoscopy is invaluable in the work-up of a suspected lung abscess, both for diagnosis and as a therapeutic tool for drainage of centrally located abscesses for the following indications:
1. To obtain specific bacteriological, fungal and TB cultures
2. For endobronchial tumor identification, biopsy, and/or cytology
3. For foreign body removal (usually by rigid bronchoscopy)
4. For dilating the appropriate bronchial communication to enhance drainage

(H) Fine-needle aspiration (FNA) is appropriate with thick-walled abscesses and where carci-noma is highly suspected.

(I) Open biopsy is rarely needed except when the diagnosis has not been established by other means. Usually the diagnostic tissue is obtained using a small intercostal space incision or by minimally invasive, video-assisted techniques (VATS). In immunocompromised patients, where a therapeutic decision may be needed quickly, surgical biopsy should be considered early in the work-up.

(J) Antibiotics and postural drainage are main-stays in the conservative treatment of typical lung abscesses. Since the introduction of antibiotics the mortality from lung abscess has dropped signif-icantly, from 60% to 70% to 5% to 10%. Surgical procedures are rarely necessary, and percutaneous drainage using small tubes inserted by interven-tional radiologists is now widely utilized. Standard therapy includes the following:
1. Antibiotics are started with clindamycin or penicillin after appropriate cultures are obtained, until offending organisms are defined and antibiotics directed according to culture sensitivities. Coverage for *Staphylococcus aureus* and Klebsiella is added in patients with necrotizing pneumonia. Therapy is usually needed for at least 4 to 6 weeks. Treatment with antifungal or antituberculous agents is often begun before definitive culture results if the clinical scenario or stains are suggestive.
As a rule, clinical improvement precedes radiological changes.
2. Physiotherapy and nutritional support are essential parts of the treatment.
3. Flexible bronchoscopy can be very helpful in draining centrally located abscesses; care must be taken not to contaminate uninvolved lung.

(K) Foreign bodies are removed by rigid bron-choscopy or operatively to open an obstructed bronchus.

(L) Tumors are treated by either endobronchial or open resection as appropriate for the par-ticular tumor cell type and stage. Unresectable tumors can initially be palliated by bronchoscopic débride-ment and then followed by external beam radio-therapy, brachytherapy, photodynamic therapy, or stent insertion.

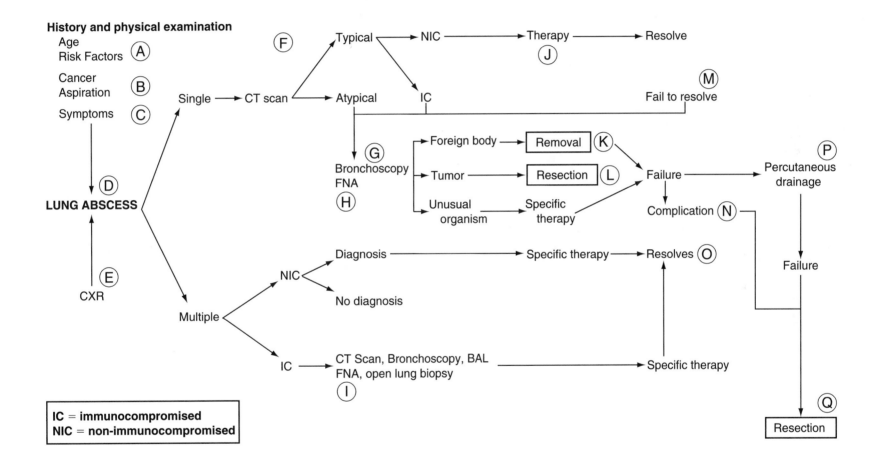

History and physical examination
Age
Risk Factors Ⓐ

Cancer
Aspiration Ⓑ

Symptoms Ⓒ

Ⓓ

LUNG ABSCESS

Ⓔ
CXR

Single → CT scan

Ⓕ Typical → NIC → Therapy → Resolve
Ⓙ

Atypical → IC

Ⓜ Fail to resolve

Ⓖ
Bronchoscopy
FNA
Ⓗ

→ Foreign body → Removal Ⓚ

→ Tumor → Resection Ⓛ

→ Unusual organism → Specific therapy

→ Failure → Percutaneous drainage Ⓟ

Complication Ⓝ

Multiple

NIC → Diagnosis → Specific therapy → Resolves Ⓞ

→ No diagnosis

IC → CT Scan, Bronchoscopy, BAL FNA, open lung biopsy Ⓘ → Specific therapy

Failure

Resection Ⓠ

IC = immunocompromised
NIC = non-immunocompromised

Ⓜ Prognostic factors associated with medical treatment failures include the following:
1. Recurrent aspiration
2. Large cavity size (greater than 6.0 cm)
3. Prolonged symptom complex before presentation
4. Abscess associated with an obstructing lesion
5. Abscess with a thick-walled cavity
6. Serious co-morbidities (e.g., advanced age, neoplasm, and other chronic medical conditions)

Ⓝ Complications of lung abscess include empyema, bronchopleural fistula, massive hemoptysis, spontaneous rupture into uninvolved lung segments, metastatic abscesses (commonly in the brain), and nonresolution of abscess cavity. Although uncommon, these complications often require prolonged medical therapy as well as surgical intervention. Tube thoracostomy, and possibly decortication, is required for empyema, whereas arterial embolization or surgical resection may be necessary for massive hemoptysis. Lung tissue preservation and a secure bronchial closure are important goals in deciding the appropriate surgical procedure.

Ⓞ Lung abscess usually resolves within 2 to 4 weeks from initiation of antibiotics. Prognosis depends on the following:
1. General condition of the patient
2. Host immune status
3. Underlying disease and etiology
4. Size of the abscess correlates with hospitalization time and mortality
5. Infection with virulent organisms such as pseudomonas, klebsiella, and HIV-related organisms

Ⓟ A persistent cavity not responding to conservative therapy may improve with radiologic percutaneous drainage. Catheter placement under CT scan guidance allows external drainage of the lung abscess.

Ⓠ Approximately 10% of lung abscesses require surgical intervention, usually as a result of one of the following:
1. Massive hemoptysis
2. Bronchopleural fistula
3. Empyema
4. Fulminant infection
5. Failure of medical management

REFERENCES

Abolhoda A, Keller SM: Thoracic surgical spectrum of HIV infection. Semin Respir Infect 14:359–365, 1999.

Bartlett JG: Antibiotics in lung abscess. Semin Respir Infect 6:103–111, 1991.

Erasmus JJ, McAdams HP, Rossi S, et al: Percutaneous management of intrapulmonary air and fluid collections. Radiol Clin North Am 38:385–493, 2000.

Furman AC, Jacobs J, Sepkowitz KA: Lung abscess in patients with AIDS. Clin Infect Dis 22:81–85, 1996.

Hirshberg B, Sklair-Levi M, Nir-Paz R: Factors predicting mortality of patients with lung abscess. Chest 115:746–750, 1999.

Cassiere HA, Fein AM: Lung abscess: Diagnosis and treatment. Medscape General Medicine [TM]. Posted 07/03/1997. http://www.medscape.com

Jeong MP, Kim WS, An SK, et al: Transbronchial catheter drainage via fiberoptic bronchoscope in intractable lung abscess. Korean J Intern Med 4:54–58, 1989.

Konishi M, Mori K, Yoshimoto E: Clinical evaluation of lung abscess diagnosed by transtracheal aspiration. Kansenshogaku Zasshi 72:1193–1196, 1998.

Mansharamani N, Balachandran D, Delaney D: Lung abscess in adults: Clinical comparison of immunocompromised to nonimmunocompromised patients. Respir Med 96:178–185, 2002.

Mwandumba HC, Beeching NJ: Pyogenic lung infections: Factors for predicting clinical outcome of lung abscess and thoracic empyema. Curr Opin Pulm Med 6:234–239, 2000.

Parker LA, Melton JW, Delany DJ, et al: Percutaneous small bore catheter drainage in the management of lung abscesses. Chest 92:213–218, 1987.

Pena Grinan N, Munoz Lucena F, Vargas Romero J: Yield of percutaneous needle lung aspiration in lung abscess. Chest 97:69–74, 1990.

Sosenko A, Glassroth J: Fiber-optic bronchoscopy in the evaluation of lung abscesses. Chest 87:489–494, 1985.

Van Sonnenberg E, D'Agostino HB, Casola G, et al: Lung abscess: CT-guided drainage. Radiology 178:347–351, 1991.

Wiedemann HP, Rice TW: Lung abscess and empyema. Semin Thorac Cardiovasc Surg 7:119–128, 1995.

Yellin A, Yellin EO, Lieberman Y: Percutaneous tube drainage: The treatment of choice for refractory lung abscess. Ann Thorac Surg 39:266–270, 1985.

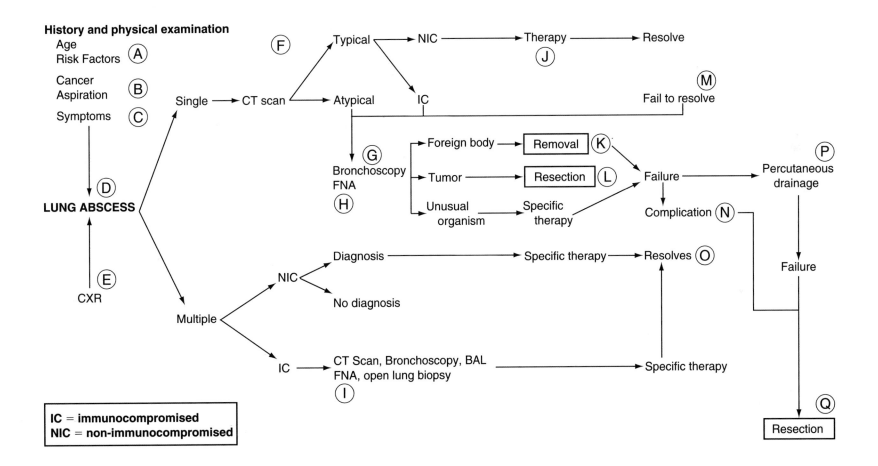

History and physical examination

Age
Risk Factors (A)

Cancer
Aspiration (B)

Symptoms (C)

(D)

LUNG ABSCESS

(E)

CXR

Single → CT scan

(F) Typical → NIC → Therapy → Resolve
(J)

Atypical → IC

(M)
Fail to resolve

(G)
Bronchoscopy
FNA
(H)

Foreign body → Removal (K)

Tumor → Resection (L)

Unusual organism → Specific therapy

Failure → Percutaneous drainage (P)

Complication (N)

Multiple

NIC → Diagnosis → Specific therapy → Resolves (O)

No diagnosis

IC → CT Scan, Bronchoscopy, BAL FNA, open lung biopsy (I) → Specific therapy

Failure

Resection (Q)

IC = immunocompromised
NIC = non-immunocompromised

Chapter 25 *Carcinoma of the Lung*

LAURENCE H. BRINCKERHOFF, MD • JOHN D. MITCHELL, MD

(A) The probability of malignancy is low in patients younger than 30 years and is significantly greater in patients older than 50 years; however, no lung nodule can be ignored. The differential diagnosis of a solitary pulmonary nodule is extensive and includes infection (e.g., tuberculosis, abscess, fungus); hamartoma; arteriovenous malformation; and malignancy (both primary lung and metastatic). Only 5% of all lung nodules prove to be malignant; however, in nodules that are resected owing to size, rapid growth, or morphology, approximately 40% are malignant. History should focus on tobacco use/exposure because this is associated with 80% to 85% of all lung cancers. In addition, exposure to chemicals, asbestos, or coal mining is noted. Shortness of breath, chest pain, cough, hemoptysis, and/or weight loss are important symptoms. Palpation for cervical, clavicular, and axillary adenopathy and thorough auscultation of all lung fields is essential.

(B) Old radiographs are essential to evaluate for interval growth or morphologic changes. Lesions greater than 3 cm in diameter, regardless of other features or time course, are almost always malignant and require a histologic diagnosis. Nodules greater than 3 cm in diameter or lesions that have a smooth contour and diffuse or popcorn calcification are probably benign and can be followed. Tumor doubling time (i.e., the period in which tumor volume increases twofold) provides the most reliable means of distinguishing between malignant and benign lesions. Malignant nodules double in size over weeks to months; benign nodules double over several years or remain unchanged. Follow-up chest x-ray should be performed annually.

(C) The initial evaluation of a worrisome pulmonary nodule is designed to better characterize the mass and, if possible, to establish a histologic diagnosis. Computed tomography (CT) of the chest and upper abdomen with intravenous contrast is the best single study in this setting, providing specific information about the location, morphology, and invasive nature of the nodule. In addition, other lung parenchymal lesions, mediastinal adenopathy, and the presence of liver or adrenal lesions can be detected. Histologic diagnosis can be obtained by sputum cytology; by fiberoptic bronchoscopy, including transbronchial needle aspiration (TBNA); or by transthoracic needle aspiration (TTNA) under CT guidance. If a pleural effusion is seen on chest x-ray or CT, diagnostic thoracentesis should be performed. If cytology shows malignant cells, a T4 lesion is present (Table 25-1).

(D) If the initial evaluation suggests a benign diagnosis, the nodule may be followed with repeat CT scanning at 6- to 12-week intervals. If there is significant change in size or character, the lesion is resected.

(E) In nodules where a malignant diagnosis is proven or strongly suspected, a thorough staging evaluation is essential in determining appropriate therapy. Positron emission tomography (PET) provides information on the metabolic activity of tissues by measuring the uptake of radioactive-labeled glucose; it is affected by the volume of tissue in question and the metabolic activity of surrounding tissues. Most, but not all, non–small-cell lung cancers (NSCLC) are hypermetabolic on PET given a sufficient volume of tumor present. PET may better characterize the initial lung mass, but the primary use of PET lies in detecting metastatic disease within the mediastinum, contralateral lung, and distant sites. PET is less useful in identifying metastatic brain lesions, and if neurologic symptoms are present a CT or MRI of the brain is obtained. PET has largely supplanted the use of bone scanning in detecting bony metastases. Mediastinoscopy remains the gold standard for evaluating ipsilateral (N2) or contralateral (N3) adenopathy of any degree. Unless obvious metastatic disease is present, mediastinoscopy should be performed in every patient with non–small-cell cancer as an integral part of the staging evaluation. The PET scan rarely obviates the need for mediastinoscopy but rather serves as a complementary study to identify targets for biopsy. Mediastinal lesions not accessible via mediastinoscopy may be approached through either mediastinotomy (A-P window nodes) or VATS, with the latter technique useful for pleural evaluation as well. If evidence of distant metastatic disease is suggested, confirmatory biopsy through a CT-guided approach may be used.

(F) All NSCLCs should be staged according to the TNM criteria (see Table 25-1, Table 25-2). The mode of therapy is directed from the clinical stage and the medical condition of the patient.

(G) Resection is indicated for stages I, II, and selected IIIA NSCLC. Appropriate patients should undergo assessment of operative risk including pulmonary function testing (PFT) and laboratory analysis. The benefit of neoadjuvant therapy in patients with early stage NSCLC is currently being evaluated in a large, nationwide cooperative trial. For patients with adequate pulmonary function, formal anatomic resection (lobectomy or, if needed, pneumonectomy) is performed. Lesser resection techniques (wedge) are reserved for patients with limited pulmonary reserve or significant comorbidities. The relative merits of lymph node sampling compared with node dissection at the time of resection are currently under study. In selected patients, the pathologic stage following surgery may suggest the need for further therapy. The routine use of adjuvant therapy for early stage NSCLC is currently not supported by published studies.

(H) Selected patients with stage IIIB or stage IV NSCLC may experience a survival benefit from resection but, in most circumstances, operative resection offers them no survival benefit. Chemotherapy and radiation therapy are options. Patients with small-cell carcinoma are treated with nonoperative therapy unless limited disease is incidentally discovered at thoracotomy. If an isolated peripheral nodule is found to be small cell carcinoma in this circumstance, lobectomy and lymph node dissection is indicated.

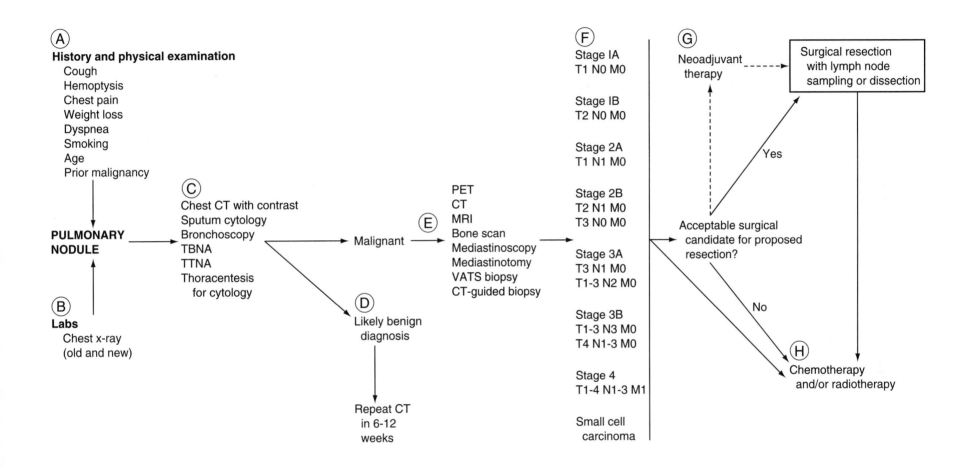

Ⓐ **History and physical examination**
  Cough
  Hemoptysis
  Chest pain
  Weight loss
  Dyspnea
  Smoking
  Age
  Prior malignancy

**PULMONARY
NODULE**

Ⓑ **Labs**
  Chest x-ray
  (old and new)

Ⓒ Chest CT with contrast
  Sputum cytology
  Bronchoscopy
  TBNA
  TTNA
  Thoracentesis
    for cytology

Malignant

Ⓓ Likely benign
  diagnosis

Repeat CT
in 6-12
weeks

Ⓔ PET
  CT
  MRI
  Bone scan
  Mediastinoscopy
  Mediastinotomy
  VATS biopsy
  CT-guided biopsy

Ⓕ Stage IA
  T1 N0 M0

  Stage IB
  T2 N0 M0

  Stage 2A
  T1 N1 M0

  Stage 2B
  T2 N1 M0
  T3 N0 M0

  Stage 3A
  T3 N1 M0
  T1-3 N2 M0

  Stage 3B
  T1-3 N3 M0
  T4 N1-3 M0

  Stage 4
  T1-4 N1-3 M1

  Small cell
  carcinoma

Ⓖ Neoadjuvant
  therapy

Acceptable surgical
candidate for proposed
resection?

Yes

No

Surgical resection
with lymph node
sampling or dissection

Ⓗ Chemotherapy
  and/or radiotherapy

TABLE 25.1
TNM Classification for Non–Small-Cell Lung Cancer

Primary Tumor (T)

T0	No evidence of primary tumor
Tis	Carcinoma in situ
T1	Tumor that is 3 cm or less in its greatest dimension, does not invade the visceral pleura, and is without bronchoscopic evidence of invasion more proximal than a lobar bronchus
T2	Tumor that has any of the following features: Size more than 3 cm in its greatest dimension Involvement of a mainstem bronchus, with a proximal extent greater than 2 cm from the carina Invasion of the visceral pleura Association with atelectasis or obstructive pneumonitis that extends to the hilar region but does not involve the entire lung
T3	Tumor of any size with any of the following features: Invasion of the chest wall, diaphragm, mediastinal pleura, or parietal pericardium Involvement of a mainstem bronchus within 2 cm of the carina but without invasion of the carina Association with atelectasis or obstructive pneumonitis of the entire lung`
T4	Tumor of any size with any of the following features: Invasion of mediastinum, heart, great vessels, trachea, esophagus, vertebral body, or carina Association with a malignant pleural or pericardial effusion Presence of satellite tumor nodule(s) within lobe of lung containing the primary tumor

Regional Lymph Node (N)

N0	No regional lymph node involvement
N1	Involvement of ipsilateral peribronchial, intrapulmonary, and/or ipsilateral hilar lymph nodes
N2	Involvement of ipsilateral mediastinal and/or subcarinal nodes
N3	Metastasis to contralateral mediastinal or contralateral hilar nodes, or either ipsilateral or contralateral involvement of scalene or supraclavicular lymph nodes

Distant Metastasis (M)

M0	No distant metastasis
M1	Distant metastasis present, including separate tumor nodule(s) in a different lobe from the primary tumor

Staging

Stage 0	Tis N0 M0
Stage IA	T1 N0 M0
Stage IB	T2 N0 M0
Stage IIA	T1 N1 M0
Stage IIB	T2 N1 M0
	T3 N0 M0
Stage IIIA	T3 N1 M0
	T1-3 N2 M0
Stage IIIB	T1-3 N3 M0
	T4 N0-3 M0
Stage IV	Any T, Any N, M1

Mountain CF: Revisions in the International System for Staging Lung Cancer. Chest 111:1710–1717, 1997.

TABLE 25.2
Staging and 5-year Survival for Non–Small-Cell Lung Cancer

TNM Stage		Survival (%)
Stage IA	T1 N0 M0	67
Stage IB	T2 N0 M0	57
Stage IIA	T1 N1 M0	55
Stage IIB	T2 N1 M0	39
	T3 N0 M0	38
Stage IIIA	T3 N1 M0	38
	T1-3 N2 M0	23
Stage IIIB	T1-3 N3 M0	3
	T4 N0-3 M0	6
Stage IV	Any T, Any N, M1	1

Mountain CF: Revisions in the International System for Staging Lung Cancer. Chest 111:1710–1717, 1997.

REFERENCES

Bonnefoi H, Smith IE: How should cancer presenting as a malignant pleural effusion be managed? Br J CA 74:832–835, 1996.

Burdine J, Joyce LD, Plunkett MB et al: Feasibility and value of video-assisted thoracoscopic surgery wedge excision of small pulmonary nodules in patients with malignancy. Chest 122:1467–1470, 2002.

Clinical Practice Guidelines for the Treatment of Unresectable Non–Small-Cell Lung Cancer: Adopted on May 16, 1997 by the American Society of Clinical Oncology. J Clin Oncol 15:2996–3018, 1997.

Cooper JD: Management of the solitary pulmonary nodule: Directed resection. Semin Thorac Cardiovasc Surg 14:286–291, 2002.

Dizendorf EV, Baumert BG, von Schulthess GK et al: Impact of whole-body 18F-FDG PET on staging and managing patients for radiation therapy. J Nuclear Med 44:24–29, 2003.

Edell ES: Diagnostic tests for lung cancer. Curr Opin Pulmon Med 3:247–251, 1997.

Ettinger DS, Cox JD, Ginsberg RJ et al: NCCN Non–Small-Cell Lung Cancer Practice Guidelines. The National Comprehensive Cancer Network. Oncology 10:81–111, 1996.

Gasparini S: Bronchoscopic biopsy techniques in the diagnosis and staging of lung cancer. Monaldi Arch Chest Dis 52:392–398, 1997.

Gridelli C, Maione P, Colantuoni G et al: Chemotherapy of non–small-cell lung cancer in elderly patients. Curr Med Chem 9:1487–1495, 2002.

Lowe VJ, Naunheim KS: Positron emission tomography in lung cancer. Ann Thorac Surg 65:1821–1829, 1998.

Machtay M, Glatstein E: Combined modality therapy for non–small-cell lung carcinoma. Cancer J 8 Suppl 1:S55–S67, 2002.

Mentzer SJ, Swanson SJ, DeCamp MM et al: Mediastinoscopy, thoracoscopy, and video-assisted thoracic surgery in the diagnosis and staging of lung cancer. Chest 112:239S–241S, 1997.

Mountain CF: Revisions in the International System for Staging Lung Cancer. Chest 111:1710–1717, 1997.

Mulshine JL: Screening for lung cancer: In pursuit of pre-metastatic disease. Cancer 3:65–73, 2003.

Naruke T, Tsuchiya R, Kondo H et al: Implications of staging in lung cancer. Chest 1112:242S–248S, 1997.

Swanson SJ, Batirel HF: Video-assisted thoracic surgery (VATS) resection for lung cancer. Surg Clin N Am 82:541–559, 2002.

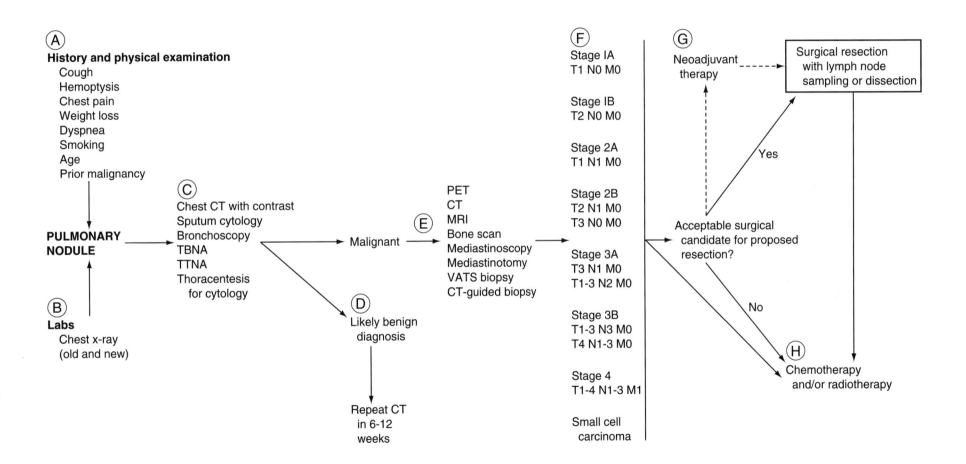

Chapter 26 *Mediastinal Tumor*

DUYKHANH T. PHAM, MD • THOMAS A. D'AMICO, MD

Ⓐ A thorough history and physical examination are integral in the evaluation of patients with newly identified mediastinal masses. Symptoms are present in 62% of patients with mediastinal masses; these include chest pain (30%), fever (20%), cough (16%), dyspnea (16%), SVC syndrome (6%), fatigue (6%), and dysphagia (4%). Patients with malignant disease are more likely to be symptomatic than are patients with benign disease (85% vs. 46%). Patients may also present with the complaint of Horner's syndrome, hoarseness, Cushing's syndrome, thyrotoxicosis, hypertension, or hypercalcemia. Importantly, 40% of patients are asymptomatic at the time of diagnosis.

Ⓑ Chest radiography remains the primary initial diagnostic examination; however, computed tomography (CT) has become standard for the characterization of mediastinal masses. CT with intravenous contrast can delineate masses from pulmonary lesions and aneurysms. Additionally, the portrayal of cross-sectional anatomy allowed by CT scan can occasionally provide a diagnosis based on classic tumor locations. Thymomas, lymphomas, germ cell tumors, and carcinomas are typically located in the anterior mediastinum. Middle mediastinal tumors are usually primary cysts. Tumors of neurogenic origin are most common in the posterior mediastinum. Other advanced imaging techniques may prove helpful for further evaluation of certain tumor types. Echocardiography, for instance, is important in the evaluation of cardiac lesions. Magnetic resonance imaging (MRI) provides excellent anatomical definition and is preferred in the evaluation of masses suspected to be of neurogenic origin to evaluate for an intraspinal component. Positron emission tomography (PET) scans can identify lesions with hypermetabolic activity and play an adjunctive role in evaluating malignant tumors. Finally, nuclear studies with [123]iodine MIBG (meta-iodo-benzyl-guanidine) can locate neoplasms of sympathetic origin.

Ⓒ Elevations of various serum markers have been associated with tumors of the mediastinum.

TABLE 26.1
Serum Markers in Germ Cell Tumors

	α-FP	β-HCG
Seminoma	–	+/–
Yolk sac		–
Choriocarcinoma	–	
Teratocarcinoma		

Elevated levels of α-fetoprotein and β-human chorionic gonadotropin are coupled with germ cell tumors (Table 26-1). Patients with neuroblastomas may have increased catecholamine levels and often excrete urine catecholamine byproducts (e.g., homovanillic acid, vanillylmandellic acid).

Ⓓ Biopsy of a mass is indicated if it will influence therapy; it is important if the mass is likely to be treated primarily by chemotherapy and/or radiation or to direct preoperative therapy. Fine-needle aspiration (CT-guided) may provide the diagnosis in some patients with mediastinal masses; however, the histopathologic differentiation among the most common mediastinal tumors, especially anterior mediastinal masses (e.g., lymphoma, thymoma, and germ cell tumors), is unreliable when based on needle biopsy alone. Minimally invasive alternatives to obtain reliable tissue for diagnosis include cervical mediastinoscopy, anterior mediastinoscopy, and thoracoscopy.

Ⓔ Neurogenic tumors account for approximately 20% of mediastinal tumor masses. They represent 20% and 35% of all adult and pediatric mediastinal neoplasms, respectively. Occurring mostly in the posterior mediastinum, these tumors usually originate from peripheral nerves; and sympathetic or, rarely, parasympathetic ganglia. Schwannoma, neurofibroma, and malignant tumor of nerve sheath origin (MTNSO; most common in adults) arise from peripheral nerves. Ganglioneuroma, ganglioneuroblastoma, and neuroblastoma arise from sympathetic ganglia. The latter three are more common

TABLE 26.2
Staging of Neuroblastoma and Ganglioneuroblastoma

Stage I	Well-circumscribed, ipsilateral tumor
Stage II	Tumor with local invasion into adjacent soft tissues, bone, spinal canal No extension across midline
Stage III	Tumor extension across midline Involvement of bilateral regional lymph nodes
Stage IV	Metastatic disease

in children. Both types of tumors should be completely resected. Schwannomas, neurofibromas, ganglioneuromas, and stage I (Table 26-2) neuroblastomas and ganglioneuroblastomas are cured by complete surgical excision. Surgical resection of MTNSO, stage II or III neuroblastomas, and ganglioneuroblastomas should be coupled with adjuvant external beam radiation therapy (EBRT) and chemotherapy. Adjuvant therapy for MTNSO has not been shown to increase survival but is thought to have utility in the treatment of metastatic disease. Radiation and chemotherapy following resection of stage III neuroblastomas and ganglioneuroblastomas have been shown to induce partial or complete response in 70% of patients.

Ⓕ Thymomas are the most common neoplasm of the anterior mediastinum and are the second most common mediastinal mass. Up to 50% of patients suffer from one or more parathymic syndromes (e.g., myasthenia gravis, hypogammaglobulinemia, or pure red cell aplasia). Although the majority of thymomas are benign, malignant disease is determined by the presence of gross invasion of adjacent structures, metastasis, or microscopic evidence of capsular invasion (Table 26-3). Complete surgical resection through a median sternotomy is sufficient treatment for Stage I. The adjuvant use of radiation therapy (50 Gy) is recommended for Stage II or III disease. Tumors greater than 5 cm or locally invasive, unresectable, or metastatic (Stage IV)

History and physical examination
    Chest pain (30%)
    Fever (20%)
    Cough (16%)
    Dyspnea (16%)

Differential diagnosis

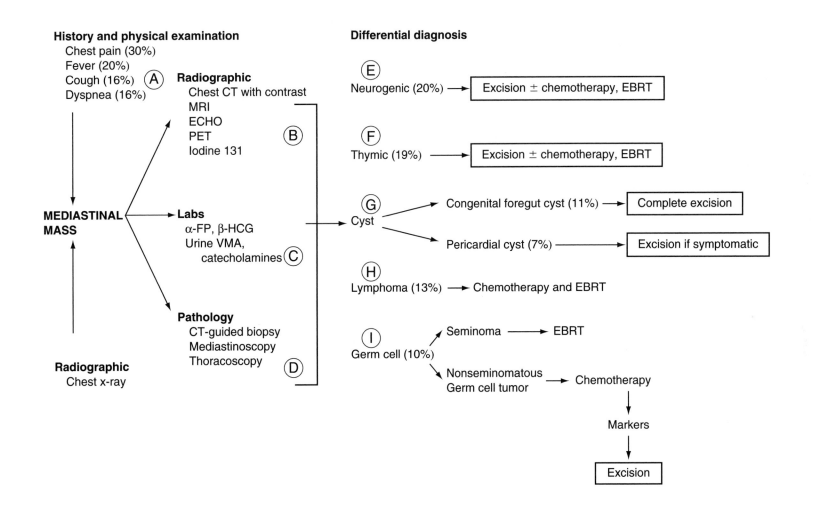

MEDIASTINAL MASS

Radiographic
    Chest x-ray

A **Radiographic**
    Chest CT with contrast
    MRI
    ECHO
    PET
    Iodine 131
    B

Labs
    α-FP, β-HCG
    Urine VMA,
        catecholamines
    C

Pathology
    CT-guided biopsy
    Mediastinoscopy
    Thoracoscopy
    D

E Neurogenic (20%) → Excision ± chemotherapy, EBRT

F Thymic (19%) → Excision ± chemotherapy, EBRT

G Cyst → Congenital foregut cyst (11%) → Complete excision
       → Pericardial cyst (7%) → Excision if symptomatic

H Lymphoma (13%) → Chemotherapy and EBRT

I Germ cell (10%) → Seminoma → EBRT
       → Nonseminomatous Germ cell tumor → Chemotherapy → Markers → Excision

TABLE 26.3
Masaoka Staging System for Thymoma

Stage I	Well-encapsulated without evidence of gross or microscopic invasion
Stage II	Pericapsular growth into adjacent fat or mediastinal pleura, or microscopic invasion of thymic capsule
Stage III	Invades adjacent organs
Stage IVa	Intrathoracic metastatic spread
Stage IVb	Extrathoracic metastatic spread

tumors should be treated by protocols that include induction chemotherapy, followed by surgical exploration and postoperative radiation.

Ⓖ Primary cysts of the mediastinum originate from the foregut (75%), or pericardium (7%), or lack specific histologic features (20%). Congenital foregut cysts are bronchogenic (50% to 60%), esophageal (5% to 10%), or neuroenteric (2% to 5%) in origin. Bronchogenic cysts are typically asymptomatic, but respiratory compromise may occur. Esophageal duplication cysts can lead to obstruction, presenting as dysphagia. Duplication cysts are commonly associated with anomalies of the vertebral column (e.g., neuroenteric cysts), and preoperative evaluation for potential spinal cord involvement is mandatory. Surgical excision is recommended in all patients with congenital foregut cysts for definitive histologic diagnosis, alleviation of symptoms, and prevention of potential complications, usually infectious.

Pericardial cysts, the second most common cyst of the mediastinum, may or may not communicate with the pericardium. Surgical excision of pericardial cysts is indicated primarily for symptomatic patients, although it may also be required for diagnosis and/or to differentiate from malignant lesions.

Ⓗ The mediastinum is commonly involved in patients with lymphoma; however, it is rarely the sole site of disease at the time of presentation. Hodgkin's lymphoma is the most common mediastinal lymphoma (Table 26-4), but both patients with Hodgkin's or non-Hodgkin's lymphoma are typically symptomatic. Lymphomas are treated aggressively with radiation therapy alone (stage I or II Hodgkin's disease), chemotherapy alone (non-Hogkin's lymphoma), or a combination of the two treatment modalities (stage III or IV Hodgkin's lymphoma). Patients in first response with poor prognosis, with refractory disease, or with recurrent lymphoma can be treated with high-dose chemotherapy and either autologous bone marrow or peripheral stem cell transplantation.

Ⓘ Teratomatous lesions are benign tumors that should be completely resected for diagnostic and therapeutic reasons. Partial resection, in the event that complete resection is not possible, has been shown to resolve symptoms and relapse is uncommon. Malignant nonteratomatous germ cell tumors are either seminomas (50%) or nonseminomatous. Nonseminomatous neoplasms, the more aggressive of the two, can be further subdivided into choriocarcinomas, embryonal cell carcinomas, immature or malignant teratomas, and yolk sac tumors. Over 90% of nonseminomatous neoplasms produce either β-HCG or α-FP (see Table 26-1). These tumors have extensive intrathoracic involvement and commonly metastasize outside the thorax by the time of presentation. Therefore serum markers

TABLE 26.4
Modified (Cotswold) Ann Arbor Staging Classification for Hodgkin's lymphoma

Stage I	Single node or lymphoid structure
Stage II	Two or more regions on the same side of the diaphragm
Stage III	Node regions involving both sides of the diaphragm
Stage IV	Diffuse or disseminated involvement of more than 1 extranodal organ

and α-FP and β-HCG levels are followed to assess response to multiagent chemotherapy. If markers remain elevated, "salvage" chemotherapy is used. Surgical resection of residual masses after normalization of tumor markers is performed because this mass may represent a teratomatous component.

REFERENCES

Davis RD, Oldham H, Sabiston DC: Primary cysts and neoplasms of the mediastinum: Recent changes in clinical presentation, methods of diagnosis, management, and results. Ann Thor Surg 44:229–237, 1987.

Grosfeld JL, Skinner MA, Rescorla FJ et al: Mediastinal tumors in children: Experience with 196 cases. Ann Surg Onc 1:121–127, 1994.

King RM, Telander RL, Smithson WA et al: Primary mediastinal tumors in children. J Pediatric Surgery 17:512–520, 1982.

Masaoka Monden Y, Nakahara Z, Tanioka T: Follow-up studies of thymomas with special reference to their clinical stages. Cancer 48:2485–2492, 1981.

Strollo DC, Rosado-de-Christenson ML, Jett JR: Primary mediastinal tumors part I: Tumors of the anterior mediastinum. Chest 112:511–522, 1997.

Strollo DC, Rosado-de-Christenson ML, Jett JR: Primary mediastinal tumors part II: Tumors of the middle and posterior mediastinum. Chest 112:1344–1357, 1997.

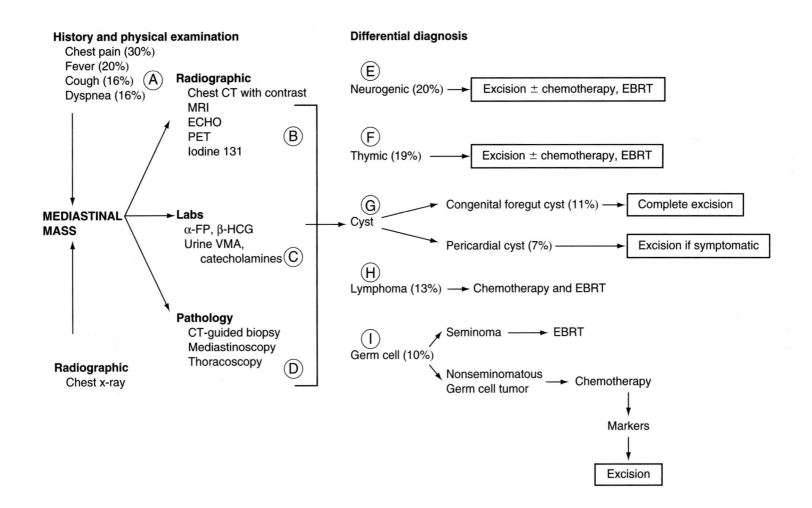

History and physical examination
Chest pain (30%)
Fever (20%)
Cough (16%) (A)
Dyspnea (16%)

Radiographic
Chest CT with contrast
MRI
ECHO
PET (B)
Iodine 131

MEDIASTINAL MASS

Labs
α-FP, β-HCG
Urine VMA,
    catecholamines (C)

Pathology
CT-guided biopsy
Mediastinoscopy
Thoracoscopy (D)

Radiographic
Chest x-ray

Differential diagnosis

(E) Neurogenic (20%) → Excision ± chemotherapy, EBRT

(F) Thymic (19%) → Excision ± chemotherapy, EBRT

(G) Cyst → Congenital foregut cyst (11%) → Complete excision
→ Pericardial cyst (7%) → Excision if symptomatic

(H) Lymphoma (13%) → Chemotherapy and EBRT

(I) Germ cell (10%) → Seminoma → EBRT
→ Nonseminomatous Germ cell tumor → Chemotherapy → Markers → Excision

Chapter 27 *Patent Ductus Arteriosus*

JAMES M. HAMMEL, MD • CHRISTOPHER A. CALDARONE, MD

(A) Patent ductus arteriosus (PDA) consists of a persistently patent connection of the central pulmonary artery to the descending aorta through the distal remnants of the embryonic left sixth arch. Its incidence is approximately 1 in 200 term births. Causes include maternal rubella, high altitude environment, polygenic inheritance, prematurity, neonatal hypoxia, and respiratory distress of the newborn.

(B) Left-to-right shunt through the PDA causes a systolic murmur in the left second intercostal space that extends into diastole as pulmonary pressure falls, eventually becoming a continuous systolic-diastolic "machinery" murmur, the hallmark of the disease. Active precordium and widened pulse pressure are present. Signs of left ventricular volume overload may also be present.

(C) In the absence of other cardiovascular anomalies, PDA is manifested by increased flow through the pulmonary vasculature. Consequently, the radiographic hallmark is increased pulmonary vascular markings and cardiomegaly. The size of the shunt dictates the prominence of the radiographic findings. Other findings include enlargement of the pulmonary artery segment, enlargement of the left atrium, and dilation of the aortic arch.

(D) Echocardiography is essential to evaluation of PDA. Echocardiographic observations include the minimum diameter of the ductus and the direction and volume of flow. Pulmonary artery pressure can be estimated from the observed flow gradient, and changes in left-heart size and function can be observed. Importantly, echocardiography can effectively screen for associated cardiovascular anomalies.

(E) Complex congenital anomalies may be associated with PDA. Patency of the ductus is necessary for survival in cases of interrupted aortic arch, critical aortic coarctation, pulmonary atresia, and hypoplastic left heart syndrome. Differential diagnoses include aortopulmonary window, pulmonary arteriovenous fistula, hemi-truncus, and peripheral pulmonary stenosis.

(F) PDA is very common in premature infants because of immaturity of the pulmonary vasculature, diminished sensitivity of ductal tissue to oxygen, and altered prostaglandin levels. Patency is present in 45% of infants with birth weight less than 1750 g and 80% of infants weighing less than 1200 g. Preterm infants may manifest signs of left-heart failure including pulmonary edema or hemorrhage and systemic hypoperfusion. The likelihood of spontaneous closure with ongoing maturation of the lungs is much higher than in term infants.

(G) In term infants, PDA is caused by abnormal ductal tissue and anatomy. Consequently, cyclooxygenase inhibition is rarely effective in term infants and the likelihood of spontaneous closure after the first few weeks of life is very small. Term infants are generally referred for surgical closure of PDA at the time of diagnosis; however, in minimally symptomatic infants, medical management may suffice until body size allows percutaneous occlusion (when they reach a weight greater than 5 kg).

(H) Initial management of premature infants with PDA is medical and consists of respiratory support, fluid restriction, and diuretics. The goal of therapy is to treat the left ventricular volume overload and subsequent congestive heart failure, allowing the ductus to close as the infant matures. There is a trend to earlier and even prophylactic medical closure of PDA in preterm infants by using cyclooxygenase inhibition.

(I) Thoracoscopic ductus ligation is performed in an increasing number of centers. Complications are similar to the open technique. Operative mortality approaches 0%. Intraoperative echocardiography can be used to demonstrate complete ductus occlusion.

(J) Occlusion of PDA can be effected via three different routes. The traditional approach, performed since 1938, is a posterolateral thoracotomy with ligation, division, or clipping of the ductus. Transaxillary and muscle-splitting techniques limit morbidity. Complications are rare but include laryngeal nerve dysfunction, incomplete occlusion, hemorrhage, and chylothorax.

(K) Transcatheter occlusion of PDA is routine in many centers. Catheter availability and local expertise prohibit applicability to patients weighing less than 5 to 10 kg. The small ductus is more easily treated. Moderate-sized shunts (i.e., 3 to 6 mm) require multiple coils and entail a greater risk of residual shunt flow and device embolization. Other concerns include distortion of the left pulmonary artery and the introduction of an intravascular foreign body.

(L) The second line of medical therapy in the preterm infant is cyclooxygenase inhibition, usually with indomethacin. Closure is produced in 85% of patients. Re-opening can occur; follow-up echocardiography is recommended. Decreased neonatal mortality, shortened mechanical ventilation, and decreased risk of intraventricular hemorrhage are associated with early indomethacin treatment. Increased incidence of necrotizing enterocolitis and impairment of renal function are rare complications.

(M) Contraindications to indomethacin therapy include necrotizing enterocolitis, impaired renal function, gastrointestinal bleeding, intraventricular hemorrhage, thrombocytopenia, and sepsis.

REFERENCES

Bhatt V, Nahata MC: Pharmacologic management of patent ductus arteriosus. Clin Pharmacol 8:17–33, 1989.

Burke RP, Jacobs JP, Cheng W et al: Video-assisted thoracoscopic surgery for patent ductus arteriosus in low–birth weight neonates and infants. Pediatrics 104:227–230, 1999.

Burke RP, Wernovsky G, van der Velde M et al: Video-assisted thoracoscopic surgery for congenital heart disease. J Thorac Cardiovasc Surg 109:499–507, 1995.

Ellison RC, Peckham GJ, Lang P et al: Evaluation of the preterm infant for patent ductus arteriosus. Pediatrics 71:364–372, 1983.

Flanagan MF, Yeager SB, Weindling SN: Cardiac Disease. In Avery GB, Fletcher MA, MacDonald MG (eds): Neonatology: Pathophysiology and Management of the Newborn. Philadelphia: Lippincott Williams & Wilkins, 1999.

Fowlie PW: Prophylactic indomethacin: Systemic review and meta-analysis. Arch Dis Child Fetal Neonatal Ed 74(2): F81–F87, 1996.

Gross RE, Hubbard JP: Surgical ligation of patent ductus arteriosus. JAMA 112:729–731, 1939.

Heyman MA: Patent ductus arteriosus. In Adams FA, Emmnouilides GC, Reimenschneider TA (eds): Moss' Heart Disease in Infants, Children, and Adolescents, 4th ed. Baltimore: Lippincott Williams & Wilkins, 1989.

Mavroudis C, Backer CL, Gevitz M: Forty-six years of patent ductus arteriosus division at Children's Memorial Hospital of Chicago: Standards for comparison. Ann Surg 220:402–409, 1994.

O'Donnell C, Neutze JM, Skinner JR et al: Transcatheter patent ductus arteriosus occlusion: Evolution of techniques and results from the 1990s. J Paediatrics Child Health. 37:451–455, 2001.

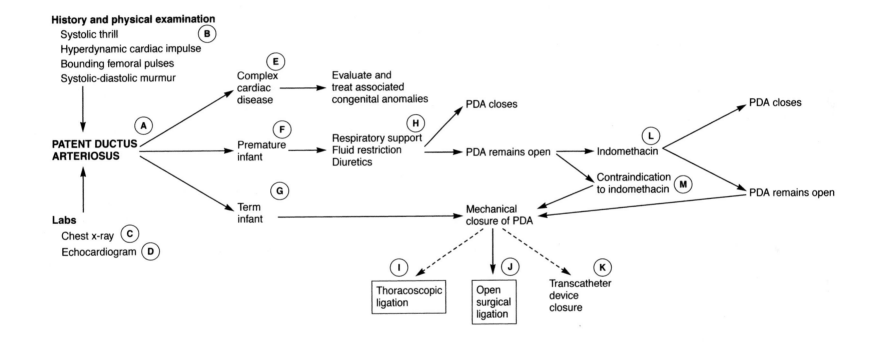

Chapter 28 **Coarctation of the Aorta**

PAUL J. CHAI, MD • JAMES JAGGERS, MD

(A) Coarctation of the aorta is a narrowing of the thoracic aorta usually occurring just distal to the left subclavian artery near the site of insertion of the ductus arteriosus. This anomaly occurs in 0.2 to 0.6 per 1000 live births and accounts for 5% to 8% of all congenital heart defects. It is commonly associated with other congenital defects such as patent ductus arteriosus, ventricular septal defect, bicuspid aortic valve, and mitral valve abnormalities.

(B) Coarctation of the aorta can present in a variety of ways. In neonates with coarctation, the peripheral perfusion may be dependent upon a patent ductus. As the ductus begins to close in the first few days of life, the child may present with poor peripheral perfusion, ventricular dysfunction, metabolic acidosis, and renal dysfunction. These children require urgent surgical repair after a short period of medical resuscitation. Coarctation may be associated with other defects of the left ventricular outflow tract. Neonates may present in shock with left ventricular dysfunction caused by the obstruction of left ventricular outflow. Pulmonary hypertension and right ventricular hypertrophy may also be present. Physical examination of the neonate with critical coarctation will often reveal cool extremities, delayed capillary refill, lethargy, and poor feeding. Tachycardia and tachypnea are common findings. The child may appear pale and have thready upper extremity pulses with markedly decreased lower extremity pulses. The liver may be enlarged secondary to right ventricular hypertrophy.

(C) In late childhood, systemic hypertension is the most common presentation. Older children may be asymptomatic and present only after discovery of an upper-to-lower extremity pulse differential or the presence of hypertension on routine examination.

(D) Chest radiograph will demonstrate cardiomegaly with evidence of congestive heart failure. Electrocardiogram may demonstrate left ventricular strain. Chest radiography may demonstrate "rib notching" from enlargement of the chest wall collateral vessels. The classic "3" sign on the left mediastinal margin results from dilatation of the subclavian artery, the coarctation site, and poststenotic dilatation of the descending aorta.

(E) Echocardiography can be diagnostic in the small child and is quite helpful in the identification of associated defects. Attention should be paid to the anatomy of the aortic arch and isthmus, patency of the ductus arteriosus, presence of the posterior coarctation shelf, and any associated cardiac lesions. Echocardiography is usually the only diagnostic test necessary in neonates and small children. Echocardiographically derived gradients across a coarctation may be misleading when the ductus is patent or when there is significant left ventricular dysfunction.

(F) Cardiac catheterization is useful in defining aortic arch anatomy and pressure gradients. Newer modalities such as spiral CT scan and MRI are less invasive and provide impressive anatomic detail.

(G) Initial management of the critical newborn requires ICU admission and resuscitation. In neonates, peripheral perfusion is often dependent on a patent ductus arteriosus. Prostaglandin E_1 infusion is utilized to maintain ductal patency. This improved distal perfusion helps to correct metabolic acidosis and restore renal perfusion. Elective endotracheal intubation and mechanical ventilation may be indicated because there is a 20% incidence of apnea associated with PGE_1. Older patients are often minimally symptomatic and can be repaired electively.

(H) Once the diagnosis of coarctation of the aorta is confirmed, surgical correction is indicated. Surgical approach is usually through a left posterolateral thoracotomy incision, entering the thorax through the third or fourth intercostal space. A median sternotomy incision may be indicated for patients with associated anomalies that require simultaneous repair on cardiopulmonary bypass (e.g., VSD). The timing for repair of isolated coarctation of the aorta in the asymptomatic individual remains controversial. Most recommend repair by 1 to 2 years of age to avoid development of significant left ventricular hypertrophy.

Methods of repair include subclavian flap repair, end-to-end or extended end-to-end anastomosis, or prosthetic patch aortoplasty. End-to-end repair is the most popular form of repair because it does not require division of the subclavian artery or the use of prosthetic material. Anatomy of the coarctation itself, however, may dictate the method of repair that is selected. Ligation of the ductus arteriosus is also performed at this time.

(I) Balloon angioplasty for native coarctation of the aorta is associated with a significant incidence of recoarctation and aneurysm formation at the coarctation site and is not recommended as treatment for native coarctation; however, it has been quite successful in the treatment of recoarctation. Incidence of recurrent coarctation can vary from 5% to 20% depending on variables such as age at repair, length of the coarctation segment, and length of follow-up period. Intervention should be considered if the peak-to-peak gradient by catheter measurement is greater than 20 mm Hg. Recurrent coarctation can often be treated with balloon angioplasty; results are quite acceptable and may be improved with the use of intra-arterial stents. If surgical correction is required, patch aortoplasty is preferred. This group of patients may be at greater risk for perioperative paraplegia because they have a less well-developed network of collateral vessels.

(J) Complications of surgical repair include hemorrhage, recurrent laryngeal nerve injury, phrenic nerve injury, chylothorax, paraplegia, aneurysm formation, hypertension, and postcoarctectomy abdominal pain.

REFERENCES

Backer CL, Paape K, Zales VR et al: Coarctation of the aorta: Repair with polytetrafluoroethylene patch aortoplasty. J Thorac Cardiovascular Surg 92(9 Suppl):32–36, 1995.

Gaynor JW: Management strategies for infants with coarctation and an associated ventricular septal defect. J Thorac Cardiovascular Surg 122:424–426, 2001.

Hijazi ZM, Geggel RL: Balloon angioplasty for postoperative recurrent coarctation of the aorta. J Interventional Card 8(5):509–516, 1995.

Hougen TJ, Sell JE: Recent advances in the diagnosis and treatment of coarctation of the aorta. Curr Opin Cardiol 10(5):524–529, 1995.

Quaegebeur JM, Jonas RA, Weinberg AD et al: Congenital Heart Surgeons Society. Outcomes in seriously ill neonates with coarctation of the aorta: A multi-institutional study. J Thorac Cardiovasc Surg 108:841–851, 1994.

Ungerleider RM: Coarctation of the Aorta. In Kaiser LR, Kron IL, Spray TL (eds): Mastery of Cardiothoracic Surgery. Philadelphia: Lippincott-Raven, 1998.

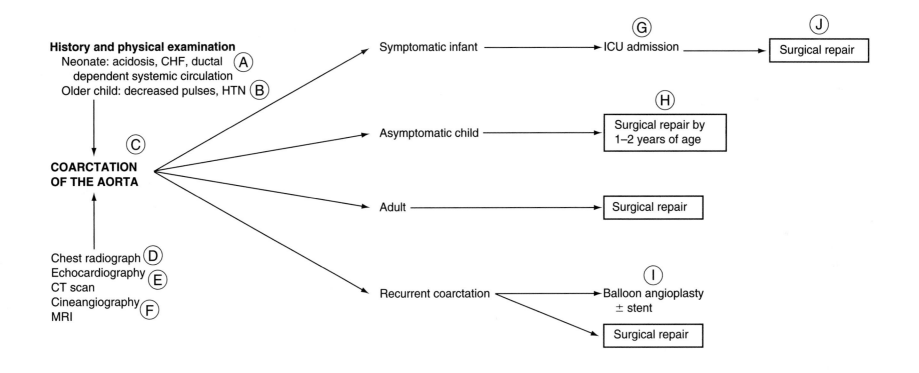

Chapter 29 **Neonatal Cyanosis**

MARK R. BIELEFELD, MD • J. MARK MORALES, MD •
DAVID R. CLARKE, MD

(A) A history of viral illness or drug use during the first trimester of pregnancy increases the likelihood of a serious congenital heart defect. Prematurity is not necessarily associated with an increased incidence of pathologic cyanosis.

(B) Cyanosis is a physical sign. A cyanotic newborn has blue discoloration of skin, nail beds, and mucous membranes. Cyanosis depends on the absolute reduced hemoglobin concentration. Reduced hemoglobin greater than 3 mg/dl produces cyanosis.

(C) The complete blood count (CBC) may imply sepsis or polycythemia as the cause of cyanosis. Methemoglobinemia, although rare, is diagnosed by absorption spectroscopy and hemoglobin electrophoresis. A prompt response to methylene blue would be expected.

(D) The chest x-ray should be examined for atelectasis, effusion, cysts, herniated bowel, cardiomegaly, and pulmonary vascular prominence.

(E) Normal PaO_2 at 5 minutes of age averages 19.5 mm Hg. It rises to an average of 56.7 mm Hg at 21 to 40 minutes. Cyanosis lasting more than 20 minutes should be investigated.

(F) Hypoglycemia can cause a readily reversible form of cyanosis and cardiomegaly. Hyperkalemia, hyponatremia, and low bicarbonate suggest Addison's disease.

(G) Echocardiography may confirm suspicions of congenital heart disease and in many instances has replaced the risks and costs of heart catheterization.

(H) Peripheral cyanosis reverses after hours to weeks and is secondary to vasomotor instability.

(I) Differential cyanosis is blue discoloration of the upper or lower half of the body. This is often caused by shunting through the ductus arteriosus.

(J) Suctioning and maintaining an airway, supporting respirations as needed, and placing the neonate in a warm incubator with 100% oxygen not only treats cyanosis caused by respiratory problems, peripheral vasomotor instability, and shock but also differentiates them from cardiac problems. PaO_2 does not increase greater than 100 mm Hg in response to 100% oxygen in cyanotic congenital heart disease.

(K) Persistent fetal circulation or pulmonary hypertension of the newborn is characterized by right-to-left shunting through a patent foramen ovale and a patent ductus arteriosus caused by elevated pulmonary pressures. Nitric oxide is the hallmark of reducing pulmonary vascular resistance. Optimization of ventilatory support and sustaining cardiac performance with inotropes are also important features of treatment.

(L) Congestive heart failure (CHF) with pulmonary edema may be caused by cardiac defects with left-to-right shunting of blood. Such defects include patent ductus arteriosus, aortopulmonary window, ventricular septal defect, and atrioventricular septal defect.

(M) Medications given to the mother at the time of delivery (e.g., narcotics and magnesium sulfate) may cause hypoventilation in the neonate.

(N) Congenital lobar emphysema is usually right sided and unilobar. Lobectomy is the treatment and is tolerated well.

(O) Cystic adenomatoid malformation is relatively rare and affects upper and lower lobes equally. Cystic adenomatoid malformation may have an appearance similar to diaphragmatic hernia on CXR.

(P) When the aortic arch is left sided (95%), a right thoracotomy and an extrapleural approach is preferred for division of the tracheoesophageal fistula and a single-layer, end-to-end anastomosis of the esophagus. Survival averages 85% and without associated anomalies can be as high as 100%.

(Q) Congenital diaphragmatic hernias involve the left hemidiaphragm 85% to 90% of the time. Morgagni's hernia is parasternal, whereas Bochdalek's hernia is posterolateral. Positioning of the nasogastric tube on chest x-ray identifies the stomach above the diaphragm. Placing the infant on the affected side and decompressing the GI tract facilitates ventilation. Ventilatory assistance with a mask should not be attempted. Endotracheal tube ventilation avoids further distention of the GI tract. Associated pulmonary hypertension may require inhaled nitric oxide or support with extracorporeal membrane oxygenation.

(R) Although a transthoracic approach may be utilized, a transabdominal approach is often preferred. The abdominal approach allows inspection of the GI tract and the use of a GI silo, if necessary. The diaphragm may be closed primarily or, in the case of large defects, with a synthetic patch. Survival is typically 50% but may be as high as 76%.

(S) A No. 10 or 12F thoracostomy tube is inserted laterally and tunneled posteriorly. Suction of 8 to 10 cm H_2O is typically applied to the tube. Chylothorax may respond to simple aspiration of the fluid.

REFERENCES

Downlard CD, Jasik T, Garza JJ et al: Analysis of improved survival rate for congenital diaphragmatic hernia. J Pediatr Surg 38:729–732, 2003.

Driscoll DJ: Evaluation of the cyanotic newborn. Pediatr Clin North Am 37:1–23, 1990.

Garson A, Bricker JT, Fischer DJ et al (eds): The Science and Practice of Pediatric Cardiology. Baltimore: Williams & Wilkins, 1998.

Kennaugh JM, Kinsella JP, Abman SH et al: Impact of new treatments for neonatal pulmonary hypertension on extracorporeal membrane oxygenation use and outcome. J Perinatol 17:366–369, 1997.

Kinsella JP, Abman SH: Recent developments in the pathophysiology and treatment of persistent pulmonary hypertension of the newborn. J Pediatr 126:853–864, 1995.

Lees MH, King DH: Cyanosis in the newborn infant. Pediatr Rev 9:36–42, 1987.

Poenaru D, Laberge JM, Nielson IR et al: A more than 25-year experience with end-to-end versus end-to-side repair for esophageal atresia. J Pediatr Surg 26:472–476, 1991.

Tingelstad J: Consultation with the specialist: Nonrespiratory cyanosis. Pediatr Rev 20:350–352, 1999.

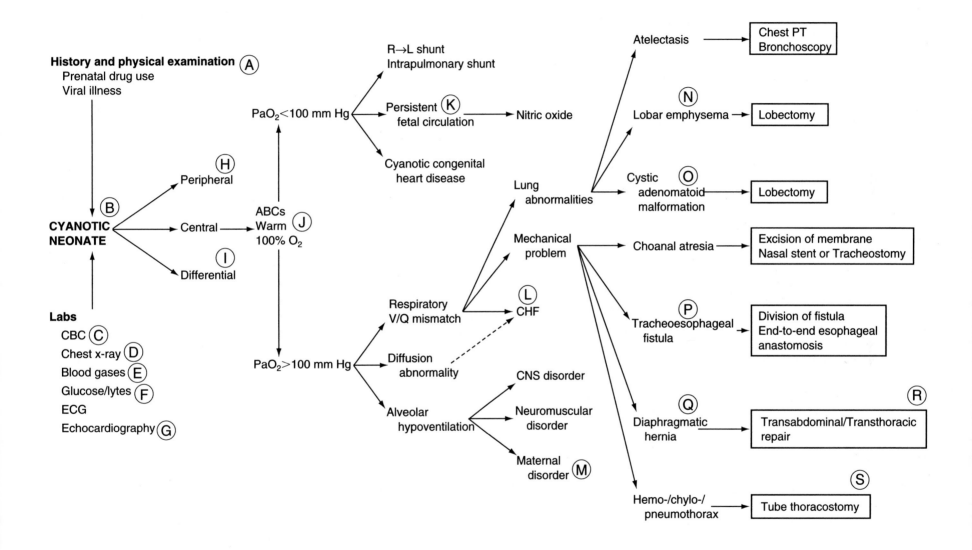

History and physical examination (A)
Prenatal drug use
Viral illness

(H)
Peripheral

(B)
**CYANOTIC
NEONATE**

Central

(I)
Differential

Labs
CBC (C)
Chest x-ray (D)
Blood gases (E)
Glucose/lytes (F)
ECG
Echocardiography (G)

ABCs
Warm (J)
100% O_2

$PaO_2 < 100$ mm Hg

R→L shunt
Intrapulmonary shunt

Persistent (K) → Nitric oxide
fetal circulation

Cyanotic congenital
heart disease

$PaO_2 > 100$ mm Hg

Respiratory
V/Q mismatch

Diffusion
abnormality

Alveolar
hypoventilation

Lung
abnormalities

Mechanical
problem

(L)
CHF

CNS disorder

Neuromuscular
disorder

Maternal
disorder (M)

Atelectasis → Chest PT
Bronchoscopy

(N)
Lobar emphysema → Lobectomy

Cystic (O)
adenomatoid → Lobectomy
malformation

Choanal atresia → Excision of membrane
Nasal stent or Tracheostomy

Tracheoesophageal (P)
fistula → Division of fistula
End-to-end esophageal
anastomosis

Diaphragmatic (Q)
hernia → Transabdominal/Transthoracic (R)
repair

Hemo-/chylo-/ (S)
pneumothorax → Tube thoracostomy

Chapter 30 Cyanotic Congenital Heart Disease

MARK R. BIELEFELD, MD • J. MARK MORALES, MD •
DAVID R. CLARKE, MD

(A) Symptoms of heart disease in the child are diverse. Inability to gain weight, feeding intolerance, easy fatigability, tachypnea, and blue discoloration of lips or appendages are common signs. Squatting to relieve cyanotic spells is found with tetralogy of Fallot (ToF).

(B) Murmurs, enlarged liver, and cardiac gallop are findings often found in children with heart disease.

(C) Cyanosis is identified when the absolute concentration of reduced hemoglobin is 3 mg/dl or greater. When Hgb is not "bound" to oxygen it remains in its reduced form. The more reduced Hgb, the more likely the clinical finding of cyanosis will be detected. Although the usually stated reduced Hgb of 5 g/dl was thought to be the lowest amount for cyanosis to be detected, this value is now felt to be as low as 3 g/dl of reduced Hgb. Therefore cyanosis is detected at 3 g/dl or more of reduced Hgb. Cyanosis may be episodic with agitation and often represents severe hypoxia (PaO$_2$ less than 30 mm Hg).

(D) Findings on chest x-ray may include increased or decreased pulmonary vascularity, cardiomegaly, dextrocardia, and lateralization of the aortic arch.

(E) The role of echocardiography has increased markedly. With heart lesions such as transposition of the great arteries (TGA), truncus arteriosus, and total anomalous pulmonary venous drainage (TAPVD), it has often obviated preoperative heart catheterization.

(F) Catheterization provides accurate diagnosis in 95% of cases, and its therapeutic role is expanding. Therapies include balloon atrial septostomy for TGA, balloon valvuloplasty for ToF and pulmonary stenosis, device closure of atrial septal defects and patent ductus arteriosus, and stenting of vessels.

(G) Evidence of increased pulmonary bloodflow includes signs of congestive heart failure, an enlarged pulmonary artery, and hypervascular lungs on chest x-ray.

(H) If cyanosis is severe and decreased pulmonary bloodflow is suspected in the newborn, immediate palliation is achieved by maintaining or increasing ductus arteriosus patency with intravenous infusion of prostaglandin E$_1$.

(I) In TGA, the aorta arises from the right ventricle and the pulmonary artery receives bloodflow from the left ventricle. Mixing of blood between the parallel pulmonary and systemic circulations is necessary for survival. Without treatment, more than 50% of patients die in the first month. A ventricular septal defect (VSD), atrial septostomy, and maintenance of ductal patency with prostaglandins help improve mixing of blood.

(J) TAPVD is a defect in which there is no direct communication between the pulmonary veins and the left atrium. Without pulmonary venous obstruction this lesion can be corrected semielectively. TAPVD with obstruction, however, represents one of the few cardiac surgical emergencies in children.

(K) A single arterial trunk supplies the systemic, pulmonary, and coronary circulations in truncus arteriosus. Untreated patients have 65% 6-month and 75% 1-year mortality. Pulmonary artery banding has such a high mortality rate (50%) that early VSD closure with right ventricle-to-pulmonary artery (PA) conduit repair is usually recommended.

(L) Other anomalies marked by increased pulmonary bloodflow include single ventricle hearts without pulmonary outflow obstruction and hypoplastic left heart syndrome and its variants. PA banding or more complex palliation is required.

(M) ToF consists of pulmonary outflow hypoplasia, malaligned VSD, overriding aorta, and right ventricular hypertrophy; it accounts for 10% of congenital heart disease. Children with ToF may have persistent cyanosis, intermittent cyanotic spells, or no cyanosis. Although complete repair can be performed at any age, the Blalock-Taussig (B-T) shunt continues to have an important role.

(N) Tricuspid atresia involves complete agenesis of the tricuspid valve, atrial septal defect (ASD), and right ventricular hypoplasia. Palliation is achieved with a B-T shunt prior to a cavopulmonary shunt and eventual completion Fontan procedure.

(O) Total interruption of the right ventricle (RV) to PA connection is characteristic of pulmonary atresia. Pulmonary atresia occurs with or without a VSD. With pulmonary atresia and an intact ventricular septum (IVS), a large ASD is almost always present. A patent ductus arteriosus (PDA) is maintained with prostaglandin E$_1$ until a palliative B-T shunt can be performed.

(P) Other examples of heart defects that decrease pulmonary bloodflow include single ventricle with pulmonic stenosis, TGA with VSD and left ventricular outflow obstruction, and pulmonary stenosis. The B-T shunt is palliative for all three. Definitive repair is achieved by creating a systemic venous-to-PA connection (Fontan), baffle closure of VSD connecting LV to aorta with a right ventricular-to-PA valve conduit (Rastelli), and pulmonary valvotomy, respectively. The latter procedure can be performed in the cardiac catheterization lab in certain cases.

(Q) Balloon atrial septostomy performed by a catheter through the femoral vein allows mixing of oxygenated and unoxygenated blood at the atrial level. This procedure is sometimes palliative for TAPVD and is usually necessary for TGA.

(R) PA banding is useful in protecting the lungs from excessive bloodflow. It can also be used to pressure load the left ventricle in TGA as preparation for an arterial switch operation.

(S) The classic B-T operation is anastomosis of the subclavian artery (SCA) to the PA. The side opposite the aortic arch is chosen for the anastomosis. The modified B-T operation is accomplished with

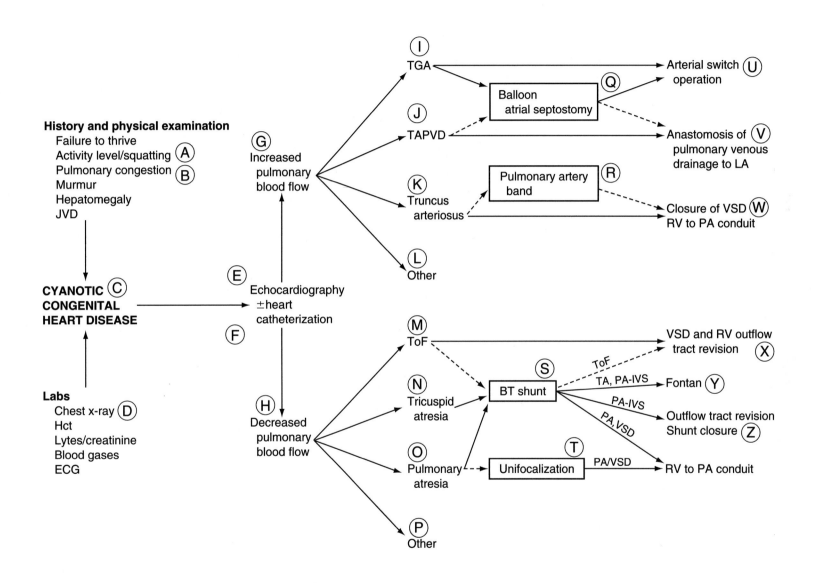

a 3- to 5-mm Goretex tube interposed between the right SCA and right PA. The resultant increase in pulmonary flow improves oxygenation and allows PA growth. It often provides palliation until the child is large enough for definitive repair.

(T) Unifocalization is the centralization of multiple sources of PA bloodflow and the elimination of aortic-to-PA collaterals in patients with pulmonary atresia and VSD. Unifocalization usually is done in preparation for complete repair.

(U) The Jatene arterial switch involves exchanging the aorta and pulmonary arteries at a supravalvular level with re-implantation of the coronary arteries.

(V) The mortality rate after operation for TAPVD ranges from 2% to 20%. The preoperative medical condition and degree of long-segment stenosis and re-stenosis determine outcome.

(W) A Rastelli operation includes baffle closure of the VSD to direct left ventricular blood into the aorta and placement of a valved conduit between the right ventricle and the PA.

(X) Single-stage definitive repair of ToF can be done in infancy. Hospital mortality after repair of ToF is 1% to 5%.

(Y) The Fontan procedure is usually staged with a cavopulmonary shunt (SVC to PA) prior to the completion Fontan (IVC routed to the PA). As a safety measure, the completed Fontan can be fenestrated into the atria. After the initial postoperative period the fenestration can be closed in the cardiac catheterization lab.

(Z) After palliation of pulmonary atresia with intact ventricular septum, the right ventricle may still become large enough to permit definitive repair by revision of the pulmonary outflow tract. If the right ventricle is unable to support venous flow to the lungs, a cavopulmonary shunt and possibly a completion Fontan may be performed.

REFERENCES

Bove EL, Mosca RS: Lessons learned in truncus arteriosus. Adv Cardiac Surg 4:91–101, 1995.

Brown JW, Park HJ, Turrentine MW: Arterial switch operation: Factors impacting survival in the current era. Ann Thorac Surg 71:1978–1984, 2001.

Castaneda AR, Jonas RA, Mayer JE et al: Cardiac Surgery of the Neonate and Infant. Philadelphia: WB Saunders, 1994.

Cobanoglu A, Menashe VD: Total anomalous pulmonary venous connection in neonates and young infants: Repair in current era. Ann Thorac Surg 55:43–49, 1993.

Garson A, Bricker JT, Fischer DJ et al (eds): The Science and Practice of Pediatric Cardiology. Baltimore, Williams & Wilkins, 1998.

Grifka RG: Cyanotic congenital heart disease with increased pulmonary bloodflow. Pediatr Clin North Am 46:405–425, 1999.

Mavroudis C, Backer CL (eds): Pediatric Cardiac Surgery, 2nd ed. St. Louis: Mosby–Year Book, 1994.

Moss AJ: Clues to diagnosing congenital heart disease. West J Med 156:392–398, 1992.

Reddy VM, Liddicoat JR, Hanley FL: Midline one-stage complete unifocalization and repair of pulmonary atresia with ventricular septal and major aortopulmonary collaterals. J Thorac Cardiovasc Surg 109:832–845, 1995.

Waldman JD, Wernly JA: Cyanotic congenital heart disease with decreased pulmonary bloodflow in children. Pediatr Clin N Am 46:385–404, 1999.

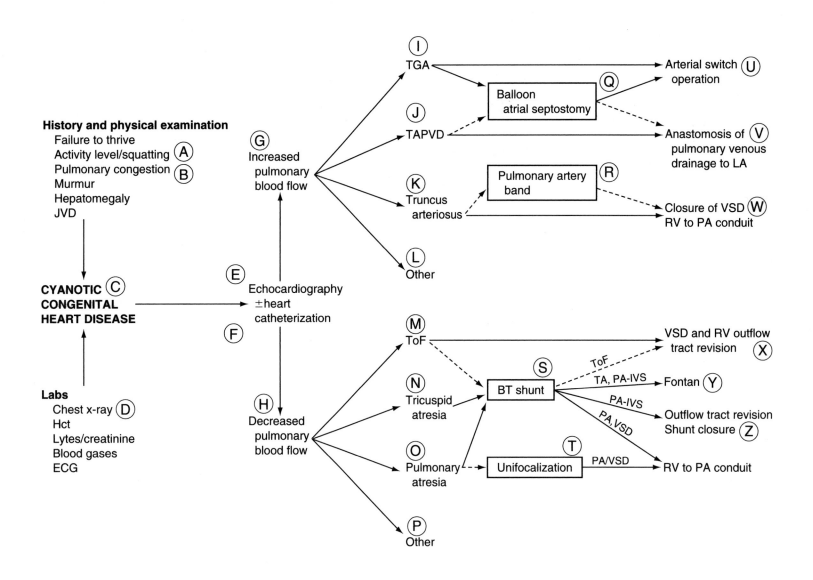

Chapter 31 *Congenital Obstructive Cardiac Anomalies*

MAX B. MITCHELL, MD • DAVID N. CAMPBELL, MD

(A) Indications for cardiac catheterization, pressure measurements, and cineangiography include systemic hypertension, dyspnea (suggesting congestive heart failure), and chest x-ray or ECG indicating increasing heart size. Investigation should be done before cardiac failure is irreversible or sudden death occurs.

(B) The most common obstructive anomalies that cause cyanosis include pulmonary atresia, tricuspid atresia, and hypoplastic left heart. Nonobstructive lesions that cause cyanosis include transposition of the great vessels, Ebstein's anomaly, total anomalous pulmonary venous return, and truncus arteriosus.

(C) Indications for repair of pulmonic stenosis include symptoms, severe right ventricular hypertrophy or strain, and systolic pressure gradient across the stenosis of greater than 50 mm Hg. The intervention of choice depends on the type of pulmonic stenosis.

(D) Indications for balloon valvuloplasty or surgical intervention in aortic stenosis include symptoms (chest pain or dyspnea), progressive left ventricular hypertrophy, and a measured gradient across the lesion greater than 50 to 60 mm Hg.

(E) Operation for congenital mitral stenosis should be delayed as long as possible. In the most severe cases presenting in the neonatal time frame, heart transplantation or univentricular palliation with the Norwood procedure is required. The Norwood procedure is a three-stage operation. Stage I is done within the first few days of life and consists of attaching the functioning right ventricle to the aorta. A Blalock-Taussig (BT) shunt is created to maintain pulmonary bloodflow. In stage II, called the Glenn or hemi-Fontan procedure, the superior vena cava is attached to the pulmonary arteries and the BT shunt is ligated. Stage III, called the Fontan procedure, involves attaching the inferior vena cava to the pulmonary arteries. This is usually performed between the ages of 2 to 3 years. In moderate cases, medical management is preferable unless cardiac decompensation occurs. Results of mitral valvuloplasty in small children have improved but remain unpredictable. Valve replacement is often required, particularly for parachute valves and patients with short chordae. The mortality rate for mitral valve replacement in children younger than 2 years with mitral stenosis is 20%. The 5-year survival rate is only 70%.

(F) Coarctation may present in the newborn as shock. Immediate operation is no longer necessary because prostaglandin E_1 opens the ductus and allows the child's condition to be stabilized. Repair is performed with an operative risk of less than 2%.

(G) Most children with interrupted aortic arch develop symptoms in the first 6 weeks of life because the ductus closes and there is no flow to the lower body. Operation is rarely emergent because prostaglandin E_1 will usually reopen the ductus and allow time for preoperative preparation. Primary repair with simultaneous repair of intracardiac lesions (e.g., ventricular septal defect) by sternotomy is the treatment of choice. If no other cardiac defect is present, primary repair is performed by left thoracotomy.

(H) Isolated peripheral pulmonary artery stenosis is uncommon and difficult to manage. Repair techniques include patch enlargement of a proximal stenosis using cardiopulmonary bypass and catheter-based balloon angioplasty. If stenosis occurs in the intraparenchymal branches, catheter-based angioplasty is preferred. Balloon dilation with stenting has become increasingly common in the proximal branch pulmonary arteries.

(I) Pure valvular pulmonary stenosis is now treated by balloon dilation at catheterization. Surgically, it can be treated by using 1 to 2 minutes of inflow occlusion, opening the main pulmonary artery, and splitting the fused commissures (valvulotomy). Valvectomy may be necessary if the valve tissue is unicuspid or if the leaflets are severely thickened. Occasionally the leaflets can be shaved or thinned. The mortality rate is low (1%). Long-term results are excellent, although asymptomatic pulmonary insufficiency is common (50%). Delayed pulmonary valve replacement may be necessary in order to prevent right ventricular failure if pulmonary insufficiency is severe.

(J) Indications for myectomy of concomitant subvalvular muscular infundibular hypertrophy include fixed scarred endothelial stenosis and right ventricular pressure greater than 200 mm Hg.

(K) Recurrence rate is 20%. Many patients require valve replacement when progressive aortic insufficiency occurs and the gradient cannot be relieved without splitting open the left ventricular outflow tract.

(L) Balloon valvuloplasty is now the procedure of choice in neonates with critical aortic stenosis unless there is coexisting aortic insufficiency. Surgical valvulotomy can be done safely in newborns using inflow occlusion, but most surgeons prefer using cardiopulmonary bypass. For older infants and children who do not have significant aortic insufficiency, balloon valvuloplasty is usually preferred. Open surgical valvotomy using cardiopulmonary bypass is recommended if balloon valvuloplasty is not available or is unsuccessful. The mortality rate is less than 3%.

(M) Extended end-to-end repair of aortic coarctation is the procedure of choice in infants and children, and recurrence rates are less than 5%. The recurrence rate when subclavian artery flap aortoplasty is used is 5% to 10%. There is a small risk of delayed aneurysm formation and a small risk of left arm underdevelopment. As an initial operation, synthetic patch aortoplasty has an unacceptably high rate of aneurysm formation on the wall opposite the prosthetic patch. Patch aortoplasty should be used only to treat recurrence. Balloon angioplasty is the procedure of choice for recoarctation following primary surgical repair. In older children with discrete coarctation, balloon angioplasty with stent insertion is now an option.

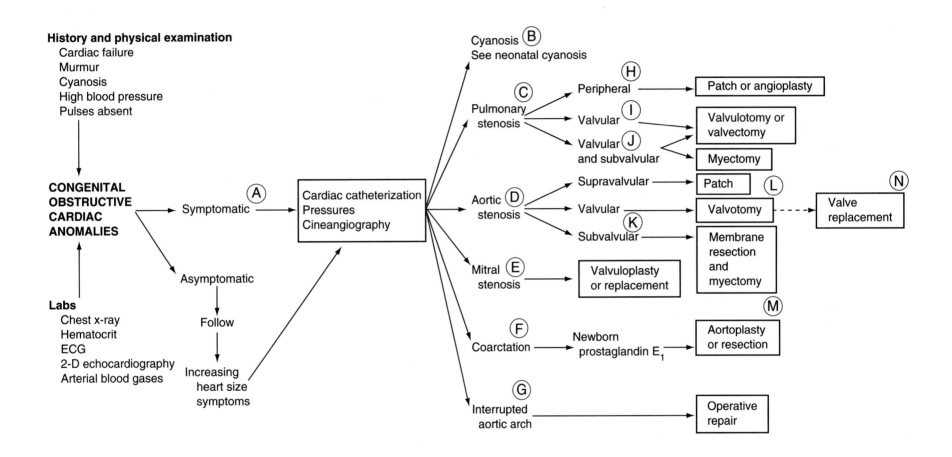

History and physical examination
 Cardiac failure
 Murmur
 Cyanosis
 High blood pressure
 Pulses absent

CONGENITAL OBSTRUCTIVE CARDIAC ANOMALIES

Labs
 Chest x-ray
 Hematocrit
 ECG
 2-D echocardiography
 Arterial blood gases

Symptomatic — Ⓐ

Asymptomatic

Follow

Increasing heart size symptoms

Cardiac catheterization
Pressures
Cineangiography

Cyanosis Ⓑ
See neonatal cyanosis

Pulmonary stenosis Ⓒ → Peripheral Ⓗ → Patch or angioplasty
 → Valvular Ⓘ → Valvulotomy or valvectomy
 → Valvular and subvalvular Ⓙ → Valvulotomy or valvectomy / Myectomy

Aortic stenosis Ⓓ → Supravalvular → Patch Ⓛ → Valve replacement Ⓝ
 → Valvular → Valvotomy
 → Subvalvular Ⓚ → Membrane resection and myectomy

Mitral stenosis Ⓔ → Valvuloplasty or replacement

Coarctation Ⓕ → Newborn prostaglandin E$_1$ → Aortoplasty or resection Ⓜ

Interrupted aortic arch Ⓖ → Operative repair

Ⓝ Reoperation is necessary in 15% of cases because of either progressive aortic insufficiency or restenosis. Most patients require valve replacement at that time. In children the operation of choice is the Ross procedure, in which the pulmonary valve and main pulmonary artery of the patient are removed and are transplanted into the aortic root position (autograft) after removal of the diseased aortic valve and aortic root. A pulmonary artery homograft is then used to replace the patient's pulmonary valve and main pulmonary artery. Other options include replacement with a mechanical valve, or aortic homograft. In a child with a small aortic annulus, a Kono aortoventriculoplasty may be used to place an adult-sized mechanical valve. Aortoventriculoplasty can also be combined with the Ross procedure using a pulmonary autograft or with a homograft aortic root replacement.

REFERENCES

Amato JJ, Douglas WI, James T et al: Coarctation of the aorta. Semin Thorac Cardiovasc Surg Pediatr Card Surg Ann 3:125–141, 2000.

Awariefe SO, Clarke DR, Pappas G: Surgical approach to critical pulmonary valve stenosis in infants less than six months of age. J Thorac Cardiovasc Surg 85:375–387, 1983.

Cheung YF, Leung MP, Lee JW et al: Evolving management for critical pulmonary stenosis in neonates and young infants. Cardiol Young 10:186–192, 2000.

Elkins RC, Knott-Craig CJ, Ward KE et al: The Ross operation in children: 10-year experience. Ann Thorac Surg 65:496–502, 1998.

Hanley FL, Sade RM, Freedom RM et al: Outcomes in critically ill neonates with pulmonary stenosis and intact ventricular septum: A multi-institutional study. Congenital Heart Surgeons Society. J Am Coll Cardiol 22:183–192, 1993.

Konno S, Imai Y, Iida Y et al: A new method for prosthetic valve replacement in congenital aortic stenosis associated with hypoplasia of the aortic valve ring. J Thorac Cardiovasc Surg 70:909–917, 1975.

Lofland GK, McCrindle BW, Williams WG et al: Critical aortic stenosis in the neonate: A multi-institutional study of management, outcomes, and risk factors. Congenital Heart Surgeons Society. J Thorac Cardiovasc Surg 121:10–27, 2001.

Mack G, Silberbach M: Aortic and pulmonary stenosis. Pediatr Rev 21:79–85, 2000.

Mitchell MB, Campbell DN, Bishop DA et al: Aortic allografts for left ventricular outflow tract replacement in children. Semin Thorac Cardiovasc Surg Pediatr Card Surg Ann 3:153–164, 2000.

van Doorn C, Yates R, Tsang V et al: Mitral valve replacement in children: Mortality, morbidity, and haemodynamic status up to medium term follow up. Heart 84:636–642, 2000.

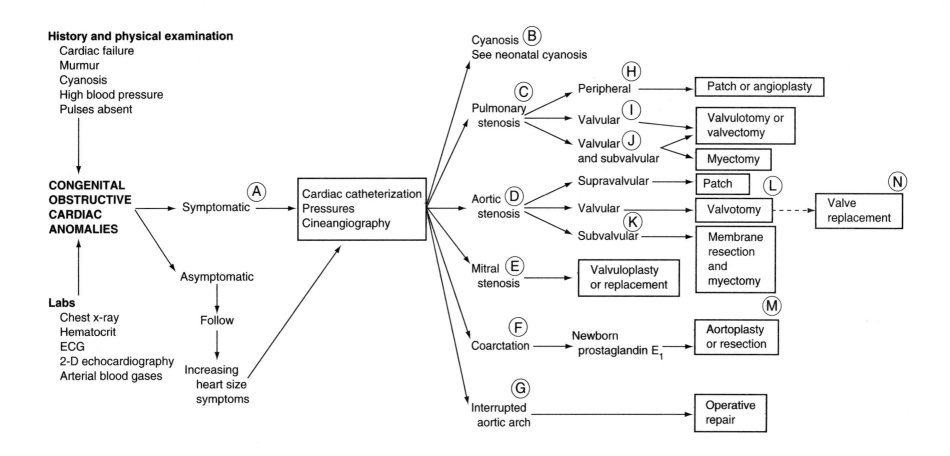

History and physical examination
Cardiac failure
Murmur
Cyanosis
High blood pressure
Pulses absent

CONGENITAL OBSTRUCTIVE CARDIAC ANOMALIES

Labs
Chest x-ray
Hematocrit
ECG
2-D echocardiography
Arterial blood gases

Symptomatic (A)

Asymptomatic

Follow

Increasing heart size symptoms

Cardiac catheterization
Pressures
Cineangiography

Cyanosis (B)
See neonatal cyanosis

Pulmonary stenosis (C)

Peripheral (H) → Patch or angioplasty

Valvular (I) → Valvulotomy or valvectomy

Valvular and subvalvular (J) → Myectomy

Aortic stenosis (D)

Supravalvular → Patch (L)

Valvular (K) → Valvotomy

Subvalvular → Membrane resection and myectomy

Valve replacement (N)

Mitral stenosis (E) → Valvuloplasty or replacement

Coarctation (F) → Newborn prostaglandin E$_1$ → Aortoplasty or resection (M)

Interrupted aortic arch (G) → Operative repair

Chapter 32 Congenital Septal Defects

IRVING SHEN, MD ● DAVID N. CAMPBELL, MD

(A) A careful history and physical examination is important in the evaluation of patients with a congenital septal defect.

(B) A large septal defect with significant left-to-right shunting can lead to poor weight gain, frequent pulmonary infections, and other symptoms of congestive heart failure (CHF).

(C) Cyanosis suggests either a mixing lesion with some degree of right-to-left shunting (truncus arteriosus) and/or inadequate pulmonary blood flow (Tetralogy of Fallot [ToF]).

(D) A loud pulmonic closure sound (P_2) suggests pulmonary hypertension. Absence of a heart murmur in a patient with a large ventricular septal defect (VSD) suggests equalization of the right and left ventricular pressure and pulmonary hypertension.

(E) Information needed for diagnosis and management for most septal defects is obtained by history, clinical examination, chest x-ray (CXR), and 2-dimensional echocardiography. Cardiac catheterization is rarely needed to confirm the diagnosis but is used when something out of the ordinary is suspected or to evaluate the reactivity of the pulmonary circulation before surgical correction.

(F) Patients with truncus arteriosus have a single arterial trunk arising from the heart supplying the systemic, pulmonary, and the coronary circulation. The truncal valve overrides a large subarterial ventricular septal defect and there is no ventricular-to-pulmonary artery continuity. Large left-to-right shunting and diastolic runoff can lead to decreased coronary perfusion and rapid development of pulmonary hypertension. Cardiac catheterization is reserved only if the anatomy is unclear by echocardiography or to check the reactivity of the pulmonary vasculature in older patients. Repair of truncus arteriosus involves separation of the pulmonary artery from the truncus, repair of the resultant defect in the aorta, VSD closure, and restoration of right ventricular-to-pulmonary artery continuity using an extracardiac conduit.

(G) In complete atrioventricular septal defect (AVSD) there is a primum atrial septal defect (ASD), an inlet VSD, and an abnormal common AV valve. This defect is usually repaired by 3 to 6 months of age or sooner if patients become symptomatic and difficult to manage. Cardiac catheterization is necessary in older patients if there is any question regarding the reactivity of their pulmonary vasculature before complete repair. Repair of complete AVSD involves closing the VSD, creating a competent right- and left-sided AV valve from the common AV valve, and closing the primum ASD.

(H) The underlying abnormality of ToF is anterior and cephalad displacement of the infundibular septum. This results in a malaligned VSD, right ventricular outflow tract obstruction (RVOTO), and overriding of the aorta. If pulmonary bloodflow is adequate, corrective surgery can be delayed until 3 to 6 months of age; otherwise, corrective repair should proceed at the onset of cyanosis or hypoxemic spells caused by worsening RVOTO, which restricts pulmonary bloodflow and increases right-to-left shunting across the VSD.

(I) Indications for repair of ASD include presence of symptoms, atrial arrhythmias, left-to-right shunt greater than 1.5 to 2:1, and pulmonary hypertension.

(J) Indications for closure of VSD include presence of symptoms, left-to-right shunt greater than 2:1, aortic valve insufficiency, and pulmonary hypertension.

(K) Secundum defect is the most common form of ASD (80%). Unless the defect causes symptoms, elective repair can be performed at any time but is preferably done before school age. Smaller defects with adequate rim of tissue can be closed percutaneously using a transcatheter ASD closure device. Operative closure, either primary or with a patch, is reserved for larger defects. Operative morbidity and mortality rates are low and long-term prognosis is excellent.

(L) Ostium primum defects account for 5% of all ASD. Some 88% of patients have an abnormal mitral valve. Repair of the abnormal mitral valve often involves closing the cleft in the septal leaflet. The ASD is usually closed with a patch. Long-term prognosis after repair is excellent.

(M) Sinus venosus defects can be associated with partial anomalous pulmonary venous return (PAPVR). Sometimes cardiac catheterization or magnetic resonance imaging before surgery is necessary to define the pulmonary venous anatomy. Repair involves using a patch to divert the anomalous pulmonary venous drainage through the ASD into the left atrium.

(N) Perimembranous VSD is the most common form of primary VSD (greater than 80%). Small pressure-restricted defects may gradually close over time. Symptomatic defects, regardless of size, or large defects should be closed surgically. Most perimembranous VSD can be closed through a right atriotomy incision. Closure of moderate and large defects requires using a prosthetic patch. Permanent heart block as a result of VSD closure should be less than 1%.

(O) Outlet VSD, also known as subarterial or supracristal VSD, is located in the outlet portion of both the right and left ventricle. Because of the proximity of this defect to the semilunar valves, the shunting of blood from the left ventricle across the VSD to the right ventricle can cause insufficiency of the aortic valve. The presence of aortic valve insufficiency is an indication for surgical repair of this defect. This defect is usually closed though an incision in the main pulmonary artery or a right ventriculotomy.

(P) Multiple muscular VSDs, also known as "Swiss cheese" VSD, can be very challenging to close surgically. Often it is difficult to locate all the defects through the thick right ventricular trabeculations. Initial palliation with pulmonary artery banding may be indicated to protect the pulmonary vasculature from overcirculation. Closure of the

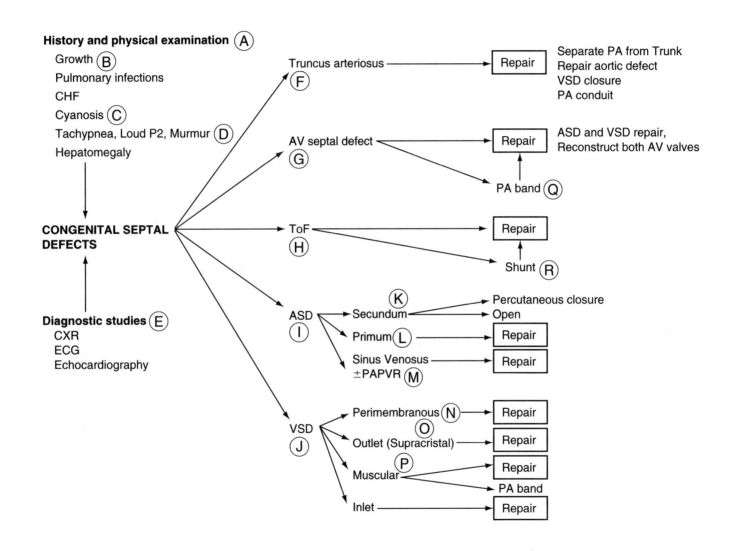

History and physical examination (A)
- Growth (B)
- Pulmonary infections
- CHF
- Cyanosis (C)
- Tachypnea, Loud P2, Murmur (D)
- Hepatomegaly

CONGENITAL SEPTAL DEFECTS

Diagnostic studies (E)
- CXR
- ECG
- Echocardiography

Truncus arteriosus → Repair
- Separate PA from Trunk
- Repair aortic defect
- VSD closure
- PA conduit

(F)

AV septal defect → Repair
- ASD and VSD repair,
- Reconstruct both AV valves

(G) → PA band (Q)

ToF → Repair

(H) → Shunt (R)

ASD (I)
- Secundum (K) → Percutaneous closure / Open
- Primum (L) → Repair
- Sinus Venosus ±PAPVR (M) → Repair

VSD (J)
- Perimembranous (N) → Repair
- Outlet (Supracristal) (O) → Repair
- Muscular (P) → Repair / PA band
- Inlet → Repair

defects is easier when the patient is older, and some defects may close spontaneously.

Ⓠ Pulmonary artery banding for complete AVSD to delay surgical repair is only indicated if there are other conditions that preclude immediate repair (e.g., sepsis and cerebral hemorrhage).

Ⓡ Initial palliation with systemic-to-pulmonary shunt to increase pulmonary bloodflow in ToF is reserved for special circumstances. This includes patients who either have a contraindication for being placed on cardiopulmonary bypass (e.g., cerebral hemorrhage) or whose repair requires a right ventricular-to-pulmonary artery conduit because of an anomalous origin of the left anterior descending coronary arising from the right coronary artery.

REFERENCES

Anderson RH, Wilcox BR: The surgical anatomy of ventricular septal defect. J Card Surg 7:17–35, 1992.

Dodge-Khatami A, Tulevski II, Hitchcock JF et al: Neonatal complete correction of tetralogy of Fallot versus shunting and deferred repair: Is the future of the right ventriculo-arterial junction at stake, and what of it? Cardiol Young 11:484–490, 2001.

Ebeid MR: Percutaneous catheter closure of secundum atrial septal defects: A review. J Invasive Cardiol 14:25–31, 2002.

Hokanson JS, Moller JH: Adults with tetralogy of Fallot: Long-term follow-up. Cardiol Rev 7:149–155, 1999.

Mavroudis C, Backer CL: Pediatric Cardiac Surgery, 3rd ed. Philadelphia: Elsevier, 2003.

Ohye RG, Bove EL: Advances in congenital heart surgery. Curr Opin Pediatr 13:473–481, 2001.

Reitz BA, Yuh DD: Congenital Cardiac Surgery. New York: McGraw-Hill, 2002.

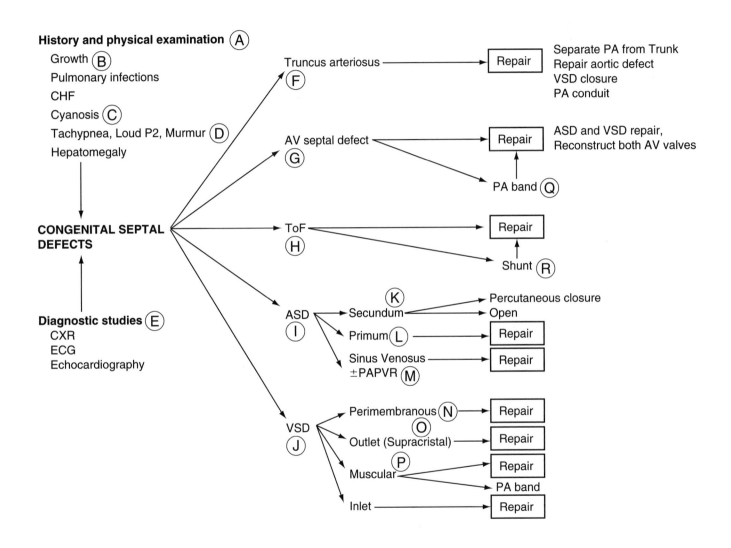

Chapter 33 *Coronary Artery Disease*

CHARLES F. SCHWARTZ, MD • AUBREY C. GALLOWAY, MD

(A) Heart disease is the major cause of death in the United States, with coronary artery disease (CAD) alone claiming 500,000 lives each year. Over 1 million people suffer a new or recurrent myocardial infarction (MI) each year in this country and, of these, more than 40% will die as a result. A thorough history and physical examination are critical in assessing a patient's risk for CAD, and this is particularly important in terms of risk assessment for patients requiring major noncardiac surgery.

(B) Asymptomatic or mildly symptomatic patients with known risk factors for CAD should undergo risk stratification with noninvasive testing. Minor cardiac risk factors are age, hypertension, peripheral vascular disease, prior stroke, and abnormal ECG, whereas intermediate risk factors are mild angina (Canadian class I or II), old myocardial infarction, diabetes, and compensated congestive heart failure (NYHA class II). Symptomatic patients should be medically optimized with β-blockers, aspirin, and nitrates or lipid-lowering drugs. Provocative stress tests include exercise or adenosine thallium studies and dobutamine echocardiography. These studies may demonstrate the presence of reversible ischemia, which would warrant further invasive evaluation with cardiac catheterization.

(C) Patients who have severe symptoms or major cardiac risk factors such as moderate to severe stable angina (Canadian class III or IV), unstable angina, recent myocardial infarction, congestive heart failure (NYHA class III or IV), or significant cardiac arrhythmias should undergo further evaluation with cardiac catheterization. Appropriate intervention for significant coronary disease is indicated in these patients before major or intermediate-risk noncardiac surgical procedures.

(D) Acute coronary syndromes include unstable angina, non–Q-wave myocardial infarction (MI), and acute transmural MI. Patients with unstable angina or acute MI require immediate, intensive medical therapy with aspirin, β-blockers, and nitrates, along with analgesia, supplemental oxygen, and close hemodynamic monitoring. Patients with unstable angina may also benefit from intravenous heparin before cardiac catheterization. Patients with an evolving MI should receive emergent thrombolytic therapy or cardiac catheterization with percutaneous coronary intervention (PCI) and coronary stenting. The mortality with acute MI has been lowered from 12% with medical therapy to 6.3% with thrombolytic therapy and 3.3% with PCI. Indications for coronary artery bypass grafting (CABG) after acute MI include cardiogenic shock or postinfarction angina with multivessel involvement. Also, the mechanical complications of MI (e.g., postinfarction ventricular septal defect, mitral insufficiency, or myocardial rupture/pseudoaneurysm) have a mortality of more than 70% with medical therapy and require emergent surgical correction.

(E) Cardiac catheterization is indicated for patients with positive provocative stress studies, Canadian class III or IV angina, unstable angina, or acute Q-wave or non–Q-wave MI. Cardiac function and valvular pathology can be assessed by catheterization, echocardiography, or cardiac magnetic resonance imaging.

(F) Patients with severe isolated disease in the left anterior descending (LAD) artery may have either PCI or surgery. Surgical techniques include MIDCAB (minimally invasive direct coronary artery bypass, with left internal mammary), OPCAB (open-chest, off-pump coronary artery bypass), or conventional CABG. MIDCAB or OPCAB may be preferable in elderly, high-risk patients.

(G) PCI is most successful in patients with single- and double-vessel disease. Short-term risks are small, but late in-stent restenosis occurs in 5% to 30% of patients within 1 to 2 years. Late results may be further improved with newer drug eluting stents.

(H) CABG is indicated for patients with left main disease, triple-vessel disease with depressed left ventricular function, and diabetic patients with double- or triple-vessel disease. Operative risk is 2% to 3% for both conventional CABG and OPCAB, and late results demonstrate improved survival and complication-free survival after surgery compared with patients undergoing medical therapy or PCI. Use of the internal mammary graft to the LAD results in a 10-year patency rate of over 95%, and use of multiple arterial grafts (e.g., right internal mammary and radial artery grafts) has further improved the late results. Reversed saphenous vein graft patency is 87% at mean follow-up of 15 months and 60% at 7 years, 4 months. The OPCAB technique, which lowers the risk of perioperative complications in patients with severe vascular or aortic arch atheromatous disease, is especially useful in elderly, high-risk patients.

REFERENCES

American Heart Association: 2001 Heart and Stroke Statistical Update. Dallas: American Heart Association, 2000.

Calafiore AM, Teodori G, DiGiammarco G et al: Minimally invasive coronary artery surgery: The last operation. Semin Thorac Cardiovasc Surg 9:305–311, 1997.

Diegeler A, Thiele H, Falk V et al: Comparison of stenting with minimally invasive bypass surgery for stenosis of the left anterior descending artery. N Engl J Med 347:561–566, 2002.

Goldman S, Zadina K, Krasnicka B et al: Predictor of graft patency 3 years after coronary artery bypass graft surgery. J Am Coll Cardiol 29:1563–1568, 1997.

The GUSTO investigators: An international randomized trial comparing four thrombolytic strategies for acute myocardial infarction. N Engl J Med 329:673–682, 1993.

Lytle BW, Loop FD, Cosgrove DM et al: Long term (5–12 years) serial studies of internal mammary and saphenous vein coronary artery bypass grafts. J Thorac Cardiovasc Surg 89:248–258, 1985.

Meharwal ZS, Mishra YK, Kohli V et al: Off-pump multivessel coronary artery surgery in high-risk patients. Ann Thorac Surg 74:S1353–S1357, 2002.

The Society of Thoracic Surgeons: Data analysis of the Society of Thoracic Surgeons National Cardiac Surgery Database. Mary C. Eiken, Director, STS National Database, www.sts.org.

Stone GW, Grines CL, Cox DA et al: Comparison of angioplasty with stenting, with or without abciximab, in acute myocardial infarction. N Engl J Med 346:957–966, 2002.

History and physical examination
   Chest pain
   Family history
   Hypertension
   Diabetes
   Smoking
   Obesity

RISK ASSESSMENT FOR CORONARY ARTERY DISEASE (CAD)

Labs
   ECG
   Lipid profiles
   Cardiac enzymes
   Chest x-ray

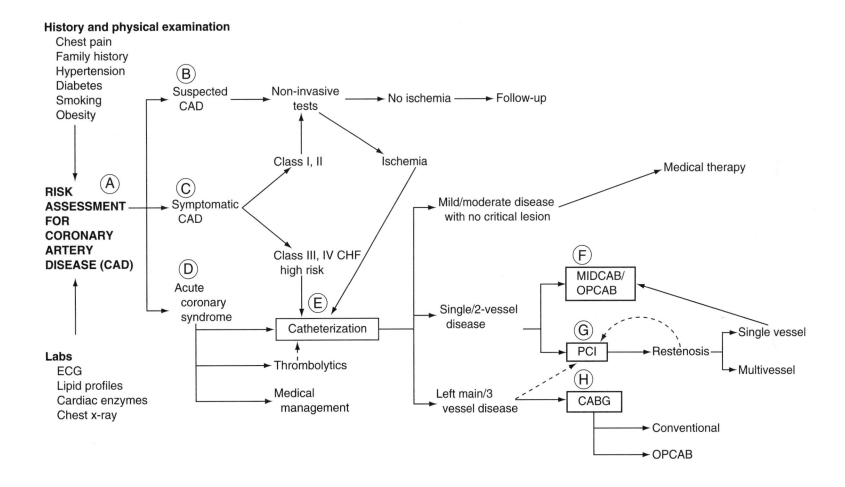

Chapter 34 *Perioperative Myocardial Ischemia and Infarction*

JAMES T. MADDUX, MD • JOHN C. MESSENGER, MD

(A) Early recognition of myocardial ischemia/infarction (MI) is imperative but may be difficult in the surgical patient. In a study by Mangano and colleagues, 94% of postoperative ischemic episodes were not associated with chest pain. Potential explanations for the absence of chest pain include the residual effect of analgesics/anesthetics and competing somatic stimuli from surgical incisions. Often perioperative ischemia/infarction presents as incidental ECG changes on telemetry, dyspnea, hypotension, hyperglycemia in diabetics, mental status changes, or positive cardiac enzymes on perioperative surveillance.

(B) Despite improvements in preoperative screening and perioperative monitoring and treatment, myocardial ischemia and infarction remain a common cause of morbidity and mortality in patients undergoing noncardiac surgery. Mortality from perioperative MI is high (40% to 70%). The incidence and severity of perioperative myocardial ischemia is greatest during the first 24 to 72 hours after surgery; this is probably related to postoperative stresses of anesthesia, surgical complications, and early postoperative ambulation. Cardiac complications after noncardiac surgery are a reflection of factors specific to the patient, the operation, and the circumstances under which the operation takes place. Preoperative risk stratification is paramount in preventing postsurgical cardiac complications. Perioperative β-blocker therapy in patients with, or at high risk for, coronary artery disease (CAD) has been shown to reduce mortality and cardiovascular complications.

(C) Assessment of the patient's cardiovascular risk (based on the patient's cardiac risk profile and the risk of the surgical procedure) is crucial in the early recognition of perioperative cardiac events. American College of Cardiology/American Heart Association (ACC/AHA) guidelines for the care of patients with cardiovascular disease undergoing noncardiac surgery state that patients at risk for perioperative MI should have an ECG obtained before surgery, another immediately after surgery, and daily for the first 2 postoperative days. In many cases, however, the ECG may be normal or reveal only subtle changes of the ST segments and T-waves. If perioperative MI is suspected, serial serum markers of myocardial injury such as cardiac troponins should be drawn.

(D) ECG changes suggestive of myocardial ischemia or infarction include ST segment elevation, ST segment depression greater than or equal to 1 mm in more than one contiguous lead, and the presence of a new LBBB or new Q-waves. The majority of perioperative MIs will be non-ST segment elevation MIs (NSTEMI). Acute ST-elevation MI (STEMI) represents a sudden thrombotic occlusion of a coronary artery, most commonly secondary to atherosclerotic plaque rupture. In many perioperative patients, NSTEMI and unstable angina result from increased myocardial demand (caused by postoperative tachycardia or hypertension) or decreased global perfusion (caused by perioperative hypotension). The distinction between the different pathophysiologic mechanisms of myocardial ischemia/infarction in the perioperative patient is important because it will influence treatment.

(E) The inability to administer medical reperfusion therapy (i.e., thrombolytics) in the postoperative patient because of the very high bleeding risk undoubtedly contributes to the high mortality associated with perioperative STEMI. Current ACC/AHA guidelines suggest that postoperative patients with STEMI who are candidates for aspirin and heparin should undergo immediate coronary angioplasty. The use of aspirin, β-blockers, and ACE inhibitors, particularly for patients with decreased ejection fractions or anterior MI, is also beneficial whether or not these patients are candidates for coronary angioplasty. Nitroglycerin is effective in decreasing pain of acute ongoing myocardial ischemia but has never been shown to improve mortality. The use of glycoprotein IIb/IIIa receptor inhibitors (e.g., ticlopidine or clopidogrel) in the setting of postoperative STEMI may increase the bleeding risk significantly but should be considered.

(F) Patients with non-ST segment elevation acute coronary syndromes (NSTACS) include patients with unstable angina (i.e., ischemic ECG changes and negative serial cardiac enzymes); and non-ST elevation myocardial infarction (i.e., no ischemic ECG changes and positive serial cardiac enzymes). Postoperative ECG changes are common, and repolarization abnormalities during this period may be nonspecific for ischemia. Up to 25% of postoperative ECGs may be uninterpretable because of the presence of left bundle branch block, a paced rhythm, or other ECG abnormalities (e.g., left ventricular hypertrophy). Serial CK-MB and/or troponin analysis is helpful in the diagnosis of MI in postoperative patients and offers some long-term or in-hospital prognostic value. Negative serial cardiac biomarkers, however, do not exclude the possibility of ongoing myocardial ischemia. Although less sensitive than serial cardiac biomarker analysis in the diagnosis of MI, transthoracic echocardiography may expedite the diagnosis of MI by identifying new segmental wall motion abnormalities.

(G) In patients without ischemic ECG changes and negative cardiac enzymes, the differential for noncardiac chest pain should be entertained. Most importantly, pulmonary embolism should be excluded. Pulmonary embolism should be considered in the differential diagnosis of patients presenting with undifferentiated chest pain or dyspnea and an elevated cardiac troponin level. Acute pulmonary embolism can be associated with ECG changes caused by right heart strain and myocardial injury.

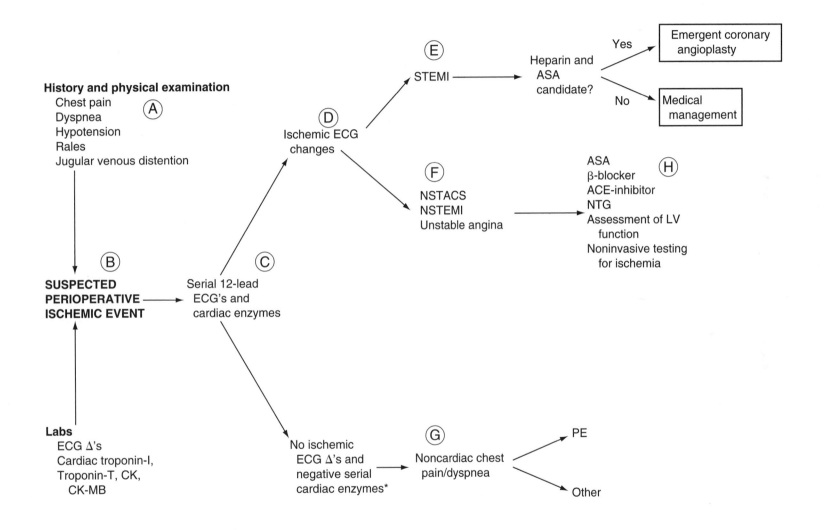

History and physical examination
Chest pain (A)
Dyspnea
Hypotension
Rales
Jugular venous distention

(B)
SUSPECTED
PERIOPERATIVE →
ISCHEMIC EVENT

(C)
Serial 12-lead
ECG's and
cardiac enzymes

Labs
ECG Δ's
Cardiac troponin-I,
Troponin-T, CK,
   CK-MB

(D)
Ischemic ECG
changes

(E)
STEMI

Heparin and
ASA
candidate?

Yes → Emergent coronary
       angioplasty

No → Medical
      management

(F)
NSTACS
NSTEMI
Unstable angina

(H)
ASA
β-blocker
ACE-inhibitor
NTG
Assessment of LV
   function
Noninvasive testing
   for ischemia

No ischemic
ECG Δ's and
negative serial
cardiac enzymes*

(G)
Noncardiac chest
pain/dyspnea

PE

Other

Similarly, an elevated cardiac troponin level can occur in patients with pulmonary embolism because of right ventricular dilation and myocardial injury.

(H) The goals for treatment in perioperative NSTACS are the same as those for treatment in the nonsurgical setting. The treatment goals include decreasing myocardial oxygen demand, stabilizing a vulnerable plaque, and preventing MI-related left ventricular remodeling. Reperfusion therapy (either with thrombolytics or coronary angioplasty) should not be performed routinely on an emergency basis in postoperative patients in whom an MI is not related to an acute coronary occlusion (STEMI). In patients with postoperative NSTACS, increased myocardial demand from tachycardia or hypertension is a likely cause, and lowering the heart rate or blood pressure is of greater benefit and less risk than immediate coronary angiography. In patients with hypotension from blood loss, improvement in global perfusion through volume resuscitation is of obvious immediate importance. Antiplatelet and antithrombotic therapy with aspirin (clopidogrel if aspirin allergic) and heparin should be administered in patients with NSTACS unless absolutely contraindicated. The risk/benefit ratio of using these agents in the postoperative period needs to be carefully assessed on a case-by-case basis. β-blockers decrease excessive reflex activation of the sympathetic nervous system in patients with myocardial infarction/ischemia and may be of particular benefit in the postoperative period. Contraindications to the use of β-blockers in the perioperative period include significant bradycardia or hypotension, severe left ventricular dysfunction, heart block, and severe bronchospastic lung disease. Nitroglycerin administration is helpful in improving symptoms of chest pain and in controlling blood pressure, thereby potentially decreasing myocardial demand. There is strong evidence supporting the early use of angiotensin-converting enzyme (ACE) inhibitors. In patients who have sustained a myocardial infarction, a transthoracic echocardiogram should be obtained to assess left ventricular systolic function. There is no evidence to support immediate angiography in patients with elevated cardiac markers who are otherwise clinically stable. Based on ACC/AHA guidelines, pharmacologic or exercise (if possible) stress testing for risk stratification before hospital discharge should be a priority to help determine who would benefit from coronary revascularization.

REFERENCES

Adams JE, Sicard GA, Allen BT et al: Diagnosis of perioperative myocardial infarction with measurement of cardiac troponin I. N Engl J Med 330:670–674, 1994.

Badner NH, Knill RL, Brown JE et al: Myocardial infarction after noncardiac surgery. Anesthesiology 88:572–578, 1998.

Douketis JD, Crowther MA, Stanton EB et al: Elevated cardiac troponin levels in patients with submassive pulmonary embolism. Arch Intern Med 14:79–81, 2002.

Eagle KA, Berger PB, Calkins H et al: ACC/AHA guideline update on perioperative cardiovascular evaluation for noncardiac surgery: A report of the American College of Cardiology/American Heart Association Task Force on Practice Guidelines (Committee to Update the 1996 Guidelines on Perioperative Cardiovascular Evaluation for Noncardiac Surgery), 2002. American College of Cardiology Website. Available at: www.acc.org/clinical/guidelines/perio/update?periupdate%5Findex.htm

Eagle KA, Brundage BH, Chaitman BR et al: Guidelines for perioperative cardiovascular evaluation for noncardiac surgery. J Am Coll Cardiol 27:910–948, 1996.

Heart Outcomes Prevention Evaluation Study Investigators: Effect of an angiotensin-converting-enzyme inhibitor, ramipril, on cardiovascular events in high-risk patients. N Engl J Med 342:145–153, 2000.

Mangano DT: Perioperative cardiac morbidity. Anesthesiology 72:153–184, 1990.

Mangano DT, Hollenberg M, Fegert G et al: Perioperative myocardial ischemia in patients undergoing noncardiac surgery: I. Incidence and severity during the 4-day perioperative period. The Study of Perioperative Ischemia (SPI) Research Group. J Am Coll Cardiol 17:843–850, 1991.

Mangano DT, Layug EL, Wallace A et al for the Multicenter Study of Perioperative Ischemia Research Group: Effect of atenolol on mortality and cardiovascular morbidity after noncardiac surgery. N Engl J Med 335:1713–1721, 1996.

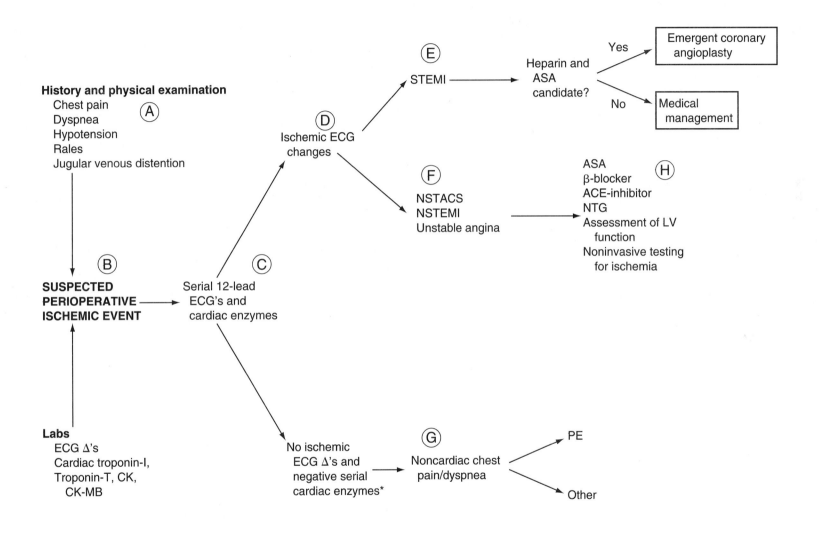

History and physical examination
Chest pain   Ⓐ
Dyspnea
Hypotension
Rales
Jugular venous distention

Ⓑ

SUSPECTED PERIOPERATIVE ISCHEMIC EVENT

Serial 12-lead ECG's and cardiac enzymes

Ⓒ

Labs
ECG Δ's
Cardiac troponin-I,
Troponin-T, CK,
CK-MB

Ⓓ Ischemic ECG changes

Ⓔ STEMI

Heparin and ASA candidate?

Yes → Emergent coronary angioplasty

No → Medical management

Ⓕ NSTACS NSTEMI Unstable angina

Ⓗ
ASA
β-blocker
ACE-inhibitor
NTG
Assessment of LV function
Noninvasive testing for ischemia

No ischemic ECG Δ's and negative serial cardiac enzymes*

Ⓖ Noncardiac chest pain/dyspnea

PE

Other

Chapter 35 *Aortic Valve Stenosis*

CHRISTOPHER D. RAEBURN, MD • ALDEN H. HARKEN, MD

(A) Although the life expectancy of patients with asymptomatic aortic stenosis is nearly normal, long-term survival is dramatically reduced once the onset of the classic symptoms of angina (50% at 5 years), syncope (50% at 3 years), or heart failure (50% at 2 years) occurs. Aortic valve replacement can restore age-corrected survival to near normal.

(B) A systolic ejection murmur in the second right intercostal space with radiation into the neck is typical. Patients with aortic stenosis may be entirely asymptomatic or may present with angina, syncope, or heart failure.

(C) Chest x-ray is commonly normal. Calcification of the aortic valve may be seen but this does not necessarily indicate stenosis. Even late, left ventricular hypertrophy (LVH) may not be apparent on chest x-ray.

(D) ECG is fairly sensitive in detecting LVH and may also reveal conduction defects (e.g., long P-R interval or bundle branch block) which can result from aortic valve calcification extending into the conducting tissues.

(E) Any symptomatic patient with a systolic murmur and any asymptomatic patient with a murmur greater than 3/6 should undergo echocardiography/Doppler ultrasound. This noninvasive, cost-effective test accurately determines aortic valve area and gradient and has all but replaced cardiac catheterization as a means of assessing the hemodynamic significance of aortic stenosis.

(F) Echocardiography/Doppler ultrasound is nearly 100% sensitive in detecting hemodynamically significant aortic stenosis; thus a negative study should prompt a search for an alternative diagnosis.

(G) Although echocardiography/Doppler ultrasound is accurate in assessing aortic valve gradient and calculating valve area, these parameters do not always correlate with the development of symptoms. The indication for aortic valve replacement is based largely on the presence or absence of symptoms. Thus the absolute valve area (or transvalvular pressure gradient) is not usually the primary determinant of the need for aortic valve replacement.

(H) In the absence of symptoms or LVH, it is safe to observe a patient with aortic stenosis, whatever the valve area/gradient. The frequency of repeat echocardiography should be based on the degree of stenosis, with yearly examinations appropriate for severe stenosis and a 5-year interval acceptable for mild stenosis.

(I) Indications for surgery in asymptomatic patients with aortic stenosis are controversial. Most clinicians agree that progressive LVH is an indication for valve repair/replacement because early intervention may reverse ventricular hypertrophy. Patients with left ventricular dysfunction, ventricular tachycardia, or an aortic valve area less than $0.6\,cm^2$ are also commonly referred for surgery.

(J) Prompt aortic valve surgery should be performed in essentially all patients with aortic stenosis who develop the classic symptoms of angina, syncope or dyspnea. Following surgery, patients improve both symptomatically and functionally and age-corrected survival is nearly normal.

(K) Patients with concomitant coronary artery disease (CAD) may require preoperative coronary angioplasty or intraoperative coronary artery bypass grafting. Thus, prior to aortic valve surgery, patients should be assessed for the need for coronary angiography. Indications for coronary angiography include age over 40 or the presence of left ventricular dysfunction or signs/risk factors for CAD in patients under the age of 40.

(L) While percutaneous, endovascular aortic valve replacement has been reported, standard aortic valve replacement via sternotomy affords excellent results with surprisingly little morbidity. Perioperative mortality of aortic valve replacement is less than 5% and restores age-corrected survival to near normal.

(M) Whether to use a mechanical vs. bioprosthetic valve is based primarily on patient age and the risk of life-long anticoagulation. Mechanical aortic valvular prostheses afford excellent, long-term relief of hemodynamic aortic stenosis but require life-long anticoagulation. Bioprosthetic valves in the aortic position do not require anticoagulation; however, in smaller sizes they provide less hemodynamic relief and 30% exhibit structural deterioration at 8-10 years.

(N) Patients with combined aortic stenosis and CAD not amenable to angioplasty/stenting should undergo concomitant aortic valve replacement and coronary artery bypass grafting because the perioperative mortality of the combined procedure is only minimally increased.

REFERENCES

Bonow RO, Carabello B, de Leon AC, et al. ACC/AHA Guidelines for the Management of Patients With Valvular Heart Disease. Executive Summary. A report of the American College of Cardiology/American Heart Association Task Force on Practice Guidelines. J Heart Valve Dis. 7:672–707, 1998.

Carabello BA. Evaluation and management of patients with aortic stenosis. Circulation. 105:1746–1750, 2002.

Filsoufi F, Aklog L, Adams DH, Byrne JG. Management of mild to moderate aortic stenosis at the time of coronary artery bypass grafting. J Heart Valve Dis. Review. 11 Suppl 1:S45–S49, 2002.

Lamb HJ, Beyerbacht HP, de Roos A, et al. Left ventricular remodeling early after aortic valve replacement: differential effects on diastolic function in aortic valve stenosis and aortic regurgitation. J Am Coll Cardiol. 40:2182–2188, 2002.

Pereira JJ, Lauer MS, Bashir M, et al. Survival after aortic valve replacement for severe aortic stenosis with low transvalvular gradients and severe left ventricular dysfunction. J Am Coll Cardiol. 39:1356–1363, 2002.

Popovic AD, Stewart WJ. Echocardiographic evaluation of valvular stenosis: the gold standard for the next millennium? Echocardiography Review 18:59–63, 2001.

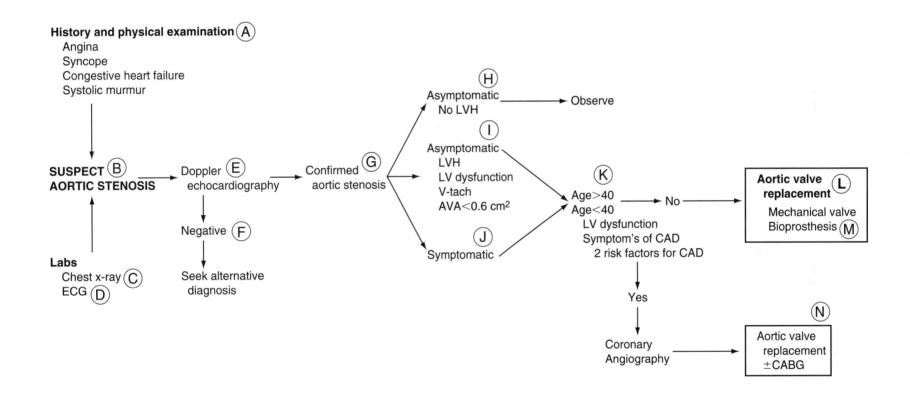

Chapter 36 *Mitral Stenosis*

DAVID A. FULLERTON, MD

(A) Mitral stenosis (MS) results from rheumatic fever. Because rheumatic fever typically occurs in early childhood, fewer than 50% of patients with MS relate a prior history of rheumatic fever. Symptoms result from elevated left atrial pressure leading to pulmonary venous congestion and, ultimately, pulmonary edema. The classic symptom is dyspnea with exertion. Other symptoms include cough, hemoptysis, and paroxysmal nocturnal dyspnea. Pulmonary hypertension is often present and results from three mechanisms: (1) retrograde transmission of hydrostatic pressure caused by left atrial hypertension; (2) reflex pulmonary arterial vasoconstriction; and (3) pulmonary vascular remodeling from long-standing pulmonary venous hypertension. Severe pulmonary hypertension may result in right heart failure (e.g., distended neck veins, hepatomegaly, ascites, or lower extremity edema). Because of left atrial hypertension and distension, patients may go into atrial fibrillation. When this happens, loss of atrial kick and shorter transit time across the stenotic mitral valve may further elevate left atrial pressure. For this reason, patients often become symptomatic when they go into atrial fibrillation. Probably because of atrial fibrillation, patients with MS are at risk for systemic embolization.

(B) The "auscultory triad" of MS includes an apical diastolic murmur, an increased first heart sound, and an opening snap. The more stenotic the valve, the longer the diastolic murmur. A loud P_2 can be heard if pulmonary hypertension is present. Patients are commonly in atrial fibrillation.

(C) There is normally no gradient across the mitral valve. Hence left atrial pressure normally approximates left ventricular diastolic pressure (LVEDP). With mitral stenosis, a gradient across the valve is created between the left atrial

pressure and LVEDP. The magnitude of the gradient is a function of two factors: (1) the size of the mitral valve orifice (mitral valve area); and (2) the flow rate across the valve during diastole. A left atrial pressure of about 15 to 20 mm Hg will produce interstitial pulmonary edema; a left atrial pressure of 35 mm Hg will produce alveolar pulmonary edema. Assuming a normal LVEDP of 5 mm Hg, a gradient across the mitral valve of 15 mm Hg will produce a left atrial pressure of 20 mm Hg and the onset of pulmonary edema. The normal cross-sectional area of the mitral valve is 4 to 6 cm^2. Mild MS (i.e., mitral valve area greater than 2 cm^2) typically produces few symptoms. Moderate MS (i.e., valve area 1 to 2 cm^2) may produce symptoms with moderate exercise. Severe MS (i.e., valve area less than 1 cm^2) produces symptoms with minimal exercise. The smallest mitral valve area compatible with life is 0.5 cm^2.

(D) The ECG may demonstrate left atrial enlargement and right and left ventricular hypertrophy. The chest x-ray is notable for several findings. First, the cardiac silhouette is typically normal; the left ventricle is not enlarged. Second, the enlarged left atrium is visible as a double density behind the cardiac silhouette. Third, the shadow of the pulmonary artery and left atrium combine to obliterate the space between the aorta and left ventricle and thereby straighten the shadow of the left heart border. Fourth, pulmonary edema may be seen. The diagnosis is confirmed by echocardiography. Echocardiography determines the mitral valve gradient and the mitral valve area by Doppler half-time and planimetry.

(E) Aymptomatic patients with mild or moderate MS should be followed with echocardiography every 3 to 5 years. Minimally symptomatic patients with left atrial pressures below 20 mm Hg may be treated with diuretics. Atrial arrhythmias

should be rate controlled with β-blockers. Atrial fibrillation will require anticoagulation (e.g., Coumadin to international normalized ratio 2 to 3). Patients should receive prophylactic antibiotics for dental and gastrointestinal procedures.

(F) Patients with moderate to severe symptoms, which typically occur with a valve area less than 1 cm^2, should undergo mechanical therapy. In addition, patients with minimal symptoms but with pulmonary hypertension or a left atrial pressure greater than 20 mm Hg despite medical therapy should have mechanical intervention. Before undergoing mechanical intervention, cardiac catheterization with coronary angiography should be performed in patients older than 40 years to exclude associated coronary artery disease.

(G) Questionable symptoms may be evaluated with an exercise stress echocardiogram. Not only may a patient's exercise capacity be quantified with a stress test, but an increased flow rate across a stenotic valve (exercise) may reveal a significant mitral valve gradient.

(H) Catheter balloon commissurotomy (CBC) is the mechanical treatment of choice. Performed in the cardiac catheterization suite, the procedure typically increases the mitral valve area to approximately 2 cm^2. In skilled hands, CBC may be performed with an initial success of 95% and less than 1% mortality. Outcomes following CBC are favorable, with a 10-year event-free survival of about 60%. The suitability of the procedure is largely determined by the morphology of the valve on echocardiography. The procedure is contraindicated if: (1) the mitral valve has 3+ to 4+ mitral regurgitation; (2) thrombus is identified in the left atrium; (3) the leaflets and/or the valve annulus is calcified; or (4) the leaflets and/or the subvalvular apparatus is significantly thickened and foreshortened.

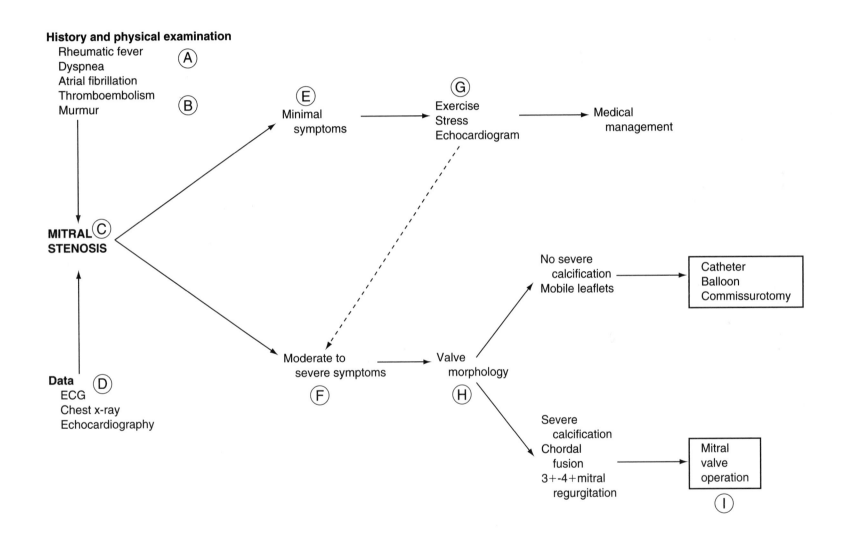

History and physical examination
Rheumatic fever (A)
Dyspnea
Atrial fibrillation
Thromboembolism (B)
Murmur

(E) Minimal symptoms

(G) Exercise Stress Echocardiogram → Medical management

MITRAL (C) **STENOSIS**

Moderate to severe symptoms (F) → Valve morphology (H)

Data (D)
ECG
Chest x-ray
Echocardiography

No severe calcification Mobile leaflets → Catheter Balloon Commissurotomy

Severe calcification Chordal fusion 3+-4+mitral regurgitation → Mitral valve operation (I)

(I)   Mitral valve surgery should be performed if CBC is contraindicated or if the patient requires additional surgical procedures (e.g., coronary artery bypass or aortic or tricuspid valve surgery). The valve may sometimes be repaired by performing an open mitral commissurotomy but will usually require replacement. If replaced, left ventricular function may be optimized if the posterior leaflet of the valve is preserved. The mitral valve area is similar following CBC or MVR. The risks of mitral valve replacement (MVR) are greater than CBC. The operative mortality rate for isolated MVR is 2% to 7%. If coronary artery bypass is also required, the operative mortality rate is 5% to 12%.

REFERENCES

Bonow RO, Carabello B, de Leon AC Jr. et al: ACC/AHA guidelines for the management of patients with valvular heart disease. J Am Coll Cardiol 32:1486–1588, 1998.

Hammermeister K, Sethi GK, Henderson WG et al: Outcomes 15 years after valve replacement with a mechanical vs. bioprosthetic valve: Final report of the VA randomized trial. J Am Coll Cardiol 36:1152–1158, 2000.

Iung B, Garbarz E, Michand P et al: Late results of percutaneous mitral commissurotomy in a series of 1024 patients: Analysis of late clinical deterioration: Frequency, anatomic findings and predictive factors. Circulation 99:3272–3278, 1999.

Palacios IF, Sanchez PL, Harrell LC et al: Which patients benefit from percutaneous mitral balloon valvuloplasty? Prevalvuloplasty and post-valvuloplasty variables that predict long-term outcome. Circulation 105:1465–1471, 2002.

Rahimtoola SH, Durairaj A, Mehra A et al: Current evaluation and management of patients with mitral stenosis. Circulation 106:1183–1188, 2002.

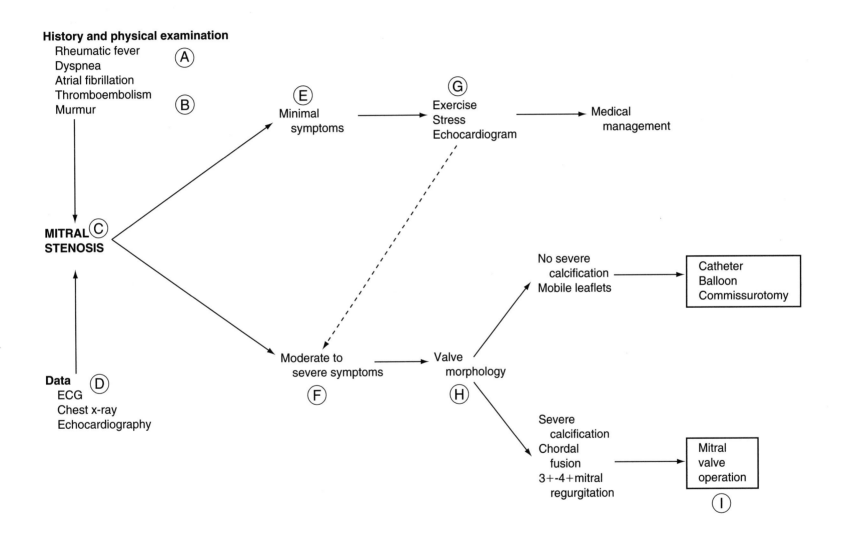

History and physical examination
Rheumatic fever (A)
Dyspnea
Atrial fibrillation
Thromboembolism
Murmur (B)

MITRAL (C)
STENOSIS

Data (D)
ECG
Chest x-ray
Echocardiography

Minimal (E)
symptoms

Exercise (G)
Stress
Echocardiogram → Medical management

Moderate to (F)
severe symptoms → Valve morphology (H)

No severe calcification
Mobile leaflets → Catheter Balloon Commissurotomy

Severe calcification
Chordal fusion
3+-4+mitral regurgitation → Mitral valve operation (I)

GASTROINTESTINAL

Chapter 37 *Achalasia*

THADEUS L. TRUS, MD

(A) The age of onset of achalasia is usually the third or fourth decade, but it can present as early as the preteens or much later in life. Symptoms include dysphagia; regurgitation, with or without aspiration; and, occasionally, chest pain.

(B) Achalasia means failure of relaxation. The mechanism is loss of vagal innervation of the esophageal body, in particular the lower esophageal sphincter (LES). Neural degeneration is seen in the visceromotor axis, which extends from the dorsal motor nucleus of the vagus to the myenteric plexus in the esophageal wall. The characteristic result is either incomplete relaxation of the LES or no relaxation at all. Peristalsis is often absent or replaced by simultaneous, low amplitude contractions. Diffuse esophageal spasm is similar to achalasia in that simultaneous, frequent contractures are seen; however, the LES is usually normal and surgical intervention is not necessary. Chagas' disease is common in South America and is caused by the parasite *Trypanosoma cruzi*, an organism that destroys the myenteric plexus. Clinically, Chagas' disease is indistinguishable from achalasia.

(C) Barium swallow shows a classic "bird's-beak" deformity of the lower esophagus with proximal esophageal dilatation.

(D) Esophagoscopy commonly reveals esophageal dilatation and retained food. The mucosa may show retention esophagitis. Passage of the scope through the LES often produces a characteristic "pop" sensation. Esophagoscopy allows for biopsy and exclusion of esophageal carcinoma.

(E) The incidence of esophageal cancer is slightly increased in patients with achalasia, and the risk is not affected by therapy.

(F) Calcium-channel blockers and long-acting nitrates may be marginally effective for short periods but they are insufficient for long-term therapy.

(G) Manometric evidence of incomplete or absent LES relaxation, usually with absence of peristalsis, is diagnostic for achalasia. Contraction, if present, is usually weak.

(H) "Vigorous achalasia" is a term used for the clinical entity marked by strong esophageal contractions, a nonrelaxing LES, and chest pain. Manometric studies are usually a brief outpatient procedure but sometimes may be difficult to perform in patients with a large, dilated esophagus because of difficulty passing the probe.

(I) Patients who have an extremely dilated esophagus (sigmoid type) generally have marginal results with myotomy and should be considered for esophageal resection with either a gastric pull-up or colon interposition. Laparoscopic myotomy outcomes for these end-stage patients appears to be better than outcomes achieved with a thoracic approach.

(J) The advantages of pneumatic dilatation are avoidance of surgery and a relatively low complication rate. The disadvantages include a perforation rate of 5% or less and variable long-term results for relief of dysphagia. Forceful pneumatic dilatation is less effective in younger persons, especially pediatric patients.

(K) Although one cannot restore normal peristaltic function to the esophageal body, the aim of therapy is to decrease the functional obstruction created by the "nonrelaxing" LES. The usual options are forceful pneumatic dilation or surgical myotomy. The great variation in results of these therapies is related to technique and experience.

	Relief of Dysphagia (%)	Reflux (%)	Perforations (%)	Mortality (%)
Forceful dilation	65–90	1–20	1–5	0–0.8
Esophago-myotomy	80–95	3–50	0–4	0–1.4

TABLE 37.1
Achalasia Treatment Outcomes

Esophagomyotomy is now easily performed through a laparoscopic approach with excellent results. A laparoscopic approach is somewhat easier than a thoracoscopic approach and affords the opportunity to perform an antireflux procedure to prevent postmyotomy reflux, although addition of an antireflux procedure remains somewhat controversial. A myotomy should extend at least 6 cm above the esophagogastric (EG) junction and at least 1 cm below the EG junction. An insufficient myotomy will not relieve dysphagia. An excessive myotomy will result in severe reflux disease. An adequate myotomy accompanied by partial fundoplication results in sustained relief of dysphagia and prevention of reflux.

(L) Botox (botulinum toxin) injection causes lower esophageal sphincter relaxation. The advantage of Botox injection is the avoidance of perforation risk. The disadvantage is that Botox injection is a transient treatment and requires multiple injections over time. Future therapy will most likely involve nerve regeneration which, to date, has eluded reproducible experimental success.

REFERENCES

Carter R, Brewer LA: Achalasia and esophageal carcinoma. Am J Surg 130:114–120, 1975.

Csendes A, Braghetto I, Henriques A et al: Late results of a prospective randomized study comparing forceful dilation and esophagomyotomy in patients with achalasia. Gut 30:299–304, 1989.

Ellis FJH, Crozier RE, Watkins E: Operation for esophageal achalasia. J Thorac Cardiovasc Surg 88:344–351, 1984.

Hunter JG, Trus TL, Branum GD et al: Laparoscopic Heller myotomy and fundoplication for achalasia. Ann Surg 225:655–665, 1997.

Pasricha PJ, Rai R, Ravich WJ et al: Botulinum toxin for achalasia: Long-term outcome and predictors of response. Gastroenterology 110:1410–1415, 1996.

Patti MG, Pellegrini CA, Horgan S et al: Minimally invasive surgery for achalasia: An 8-year experience with 168 patients. Ann Surg 230:587–594, 1999.

Richter JE: Surgery or pneumatic dilation for achalasia: A head to head comparison. Now are all the questions answered? Gastroenterology 97:1340–1341, 1989.

Spiess AE, Kahrilas PJ: Treating achalasia: From whalebone to laparoscope (review). JAMA 280:638–642, 1998.

Traube M, Hongo M, Magyar L et al: Effects of nifedipine in achalasia and in patients with high-amplitude peristaltic esophageal contractions. JAMA 252:1733–1766, 1984.

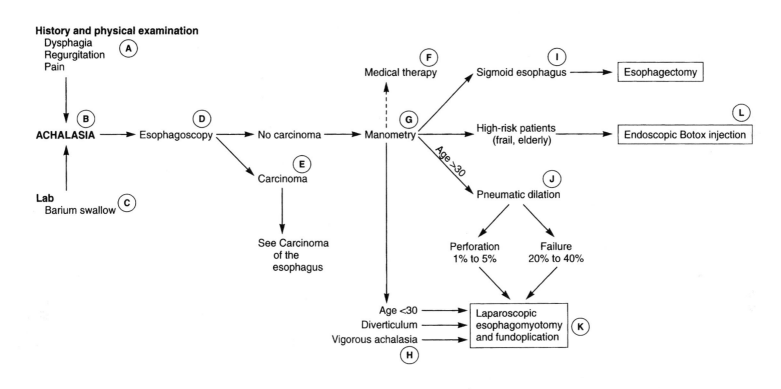

Chapter 38 *Carcinoma of the Esophagus*

NATHAN W. PEARLMAN, MD

(A) Dysphagia and/or odynophagia are classic signs of esophageal cancer but often represent advanced disease. A less common sign is anemia caused by slow blood loss from the tumor. Significant hemorrhage denotes erosion into a major vessel and is often fatal. More recently, increasing numbers of asymptomatic patients are being detected during screening endoscopy for Barrett's esophagus.

(B) Barium studies will occasionally detect an otherwise occult cancer of the esophagus or stomach; however, endoscopy and biopsy are still needed to prove the presence of such disease.

(C) Patients with Barrett's esophagus are at increased risk of cancer of the gastroesophageal junction and need periodic (every 2 to 3 years) screening to detect disease at an early stage, when it is highly curable.

(D) Upper GI endoscopy and biopsy and/or brushings are the gold standard for diagnosing esophageal cancer.

(E) Once cancer is diagnosed, endoscopic ultrasound will accurately determine depth of wall penetration and status of regional nodes in 70% to 80% of patients, as opposed to 50% to 60% with CT scan.

(F) Most patients with esophageal cancer have chronic lung disease of some kind. Chest x-ray will help evaluate that. Chest CT scan will help detect lung metastases (common site of spread) and/or tumor invasion of the trachea, left main stem bronchus, or aorta. Any of these findings makes the patient inoperable for cure. CT scan of the abdomen will help detect liver metastases or invasion of the celiac axis–again, signs of incurability. Routine blood chemistries are needed before any major operation.

(G) Most esophageal cancers are aymptomatic until at least 80% of the lumen is occluded and only liquids can be taken in. Many patients are malnourished at diagnosis and require preoperative nutritional therapy.

(H) Patients with esophageal cancer often have a long history of alcohol and tobacco use.

Evaluation of cardiopulmonary and hepatic reserve is, consequently, vital prior to surgery.

(I) Current staging of esophageal cancer is as follows:

Tis	Carcinoma in situ
T1	Tumor invades lamina propria or sub-mucosa
T2	Tumor invades muscularis propria
T3	Tumor invades adventitia
T4	Tumor invades adjacent structures
N0	No regional node metastases
N1	Regional node metastases
M0	No distant metastases
M1	Distant metastases
Stage 0	Tis N0 M0
Stage I	T1 N0 M0
Stage II	T2-3 N0 M0, or T1-2 N1 M0
Stage III	T3 N1 M0, or T4 NX M0
Stage IV	TX NX M1

(J) Some patients with early disease limited to mucosa can probably be cured with endoscopic mucosectomy or photodynamic therapy, but this treatment is experimental at present.

(K) Radiation, combined with chemotherapy, will cure about 20% of patients with early disease, and is a reasonable approach for high-risk patients with stage I tumors.

(L) For most patients, the best chance of cure lies with esophageal resection, either alone or in combination with neoadjuvant (preoperative) chemoradiotherapy. Surgery cures 60% to 80% of patients with true stage 0-I disease; but only 10% to 30% of stage II-III cancers, and only rare stage IV patients. Neoadjuvant chemoradiotherapy will sterilize 20% to 30% of localized esophageal cancer–generally the early lesions. When added to surgery, preliminary results of some studies suggest a 3- to 4-year survival rate of 30% to 40% overall,

and 80% to 90% for those with no viable tumor in the specimen. Other reports, however, are less encouraging. Thus management of stage II-III disease is still in a state of flux.

(M) The goal of palliation is to provide normal or near-normal swallowing for as long as possible when cure is not feasible. Approaches include palliative resection of bulk disease, and substernal gastric or colonic bypass of the obstructing tumor. There is generally complete relief of dysphagia, but operative mortality is 5% to 10%, with survival about 7 months. Dilating the tumor with self-expanding metallic stents will also relieve dysphagia with no treatment-related deaths; however, survival is also short, about 3 to 4 months.

(N) Cancers of the upper third (cervical) esophagus do not lend themselves to "radical" resection because of their proximity to vital structures (e.g., trachea and aorta). Obtaining adequate proximal margins also may be difficult with the larynx in place. If surgery is chosen for such tumors, it often entails removing the entire thoracic and cervical esophagus and larynx, bringing the stomach (or colon) up to the pharynx.

(O) For middle and distal third lesions, surgery entails removal of most or all of the thoracic and abdominal esophagus. Reconstruction is by way of esophagogastric/colic anastomosis high in the chest or low in the neck. The role of extended regional lymphadenectomy is not established.

(P) The traditional approach to near-total esophagectomy is a combined abdominal-thoracic approach (two incisions), and occasionally a third incision in the neck. Generally, this is done via the right chest although, on occasion, it may be necessary to use the left chest. The advantage is good exposure for esophageal mobilization in the chest; the disadvantage is the thoracic incision.

(Q) An alternative technique is the transhiatal, or "blunt" esophagectomy using only abdominal and cervical incisions. Exposure in the mid- to upper

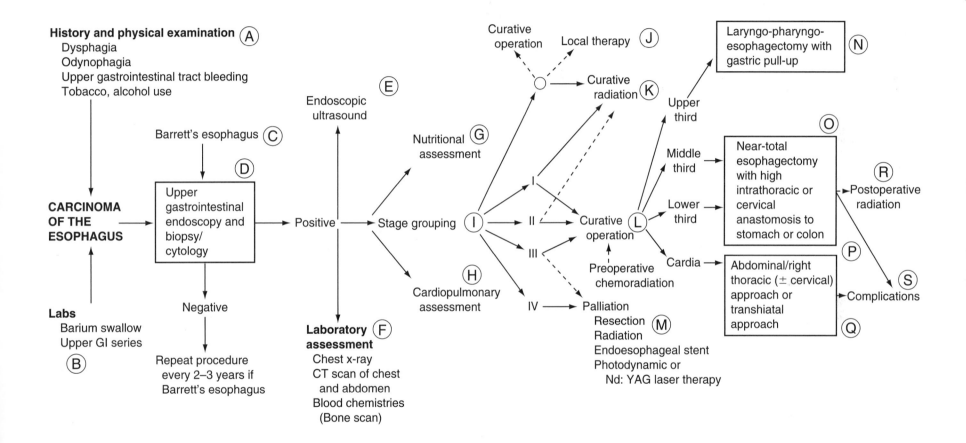

History and physical examination (A)
  Dysphagia
  Odynophagia
  Upper gastrointestinal tract bleeding
  Tobacco, alcohol use

Barrett's esophagus (C)

(D)

CARCINOMA OF THE ESOPHAGUS

Upper gastrointestinal endoscopy and biopsy/cytology

Labs
  Barium swallow
  Upper GI series
(B)

Negative

Repeat procedure every 2–3 years if Barrett's esophagus

Endoscopic ultrasound (E)

Positive

Laboratory assessment (F)
  Chest x-ray
  CT scan of chest and abdomen
  Blood chemistries
  (Bone scan)

Nutritional assessment (G)

Stage grouping

Cardiopulmonary assessment (H)

(I)

I

II

III

IV

Curative operation

Local therapy (J)

Curative radiation (K)

Curative operation

Preoperative chemoradiation

Palliation (M)
  Resection
  Radiation
  Endoesophageal stent
  Photodynamic or
    Nd: YAG laser therapy

Upper third

Middle third

Lower third

Cardia

(L)

Laryngo-pharyngo-esophagectomy with gastric pull-up (N)

Near-total esophagectomy with high intrathoracic or cervical anastomosis to stomach or colon (O)

Abdominal/right thoracic (± cervical) approach or transhiatal approach

(P)

(Q)

Postoperative radiation (R)

Complications (S)

chest is basically nonexistent, but one avoids a thoracotomy. Despite that, morbidity, mortality, and cure rates are the same with each approach.

Ⓡ   If neck dissection is not done for cancer of the cervical esophagus, the patient should receive postoperative neck irradiation.

Ⓢ   The overall nonfatal complication rate of esophagectomy (e.g., anastomostic leak, wound infection, or pneumonia) is about 20%. Operative mortality is 3% to 5%.

REFERENCES

Chu K-M, Law SYK, Fok M: A prospective comparison of transhiatal and transthoracic resection for lower third esophageal carcinoma. Am J Surg 174:320–324, 1997.

Cooper JS, Guo MD, Herskovic A et al: Chemoradiotherapy of locally advanced esophageal cancer. JAMA 281:1623–1627, 1999.

Goldmine M, Maddern G, Le-Prise et al: Oesophagectomy by a transhiatal approach or thoracotomy: A prospective randomized trial. Br J Surg 80:367–370, 1993.

Martin IG: Staging of esophageal and gastric carcinoma. In Daly JM, Hennessey TPJ, Reynolds JV (eds): Management of Upper Gastrointestinal Cancer. Philadelphia: WB Saunders/Harcourt Brace, 1999.

Mitani M, Kuwabara Y, Shinoda N et al: The effectiveness of palliative resection for advanced esophageal carcinoma: Analysis of 24 consecutive cases. Surg Today 32:784–788, 2002.

O'Donnell CA, Fullarton GM, Watt E et al: Randomized clinical trial comparing self-expanding metallic stents with plastic endoprosthesis in the palliation of oesophageal cancer. Br J Surg 89:985–992, 2002.

Pommier RF, Vetto JR, Ferris BL et al: Relationships between operative approaches and outcomes in esophageal surgery. Am J Surg 175:422–425, 1998.

Tenevieve P, Hay IM, Fingerhut A et al: Postoperative radiation therapy does not increase survival after curative resection for squamous cell carcinoma of the middle and lower esophagus, as shown by a multicenter controlled trial. Surg Gynecol Obstet 173:123–127, 1991.

Urba SG, Orringer MB, Turrisi et al: Randomized trial of preoperative chemoradiation versus surgery alone in patients with locoregional esophageal carcinoma. J Clin Oncol 19:305–313, 2001.

Walsh TN, Noonon N, Hollywood D et al: A comparison of multimodal therapy and surgery for esophageal adenocarcinoma. N Engl J Med 335:462–467, 1996.

Wright TA: High-grade dysplasia in Barrett's oesophagus. Br J Surg 84:760–766, 1997.

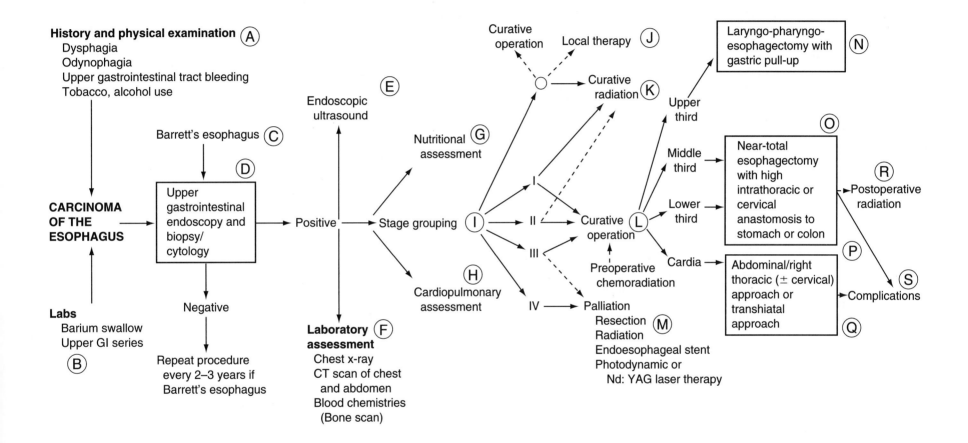

History and physical examination Ⓐ
Dysphagia
Odynophagia
Upper gastrointestinal tract bleeding
Tobacco, alcohol use

Barrett's esophagus Ⓒ

CARCINOMA OF THE ESOPHAGUS

Ⓓ
Upper gastrointestinal endoscopy and biopsy/cytology

Labs
Barium swallow
Upper GI series
Ⓑ

Negative

Repeat procedure every 2–3 years if Barrett's esophagus

Positive

Endoscopic ultrasound Ⓔ

Laboratory assessment Ⓕ
Chest x-ray
CT scan of chest and abdomen
Blood chemistries
(Bone scan)

Nutritional assessment Ⓖ

Stage grouping

Cardiopulmonary assessment Ⓗ

Ⓘ

I

II

III

IV

Curative operation

Local therapy Ⓙ

Curative radiation Ⓚ

Preoperative chemoradiation

Curative operation Ⓛ

Palliation Ⓜ
Resection
Radiation
Endoesophageal stent
Photodynamic or
    Nd: YAG laser therapy

Upper third

Middle third

Lower third

Cardia

Laryngo-pharyngo-esophagectomy with gastric pull-up Ⓝ

Ⓞ
Near-total esophagectomy with high intrathoracic or cervical anastomosis to stomach or colon

Abdominal/right thoracic (± cervical) approach or transhiatal approach Ⓠ

Ⓟ

Ⓡ
Postoperative radiation

Complications Ⓢ

Chapter 39 *Esophageal Perforation*

JOSEPH B. ZWISCHENBERGER, MD • CLARE SAVAGE, MD

(A) Esophageal perforation presents as an emergency because treatment delay reduces survival. Iatrogenic perforation, spontaneous perforation, and trauma account for the majority of esophageal perforations. Symptoms (e.g., pain, vomiting, hematemesis, dysphagia, and tachypnea) and signs (e.g., tachycardia, fever, subcutaneous emphysema, cardiac crunch, chest hypersonarity, and dullness) of esophageal perforation vary with cause and location (i.e., cervical, thoracic, or abdominal). Pain is the most common symptom, present in 70% to 90% of patients, usually referring directly to the site of perforation. Cervical perforation is characterized by neck ache and stiffness. In the abdomen, subxyphoid pain is present with anterior perforations, and dull epigastric pain radiating to the back may occur if the perforation is posterior and communicates with the lesser sac. Severe retrosternal or chest pain lateralizing to the side of perforation is seen with thoracic perforation. Severe chest pain after straining and hematemesis occur with postemetic ruptures. Tachycardia and tachypnea are documented in most patients with perforation. Subcutaneous emphysema is seen often with cervical perforations but less often with thoracic or abdominal perforations.

(B) Chest x-ray is suggestive of the diagnosis in 90% of patients but may be normal immediately after perforation. Pneumomediastinum, subcutaneous emphysema, mediastinal widening, or a mediastinal air-fluid level prompt investigation to rule out esophageal perforation. Hydropneumothorax on the left is seen in patients with distal third esophageal perforations. Initially, a water-soluble contrast esophagram identifies the site of esophageal perforation. For perforations contained within the chest, a barium esophagram may be performed for additional mucosal detail. For perforations that communicate with the peritoneal cavity, a water-soluble contrast is used for further evaluation.

(C) Nonoperative management of esophageal perforations may be applied to carefully selected patients. Criteria for nonoperative management include a well-contained leak in a stable patient without evidence of sepsis or communication with the pleural or peritoneal cavity. The perforation must easily drain back into the esophagus. Signs and symptoms of sepsis during nonoperative management warrant immediate surgical treatment. Pneumothorax, mediastinal emphysema, and respiratory failure are also indications for early surgical intervention.

(D) Conservative management includes NPO, cautious passage of a nasogastric tube for gastric decompression, administration of intravenous fluids with hyperalimentation, and an H_2-blocker or proton pump inhibitor to block acid reflux.

(E) Surgery, including primary repair, exclusion and diversion, or resection (esophagectomy), remains the mainstay of treatment for free perforations. Preoperative preparation includes nasogastric intubation for gastric decompression, broad-spectrum antibiotics, and intravenous fluid resuscitation.

(F) Esophagectomy, with or without immediate reconstruction, should be considered a first line procedure for perforations in patients with megaesophagus, severe undilatable reflux strictures, caustic ingestion, or resectable esophageal carcinoma.

(G) If esophageal perforation occurs during palliative treatment of unresectable esophageal carcinoma, a covered stent usually prevents leakage. If a stent is inadequate, exclusion and diversion with gastrostomy and jejunostomy may be necessary.

(H) Esophageal perforations recognized within 72 hours can usually be treated with primary repair reinforced by the gastric fundus, pleural flap, or muscle flap to decrease fistula formation. Cervical perforations are treated by primary closure and drainage of the neck. Thoracic esophageal perforations require a right thoracotomy for exposure of the upper two-thirds and left thoracotomy for the lower third. Lesions at the esophagogastric junction are approached by upper midline celiotomy (preferred) or left thoracotomy. Thoracic esophageal perforations require wide mediastinal drainage by opening the parietal pleura the entire length of the esophagus. Nonviable and grossly contaminated tissue in the mediastinum and parietal pleura is debrided. The esophagus (and, often, esophagogastric junction) must be dissected completely to identify the site of perforation and to mobilize the esophagus for a tension-free repair. Esophagomyotomy is often necessary to visualize the mucosal injury. Primary repair is often accomplished with closure of the mucosal defect over a bougie and reapproximation of both muscle layers. Thoracic esophageal perforations can be reinforced by an autologous pleural flap or by pedicled muscle flaps from the intercostal muscles, chest wall musculature, diaphragm, or a mobilized pedicle of omentum. Perforations at the esophagogastric junction are reinforced by gastric fundoplication.

(I) Late perforations can usually be repaired primarily and reinforced by muscle or pleura if severe inflammation and mediastinitis are absent.

(J) If primary reinforced repair is not possible because of either severe inflammation or mediastinitis, options include esophageal resection or exclusion and diversion. Exclusion and diversion entails cervical esophagostomy (diversion of the cervical esophagus, creating a salivary fistula); gastric decompression with a gastrostomy; and jejunostomy with delayed (6 months) reconstruction. An alternative to exclusion and diversion is T-tube drainage of the perforation, creating a controlled esophagocutaneous fistula. T-tube placement can be used in high-risk patients, but continued leakage can progress to sepsis and is not recommended as a routine procedure.

REFERENCES

Altorjay A, Kiss J, Voros A et al: Nonoperative management of esophageal perforations: Is it justified? Ann Surg 225:415–421, 1997.

Altorjay A, Kiss J, Voros A et al: The role of esophagectomy in the management of esophageal perforations. Ann Thorac Surg 65:1433–1436, 1998.

Bufkin BL, Miller JI Jr., Mansour KA: Esophageal perforation: Emphasis on management. Ann Thorac Surg 61:1447–1451, 1996.

Cameron JL, Kieffer RF, Hendrix TR et al: Selective nonoperative management of contained intrathoracic esophageal disruptions. Ann Thorac Surg 27:404–408, 1979.

Gouge TH, Depan HJ, Spencer FC: Experience with the Grillo pleural wrap procedure in 18 patients with perforation of the thoracic esophagus. Ann Surg 209:612–617, 1989.

Jones WG II, Ginsberg RJ: Esophageal perforation: A continuing challenge. Ann Thorac Surg 53:534–543, 1992.

Richardson JD, Martin LF, Borzotta AP et al: Unifying concepts in treatment of esophageal leaks. Am J Surg 149:157–162, 1985.

Shields TW: Esophageal Trauma. In Shields TW, LoCicero J III, Ponn RB (eds): General Thoracic Surgery, 5th ed. Philadelphia: Lippincott Williams & Wilkins, 2000.

White RK, Morris DM: Diagnosis and management of esophageal perforations. Am Surg 58:112–119, 1992.

Whyte RI, Iannettoni MD, Oringer MB: Intrathoracic esophageal perforation: The merit of primary repair. J Thorac Cardiovasc Surg 109:140–144, 1995.

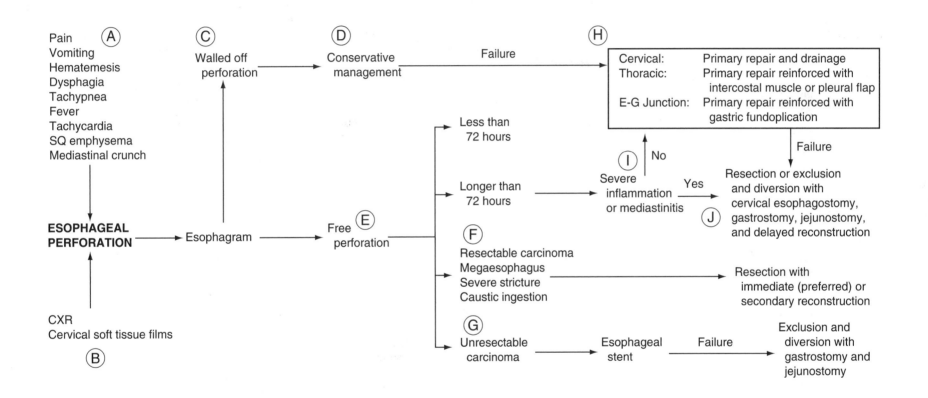

Chapter 40 **Caustic Ingestion**

JOSEPH B. ZWISCHENBERGER, MD • CLARE SAVAGE, MD

(A) Management of caustic ingestion involves immediate verification of the etiologic agent (i.e., alkali vs. acid, solid vs. liquid, and concentration). Alkali causes liquefactive necrosis and results in a deep burn, whereas acids cause coagulative necrosis, forming an eschar that limits tissue penetration. Solid alkali tends to adhere to and burn the oropharynx, whereas liquid alkali is rapidly swallowed, causing less oropharyngeal but more esophageal and/or gastric injury. Symptoms of caustic ingestion include oral pain, hematemesis, drooling, and inability or refusal to swallow. Absence of symptoms or evidence of oropharyngeal burns, however, does not exclude esophageal injury.

(B) If the physical examination and chest or abdominal x-rays indicate a perforation has occurred, abdominal exploration is mandatory with resection of all necrotic areas to prevent extension of the injury.

(C) Hoarseness, stridor, and dyspnea suggest laryngeal edema or epiglottic injury, prompting thorough airway evaluation with bronchoscopy and laryngoscopy and possible intubation or tracheostomy to maintain airway patency. Steroids may be administered to relieve airway obstruction caused by mucosal edema or bronchospasm.

(D) Esophagoscopy is recommended 12 to 24 hours postinjury to allow gastric emptying and stabilization of the patient unless esophageal or gastric perforation is suspected. The endoscope is advanced only to the area of the first severe burn to avoid iatrogenic perforation, often precluding full assessment of the esophagus and stomach.

(E) Patients with second- or third-degree burns without evidence of perforation are placed in the intensive care unit (ICU), kept nil per os (NPO), and given intravenous fluids and antibiotics to decrease the risk of aspiration and bacterial contamination of the mediastinum through the injured esophageal wall. Because acid reflux may increase stricture formation, prophylactic H_2-receptor antagonists (H_2-RA), proton-pump inhibitors (PPI), or antacids (AA) are recommended. Steroids have not been shown to be efficacious in preventing stricture formation and may mask signs of peritonitis.

(F) Treatment of first-degree esophageal burns, which do not perforate or form strictures, is usually observation for up to 48 hours.

(G) Caustic esophageal perforations are best treated by esophagectomy, with the transhiatal route preferred. Extensive, full-thickness esophageal and gastric necrosis is treated with urgent radical total esophagogastrectomy with delayed (6 months) reconstruction. All patients receive a cervical esophagostomy and feeding jejunostomy.

(H) Treatment alternatives for second- or third-degree injuries include an elective gastrostomy for feeding with passage of a nasogastric string for retrograde dilatation of strictures; this is commonly used in pediatric patients.

(I) A second alternative is intraluminal stent placement for prevention of strictures plus gastrostomy.

(J) A third option is to continue antibiotics and initiate feeding via a Dobhoff tube or total parenteral nutrition. In each of these options, patients are kept NPO until they can swallow their saliva without pain, after which the diet is advanced as tolerated. Esophagogastroduodenoscopy is performed at 3 weeks for full evaluation. The stomach and esophagus are also evaluated with a barium swallow at 3 weeks, 3 months, and 6 months to rule out stricture formation (the most common complication of second- or third-degree burns), gastric outlet obstruction, or the development of either an hourglass or linitis plastica-like appearance.

REFERENCES

Anderson KD, Rouse TM, Randolph JG: A controlled trial of corticosteroids in children with corrosive injury of the esophagus. N Engl J Med 323:637–640, 1990.

Anderson KD: Corrosive injury. In Pearson FG, Deslauriers J, Ginsberg RJ et al (eds): Esophageal Surgery. New York: Churchill Livingstone, 1995.

Cattan P, Munoz-Bongrand N, Berney T et al: Extensive abdominal surgery after caustic ingestion. Ann Surg 231:519–523, 2000.

DiPalma JA: Esophageal disorders. In Civetta JM, Taylor RW, Kirby R et al (eds): Critical Care, 3rd ed. Philadelphia: Lippincott-Raven, 1997.

Estrera A, Taylor W, Mills LJ et al: Corrosive burns of the esophagus and stomach: A recommendation for an aggressive surgical approach. Ann Thorac Surg 41:276–283, 1986.

Greenberg RE, Bank S, Blumstein M et al: Common Gastrointestinal Disorders in the Intensive Care Unit. In Bone RC, Bone RC (eds): Pulmonary and Critical Care Medicine, 2nd ed. Chicago: Mosby, 1993.

Gunnarsson M: Local corticosteroid treatment of caustic injuries of the esophagus: A preliminary report. Ann Otol Rhinol Laryngol 108:1088–1090, 1999.

Kirsh MM, Ritter F: Caustic ingestion and subsequent damage to the oropharyngeal and digestive passages. Ann Thorac Surg 21:74–82, 1976.

Lamireau T, Rebouissoux L, Denis D et al: Accidental caustic ingestion in children: Is endoscopy always mandatory? J Pediatr Gastroenterol Nutr 33:81–84, 2001.

Symbas PN, Vlasis SE, Hatcher CR Jr.: Esophagitis secondary to ingestion of caustic material. Ann Thorac Surg 36:73–77, 1983.

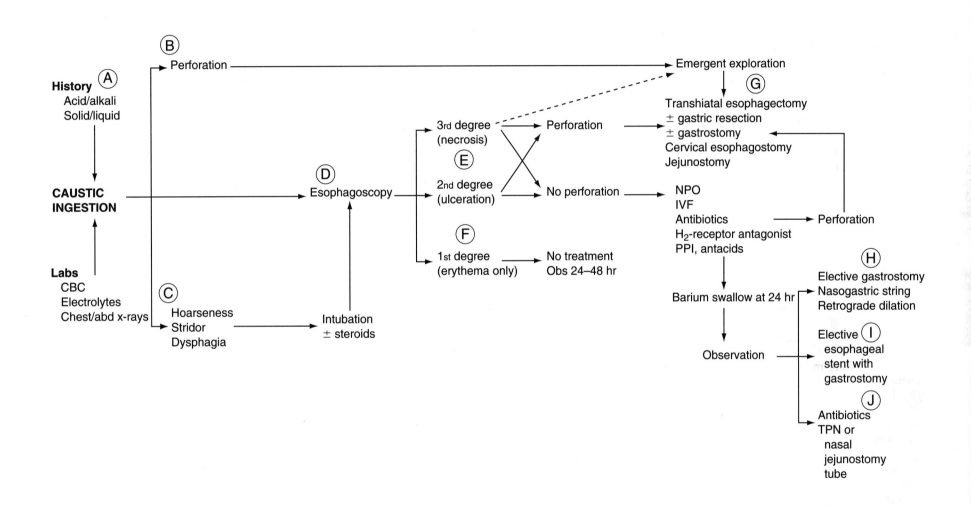

Ⓐ History
Acid/alkali
Solid/liquid

CAUSTIC INGESTION

Labs
CBC
Electrolytes
Chest/abd x-rays

Ⓑ Perforation → Emergent exploration

Ⓒ Hoarseness
Stridor → Intubation
Dysphagia ± steroids

Ⓓ Esophagoscopy

Ⓔ 3rd degree
(necrosis) → Perforation

2nd degree
(ulceration) → No perforation

Ⓕ 1st degree
(erythema only) → No treatment
Obs 24–48 hr

Ⓖ Transhiatal esophagectomy
± gastric resection
± gastrostomy
Cervical esophagostomy
Jejunostomy

NPO
IVF
Antibiotics → Perforation
H_2-receptor antagonist
PPI, antacids

Barium swallow at 24 hr

Observation

Ⓗ Elective gastrostomy
Nasogastric string
Retrograde dilation

Ⓘ Elective
esophageal
stent with
gastrostomy

Ⓙ Antibiotics
TPN or
nasal
jejunostomy
tube

Chapter 41 *Gastroesophageal Reflux Disease*

THOMAS N. ROBINSON, MD

(A) Gastroesophageal reflux disease (GERD) clinically presents with both typical and atypical symptoms. Typical reflux symptoms include heartburn and regurgitation. A recumbent position usually exacerbates typical symptoms. Atypical reflux symptoms include reflux laryngitis, substernal chest pain, cough, reactive airway disease, and loss of dental enamel.

(B) GERD is defined as the reflux of gastric contents into the esophagus. More than 40 million people in the United States have symptoms of GERD. The pathophysiology of GERD includes dysfunction of the lower esophageal sphincter, impaired ability of the esophagus to clear reflux with peristalsis, elevated intra-abdominal pressures, gastric distension, and duodenal reflux. Medical treatment is aimed at neutralizing gastric acid to prevent the symptoms of acid exposure in the esophagus. Surgical treatment is aimed at creating a new valve at the gastroesophageal junction, which prevents gastric reflux into the esophagus.

(C) Lifestyle modifications are the first line of treatment of GERD. Lifestyle modifications include avoiding recumbency following meals; elevating the head of bed for sleeping; avoiding foods that exacerbate reflux (e.g., chocolates, coffee, alcohol, and fatty meals); smoking cessation; and weight loss.

(D) Medical therapy is the second line of treatment of GERD. The mainstays of medical management include antacids, histamine type 2 receptor antagonists, proton pump inhibitors, and prokinetic agents. Empiric therapy for patients with GERD symptoms is appropriate; however, chronic treatment of GERD without further evaluation is not appropriate. Diagnostic evaluation is indicated when symptoms do not improve with medical treatment, when symptoms recur after discontinuation of medical treatment leading to chronic medical treatment, or when complications of GERD (e.g., dysphagia, bleeding, or aspiration) occur.

(E) Medical treatment of GERD without resolution of symptoms suggests a different etiology of the pain. Other potential causes of epigastric abdominal pain are symptomatic cholelithiasis, peptic ulcer disease, and pancreatitis. Appropriate evaluations for each disease process should be performed.

(F) Indications for antireflux surgery include the following: (1) a healthy patient who prefers surgery to lifelong medical treatment; (2) complications of GERD (e.g., stricture, bleeding, or refractory esophagitis); and (3) failure of improvement of extra-esophageal symptoms (e.g., airway disease or laryngitis). An operation is not reserved solely for patients who fail medical management. The American College of Gastroenterology guideline statement on GERD reads: "Antireflux surgery ... is a maintenance option for the patient with well-documented reflux."

(G) Esophagogastroduodenoscopy (EGD) is the initial diagnostic test for patients with GERD. EGD provides visualization of the esophagus to determine the extent of injury. Biopsy with subsequent histology identifies esophagitis, strictures, Barrett's syndrome, dysplasia, and carcinoma. EGD is required before surgical repair.

(H) Adenocarcinoma of the esophagus is associated with GERD. The finding of carcinoma should lead to esophageal cancer staging and surgical resection if indicated.

(I) High-grade dysplasia is a finding concerning for malignancy. Studies have shown that 40% of patients with high-grade dysplasia have carcinoma found in the surgically resected specimen. Repeated EGD with four-quadrant biopsies using jumbo forceps at 2-cm intervals along the segment of dysplasia may be helpful in determining which patients with dysplasia have carcinoma.

(J) A 24-hour ambulatory pH study quantifies the acid exposure in the esophagus; it is sensitive and specific for GERD. An abnormal 24-hour esophageal pH study is the single best predictor of a successful outcome following antireflux surgery. Acid-suppressing medications must be discontinued before the pH study. Esophageal manometry quantifies esophageal peristalsis. Peak amplitudes of primary peristaltic waves of less than 40 mm Hg define esophageal dysmotility.

(K) Upper gastrointestinal swallow study, or esophagogram, defines esophageal anatomy. Anatomic abnormalities include hiatal hernia, paraesophageal hernia, and shortened esophagus.

(L) Successful antireflux surgery requires appropriate patient selection. Multi-variant analysis reveals three factors that reliably predict successful outcome following laparoscopic Nissen (360-degree) fundoplication: (1) typical reflux symptoms; (2) an abnormal 24-hour ambulatory esophageal pH study; and (3) clinical improvement of symptoms with acid-suppressing medications. If all three predictors are favorable, then there is a greater than 90% chance of a successful outcome following surgery. Preoperative evaluation includes history/physical, EGD, 24-hour esophageal pH probe, and upper gastrointestinal swallow study.

(M) Laparoscopic Nissen fundoplication is the procedure of choice for virtually all patients with GERD. Greater than 90% patient satisfaction is achieved following a technically sound procedure. The key points of a successful procedure include adequate mediastinal dissection to mobilize the lower esophagus into the abdominal cavity, division of the short gastric vessels, posterior crural reconstruction, and a loose (or floppy) fundoplication over the distal esophagus. Creation of the fundoplication over a 56 Fr. bougie facilitates a loose wrap.

Complications of antireflux surgery include short-term and long-term problems. Approximate perioperative mortality is 1% and morbidity (i.e., pneumothorax, bleeding, or esophageal or gastric perforation) is 10%. Technical failures of antireflux surgery result from failure to perform a crural repair

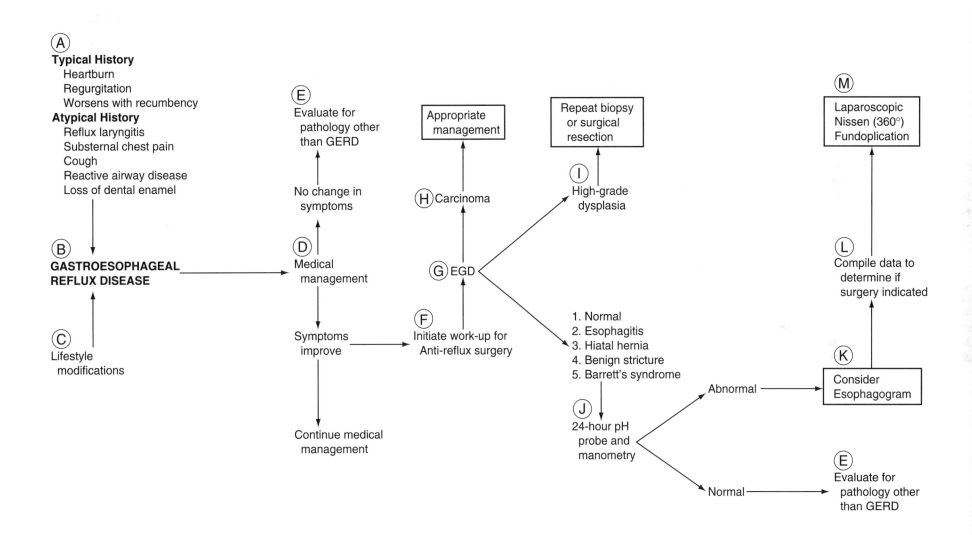

(A)
Typical History
  Heartburn
  Regurgitation
  Worsens with recumbency
Atypical History
  Reflux laryngitis
  Substernal chest pain
  Cough
  Reactive airway disease
  Loss of dental enamel

(B)
GASTROESOPHAGEAL REFLUX DISEASE

(C)
Lifestyle modifications

(E)
Evaluate for pathology other than GERD

No change in symptoms

(D)
Medical management

Symptoms improve

Continue medical management

(F)
Initiate work-up for Anti-reflux surgery

Appropriate management

(H) Carcinoma

(G) EGD

1. Normal
2. Esophagitis
3. Hiatal hernia
4. Benign stricture
5. Barrett's syndrome

(J)
24-hour pH probe and manometry

Repeat biopsy or surgical resection

(I)
High-grade dysplasia

Abnormal

Normal

(K)
Consider Esophagogram

(E)
Evaluate for pathology other than GERD

(L)
Compile data to determine if surgery indicated

(M)
Laparoscopic Nissen (360°) Fundoplication

resulting in herniation, creation of a wrap that is too tight resulting in dysphagia, and malformation of the fundoplication by using the body of the stomach rather than the fundus to create the wrap.

The tailored approach to antireflux surgery based on esophageal motility is antiquated. In the 1990s, partial (Toupet or 270-degree) fundoplication was used in cases of esophageal dysmotility. The rationale was that the incidence of dysphagia was reduced by avoiding a 360-degree fundoplication in patients with weak esophageal motility. Long-term results of multiple studies have shown a higher incidence of recurrent reflux following partial fundoplication in comparison to 360-degree fundoplication with equal rates of dysphagia. A floppy 360-degree fundoplication is the most durable form of antireflux surgery. Indications for partial fundoplication are limited to named esophageal motility disorders (i.e., achalasia and diffuse esophageal spasm).

REFERENCES

Campos GM, Peters JH, DeMeester TR et al: Multivariate analysis of factors predicting outcome after laparoscopic Nissen fundoplication. J Gastrointest Surg 3:292–300, 1999.

DeVault KR, Castell DO: Updated guidelines for the diagnosis and treatment of gastroesophageal reflux disease. The Practice Parameters Committee of the American College of Gastroenterology. Am J Gastroenterol 94:1434–1442, 1999.

Horgan S, Pohl D, Bogetti D et al: Failed antireflux surgery: What have we learned from reoperations? Arch Surg 134:809–815; discussion 815–817, 1999.

Horvath KD, Jobe BA, Herron DM et al: Laparoscopic Toupet fundoplication is an inadequate procedure for patients with severe reflux disease. J Gastrointest Surg 3:583–591, 1999.

Oleynikov D, Eubanks TR, Oelschlager BK et al: Total fundoplication is the operation of choice for patients with gastroesophageal reflux and defective peristalsis. Surg Endosc 16:909–913, 2002.

SAGES Guidelines: Guidelines for surgical treatment of gastroesophageal reflux disease (GERD). Surg Endosc 12:186–188, 1998.

Terry M, Smith CD, Branum GD et al: Outcomes of laparoscopic fundoplication for gastroesophageal reflux disease and paraesophageal hernia. Surg Endoscop 15:691–699, 2001.

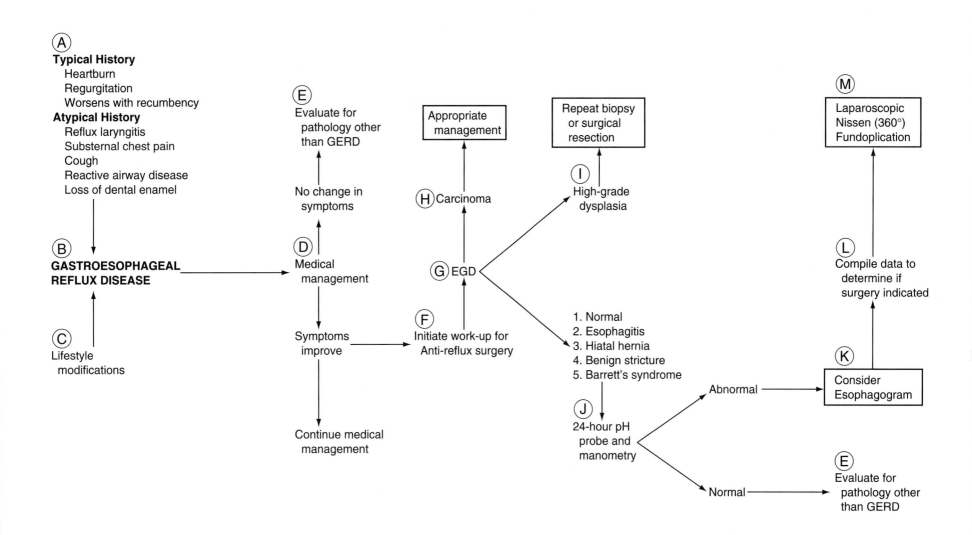

(A) **Typical History**
 Heartburn
 Regurgitation
 Worsens with recumbency
Atypical History
 Reflux laryngitis
 Substernal chest pain
 Cough
 Reactive airway disease
 Loss of dental enamel

(B) **GASTROESOPHAGEAL REFLUX DISEASE**

(C) Lifestyle modifications

(E) Evaluate for pathology other than GERD

No change in symptoms

(D) Medical management

Symptoms improve

Continue medical management

(F) Initiate work-up for Anti-reflux surgery

(H) Carcinoma

(G) EGD

Appropriate management

(I) High-grade dysplasia

Repeat biopsy or surgical resection

1. Normal
2. Esophagitis
3. Hiatal hernia
4. Benign stricture
5. Barrett's syndrome

(J) 24-hour pH probe and manometry

Abnormal

Normal

(K) Consider Esophagogram

(L) Compile data to determine if surgery indicated

(M) Laparoscopic Nissen (360°) Fundoplication

(E) Evaluate for pathology other than GERD

Chapter 42 *Gastric Ulcer*

DAVID W. MERCER, MD • EMILY K. ROBINSON, MD

(A) Gastric ulcers, unlike erosions, extend through the muscularis mucosa and tend to occur near mucosal junctions. Gastric acid was long considered a prerequisite for ulcer formation. In fact, most ulcers are caused by *Helicobacter pylori* infection or by ingestion of nonsteroidal anti-inflammatory drugs (NSAIDs).

(B) Epigastric pain, the most common symptom, occurs in 70% of patients; it is nocturnal in 30% to 45% and is often relieved by eating.

(C) Dyspepsia is manifested as epigastric discomfort, nausea, belching, and bloating. The majority of patients with dyspepsia do not have peptic ulcer disease. Other causes of dyspepsia are gastroesophageal reflux, drugs, pregnancy, delayed gastric emptying, biliary or pancreatic diseases, and mesenteric ischemia.

(D) Decreased appetite is present in 40% to 60% of patients. It may be accompanied by belching or bloating.

(E) Vomiting can occur with gastric outlet obstruction from prepyloric ulcers. Weight loss is suggestive of malignancy but can also occur with chronic outlet obstruction.

(F) Anemia may be the only sign or symptom of a malignant gastric ulcer.

(G) All NSAIDs produce mucosal damage. The risk of ulcer is dose related. Each year some 2% to 4% of NSAID users have GI complications. About 1 patient in 10 who takes NSAIDs daily develops an acute ulcer. Other medications, such as aspirin and steroids, can also cause acute gastric ulcers or erosions.

(H) Guaiac-positive stools detected on rectal examination are an important clue to gastric disease. A rectal mass anteriorly on rectal examination (Blumer shelf) suggests metastatic gastric cancer.

(I) A complete blood count (CBC) may demonstrate anemia, and a chemistry panel may reveal hypokalemic metabolic alkalosis in the presence of gastric outlet obstruction.

(J) Gastric analysis can demonstrate achlorhydria, which is suggestive of malignancy. Barium contrast studies (in the absence of perforation) are 90% accurate in diagnosing gastric ulcer. Such studies are complementary to, not a substitute for, endoscopy.

(K) Perforation carries a mortality rate of 10% to 40% depending on the presence of preoperative shock, significant underlying medical illness, and perforation of greater than 24 hours' duration. Plain x-rays of the abdomen are necessary when perforation is suspected. Free air is seen in about 70% of cases.

(L) Endoscopy is 90% accurate in diagnosing gastric ulcer. It can define five types of ulcers:

Type 1	Incisura or inferior lesser curvature
Type 2	Gastric and duodenal
Type 3	Pyloric or prepyloric
Type 4	Juxtacardial
Type 5	Occurs anywhere in the stomach and is a direct result of chronic ingestion of aspirin or NSAID

Endoscopy permits four-quadrant margin and central biopsy of the ulcer and brushing of all chronic gastric ulcerations to exclude malignancy. Brush cytology findings may be positive when biopsy is negative.

(M) Optimal management requires excision of the ulcer, usually best accomplished by distal gastrectomy. In hemodynamically unstable patients, excision of the perforation site is advisable with closure or four-quadrant biopsy and omental closure. Recurrence rates approximate 40% to 90% after closure; thus the addition of truncal vagotomy and pyloroplasty may be of benefit. For obstruction, the patient can be treated with antrectomy and gastroduodenostomy, although if scarring is so severe as to preclude a safe anastomosis, a gastrojejunostomy in conjunction with a truncal vagotomy should be performed.

(N) *H. pylori* is present in most gastric ulcer patients (60% to 90%). Gastric ulcer patients who are not infected tend to be NSAID users. All tests currently available for diagnosing *H. pylori* have good sensitivity and specificity. Noninvasive tests include serologic tests (sensitivity 90%, specificity 95%; cost is $15 in the office and $75 in the lab) and the urea breath test (sensitivity 95%; specificity 98%; cost $200). Invasive tests include the rapid urease assay (sensitivity 90%, specificity 98%, cost $10) and histology and culture (sensitivities 95% and 80%, respectively: specificities, 99% and 100%, respectively; the two tests cost roughly $150 each). It is not necessary to perform endoscopy to diagnose *H. pylori*. For initial diagnosis without endoscopy, serology is the test of choice. With endoscopy, rapid urease assay and histologic examination are both excellent options, although the rapid urease test is less expensive. The urea breath test is the test of choice to document eradication after treatment.

(O) Patients with ulcer disease whose *H. pylori* infection is successfully cured or eradicated virtually never develop recurrent ulcers. With persistent *H. pylori* infection, the annual relapse rate is roughly 58%, as opposed to roughly 2% when *H. pylori* has been eradicated. In general, triple therapy is more successful than dual therapy or monotherapy for eradicating *H. pylori*. Three promising triple regimens are currently available: OAC, OMC, and OAM. O represents omeprazole; A represents amoxicillin; C represents clarithromycin; and M represents metronidazole. These treatments last 2 weeks. The drugs contain no bismuth, and twice-daily dosing is an advantage.

(P) Drugs can heal ulcers by neutralizing acid secretion or by restoring mucosal defenses. Prostaglandins increase mucus, bicarbonate, and bloodflow. Sucralfate and low-dose antacids promote ulcer healing by unknown mechanisms. The histamine-(H_2) receptor antagonists are structurally similar to histamine and differ in potency, half-life,

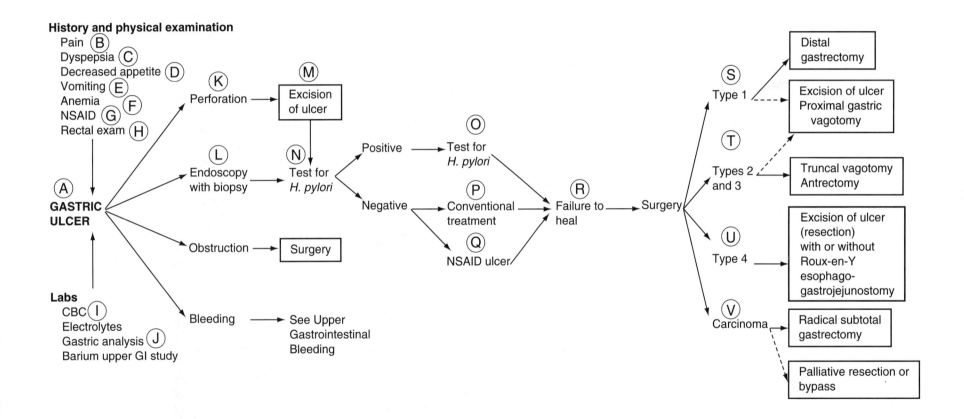

History and physical examination
- Pain Ⓑ
- Dyspepsia Ⓒ
- Decreased appetite Ⓓ
- Vomiting Ⓔ
- Anemia Ⓕ
- NSAID Ⓖ
- Rectal exam Ⓗ

Ⓐ **GASTRIC ULCER**

Labs
- CBC Ⓘ
- Electrolytes
- Gastric analysis Ⓙ
- Barium upper GI study

Ⓚ Perforation → Ⓜ Excision of ulcer

Ⓛ Endoscopy with biopsy → Ⓝ Test for *H. pylori*

Obstruction → Surgery

Bleeding → See Upper Gastrointestinal Bleeding

Positive → Ⓞ Test for *H. pylori*

Negative → Ⓟ Conventional treatment

Ⓠ NSAID ulcer

Ⓡ Failure to heal → Surgery

Ⓢ Type 1 → Distal gastrectomy

Ⓣ Types 2 and 3 → Excision of ulcer Proximal gastric vagotomy

Truncal vagotomy Antrectomy

Ⓤ Type 4 → Excision of ulcer (resection) with or without Roux-en-Y esophago-gastrojejunostomy

Ⓥ Carcinoma → Radical subtotal gastrectomy

Palliative resection or bypass

and bioavailability. Oral doses produce equivalent inhibition of parietal cell secretion. Continuous IV infusion of H_2-receptor antagonists produces more uniform acid inhibition than does intermittent administration. The H^+-K^+-adenosine triphosphatase (ATPase) is the gastric pump responsible for the final step in parietal cell acid secretion. This pump requires large amounts of energy supplied by intracellular ATP and is the final transport pathway for parietal cell hydrogen ion secretion. Because of this, inhibitors of the pump block all types of acid secretion. A proton-pump inhibitor like omeprazole inhibits acid secretion more completely than an H_2-receptor antagonist, and it produces more prolonged inhibition of acid secretion than H_2-blockers. Smoking cessation should be encouraged. Ulcer recurrence is increased by heavy alcohol use.

(Q) Once an NSAID-induced ulcer has developed, it is best to discontinue the NSAID, if possible, while the ulcer is being treated. Ulcer therapy is initiated with an antisecretory agent such as an H_2-receptor antagonist or, preferably, with a proton-pump inhibitor such as omeprazole. *H. pylori* infection should be treated. For NSAID-dependent patients, cotherapy with misoprostol, a prostaglandin analog, or switching to a safer NSAID that inhibits the inducible isoform of cyclooxygenase (COX-2) is recommended.

(R) The gastric ulcer should be treated for 8 to 12 weeks and then evaluated for healing. If the ulcer has healed, maintenance therapy should be considered if the patient is not taking NSAIDs and does not have *H. pylori* infection. The indications for operation are intractability, hemorrhage, perforation, and obstruction. Intractability is rarely a reason for operation today because of the relatively effective medications available. Historically, incomplete healing by 12 weeks was almost an absolute indication for operation;

however, most gastroenterologists no longer follow these guidelines.

(S) Type 1 is the most common form of gastric ulcer (55% to 60%). Optimal treatment is distal gastrectomy that includes the ulcer followed by gastroduodenal anastomosis (Billroth I). Truncal vagotomy is not indicated because these ulcers are not generally associated with excessive acid secretion. Elective gastrectomy has mortality and recurrence rates of 2% each. Proximal gastric vagotomy with excision of the ulcer is associated with lower mortality and morbidity rates, but recurrence rates are high (8% to 25%).

(T) Types 2 and 3 gastric ulcers are associated with acid hypersecretion and comprise 20% to 25% of cases of benign disease. Treatment is directed at reducing acid secretion. Vagotomy decreases peak hydrogen ion output by approximately 50%, and vagotomy plus antrectomy by approximately 85%. Truncal vagotomy with antrectomy incorporating the ulcer in the resection has been the treatment of choice. Proximal gastric vagotomy (highly selective vagotomy or parietal cell vagotomy) is an acceptable alternative provided the ulcer is also excised. It is as effective as truncal vagotomy in decreasing acid secretion and produces less severe side effects but has a higher recurrence rate.

(U) A gastric ulcer at the gastroesophageal junction is type 4. These ulcers are uncommon in the United States. Resection ensures the lowest long-term recurrence rate but introduces technical problems. The resection must be carried as a tongue high onto the lesser curvature. To avoid narrowing the gastric inlet, reconstruction with a Roux-en-Y esophagogastrojejunostomy (Csendes' procedure) is recommended for ulcers within 2 cm of the gastroesophageal junction.

(V) A radical subtotal gastrectomy with antecolic Billroth II reconstruction or Roux-en-Y is

preferred treatment for a malignant gastric ulcer. Distant metastases indicate unresectability for cure, although a palliative resection or bypass may be required.

REFERENCES

Buckner JW III, Austin JC, Steinberg JB et al: Factors predicting failure of medical therapy of gastric ulcers. Am J Surg 158:570–573, 1989.

Csendes A, Braghetto I, Smok G: Type IV gastric ulcer: A new hypothesis. Surgery 101:361–366, 1987.

Donahue PE: Parietal cell vagotomy versus vagotomy-antrectomy: Ulcer surgery in the modern era. World J Surg 24:264–269, 2000.

Freston JW: Management of peptic ulcers: Emerging issues. World J Surg 24:250–255, 2000.

Fries JF, Miller SR, Spitz PW et al: Toward an epidemiology of gastropathy associated with nonsteroidal anti-inflammatory drug use. Gastroenterology 96:647–655, 1989.

Hodnett RM, Gonzalez F, Lee WC et al: The need for definitive therapy in the management of perforated gastric ulcers: Review of 202 cases. Ann Surg 209:36–39, 1989.

NIH Consensus Conference: Helicobacter pylori in peptic ulcer disease. JAMA 272:65–69, 1994.

Richardson CT: Gastric Ulcer. In Slesinger M, Fordtran J (eds): Gastrointestinal Disease: Pathophysiology, Diagnosis, and Management. Philadelphia: WB Saunders, 1989.

Ross P, Dutton AM: Computer analysis of symptom complexes in patients having upper gastrointestinal examinations. Am J Dig Dis 17:248–254, 1977.

Sachs G, Carlsson E, Lindberg P et al: Gastric H^+K^+ATPase as a therapeutic target. Ann Rev Pharmacol Toxicol 28:269–284, 1988.

Sachs G, Wallmark B: The gastric H^+K^+ATPase: The site of action of omeprazole. Scand J Gastroenterol Suppl 166:3–11, 1989.

Soll AH: Pathogenesis of peptic ulcer and implications for treatment. N Engl J Med 322:909–916, 1990.

Sonnenberg A: Changes in physician visits for gastric and duodenal ulcer in the United States during 1958–1984 as shown by National Disease and Therapeutic Index (NDTI). Dig Dis Sci 32:1–7, 1987.

Tytgat GNJ: Treatments that impact favorably upon the eradication of Helicobacter pylori and ulcer recurrence. Aliment Pharmacol Ther 8:359–368, 1994.

Wolfe MM, Soll AH: The physiology of gastric acid secretion. N Engl J Med 319:1707–1715, 1988.

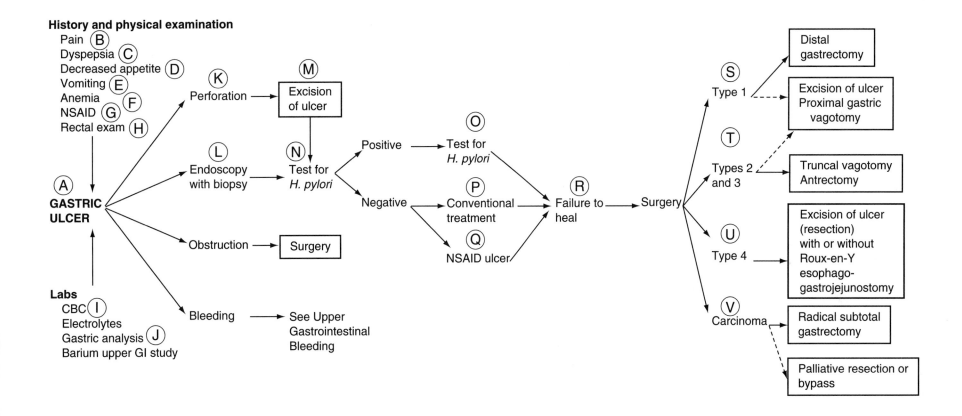

History and physical examination
Pain (B)
Dyspepsia (C)
Decreased appetite (D)
Vomiting (E)
Anemia (F)
NSAID (G)
Rectal exam (H)

(A)

**GASTRIC
ULCER**

Labs
CBC (I)
Electrolytes
Gastric analysis (J)
Barium upper GI study

(K) Perforation

(L) Endoscopy
with biopsy

Obstruction

Bleeding

(M)
Excision
of ulcer

(N)
Test for
H. pylori

Surgery

See Upper
Gastrointestinal
Bleeding

Positive

Negative

(O) Test for
H. pylori

(P) Conventional
treatment

(Q) NSAID ulcer

(R) Failure to
heal

Surgery

(S) Type 1

(T) Types 2
and 3

(U) Type 4

(V) Carcinoma

Distal
gastrectomy

Excision of ulcer
Proximal gastric
vagotomy

Truncal vagotomy
Antrectomy

Excision of ulcer
(resection)
with or without
Roux-en-Y
esophago-
gastrojejunostomy

Radical subtotal
gastrectomy

Palliative resection or
bypass

Chapter 43 *Duodenal Ulcer*

GEORGE B. KAZANTSEV, MD, PhD • WAYNE H. SCHWESINGER, MD

(A) Peptic ulcer disease of the duodenum continues to be a serious health problem that causes about 1 million hospital admissions and nearly 15,000 deaths annually. The majority of duodenal ulcers are caused either by infection of the stomach with *Helicobacter pylori* (90%) or by long-term use of nonsteroidal anti-inflammatory drugs (NSAIDs).

(B) Although healing rates of 95% can be achieved with the use of H$_2$-receptor blockers or proton-pump inhibitors alone, most ulcers recur within 2 years once antisecretory therapy is stopped. Noninvasive testing with serologic or breath tests accurately identifies those patients who have an underlying *H. pylori* infection. Subsequent therapy in these patients with a variety of short-term, multiple-drug regimens can eradicate most such infections and produces a cost-effective, durable cure of the ulcer in 85% to 95% of treated cases. A recent meta-analysis confirms recurrence rates for duodenal ulcer following *H. pylori* eradication of only 6% compared with 67% without eradication. Failure to eradicate *H. pylori* infection may result from the emergence of resistant strains or from poor patient compliance. Any complementary role of NSAID use is still undefined.

(C) Serum gastrin levels should be measured when the diagnosis of gastrinoma is suggested by massive hypersecretion (diarrhea), prominent rugae, multiple and/or distal ulcers, or medical/surgical refractory ulcer. Fasting gastrin levels may be slightly elevated in patients who are taking antisecretory medications. If a patient is able to stop PPI without difficulty for 1 week, then a fasting serum gastrin and a gastric fluid pH is measured after 1 week. If the patient has severe symptoms with discontinuation of PPI, a H$_2$-receptor antagonist (H$_2$RA) can be used for 1 week. Then the H$_2$RA is discontinued for 30 hours and the fasting gastrin and gastric fluid pH obtained. The diagnosis of gastrinoma is made if the gastric fluid pH is less than 2.5 and the gastrin is greater than 1000 pg/ml. Gastrinoma is excluded in a patient with a serum gastrin level lower than 100 pg/ml or pH greater than 2.5 (hypochlorhydria/achlorhydria). If the patient has moderate gastrin elevation (i.e., 101 to 999 pg/ml) and a pH lower than 2.5, then a secretin stimulation test should be performed.

(D) Hemorrhage is the most serious and common complication of peptic ulcer disease (overall mortality 2% to 10%). When aggressively treated, ulcer bleeding is self-limited in 80% of patients. Initial medical therapy includes the administration of appropriate transfusions, infusion of antisecretory drugs, and correction of coagulopathies.

(E) Gastric outlet obstruction has been reported in 6% to 8% of patients with duodenal ulcers. It results from edema or scarring adjacent to prepyloric or channel ulcers. Endoscopy confirms the benign nature of the lesion and affords appraisal of the severity of obstruction. Endoscopic balloon dilation has been used with limited success in certain very special cases but is associated with a modest risk of perforation. A short-term trial of nasogastric tube decompression, combined with medical management of the ulcer, relieves the obstruction in some patients; the remainder require surgical correction.

(F) Most patients with perforated duodenal ulcer present with the abrupt onset of severe abdominal pain and rigidity. The symptoms tend to be subtler in elderly patients and in persons who take steroids.

(G) When patients remain symptomatic after 6 to 8 weeks of optimal therapy, endoscopy should be used to confirm the diagnosis and redirect therapy. Other serious lesions should be sought, including gastrinomas, gastric ulcers or tumors, inflammatory bowel disease, and hepatobiliary or pancreatic disorders. A persistent but partially healed duodenal ulcer may benefit from further medical management using higher doses or more potent agents. Renewed attention should also be given to the avoidance of risk factors such as smoking, ethanol, aspirin, and NSAIDs.

(H) Endoscopy should be performed once the patient has stabilized. The endoscopic appearance of the ulcer helps to predict its course. Clean-based ulcers rarely rebleed and do not require intervention, whereas ulcers with an adherent clot or a nonbleeding visible vessel have higher risks of rebleeding (22% and 43%, respectively) and require aggressive intervention. Multipolar and monopolar electrocoagulation, as well as heater probe and injection therapy, have been shown to control the majority of bleeding episodes and to decrease their associated mortality. Bleeding may persist or recur in up to 20% of higher-risk patients; at least half eventually require emergency operation. Eradication of *H. pylori* has been shown to significantly reduce the frequency of recurrent bleeding.

(I) Simple closure of the perforation with a Graham patch and subsequent *H. pylori* eradication is associated with recurrence rate of only 4.8%, obviating the need for more extensive ulcer surgery in the majority of patients. Laparoscopic methods have been shown to be highly effective and well-tolerated when combined with appropriate medical therapy.

(J) Definitive operation should be considered in patients who are *H. pylori* negative, who have failed adequate *H. pylori* therapy, or who are NSAID-dependent. Highly selective vagotomy is the treatment of choice and may be performed using an open or laparoscopic approach. Hemodynamic instability and heavy peritoneal contamination are recognized as contraindications.

(K) In a high-risk patient, when endoscopic control of ulcer bleeding has failed, angiography can localize the bleeding site by demonstrating extravasation from the gastroduodenal artery or the anterior superior or posterior superior pancreaticoduodenal arteries. Hemostasis can be induced in 60% to 90% of patients by transcatheter embolization of the vessel.

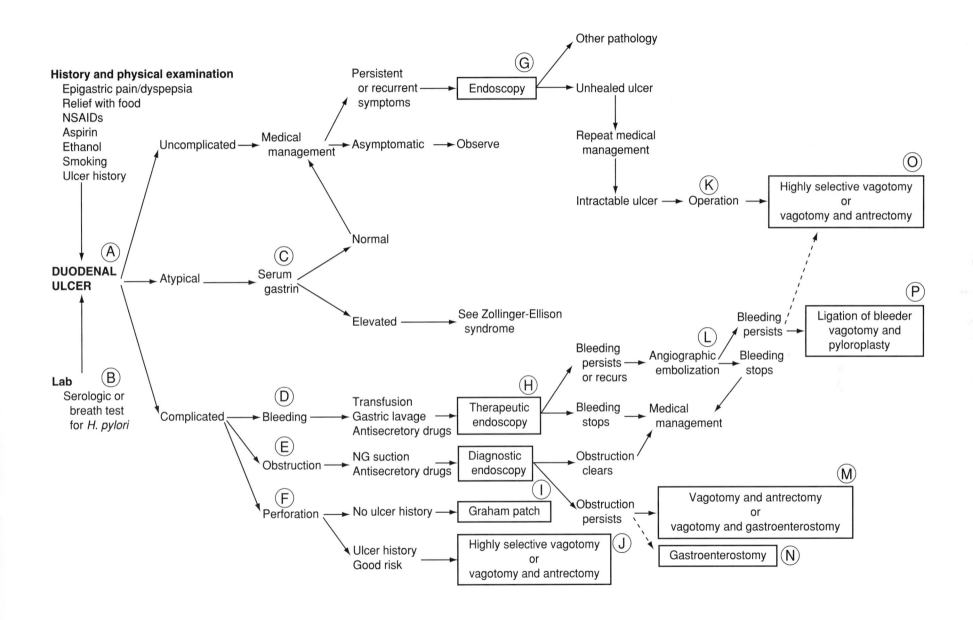

History and physical examination
Epigastric pain/dyspepsia
Relief with food
NSAIDs
Aspirin
Ethanol
Smoking
Ulcer history

Lab
Serologic or
breath test
for *H. pylori*

(L) Open vagotomy with antrectomy is recommended for severe obstruction and for giant ulcers (greater than 2 cm). As an alternative, the laparoscopic approach with highly selective vagotomy and gastrojejunostomy also yields satisfactory results.

(M) Gastroenterostomy without vagotomy may be advisable in elderly patients, especially men, to avoid postoperative gastric atony.

(N) Operations for duodenal ulcer have become less common as nonoperative measures have improved. Nonetheless, surgical therapy may become necessary if ulcer disease is complicated or intractable. Most operative approaches have two major objectives: (1) to relieve specific ulcer-related problems and (2) to prevent recurrence. The defined risks and benefits of the different procedures vary and can be used to determine their respective roles (see following). All such procedures can be successfully performed laparoscopically, but this approach should be limited to specialized centers and/or to surgeons who have completed advanced laparoscopic training.

Vagotomy/Pyloroplasty
Recurrence   12%
Mortality   1%
Morbidity   15% to 20%

Vagotomy/Antrectomy
Recurrence   1%
Mortality   1% to 2%
Morbidity   15% to 20%

Highly Selective Vagotomy
Recurrence   10% to 15%
Mortality   0.5%
Morbidity   5%

(O) Highly selective vagotomy is the treatment of choice for intractability. Laparoscopic methods can reliably reproduce the results achieved with open procedures.

(P) Vagotomy with pyloroplasty is usually preferred for the management of acute bleeding ulcer. Oversewing of the bleeding site is essential.

REFERENCES

Awad W, Csendes A, Braghetto I et al: Laparoscopic highly selective vagotomy: Technical considerations and preliminary results in 119 patients with duodenal ulcer or gastroesophageal reflux disease. World J Surg 21:261–269, 1997.

Chung SC: Surgery and gastrointestinal bleeding. Surg Clin North Am 7:687–701, 1997.

Dubois F: New surgical strategy for gastroduodenal ulcer: Laparoscopic approach. World J Surg 24:270–276, 2000.

Hopkins RJ, Girardi LS, Turney EA: Relationship between Helicobacter pylori eradication and reduced duodenal and gastric ulcer recurrence: A review. Gastroenterology 110: 1244–1252, 1996.

Katkhouda N, Mavor E, Mason RJ et al: Laparoscopic repair of perforated duodenal ulcers: Outcome and efficacy in 30 consecutive patients. Arch Surg 134:845–850, 1999.

Ng E, Lam YH, Sung JJY et al: Eradication of Helicobacter pylori prevents recurrence of ulcer after simple closure of duodenal ulcer perforation: Randomized controlled trial. Ann Surg 231:153–158, 2000.

Schwesinger WH, Page CP, Sirinek KR et al: Operations for peptic ulcer disease: Paradigm lost. J Gastrointest Surg 5:438–443, 2001.

Siu WT, Leong HT, Law BKB et al: Laparoscopic repair for perforated peptic ulcer: A randomized controlled trial. Ann Surg 235:313–319, 2002.

Soll AH: Medical treatment of peptic ulcer disease. JAMA 275:622–629, 1996.

Van der Hulst RW, Rauws EA, Koycu B et al: Prevention of ulcer recurrence after eradication of Helicobacter pylori: A prospective long-term follow-up study. Gastroenterology 113:1082–1086, 1997.

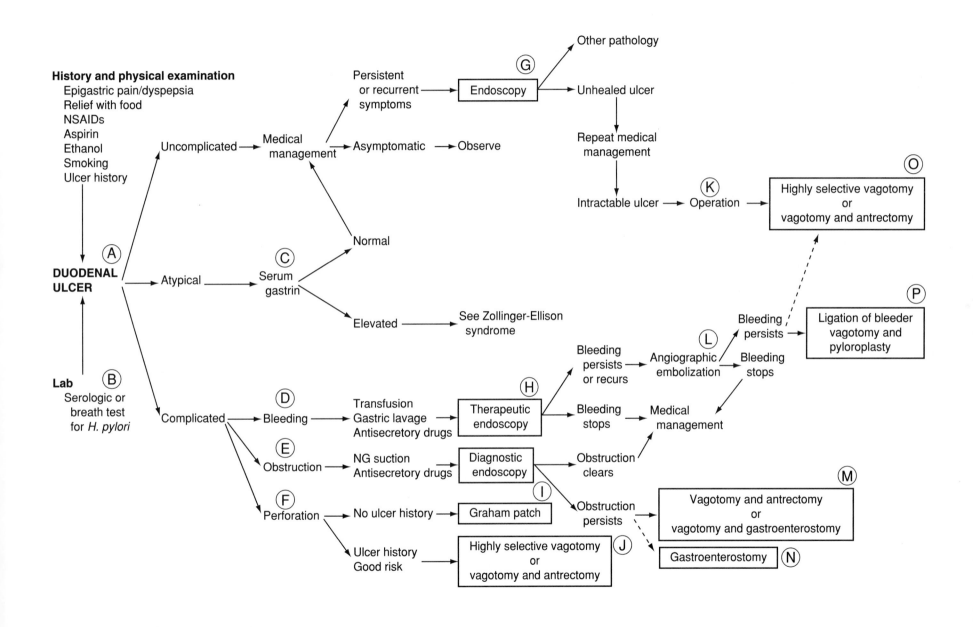

Chapter 44 *Morbid Obesity*

ADOLFO Z. FERNANDEZ, JR., MD • DAVID S. TICHANSKY, MD •
HARVEY J. SUGERMAN, MD

(A) The initial history and physical examination determines a person's eligibility for surgical treatment of obesity. The patient must meet the weight criteria set by the 1991 National Institutes of Health (NIH) consensus conference. Endocrine disorders that cause obesity (e.g., hypothyroidism and Cushing's syndrome) must be ruled out. A detailed history of the failed, prior weight loss attempts through dietary or medical interventions must be reviewed along with a weight log demonstrating that obesity has been a chronic problem. Inadequate medical attempts at weight loss may require additional nonsurgical attempts. Occasionally, obesity comorbidity may be so severe (e.g., venous stasis ulcer, severe pseudotumor cerebri, or obesity hypoventilation) that one should proceed with bariatric surgery without a prolonged medical weight loss trial. Last, but most importantly, a basic understanding by the patient of the procedure, its risks, and its benefits is necessary before any further evaluation for surgery.

(B) Morbid obesity is reaching epidemic proportions in the United States. Western society has championed a fast food diet and sedentary lifestyle. Approximately 300,000 Americans die each year from causes related to obesity, and close to 10% of U.S. healthcare expenditures result from obesity and physical inactivity. The 1991 NIH consensus conference on GI surgery for severe obesity established the current weight guidelines for obesity surgery. To be candidates for obesity surgery, patients must have a body mass index (BMI) between 35 and $40 \, kg/m^2$ and either high-risk or lifestyle-limiting comorbid conditions; or a BMI greater than $40 \, kg/m^2$. Obesity-related comorbidities include pseudotumor cerebri, depression, hypertension (HTN), coronary artery disease (CAD), obstructive sleep apnea (OSA), obesity hypoventilation syndrome (Pickwickian syndrome), gastroesophageal reflux disease, cholelithiasis, nonalcoholic steatohepatitis (NASH), cirrhosis, diabetes mellitus (DM), hyperlipidemia, uterine cancer, breast cancer, colon cancer, venous stasis disease, venous stasis ulcers, hypercoagulability, peripheral vascular disease, degenerative joint disease, skin infections, dysmenorrhea, hirsutism, infertility, and stress urinary incontinence. Bariatric surgery is a rapidly growing field because of the effectiveness of surgically induced weight loss in correcting most of these obesity comorbidities, improved techniques and technology, and increased national media attention.

(C) Evaluation of the gallbladder, either before or during the operation, is essential. If gallstones are present, a cholecystectomy should be performed at the time of surgery. If gallstones are not present, then prophylactic treatment with ursodiol acid has been shown to significantly decrease the rate of gallstone formation in the rapid weight loss period.

(D) Patients who fail the initial evaluation may be counseled in other weight loss programs such as medically supervised diets, drug therapy, or diet and exercise programs. Unfortunately the reported rates of long-term success with medical weight loss programs are less than 10%.

(E) Morbid obesity has multiple comorbidities that can affect the outcome of surgery. A multidisciplinary approach to the care of the patient is needed. The initial evaluation should be a cooperative effort of all the disciplines necessary to best prepare the patient for surgery.

(F) The nutritionist is instrumental before and after operation. Initially, the nutritionist can reinforce the basic understanding of the procedure and the lifestyle changes necessary for success (e.g., the supplements necessary after malabsorptive procedures). After proximal gastric bypass, patients will require a daily multivitamin, calcium, and B_{12} supplements at a minimum. In addition, menstruating women will require iron supplementation. Patients with the more malabsorptive procedures will require all of the above plus fat-soluble vitamin supplementation. After the surgery, nutritionists can counsel patients on their dietary changes and alternatives, and help patients maintain their weight loss over the long term with additional dietary interventions.

(G) Routine psychological screening is important in all cases to establish the stability of the patient. Patients should be carefully questioned about substance abuse or alcoholism. Formal psychiatric evaluation is necessary in cases of active ongoing psychiatric disease or prior psychiatric hospitalizations. Adolescents planning to undergo bariatric surgery will benefit from a formal evaluation to establish their level of maturity and to provide them with postoperative care and support.

(H) Cardiac evaluation should be reserved for those patients with a history of chest pain, abnormal ECGs, CAD, or myocardial infarction; or for older patients with a long history of HTN or DM. Proper evaluation may require an echocardiogram or a cardiac stress test.

(I) A sleep study and arterial blood gas study is required for all patients with symptoms of sleep apnea (e.g., multiple night waking episodes, early morning headaches, loud snoring, somnolence while driving, or daily afternoon naps). All patients with a BMI of $50 \, kg/m^2$ or greater should have an arterial blood gas determination. An echocardiogram should be considered in patients with severe obesity hypoventilation or Pickwickian syndrome to rule out pulmonary hypertension. Involvement of a pulmonologist in the perioperative care of these patients may be helpful, along with an intraoperative pulmonary artery catheter.

(J) Morbidly obese patients are at high risk for the development of venous thromboembolism. All of the patients should routinely get thigh-high intermittent compression boots or foot pumps placed at the beginning of surgery, and preoperative as well as postoperative regular or low–molecular weight heparin prophylaxis. Prophylactic inferior vena caval (IVC) filters are placed in patients with Pickwickian

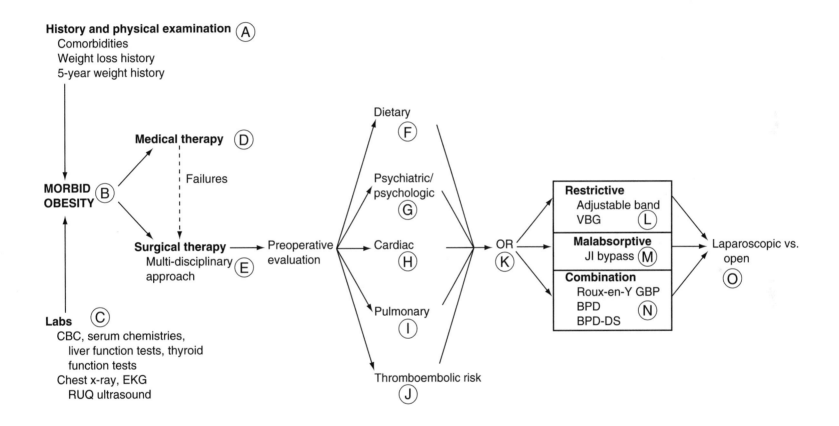

History and physical examination (A)
Comorbidities
Weight loss history
5-year weight history

Medical therapy (D)

Failures

**MORBID
OBESITY** (B)

Surgical therapy (E)
Multi-disciplinary
approach

Preoperative
evaluation

Dietary (F)

Psychiatric/
psychologic (G)

Cardiac (H)

Pulmonary (I)

Thromboembolic risk (J)

OR (K)

Labs (C)
CBC, serum chemistries,
liver function tests, thyroid
function tests
Chest x-ray, EKG
RUQ ultrasound

Restrictive
Adjustable band
VBG (L)

Malabsorptive
JI bypass (M)

Combination
Roux-en-Y GBP
BPD
BPD-DS (N)

Laparoscopic vs.
open
(O)

syndrome and pulmonary hypertension because of the significant potential danger of a fatal pulmonary embolus (PE). Prophylactic IVC filters are also routinely placed at the time of obesity surgery in patients with severe venous stasis disease because of a higher risk for a fatal PE.

(K) In the operating room, the morbidly obese patient requires special considerations. The positioning of these patients is critical. Care must be taken to reduce the risk of pressure ulcers or neurologic deficits. Intraoperative monitoring is a key component. All patients require a Foley catheter. In the more complex cases, a pulmonary artery catheter and/or radial artery line may be helpful. Intraoperative ultrasound may also be useful in evaluating the gallbladder of patients in which preoperative routine sonography is inadequate.

(L) The most commonly performed restrictive procedures include the vertical banded gastroplasty (VBG) and the adjustable gastric bands. The VBG does not produce as much excess weight loss (EWL) and is not as durable as the gastric bypass procedure (GBP). Compared with the GBP, it is simpler to perform, has less operative and micronutritional risk, and maintains the continuity of the gastrointestinal tract. The adjustable band works much the same as the VBG. Like the VBG, gastric banding does not appear to produce as much EWL and is not as durable as GBP. Furthermore, 25% to 30% of bands are removed by 3 years because of inadequate weight loss, band slippage/pouch dilation, obstruction, or infection.

(M) The first malabsorptive procedure was the jejunoileal bypass (JIB). The JIB had significant late complications including protein-calorie malnutrition, cirrhosis, severe osteoporosis, and interstitial nephritis. Some of these complications were attributed to the long segment of small intestine left without any flow of food or biliopancreatic secretions. This procedure is no longer approved for the treatment of morbid obesity.

(N) The Roux-en-Y gastric bypass procedure (GBP), the biliopancreatic diversion (BPD) and the biliopancreatic diversion–duodenal switch (BPD-DS) are both restrictive and malabsorptive. The GBP, a derivative of the VBG, is composed of a small, lesser-curved based gastric pouch holding about 20 milliliters. Description of the malabsorptive component varies from author to author. The most serious of its complications are leaks (about 2%), pulmonary embolus (less than 1%), and death (0.5% to 1.5%). It is the most common bariatric surgery performed in the United States. The average patient will lose about two-thirds of his or her EWL after the first 12 to 18 months and maintain this weight loss for the first 5 years. There is some long-term weight regain, but its most important benefit is the improvement in the patient's comorbidities. From the JIB the biliopancreatic diversion (BPD) was developed. The BPD is a horizontal gastrectomy and long Roux limb that connects 50 cm from the ileocecal valve. The common channel is short and induces a significant amount of malabsorption. Scopinaro reports an EWL of 70% that is maintained after 20 years of follow-up. The BPD may be complicated by osteoporosis, protein malnutrition, and anemia. The BPD-DS is a modification of the Scopinaro procedure in that a sleeve gastrectomy is performed and the pylorus is preserved. This eliminates the dumping syndrome and allows more freedom with the diet. The complications are similar to those of the BPD.

(O) All bariatric procedures can be done laparoscopically. The advantages of laparoscopy are the decreased rate of wound complications (e.g., incisional hernias and wound infections), decreased pulmonary sequella, and quicker recovery from surgery. Weight loss results appear to be equivalent to the open approach, although the data are still lacking.

REFERENCES

Brolin RE: Gastric bypass. Surg Clin North Am 81:1077–1095, 2001.

Brolin RL, Robertson LB, Kenler HA et al: Weight loss and dietary intake after vertical banded gastroplasty and Roux-en-Y gastric bypass. Ann Surg 220:782–790, 1994.

Ceelen W, Walder J, Cardon A et al: Surgical treatment of severe obesity with a low-pressure adjustable gastric band: Experimental data and clinical results in 625 patients. Ann Surg 237:10–16, 2003.

DeMaria EJ, Sugerman HJ, Meador JG et al: High failure rate after laparoscopic adjustable silicone gastric banding for treatment of morbid obesity. Ann Surg 233:809–818, 2001.

Doherty C, Maher JW, Heitshusen DS: Long-term data indicate a progressive loss in efficacy of adjustable silicone gastric banding for the surgical treatment of morbid obesity. Surgery 132:724–728, 2002.

Gastrointestinal surgery for severe obesity. National Institutes of Health consensus development conference statement. Am J Clin Nutr 55:615S–619S, 1992.

Mokdad AH, Bowman BA, Ford ES et al: The continuing epidemics of obesity and diabetes in the United States. JAMA 286:1195–1200, 2001.

Nguyen NT, Ho HS, Palmer LS et al: A comparison study of laparoscopic versus open gastric bypass for morbid obesity. J Am Coll Surg 191:149–157, 2000.

Schauer PR, Ikramuddin S, Gourash W et al: Outcomes after laparoscopic Roux-en-Y gastric bypass for morbid obesity. Ann Surg 232:515–529, 2000.

Scopinaro N, Gianetta E, Adami GF: Biliopancreatic diversion for obesity at 18 years. Surgery 119:261–268, 1996.

Sugerman HJ, DeMaria EJ: Gastric Surgery for Morbid Obesity. In Nyhus LM, Fischer JE, Baker RE (eds): Mastery of Surgery. Boston: Little, Brown & Co, 1997.

Sugerman HJ, Starkey JV, Birkenhauer R: A randomized prospective trial of gastric bypass versus vertical banded gastroplasty for morbid obesity and their effects on sweets versus nonsweets eaters. Ann Surg 205:613–624, 1987.

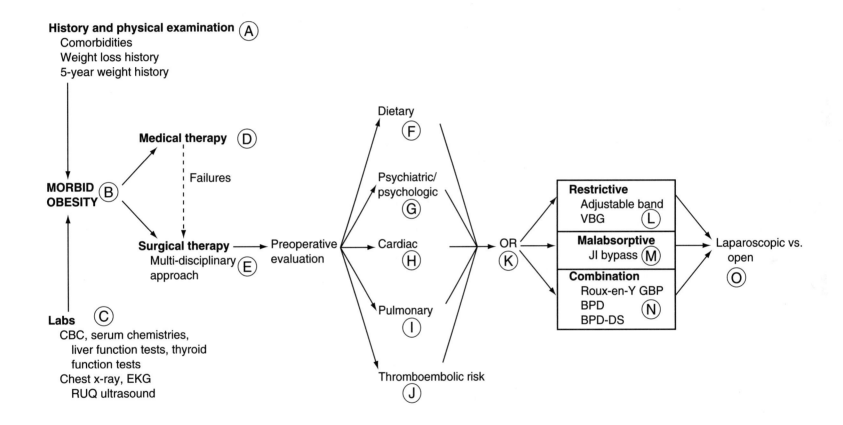

Chapter 45 *Upper Gastrointestinal Bleeding*

CHOICHI SUGAWA, MD, PhD

(A) Hematemesis signifies acute upper GI bleeding (UGIB); melena usually indicates moderate UGIB. The most common cause of UGIB is peptic ulcer disease. Recent ingestion of aspirin, nonsteroidal anti-inflammatory drugs (NSAIDs), or alcohol raises the possibility that erosive gastritis or an acute ulcer has developed. Other diseases that present with acute UGIB include portal hypertension (esophageal varices), mucosal tears of the gastroesophageal junction caused by severe retching or vomiting (Mallory-Weiss tears), esophagitis, gastric cancer, marginal ulcers, angiodysplasia, hemobilia, and aortoenteric fistula.

(B) Laboratory studies should include CBC; liver function studies (ALT, AST, bilirubin, albumin, total protein); prothrombin time (PT); partial thromboplastin time (PTT); and platelet counts. The hematocrit may significantly underestimate the amount of blood lost during an acute bleed. Immediately, type and cross-match should be ordered in case of massive bleeding. Serial hematocrits may be an indicator of ongoing bleeding or rebleeding and can help guide transfusions.

(C) Prompt attention to the ABCs (airway, breathing, and circulation) is required for patients with acute upper GI bleeding. A nasogastric tube (18 Fr) is passed to determine if bleeding is active. Crystalloid fluid is infused with a large-bore IV cannula. Blood is transfused in the presence of ongoing hemorrhage if greater than 1 L of blood is estimated to have been lost or if the patient fails to improve with crystalloid resuscitation.

(D) The stomach is irrigated with room temperature water or saline until the aspirate is clear. In massive, active bleeding, an orogastric tube is passed (32 to 36 Fr). In addition, an H_2-receptor antagonist is given IV. Endotracheal or nasotracheal intubation is recommended before emergency endoscopy for patients with massive bleeding, severe agitation, or impaired respiratory status. This facilitates both diagnostic and therapeutic endoscopy while minimizing the risk of aspiration.

(E) Endoscopy is the investigation method of choice for UGIB, identifying the bleeding site in 90% of patients. For massive UGIB, the esophagus should be irrigated well and examined for varices because bleeding from this source may be controlled without laparotomy. Deep, bleeding ulcers on the posterior duodenal bulb or high lesser curvature also carry high risk for major hemorrhage. Mallory-Weiss tears, acute erosive gastritis, and esophagitis rarely bleed persistently. When they do, there is usually an associated discrete ulcer with arterial bleeding or an overlying sentinel clot. Endoscopy should be performed with a large-channel therapeutic endoscope whenever possible. Patients with a nonbleeding Mallory-Weiss tear, erosive gastritis, esophagitis, or ulcers that have a clean white base can be discharged without hospital admission.

(F) Hemostatic methods include thermal therapy (e.g., heater probe, multipolar or bipolar electrocoagulation); injection of ethanol or epinephrine solutions; hemoclips; and argon plasma coagulator. For nonvariceal bleeding, the author currently favors the use of epinephrine injection, heater probe, multipolar coagulation, and combination therapy with epinephrine and thermal therapy.

Combination therapy is now the method generally used to control upper GI bleeding in the United States. Permanent hemostasis is obtained in about 90% of patients. In addition, the overall mortality from bleeding ulcers has decreased from 10% to approximately 7% over the past 30 years. Most feel this is related to better management with intensive care as well as endoscopic evaluation and therapy. Advanced age and concurrent illness are important predictors of death.

(G) Even when the exact diagnosis cannot be made, the endoscopist can give the surgeon a rough idea of the location of the bleeding lesions (i.e., esophagus, proximal or distal stomach, or duodenum). The options at this point include waiting for stabilization and cessation of bleeding or, failing that, proceeding to selective angiography. This modality can diagnose and treat bleeding in approximately 70% of patients with intra-arterial Gelfoam, metal coil springs, or clot. Arterial vasopressin stops bleeding in some patients with gastric or duodenal ulcers.

(H) When the bleeding is controlled, long-term medical treatment includes antacids, sucralfate, H_2-blockers, and proton-pump inhibitors. In addition, eradication of *H. pylori* almost completely eliminates recurrence of gastric and duodenal ulcers in infected patients and prevents recurrent bleeding. NSAIDs should be stopped, if possible. A prostaglandin analog (misoprostol) helps prevent NSAID-related gastric and duodenal ulcers and reduces the incidence of ulcer complications by 40%.

(I) If the bleeding continues or recurs, and repeated endoscopic treatment is not possible or successful, surgery may be indicated. It is usually reserved for complicated peptic ulcer disease with massive, persistent, or recurrent UGIB and nonhealing or giant ulcers. A bleeding gastric ulcer is best controlled by excision, either as a local procedure or as part of gastrectomy. Vagotomy and pyloroplasty after ligation of a bleeder is usually effective for an ulcer at the esophagogastric junction. Bleeding duodenal ulcers require suture ligation of the vessel followed by vagotomy and pyloroplasty or vagotomy and antrectomy.

REFERENCES

Beejay U, Wolfe MM: Acute gastrointestinal bleeding in the intensive care unit. Gastroenterol Clin N Am 29:309–336, 2000.

Eisen GM, Dominitz JA, Faigel DO et al: An annotated algorithmic approach to upper gastrointestinal bleeding. Gastrointestinal Endoscopy 53:853–858, 2001.

Lau JYW, Sung JJY, Lam YH et al: Endoscopic retreatment compared with surgery in patients with recurrent bleeding after initial endoscopic control of bleeding ulcers. N Engl J Med 340:751–756, 1999.

Lau JYW, Sung JJY, Lee KKC et al: Effect of intravenous omeprazole on recurrent bleeding after endoscopic treatment of bleeding peptic ulcers. N Engl J Med 343:310–316, 2000.

Lefkovitz Z, Cappell MS, Lefkovitz Kaplan M et al: Radiology in the diagnosis and therapy of gastrointestinal bleeding. Gastroenterol Clin N Am 29:489–511, 2000.

Longstreth GF, Feitelberg SP: Successful outpatient management of acute upper gastrointestinal hemorrhage: Use of practice guidelines in a large patient series. Gastrointestinal Endoscopy 47:219–221, 1998.

NIH Consensus Conference: Therapeutic endoscopy and bleeding ulcers. JAMA 262:1369–1372, 1989.

Ohmann C, Imhof M, Roher HD: Trends in peptic ulcer bleeding and surgical treatment. World J Surg 24:284–293, 2000.

Soehendra N, Sriram PVJ, Ponchon T et al: Hemostatic clip in gastrointestinal bleeding. Endoscopy 33:172–180, 2001.

Steffes CP, Sugawa C: Endoscopic management of nonvariceal gastrointestinal bleeding. World J Surg 16:1025–1033, 1992.

Sugawa C: Control of Nonvariceal Upper GI Bleeding. In Scott-Conner CEH (ed): The SAGES Fundamental Manual of Laparoscopy and GI Endoscopy. New York, Springer 1998.

Sugawa C, Joseph AL: Endoscopic interventional management of bleeding duodenal and gastric ulcers. Surg Clin N Am 72:317–334, 1992.

Sugawa C, Joseph AL: Management of Nonvariceal Upper Gastrointestinal Bleeding. In Greene FL, Ponsky JL (eds): Endoscopic Surgery. Philadelphia: WB Saunders, 1994.

Sugawa C, Steffes CP, Nakamura R et al: Upper GI bleeding in an urban hospital. Ann Surg 212:521–527, 1990.

Sugawa C, Takekuma Y, Lucas CE et al: Bleeding esophageal ulcers caused by NSAIDs. Surg Endosc 11:143–146, 1997.

van Leerdam ME, Tytgat GN: *Helicobacter pylori* infection in peptic ulcer haemorrhage. Aliment Pharmacol Ther 16(suppl 1):66–78, 2002.

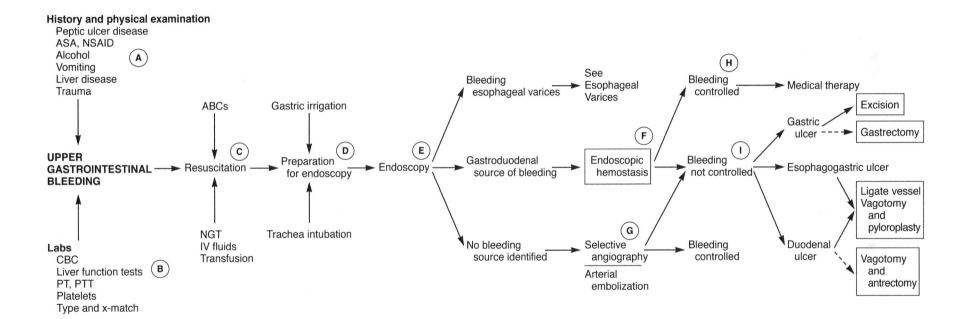

Chapter 46 *Bleeding Esophageal Varices*

GREGORY VAN STIEGMANN, MD

A The prognosis for patients bleeding from esophageal varices is directly related to liver function. In patients with advanced cirrhosis who bleed from varices, mortality can be as high as 60% in 1 year.

B Vasoactive drug therapy (e.g., IV octreotide 25 to 50 µg/hour) should be initiated before endoscopy and as soon as the patient is hemodynamically stable. Vasoactive drug administration combined with endoscopic therapy results in better control of acute hemorrhage from varices than does endoscopic treatment alone. Broad-spectrum antibiotic treatment (e.g., fluoroquinolone given IV and switched to PO when possible) should also be started and continued for 7 days. Antibiotic therapy has been shown to diminish the incidence of recurrent bleeding and other serious infections in cirrhotic patients.

C Endoscopy is performed after hemodynamic stabilization is achieved. Up to 25% of patients with varices have a nonvariceal source of hemorrhage (e.g., Mallory-Weiss tear or gastritis). The presence of varices and no other potential bleeding site is adequate evidence that the bleeding was from varices.

D Endoscopic treatment (e.g., band ligation or sclerotherapy) should be instituted as soon as a variceal source of bleeding is confirmed. Vasoactive drug therapy should be continued for 3 to 5 days after endoscopic treatment. Control of acute variceal bleeding can be achieved in up to 90% of patients with this approach.

E Balloon tamponade temporarily halts bleeding in 80% to 90% of patients, but 60% rebleed. Significant morbidity, including aspiration and perforation, is associated with this therapy.

F Liver transplantation is the best eventual treatment for patients with advanced cirrhosis who bleed from varices. Patients at lower risk (Child A and Child B) may be maintained using endoscopic therapy until liver function deteriorates.

G Endoscopic ligation or sclerotherapy is repeated at 1- or 2-week intervals until varices in the distal esophagus are small or eradicated. Endoscopic ligation is associated with fewer complications, fewer treatment sessions to eradicate varices, and a lower incidence of rebleeding in most series. Repeat treatments aimed at eradication of varices are performed in an outpatient setting.

H Elective shunt operations may be indicated for patients who have good liver function or who live in geographically remote areas. Portacaval shunts should probably be avoided in liver transplant candidates. Surgical options include selective splenorenal shunt, standard central portacaval shunt, and small-diameter portacaval H-graft shunt.

I Emergency shunt operations are generally central portacaval anastomoses with or without a prosthetic graft. Operative esophageal transection or devascularization of the stomach and distal esophagus combined with splenectomy may be better suited for patients who are liver transplant candidates. Patients who undergo the latter operation require endoscopic surveillance and institution of endoscopic therapy if varices recur.

J Transjugular intrahepatic portacaval shunt (TIPS) has supplanted emergency surgery for uncontrollable variceal bleeding in most institutions. TIPS can be performed successfully in approximately 90% of patients, and procedure-related mortality is low. Portal decompression is often combined with trans-shunt embolization of the feeding esophageal veins. Control of acute bleeding with TIPS is excellent, and bleeding recurs in 15% to 20% of patients over 2-year follow-up. The patient with a TIPS needs continuous follow-up because of the high rates of shunt narrowing and occlusion. Narrowed shunts can be revised as needed; the revision rate in many series approaches 50% 18 months after insertion.

K Definitions for failure of endoscopic therapy vary. The author believes that patients who experience two or more portal hypertension–related bleeds after endoscopic therapy is instituted should be considered for operative treatment or transplantation.

L Surveillance endoscopy is performed at 3- or 6-month intervals to detect and treat any varices that recur.

REFERENCES

Banares R, Albillos A, Rincon D et al: Endoscopic treatment vs. endoscopic plus pharmacologic treatment for acute variceal bleeding: A meta-analysis. Hepatology 35:609–615, 2002.

Bernard B, Grange JD, Khac EN et al: Antibiotic prophylaxis for prevention of bacterial infections in cirrhotic patients with gastrointestinal bleeding: A meta-analysis. Hepatology 29:1655–1661, 1999.

Chung S. Management of bleeding in the cirrhotic patient. J Gastroenterol Hepatol 17:355–360, 2002.

Gulberg V, Schepke M, Geigenberger G et al: Transjugular intrahepatic portosystemic shunting is not superior to endoscopic variceal band ligation for prevention of variceal rebleeding in cirrhotic patients: A randomized, controlled trial. Scand J Gastroenterol 37:338–343, 2002.

Helton WS, Maves R, Wicks K et al: Transjugular intrahepatic portasystemic shunt vs. surgical shunt in good-risk cirrhotic patients: A case-control comparison. Arch Surg 136: 17–20, 2001.

Sarfeh IJ, Rypins EB: Partial versus total portacaval shunt in alcoholic cirrhosis. Ann Surg 18:233–239, 1994.

Wu YK, Wang YH, Tsai CH et al: Modified Hassab procedure in the management of bleeding esophageal varices: A two-year experience. Hepatogastroenterology 49:205–207, 2002.

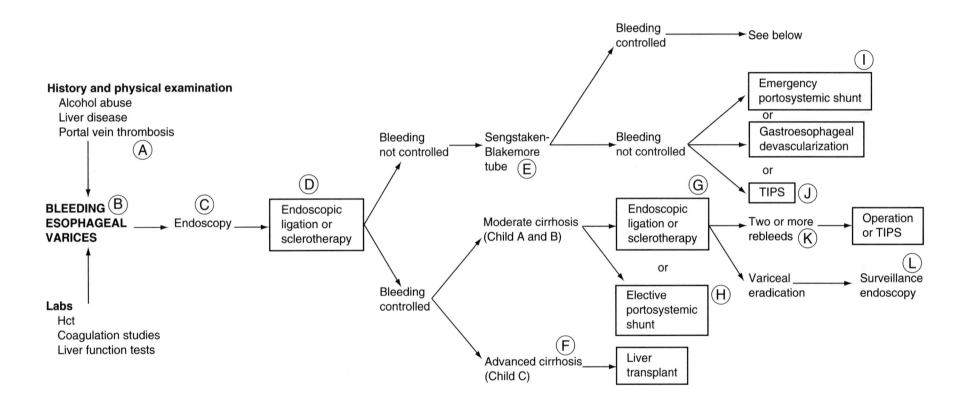

Chapter 47 *Jaundice*

KIAN A. MODANLOU, MD • MICHAEL E. WACHS, MD •
IGAL KAM, MD • THOMAS E. BAK, MD

(A) Normal serum bilirubin ranges from 0.5 to 1.3 mg/dl; when levels exceed 2.0 mg/dl, the bilirubin staining of the tissues becomes clinically apparent as jaundice. The diagnosis of jaundice can be made in the majority of cases by the history and physical examination alone. Jaundice caused by choledocholithiasis is usually transient and associated with pain and, sometimes, fever (cholangitis). The gradual onset of jaundice without pain (and, possibly, with weight loss) is suggestive of malignancy. Jaundice occurring after cholecystectomy would be suggestive of either retained bile stones or injury to the bile duct. A careful review of medications may reveal drugs prone to toxic side effects, whereas a recent blood transfusion may put the patient at risk for hemolysis.

(B) Liver function tests routinely combine markers of function (i.e., albumin, indirect and direct bilirubin) with markers of liver damage (i.e., alanine aminotransferase [ALT], aspartate aminotransferase [AST], and alkaline phosphatase) and can be used to differentiate medical problems (e.g., intrahepatic cholestasis) from surgical problems (e.g., extrahepatic or obstructive cholestasis). A low serum albumin concentration suggests chronic liver disease. Unconjugated (indirect) hyperbilirubunemia occurs when there is either an increase in bilirubin production or a decrease in hepatocyte uptake and conjugation. Defects in bilirubin excretion or extrahepatic biliary obstruction result in a predominantly conjugated (direct) hyperbilirubinemia. Choledocholithiasis is usually associated with a moderate increase in bilirubin (10 to 12 mg/dl), whereas malignant obstruction can lead to higher elevations (greater than 20 mg/dl). Rises in the transaminase activity are indicative of a hepatic process. Alkaline phosphatase is a sensitive marker for biliary tract pathology. A complete blood count may show red blood cell abnormalities or evidence of an inflammatory process. A decreased white blood cell count may be an indicator of chronic liver disease. Pregnancy may precipitate certain forms of liver disease.

(C) Ultrasonography (US) is usually the first-line imaging modality for patients with jaundice. The diagnosis of mechanical jaundice is based on the visualization of dilated extrahepatic (greater than 10 mm) or intrahepatic (greater than 4 mm) bile ducts (sensitivity 87%, specificity 99%). US is also accurate in identifying gallstones, liver masses, fluid collections, and pancreatic masses, although visualization of the distal common bile duct (CBD) and pancreas may be inadequate. Computed tomography (CT) is usually complementary to US and is better at determining the level and character of biliary obstruction. It is also useful in characterizing smaller lesions of the liver and pancreas as well as providing staging information, including vascular involvement of periampullary tumors. Magnetic resonance cholangiopancreatography (MRCP) has made it possible to obtain images similar to those of endoscopic retrograde cholangiopancreatography (ERCP) without the administration of contrast material. The overall accuracy of MRCP is 95% for identifying a normal biliary tract, 93% for a dilated main bile duct, 93% for stones 3 mm or smaller, and greater than 90% for both benign and malignant stricture. It is indicated when the patient is too high risk for ERCP or when cannulation of the bile duct is not technically feasible. Its other main advantage is evaluation of the bile ducts situated above the obstruction.

(D) A radiologic evaluation that shows no evidence of obstructive jaundice leads to further delineation of causes of medical jaundice. A predominantly indirect hyperbilirubinemia is indicative of increased production of bilirubin or of decreased hepatocyte uptake or conjugation. Common causes of increased production include multiple transfusions, transfusion reaction, sepsis, burns, congenital hemoglobinopathies, and hemolysis of congenital red call variants. Common causes of decreased transport or conjugation include Gilbert's disease, Crigler-Najjar syndrome, neonatal jaundice, viral hepatitis, drug inhibition, total parenteral nutrition and sepsis. Normal sized bile ducts and a predominantly direct hyperbilirubinemia can result from Dubin-Johnson syndrome; Rotor's syndrome; cirrhosis; amyloidosis; cancer; hepatitis (viral, drug-induced, or alcoholic); and pregnancy. Decreased secretion of bile with the subsequent finding of small bile ducts may result from primary biliary cirrhosis, primary sclerosing cholangitis, autoimmune cholangiopathy, idiopathic adult ductopenia, or sarcoidosis.

(E) Suspicion of hepatocellular dysfunction prompts further testing to identify the specific cause of jaundice and to guide any subsequent therapy. Hematologic testing (e.g., peripheral smear, hemoglobin electrophoresis, red cell antibodies, or osmotic fragility) can delineate causes of increased production of bilirubin. Viral serologies for hepatitis A, B, and C; as well as tests for antinuclear antibody, antimitochondrial antibody, ceruloplasmin, serum copper, and α-1 antitrypsin can identify potential causes of parenchymal liver damage and cirrhosis. Either percutaneous or transjugular liver biopsy is essential to diagnose chronic hepatitis and establish the cause of cirrhosis.

(F) Jaundice with confirmation of dilated ducts and gallstones by radiologic examination requires further invasive diagnosis and therapy. The sensitivity of ERCP in the detection of

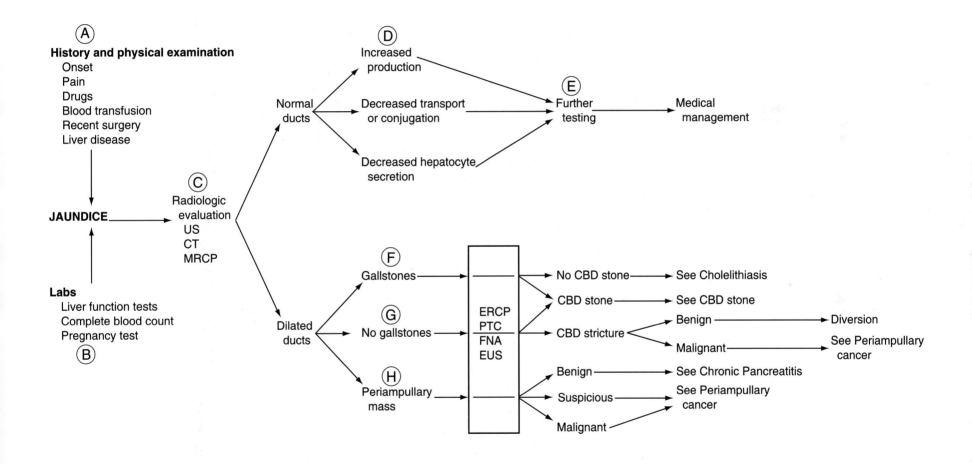

choledocholithiasis is about 90% and offers the possibilities of simultaneous endoscopic sphincterotomy, stone retrieval, or stenting. If not already done, the patient should be evaluated for cholecystectomy.

Ⓖ The finding of dilated ducts and no evidence of gallstones also requires more advanced testing. ERCP is useful in diagnosing a biliary stricture or in finding a stone missed by ultrasound. Brushings can be taken to determine the etiology of the stricture, either benign (secondary to trauma) or malignant (cholangiocarcinoma). If the obstruction is located at or above the hilum, a percutaneous transhepatic cholangiogram (PTC) may be necessary to plan for subsequent management. In either case, a stent can be placed to increase bile drainage.

Ⓗ The identification of a periampullary mass as the cause of obstructive jaundice warrants further characterization of the lesion's etiology and extent. ERCP is the preferred method of evaluation, given that a biopsy can be followed by palliation of the obstruction via stent placement. If ERCP is not feasible, a CT or US-guided fine needle aspiration (FNA) of the mass can be done. Endoscopic ultrasound (EUS) is a newer modality that can be used to distinguish between benign and malignant strictures and to evaluate the local extent of a neoplastic process as well as vascular invasion. Overall more accurate than CT, EUS is especially helpful in tumors smaller than 3 cm.

REFERENCES

Beckingham IJ, Ryder SD: Investigation of liver and biliary disease. BMJ 322:33–36, 2001.

Benson MD, Ghandi MR: Ultrasound of the hepatobiliary-pancreatic system. World J Surg 24:166–170, 2000.

Cieszanowski A, Chomicka D, Andrzejewska M et al: Imaging techniques in patients with biliary obstruction. Med Sci Monit 6:1197–1202, 2000.

Lucas WB, Chuttani R: Pathophysiology and current concepts in the diagnosis of obstructive jaundice. Gastroenterologist 3:105–118, 1995.

Mallery S, Van Dam J: Advances in diagnostic and therapeutic endoscopy. Med Clin N Am 84:1059–1083, 2000.

McGill JM, Kwiatkowski AP: Cholestatic liver diseases in adults. Am J Gastroenterol 93:684–691, 1998.

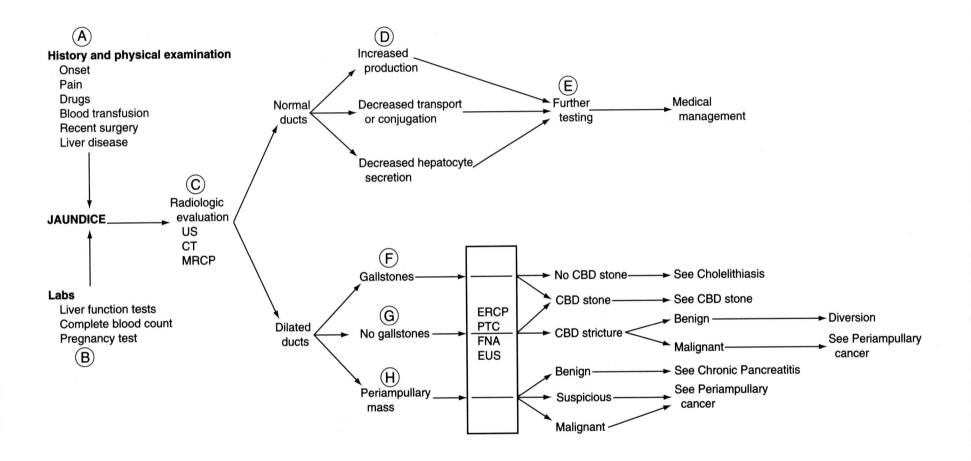

Ⓐ

History and physical examination
Onset
Pain
Drugs
Blood transfusion
Recent surgery
Liver disease

JAUNDICE

Labs
Liver function tests
Complete blood count
Pregnancy test

Ⓑ

Ⓒ
Radiologic
evaluation
US
CT
MRCP

Normal
ducts

Ⓓ
Increased
production

Decreased transport
or conjugation

Decreased hepatocyte
secretion

Ⓔ
Further
testing

Medical
management

Dilated
ducts

Ⓕ
Gallstones

Ⓖ
No gallstones

Ⓗ
Periampullary
mass

ERCP
PTC
FNA
EUS

No CBD stone —→ See Cholelithiasis

CBD stone —→ See CBD stone

CBD stricture
 Benign —————————→ Diversion
 Malignant ————→ See Periampullary cancer

Benign —→ See Chronic Pancreatitis

Suspicious —→ See Periampullary cancer

Malignant

Chapter 48 *Obstructive Jaundice: Interventional Options*

JANETTE D. DURHAM, MD • BERNARD E. ZELIGMAN, MD

(A) A history of cholelithiasis or previous biliary tract surgery suggests the cause of jaundice is obstruction.

(B) Obstruction of the extrahepatic duct or of both the right and the left hepatic ducts results in jaundice. Isolated obstruction of either the main right or left hepatic duct does not cause jaundice if the liver is otherwise normal.

(C) Obstructive jaundice results in direct hyperbilirubinemia. *Serum total bilirubin levels greater than 10 mg/dl suggest malignant obstruction.* Serum alkaline phosphatase greater than three times normal and elevated serum γ-glutamyl transferase favor obstructive jaundice over hepatocellular disease.

(D) Transabdominal ultrasound (US) is the preferred initial imaging study for detection of extrahepatic or intrahepatic bile duct dilation. Patients who have had a previous bile duct obstruction may have persistent dilatation of their bile duct. Absence of bile duct dilatation by US usually excludes obstruction unless of very recent onset. If US is technically inadequate, equivocal for dilatation, or negative when clinical suspicion of obstruction is high, magnetic resonance cholangiopancreatography (MRCP) should be done. Diagnostic endoscopic retrograde cholangiography (ERC) may be indicated in some cases.

(E) The most common cause of extrahepatic obstructive jaundice is ductal stones.

(F) Endoscopic stone extraction is done at ERC and usually requires endoscopic sphincterotomy. Endoscopic management of extrahepatic duct stones is as effective as surgical duct exploration.

(G) Percutaneous extraction via a transhepatic route or a mature T-tube track is needed for duct stones if surgically altered anatomy precludes endoscopic access to the biliary tract or if surgical or endoscopic therapy has failed. Percutaneous extraction is preferable to endoscopic extraction for some cases of intrahepatic stones. A simultaneous percutaneous and endoscopic approach is required in some cases.

(H) Open bile duct exploration is indicated when endoscopic or percutaneous therapy has failed or if cholecystectomy will be performed by laparotomy. Laparoscopic bile duct exploration, done at the time of laparoscopic cholecystectomy, may be more efficient than preoperative endoscopic stone extraction.

(I) Biliary strictures may be benign or malignant. The location of a stricture suggests the following possible causes: (1) hepatic duct confluence—cholangiocarcinoma, gallbladder carcinoma, porta hepatis lymphadenopathy (often from metastatic cancer), or injury from laparoscopic cholecystectomy; (2) intrapancreatic common bile duct—pancreatic cancer or pancreatitis; or (3) at the papilla of Vater—adenoma or adenocarcinoma of the papilla or contiguous duodenum. Cholangiocarcinoma, metastasis, lymphoma, and primary and secondary sclerosing cholangitis can cause strictures at any location.

(J) Magnetic resonance cholangiopancreatography (MRCP) has replaced diagnostic ERC for initial assessment of strictures except when endoscopic intervention is likely. The most efficient way to establish the location and determine if the obstruction is cancer is to combine MRCP with magnetic resonance imaging (MRI). If high-quality MRI is unavailable, multidetector CT scanning can be used in conjunction with direct cholangiography (ERC or PTC). Endoscopic ultrasound (EUS) accompanied by FNA of a mass lesion or suspicious lymph nodes may be indicated after noninvasive imaging and/or ERCP to establish the diagnosis of, and to stage cancer.

(K) Common malignant causes of obstructive jaundice are adenocarcinoma of the pancreatic head and cholangiocarcinoma. If imaging studies suggest malignant obstruction, a diagnosis may be made using intraductal brush cytology, intraductal forceps biopsy, or percutaneous or EUS-guided FNA cytology. These techniques, even when used in combination, cannot exclude malignancy because of a significant incidence of false negative results.

(L) Only 10% to 20% of pancreatic cancers presenting with obstructive jaundice are resectable. Approximately one third of cholangiocarcinomas (up to 50% of those in the inferior third of the bile duct) are resectable.

(M) Routine use of preoperative biliary drainage does not improve surgical outcome. Assessment for resectability should precede nonoperative biliary drainage procedures. Preoperative drainage is valuable when used selectively to improve clinical status, to manage obstruction when surgery is delayed, or to facilitate identification of ducts during the operation.

(N) Endoscopic drainage (by plastic or metal stent insertion) is indicated for unresectable malignant strictures in patients with limited life expectancy.

(O) Intrahepatic and hilar strictures are difficult to manage endoscopically. They often require percutaneous cholangiography to delineate the intrahepatic ductal anatomy and percutaneous transhepatic biliary drainage (PTBD) to relieve obstruction.

(P) Biliary bypass surgery is appropriate palliation for patients with unresectable cancers who have a life expectancy of more than 1 year or for those whose cancer is found to be unresectable at laparotomy. Surgical biliary bypass avoids the multiple interventions (stent changes) required to maintain endoscopic or percutaneous drainage.

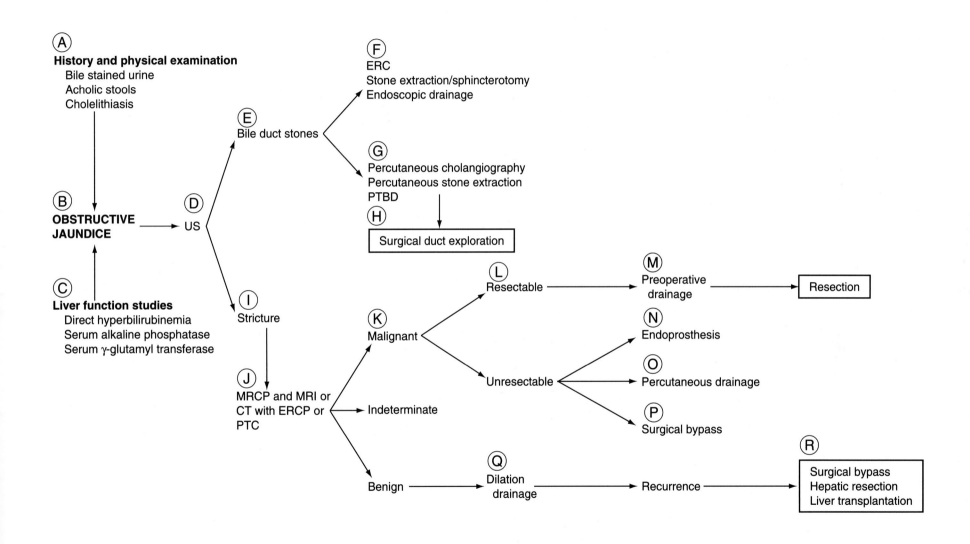

(A) **History and physical examination**
Bile stained urine
Acholic stools
Cholelithiasis

(B) **OBSTRUCTIVE JAUNDICE**

(C) **Liver function studies**
Direct hyperbilirubinemia
Serum alkaline phosphatase
Serum γ-glutamyl transferase

(D) US

(E) Bile duct stones

(F) ERC
Stone extraction/sphincterotomy
Endoscopic drainage

(G) Percutaneous cholangiography
Percutaneous stone extraction
PTBD

(H) Surgical duct exploration

(I) Stricture

(J) MRCP and MRI or
CT with ERCP or
PTC

Indeterminate

Benign

(K) Malignant

Resectable

Unresectable

(L) Resectable

(M) Preoperative drainage

Resection

(N) Endoprosthesis

(O) Percutaneous drainage

(P) Surgical bypass

(Q) Dilation drainage

Recurrence

(R) Surgical bypass
Hepatic resection
Liver transplantation

Q Endoscopic or percutaneous stricture dilatation and stent placement may successfully treat some benign biliary strictures. These procedures usually need to be repeated several times over a course of months. Strictures that develop at biliary-enteric anastomosis are the most likely to respond.

R Biliary-enteric anastomosis is successful in most patients with benign bile duct stricture. Partial hepatectomy and occasionally liver transplantation may be necessary in a small number of patients.

REFERENCES

Anderson JR, Sørensen SM, Kruse A et al: Randomized trial of endoscopic endoprosthesis versus operative bypass in malignant obstructive jaundice. Gut 30:1132–1135, 1989.

Jung G, Huh J, Lee SU et al: Bile duct: Analysis of percutaneous transluminal forceps biopsy in 130 patients suspected of having malignant biliary obstruction. Radiology 224:725–730, 2002.

Lopera JE, Soto JA, Munera F: Malignant hilar and perihilar biliary obstruction: Use of MR cholangiography to define the extent of biliary ductal involvement and plan percutaneous interventions. Radiology 220:90–96, 2001.

Mark DH, Flamm CR, Aronson N: Evidence-based assessment of diagnostic modalities for common bile duct stones. Gastrointestinal endoscopy 56:S190–S194, 2002.

Patel AP, Lokey JS, Harris JB et al: Current management of common bile duct stones in a teaching community hospital. The American Surgeon 69:555–561, 2003.

Reding R, Buard J, Lebeau G et al: Surgical management of 552 carcinomas of the extrahepatic bile ducts (gallbladder and periampullary tumors excluded). Results of the French Surgical Association Survey. Ann Surg 213:236–241, 1991.

Sarli L, Iusco DR, Roncoroni L: Preoperative endoscopic sphincterotomy and laparoscopic cholecystectomy for the management of cholecystocholedocholithiasis: 10-year experience. World J Surg 27:180–186, 2003.

Schoder M, Rossi P, Uflacker R et al: Malignant biliary obstruction: Treatment with ePTFE-FEP covered endoprostheses—initial technical and clinical experiences in a multicenter trial. Radiology 225:35–42, 2002.

Wright BE, Freeman ML, Cumming JK et al: Current management of common bile duct stones: Is there a role for laparoscopic cholecystectomy and intraoperative endoscopic retrograde cholangiopancreatography as a single-stage procedure? Surgery 132:729–737, 2002.

Zidi SH, Prat F, Le Guen O et al: Performance characteristics of magnetic resonance cholangiography in the staging of malignant hilar strictures. Gut 46:103–106, 2000.

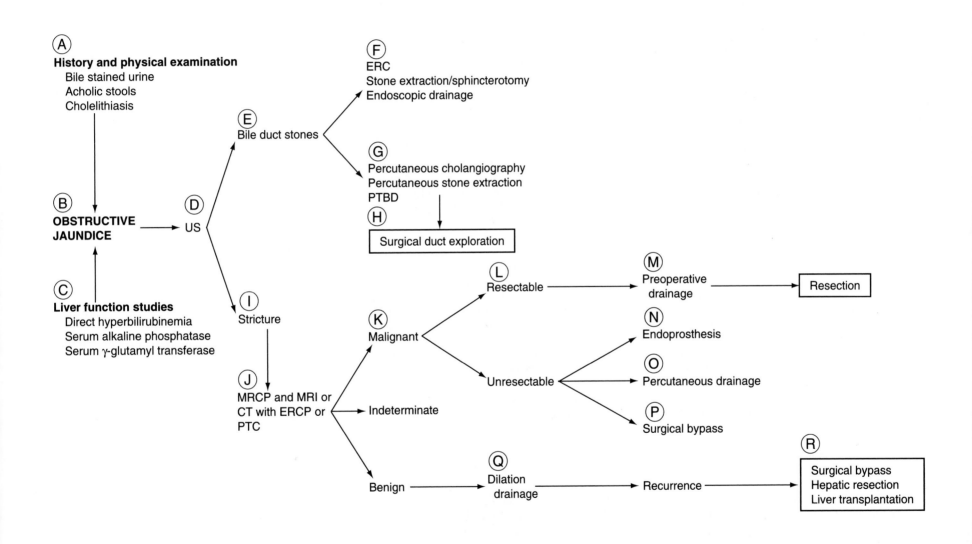

(A) **History and physical examination**
  Bile stained urine
  Acholic stools
  Cholelithiasis

(B) **OBSTRUCTIVE JAUNDICE**

(C) **Liver function studies**
  Direct hyperbilirubinemia
  Serum alkaline phosphatase
  Serum γ-glutamyl transferase

(D) US

(E) Bile duct stones

(F) ERC
  Stone extraction/sphincterotomy
  Endoscopic drainage

(G) Percutaneous cholangiography
  Percutaneous stone extraction
  PTBD

(H) Surgical duct exploration

(I) Stricture

(J) MRCP and MRI or
  CT with ERCP or
  PTC

Indeterminate

(K) Malignant

Resectable

Benign

(L) Resectable

(M) Preoperative drainage

Resection

(N) Endoprosthesis

(O) Percutaneous drainage

(P) Surgical bypass

Unresectable

(Q) Dilation drainage

Recurrence

(R) Surgical bypass
  Hepatic resection
  Liver transplantation

Chapter 49 Cholelithiasis (Gallstones)

FRANK H. CHAE, MD, CM

A Gallstones are found in more than 1 million American adults each year; 80% of these adults experience no symptoms. The incidence of gallstones increases with age and female gender, being found in 20% of females and 5% of males in the 50 to 65 year age-group. Most gallstones (75%) contain a mixture of bile pigments and cholesterol. Cholesterol stone formation is attributed to the bile saturation with cholesterol, gallbladder stasis, and debris aggregation. Risk factors include obesity, multiparity, oral contraceptives, family history, and Native American ancestry. Black pigmented stones (10% to 20% of gallstones in the United States) tend to be associated with hemolytic anemia, cirrhosis, or bile stasis. Calcium bilirubinate stone (light brown-orange) is associated with infection.

B Ultrasound (US) detects gallstones in 90% to 95% of patients and may also be used in patients with jaundice to detect bile duct dilation. Oral cholecystography is slightly more accurate but requires more time to perform and should be avoided in jaundiced patients. For equivocal diagnosis of cholecystitis, radionuclide scan imaging using technetium 99m–labeled derivatives of iminodiacetic acid (HIDA scan) may be used. Failure of the radionuclide marker to enter the gallbladder suggests cholecystitis. Accuracy is about 90%. False-positive findings may be caused by alcohol ingestion, a recent meal, or failure of the liver to take up and excrete the radionuclide (critical illness). Magnetic resonance cholangio-pancreatography (MRCP) shows promise as a noninvasive diagnostic test for detecting common bile duct stones (see Chapter 50).

C About 20% to 40% of patients with asymptomatic gallstones develop symptoms within 10 years and require cholecystectomy. Another 5% to 18% undergo emergency cholecystectomy for complications of gallstones. Clinical management depends on symptoms. Strong indications for prophylactic cholecystectomy in asymptomatic cholelithiasis include sickle cell disease in children; nonfunctioning gallbladder; calcified gallbladder; stones greater than 2.5 cm; and a bariatric operation. An occupation involving remote access to medical care (e.g., Antarctic explorers, pilots, or astronauts) is a relative indication. Diabetes, by itself, is not an absolute indication, although nearly 50% eventually develop symptoms with high complication rates. Death from acute cholecystitis in diabetics may be as high as 10%.

D Chronic cholecystitis implies nonemergent symptoms (usually intermittent, postprandial, epigastric, or right upper quadrant abdominal pain) caused by gallstones. Symptoms are often vague (e.g., dyspepsia). Within 10 years, about 50% of patients with chronic cholecystitis will need cholecystectomy or hospitalization without surgery. Because of this risk, elective cholecystectomy is recommended. Mildly elevated white blood count, alkaline phosphatase, and/or amylase may be present. Ultrasonography reveals gallstones in 95% of cases; if US is negative, proceed to HIDA scan. If still equivocal, consider a cholecystokinin-provocative HIDA scan to evaluate for biliary dyskinesia. Acalculous chronic cholecystitis (6% to 10%) such as cholesterosis of the gallbladder or adenomyomatosis may be difficult to diagnose but, if suspected, is often treated by elective cholecystectomy.

E Acute cholecystitis is characterized by right upper quadrant abdominal pain, nausea, fever, and leukocytosis. Jaundice may manifest (10%). The usual age range is 30 to 70 years with female predominance. Obstruction of cystic duct is either from stone or sludge. Laboratory results may show elevated white blood count, alkaline phosphatase, bilirubin, liver function enzymes, and/or amylase. HIDA scan is ideal, but US is usually sufficient. Immediate treatment should involve antibiotic(s) to cover gram-negatives and anaerobes (60% to 90% resolution). Acalculous acute cholecystitis (5%) is often a complication of sepsis and is associated with multiple organ failure or prolonged total parenteral hyperalimentation. Collagen vascular disease and diabetes appear to increase the risk. The risk of gallbladder gangrene or perforation from acute cholecystitis is 15% to 20% with stones and 25% to 30% without stones. Diagnosis may be difficult and is usually suspected in cases of persistent sepsis of unknown origin. US typically reveals distended thick-walled gallbladder with sludge, no stones, and pericholecystic fluid. Treatment is cholecystectomy; or, if the patient is a poor surgical candidate, cholecystostomy.

F Cholecystoenteric fistula may arise from chronic gallbladder inflammation. A tract may develop from gallbladder to duodenum, colon, or stomach. Most are found incidentally during gallbladder surgery. Cholecystocolonic fistula may cause malabsorption and steatorrhea. Large stones (larger than 2 cm) may lead to gallstone ileus (average age 70 years, more often in females). Up to 25% of these patients had acute cholecystitis before small bowel obstruction (SBO). On presentation, about 40% with x-ray films demonstrate gas in the biliary tree. Upper GI series may demonstrate gallbladder-duodenal fistula. The safest approach (less mortality) may be to surgically treat the intestinal obstruction followed by delayed expectant treatment of fistula because most close spontaneously.

G Serum amylase levels are commonly elevated with acute cholecystitis. In 1% to 3% of patients, passage of a common bile duct stone causes clinical pancreatitis. Gallbladder should be removed after resolution of pancreatitis and before hospital discharge.

H Elective laparoscopic cholecystectomy is applicable in 95% of patients with symptomatic cholelithiasis. Although the indication for resection has not changed, the rate of cholecystectomy has increased over the years (largely attributed to increased recognition of chronic cholecystitis and laparoscopic technique). The rate of bile duct injury for laparoscopic cholecystectomy used to be as high as 1% but is now approaching the rate for open procedure at 0.1% or less. Acute cholecystitis

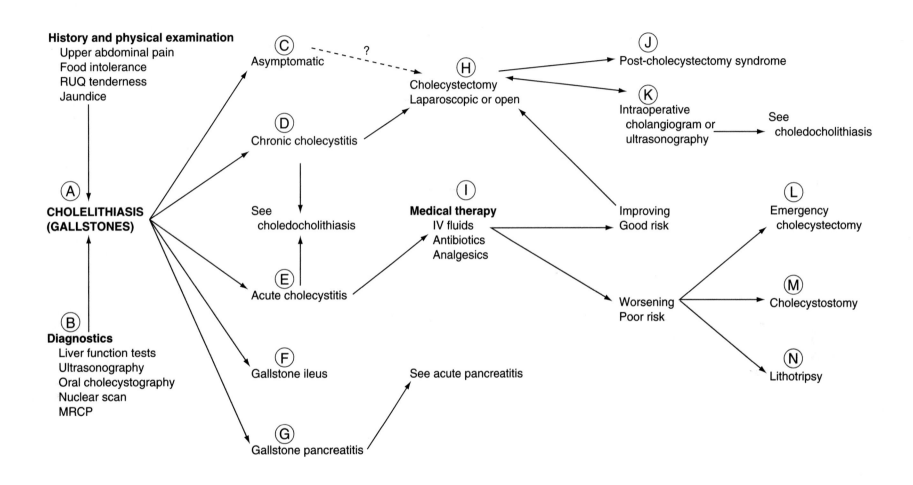

History and physical examination
  Upper abdominal pain
  Food intolerance
  RUQ tenderness
  Jaundice

Ⓐ

**CHOLELITHIASIS
(GALLSTONES)**

Ⓑ

Diagnostics
  Liver function tests
  Ultrasonography
  Oral cholecystography
  Nuclear scan
  MRCP

Ⓒ Asymptomatic

Ⓓ Chronic cholecystitis

See
choledocholithiasis

Ⓔ Acute cholecystitis

Ⓕ Gallstone ileus

Ⓖ Gallstone pancreatitis

?

Ⓗ Cholecystectomy
Laparoscopic or open

Ⓘ **Medical therapy**
  IV fluids
  Antibiotics
  Analgesics

See acute pancreatitis

Ⓙ Post-cholecystectomy syndrome

Ⓚ Intraoperative
cholangiogram or
ultrasonography

See
choledocholithiasis

Improving
Good risk

Worsening
Poor risk

Ⓛ Emergency
cholecystectomy

Ⓜ Cholecystostomy

Ⓝ Lithotripsy

and gallstone pancreatitis are associated with increased risk for bile duct injury. Open cholecystectomy is advised when the anatomic structures of Calot's triangle are indeterminate. Conversion to open cholecystectomy is not considered a complication; rather, it is an alternative approach. Mortality rates are less than 0.1% for ages under 50 years, 0.5% for ages over 50 years, and about 5% for those with acute cholecystitis.

Ⓘ   Antibiotic(s) to cover gram-negatives (e.g., *E. coli*) and anaerobes (e.g., clostridia) are given to patients with evidence of sepsis or severe cholecystitis. Early cholecystectomy (within 72 hours of onset) is generally recommended. Surgery may be delayed if presentation is more than 72 hours and antibiotics are showing good response. Most patients (more than 85%) with acute cholecystitis respond rapidly to medical treatment (i.e., pain, fever, and leukocytosis typically resolve within 2 to 3 days). When compared to deferment beyond 72 hours, laparoscopic cholecystectomy performed within 72 hours of symptom is associated with a lower conversion rate (12% vs. 30%), less technical difficulty, less operative time, shorter recovery time, and lower overall cost. If the 72-hour window is missed, a delayed elective surgery may be planned after acute inflammation has resolved. If symptoms worsen during treatment (particularly in the elderly or in diabetics), emergent surgery is indicated to prevent empyema, gangrene, emphysematous cholecystitis, or perforation, any one of which may triple the mortality rate. Initial treatment for emphysematous cholecystitis is high-dose antibiotics (to cover anaerobes and gram-negatives) and resuscitation, followed by surgery.

Ⓙ   Residual biliary tract disease after gallbladder removal may be associated with persistent symptoms of dyspepsia or RUQ pain, coupled with abnormal liver function test, jaundice, or cholangitis. ERCP or MRCP may reveal cystic duct leak, long cystic duct remnant, common bile duct stones, biliary stricture, pancreatitis, ampullary stenosis, or sphincter of Oddi dysmotility (via manometry). ERCP sphincterotomy may be performed for residual stone.

Clinically significant bile leak from cystic duct should be treated by ERCP and sphincterotomy with stenting. Extra-biliary causes may include peptic ulcer disease, gastroesophageal reflux disease, irritable bowel syndrome, or food intolerance.

Ⓚ   Intraoperative transcystic cholangiography (80% sensitivity, 97% specificity, 95% accuracy) may be performed to detect unsuspected bile duct stones (5%) and to outline the biliary tree. An alternative is intraoperative ultrasonography (80% sensitivity, 98% specificity, and 97% accuracy). The use of cholangiography may lessen the severity of bile duct injury during laparoscopic cholecystectomy. If cholangiography reveals a minor partial bile duct injury that appears readily correctable, an open primary duct repair over a T-tube may be attempted. For extensive injury or complete transection, the biliary tree should be drained and definitive choledochoenteric or hepaticoenteric bypass (with or without stents) should be planned at another time.

Ⓛ   Emergency cholecystectomy increases perioperative risk considerably. Mortality rates approach 10% or greater in patients aged more than 60 years. All patients with clinical evidence of peritonitis or diagnostic evidence of gas in the gallbladder and biliary tract should undergo immediate laparotomy after resuscitation. Mortality rate in Child's class C cirrhotics may be as high as 40%; therefore, to minimize major hemorrhage from the gallbladder fossa, most of the gallbladder may be removed with the portion of the wall adjacent to the liver bed left intact and the cystic duct suture ligated.

Ⓜ   In poor surgical risk patients, cholecystostomy may precede cholecystectomy. Minimally invasive approaches include ultrasound-guided percutaneous or laparoscopic catheter drainage of gallbladder. Other options include small-incision open cholecystostomy and cholecystectomy under local anesthesia. Despite minimally invasive intervention, mortality (6% to 13%) and morbidity (35%) rates are still high in poor risk patients. When possible, eventual removal of gallbladder is advised

after patient recovery (only a third of the patients after cholecystostomy remain asymptomatic after resolution of cholecystitis).

Ⓝ   Electrohydraulic extracorporeal shock wave lithotripsy may fragment small gallstones (ideal if single stone smaller than 2 cm), but only half of patients remain stone free at 2 years because of retained fragments or new stones. The addition of oral medication (e.g., chenodeoxycholate and ursodeoxycholate) promotes dissolution of fragments and prevents new stone formation. This procedure may be considered for poor surgical risk patients.

REFERENCES

Barwood NT, Valinsky LJ, Hobbs MS et al: Changing methods of imaging the common bile duct in the laparoscopic cholecystectomy era in Western Australia: Implications for surgical practice. Ann Surg 235:41–50, 2002.

Berber E, Engle KL, Garland A et al: A critical analysis of intraoperative time utilization in laparoscopic cholecystectomy. Surg Endosc 15:161–165, 2001.

Biffl WL, Moore EE, Offner PJ et al: Routine intraoperative laparoscopic ultrasonography with selective cholangiography reduces bile duct complications during laparoscopic cholecystectomy. J Am Coll Surg 193:272–280, 2001.

Brockmann JG, Kocher T, Senninger NJ et al: Complications due to gallstones lost during laparoscopic cholecystectomy. Surg Endosc 16:1226–1232, 2002.

Cameron IC, Chadwick C, Phillips J et al: Acute cholecystitis—room for improvement? Ann R Coll Surg Engl 84:10–13, 2002.

National Institutes of Health consensus development conference statement on gallstones and laparoscopic cholecystectomy. Am J Surg 165:390–398, 1993.

Madan AK, Aliabadi-Wahle S, Tesi D et al: How early is early laparoscopic treatment of acute cholecystitis? Am J Surg 183:232–236, 2002.

Robinson TN, Stiegmann GV, Durham JD et al: Management of major bile duct injury associated with laparoscopic cholecystectomy. Surg Endosc 15:1381–1385, 2001.

Spira RM, Nissan A, Zamir O et al: Percutaneous transhepatic cholecystostomy and delayed laparoscopic cholecystectomy in critically ill patients with acute calculus cholecystitis. Am J Surg 183:62–66, 2002.

Zacks SL, Sandler RS, Rutledge R et al: A population-based cohort study comparing laparoscopic cholecystectomy and open cholecystectomy. Am J Gastroenterol 97:334–340, 2002.

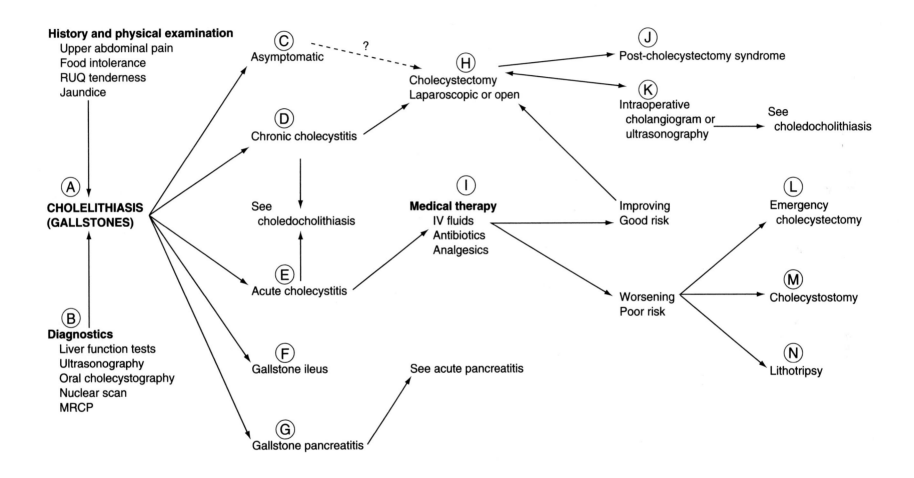

History and physical examination
    Upper abdominal pain
    Food intolerance
    RUQ tenderness
    Jaundice

(A)

CHOLELITHIASIS
(GALLSTONES)

(B)

Diagnostics
    Liver function tests
    Ultrasonography
    Oral cholecystography
    Nuclear scan
    MRCP

(C) Asymptomatic

(D) Chronic cholecystitis

See
    choledocholithiasis

(E) Acute cholecystitis

(F) Gallstone ileus

(G) Gallstone pancreatitis

See acute pancreatitis

?

(H)
Cholecystectomy
Laparoscopic or open

(I)
Medical therapy
    IV fluids
    Antibiotics
    Analgesics

Improving
Good risk

Worsening
Poor risk

(J)
Post-cholecystectomy syndrome

(K)
Intraoperative
cholangiogram or
ultrasonography

See
    choledocholithiasis

(L)
Emergency
cholecystectomy

(M)
Cholecystostomy

(N)
Lithotripsy

Chapter 50 *Choledocholithiasis (Common Bile Duct Stones)*

FRANK H. CHAE, MD, CM

(A) Common bile duct (CBD) stones are primarily (95%) from the gallbladder (usually cholesterol stones) and are present in about 10% to 15% of patients undergoing cholecystectomy (25% for age greater than 60 years). Conversely, 5% of CBD stones are associated with no stones in the gallbladder. Primary duct stones (pigmented calcium bilirubinate) are rare and usually result from biliary stasis. About 50% of patients with CBD stones remain asymptomatic. Presentation may range from no symptoms to toxic sepsis (e.g., cholangitis and pancreatitis). Typical symptoms are indistinguishable from cholelithiasis (see Chapter 49), but the presence of fever or jaundice suggests CBD stone. Other differentials include alcoholic cirrhosis, hepatitis, and primary biliary cirrhosis.

(B) CBD stones characteristically result in elevation of liver enzymes (5% to 7% of cases reveal normal liver function tests). A high white blood cell count points to cholangitis. In chronic biliary obstruction, vitamin K malabsorption may occur, leading to coagulopathy. Preoperative ultrasonography (US) is 55% to 80% accurate for detecting CBD stones or dilated ducts. CT scan may also reveal dilated ducts. Preoperative endoscopic retrograde pancreato-cholangiography (ERCP) may be reserved for cases of elevated bilirubin, jaundice, or evidence of dilated ducts to search for tumor or stone (especially with history of prior gallbladder removal). Bile duct obstruction from tumor tends to cause less pain and more ductal dilatation when compared with obstruction from stone. Magnetic resonance cholangio-pancreatography (MRCP) shows promise in detecting CBD stones before laparoscopic cholecystectomy. If CBD stone is suspected, noninvasive MRCP may be an ideal alternative to the invasive diagnostic ERCP, thereby determining the need for either a CBD exploration or preoperative ERCP and sphincterotomy.

(C) In the era of laparoscopic cholecystectomy, selective vs. routine intraoperative cholangiography remains debatable. Another option is either pre- or postoperative ERCP. Typical indication for laparoscopic cholangiography to detect CBD stones includes history of pancreatitis or jaundice, multiple gallstones, dilated cystic duct or CBD, or elevated liver enzymes. Overall, CBD stones should be anticipated in about 15% of cholecystectomies. If available, laparoscopic US is an alternative to cholangiography. A single small (less than 5 mm in diameter) CBD stone visualized by cholangiography usually passes spontaneously; however, for patients with history of pancreatitis or jaundice, all stones should be removed. Saline irrigation through the cholangio-catheter, coupled with intravenous glucagon for ampullary relaxation, may clear the stone (see H).

(D) In the presence of Charcot's triad (right upper quadrant pain, fever, and jaundice) or Reynold's pentad (Charcot's triad plus hypotension and CNS changes), initial management of acute cholangitis should be aggressive fluid resuscitation and antibiotic therapy. Emergent ERCP is indicated if the patient fails to improve. If no response is seen with tumor obstruction, transhepatic drainage may be added.

(E) Antibiotics, either a triple combination (ampicillin, gentamicin, metronidazole) or a broad-spectrum agent (imipenem), should cover gram-negatives (*E. coli*, Klebsiella) and anaerobes (bacteroides, clostridia). Most cases respond to antibiotics. In the presence of cholangitis, about 5% to 10% of patients progress to septic shock, a condition that demands aggressive fluid resuscitation with hemodynamic monitoring in addition to antibiotics. After the resolution of toxic sepsis, ERCP may be followed by cholecystectomy. If no response, proceed to emergent decompression.

(F) Before gallbladder removal, ERCP and sphincterotomy may be performed in patients with history of jaundice, cholangitis, pancreatitis, markedly elevated liver enzymes, or dilated CBD. If gallbladder was removed in the past, ERCP and sphincterotomy alone may be sufficient.

(G) If advanced laparoscopic experience is available, preoperative ERCP may be omitted in favor of laparoscopic cholecystectomy and CBD exploration. Postoperative ERCP is another option.

(H) CBD stones should be flushed out with saline irrigation and sphincter relaxation obtained with IV glucagon. By laparoscopic transcystic CBD exploration, 80% to 90% of the stones may be removed with minimal morbidity. Either a helical basket or Fogarty balloon catheter may be inserted via the cystic duct to retrieve or push the CBD stones. A laparoscopic choledochoscope may be introduced into the CBD over a guide wire. With the ductal lumen under video monitoring, the stone is either retrieved or pushed using a No. 3 French helical basket. Another option is dilation of the sphincter of Oddi using a transcystic balloon catheter under fluoroscopic guidance (catheter is positioned and inflated to a pressure of 12 atmospheres for 5 minutes). The CBD stone is either flushed with irrigation or pushed with instruments as mentioned previously. There is a 10% risk of pancreatitis. Intracorporeal lithotripsy has shown only limited success.

(I) Postoperative ERCP with sphincterotomy and stone extraction fail in about 5% to 10% of cases depending on local expertise. One option is intraoperative ERCP so that, in case of failure, open CBD exploration may be performed.

(J) ERCP and sphincterotomy with stone extraction is done at the time of stones detection. If the stones cannot be extracted (5% to 10%), or if

History and physical examination
- Pain
- Fever
- Jaundice
- Septic shock

Ⓐ

CHOLEDOCHOLITHIASIS (COMMON BILE DUCT STONES)

Ⓑ

Diagnostics
- WBC
- Liver function studies
- Amylase
- Coagulation studies
- US/CT
- Cholangiography
- MRCP

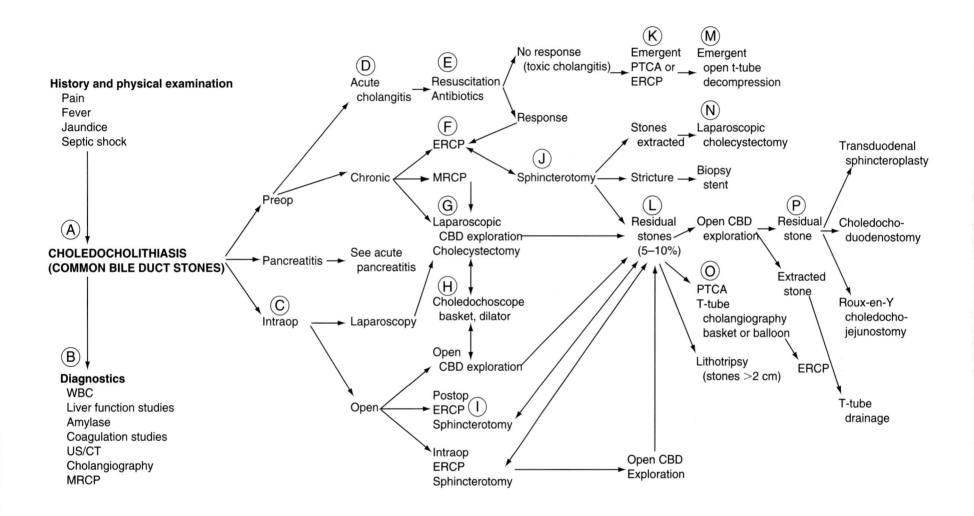

a biliary stricture from tumor is encountered, an endoscopic stent is placed to bypass the obstruction.

(K) Toxic cholangitis unresponsive to antibiotics requires emergent decompression by percutaneous transhepatic cholangiography (PTCA) or ERCP stenting (with or without sphincterotomy).

(L) Residual CBD stones may be followed for 6 weeks to permit spontaneous passage. A T-tube should be placed at the time of initial surgery and allowed to mature during the wait. If unsuccessful, radiographically directed extraction via the T-tube is next. Extracorporeal shockwave lithotripsy may be added for large stones (greater than 2 cm) or for patients who failed ERCP and have prior history of gallbladder removal.

(M) Emergency CBD exploration for acute cholangitis is rarely necessary and should be deferred until resolution of septic shock (the associated mortality is 30%). If no other course is available, consider open drainage with T-tube only.

(N) Laparoscopic cholecystectomy may be performed within 24 to 48 hours of ERCP.

(O) Radiographically directed removal of CBD stones (PTCA or T-tube cholangiography) using a basket or balloon has an overall success rate of 95% and morbidity of 5%. A third of the cases will require repeated attempts. Choledochotomy in small bile ducts (smaller than 6 mm) may lead to duct stenosis; therefore either ERCP or PTCA should be attempted first for normal sized ducts. If the repeat cholangiogram shows no stone, clamp T-tube 10 days postoperatively and remove 3 weeks later; if not, repeat T-tube stone extraction. Proceed to ERCP if unsuccessful.

(P) Most impacted stones may be removed through a choledochotomy, but a transduodenal sphincteroplasty is necessary in about 15% of cases to gain access to the area of impaction. Another option is a CBD drainage procedure (choledochoduodenostomy or Roux-en-Y choledochojejunostomy). The indications for a drainage procedure include multiple (more than 5) impacted stones, marked ductal dilatation (greater than 2 cm), or previous CBD surgery. Finally, if intrahepatic stone completely obstructs one side and is impossible to remove, lobectomy may be necessary.

REFERENCES

Adamek HE, Kudis V, Jakobs R et al: Impact of gallbladder status on the outcome in patients with retained bile duct stones treated with extracorporeal shockwave lithotripsy. Endoscopy 34:624–627, 2002.

Boerma D, Rauws EA, Keulemans YC et al: Wait and see policy or laparoscopic cholecystectomy after endoscopic sphincterotomy for bile duct stones: A randomized trial. Lancet 360:761–765, 2002.

Costamagna G, Tringali A, Shah SK et al: Long-term follow-up of patients after endoscopic sphincterotomy for choledocholithiasis and risk factors for recurrence. Endoscopy 34:273–279, 2002.

Liu Th, Consorti ET, Kawashima A et al: Patient evaluation and management with selective use of magnetic resonance cholangiography and endoscopic retrograde cholangiopancreatography before laparoscopic cholecystectomy. Ann Surg 234:33–40, 2001.

Schreurs WH, Juttmann JR, Stuifbergen WN et al: Management of common bile duct stones: Selective endoscopic retrograde cholangiography and endoscopic sphincterotomy: Short and long-term results. Surg Endosc 16:1068–1072, 2002.

Stiegmann GV, Soper NJ, Filipi CJ et al: Laparoscopic ultrasonography as compared with static or dynamic cholangiography at laparoscopic cholecystectomy: A prospective multicenter trial. Surg Endosc 9:1269–1273, 1995.

Sugiyama M, Atomi Y: Risk factors predictive of late complications after endoscopic sphincterotomy for bile duct stones: Long-term (more than 10 years) follow-up study. Am J Gastroenterol 97:2699–2701, 2002.

Wright BE, Freeman ML, Cummings JK et al: Current management of common bile duct stones: Is there a role for laparoscopic cholecystectomy and intraoperative endoscopic retrograde cholangio-pancreatography as a single-stage procedure? Surgery 132:729–735, 2002.

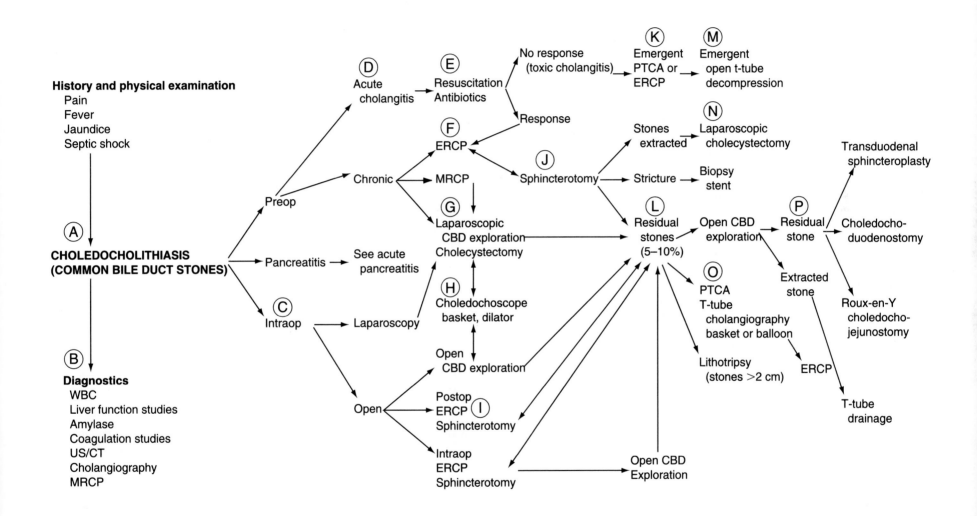

History and physical examination
Pain
Fever
Jaundice
Septic shock

Ⓐ

**CHOLEDOCHOLITHIASIS
(COMMON BILE DUCT STONES)**

Ⓑ

Diagnostics
WBC
Liver function studies
Amylase
Coagulation studies
US/CT
Cholangiography
MRCP

Preop

Pancreatitis → See acute pancreatitis

Ⓒ Intraop

Ⓓ Acute cholangitis

Chronic

Ⓔ Resuscitation Antibiotics

No response (toxic cholangitis)

Response

Ⓚ Emergent PTCA or ERCP

Ⓜ Emergent open t-tube decompression

Ⓕ ERCP

MRCP

Ⓖ Laparoscopic CBD exploration Cholecystectomy

Ⓙ Sphincterotomy

Stones extracted

Ⓝ Laparoscopic cholecystectomy

Stricture → Biopsy stent

Laparoscopy

Ⓗ Choledochoscope basket, dilator

Open CBD exploration

Open

Postop ERCP Ⓘ Sphincterotomy

Intraop ERCP Sphincterotomy

Open CBD Exploration

Ⓛ Residual stones (5–10%)

Ⓞ PTCA T-tube cholangiography basket or balloon

Lithotripsy (stones >2 cm)

Open CBD exploration

Ⓟ Residual stone

Extracted stone

ERCP

Transduodenal sphincteroplasty

Choledocho-duodenostomy

Roux-en-Y choledocho-jejunostomy

T-tube drainage

Chapter 51 *Liver Tumor*

CHRISTOPHER D. ANDERSON, MD • MARK P. CALLERY, MD •
RAVI S. CHARI, MD

(A) As a general rule, a lesion seen as a discrete nodule in the liver should be presumed to be a neoplastic lesion and should be investigated. Symptoms often reflect complications of the mass.

(B) Metastatic cancer is the most common cause of malignant liver tumors. Bronchogenic carcinoma is the most common cause of hepatic metastases, followed by cancers of the prostate, colon, breast, pancreas, stomach, kidney, and cervix.

(C) Male sex, age over 53 years, and alphafetoprotein greater than 20 ng/ml are all independent predictors of hepatocellular carcinoma (HCC) in patients with cirrhosis. An elevation of carcinoembryonic antigen (CEA) level in the patient with a history of colorectal carcinoma usually indicates recurrence.

(D) Ultrasonography (US) is commonly the first imaging modality used for screening and follow-up of liver tumors, but triple-phase helical computed tomography (CT) is superior for determination of size, number, and location of lesions. When further definition of hepatic lesions is required, magnetic resonance imaging (MRI) is useful. Radionucleotide studies have little role in the evaluation of liver masses.

(E) A metastatic screen including a chest CT should be performed to rule out metastatic disease. For patients with a history of colorectal carcinoma, positron emission tomography (PET) is useful for the evaluation of extrahepatic metastatic disease.

(F) Biopsy of a liver nodule is almost never indicated. In an adequate surgical candidate, resection of an occult liver mass should be considered without a biopsy. Laparoscopy can offer intra-abdominal staging and biopsy and should be performed before laparotomy when the lesion is a suspected primary liver tumor.

(G) Hemangiomas occur in all age groups, often grow during pregnancy, and are usually diagnosed by CT or MRI. They are rarely large, and spontaneous rupture is reported. The decision for resection should consider the presence of symptoms or if there is a danger of traumatic rupture (e.g., large lesions located below the costal margin). Occasionally, large lesions may present as dull, right upper quadrant discomfort that is relieved only by surgical resection; these lesions are usually larger than 5 cm.

(H) Hepatic adenomas occur primarily in young women, are associated with the use of oral contraceptives, and are usually solitary masses. They are prone to hemorrhage, necrosis, and tumor rupture in approximately one third of patients. Malignant change is possible. Resection is the treatment of choice when diagnosed. Excisional biopsy is the only reliable method to distinguish FNH, adenoma, and HCC; however, it should be noted that radiological evaluation is more than 90% accurate in distinguishing between benign and malignant lesions. Adenoma and FNH can be differentiated by biopsy: adenomas lack biliary elements.

(I) Focal nodular hyperplasia rarely produces symptoms (less than 10%). Hemorrhage, rupture, and malignant change are exceedingly rare. Central stellate-scarring detectable by US or CT is possible in lesions greater than 5 cm in diameter. Resection is unnecessary in the absence of symptoms.

(J) Gallbladder carcinoma is most commonly detected during or following cholecystectomy; it can often involve the liver via local extension or metastasis. If it is suspected during laparoscopic cholecystectomy, the procedure should be converted to open, and liver resection should be contemplated if appropriate. Radical resection (i.e., resection of segments 4B and 5) portends a survival advantage and remains the only chance of cure; it is indicated for stage II and III disease. After screening for distant metastases, a planned resection should begin with a staging laparoscopy to rule out advanced disease. Unresectable patients can be evaluated for palliative chemotherapy or supportive care.

(K) Intrahepatic cholangiocarcinoma is much less common than extrahepatic cholangiocarcinoma. Aggressive resection is the only chance of cure. Staging laparoscopy may be useful before laparotomy.

(L) Hepatoblastoma is a malignant tumor of embryonic or fetal hepatocytes that occurs in children younger than 3 years. Resection is the principal treatment. Primary hepatic angiosarcoma is rare, and there are no reported cases of 5-year survival. Cystadenocarcinoma may rarely arise from a cystadenoma; resection is beneficial.

(M) Neuroendocrine metastases are the second-most common indication for resection of secondary liver tumors. The indication for resection is palliation of symptoms. Medical palliation includes octreotide, embolization, and chemotherapy.

(N) Approximately 30% of patients with colorectal carcinoma will have synchronous liver metastases. Between 10% and 20% of patients with colorectal liver metastases have potentially resectable disease. Resection is the treatment of choice. Resection of a solitary colorectal metastatic lesion can give up to a 40% to 60% 5-year survival rate. Clinical trials are ongoing to evaluate adjuvant and neoadjuvant therapies. Favorable factors associated with improved survival include metachronous lesions, unilobar distribution of lesions, fewer that three lesions, having a largest lesion less than 5 cm in diameter, and CEA elevation less than 200 ng/dl.

(O) Solitary hepatic metastases from breast or renal cell carcinoma are rare. There are few data evaluating aggressive resection with or without adjuvant chemotherapy. Resection of hepatic metastases (in the absence of detectable extrahepatic disease) remains controversial, but may be beneficial in selected cases.

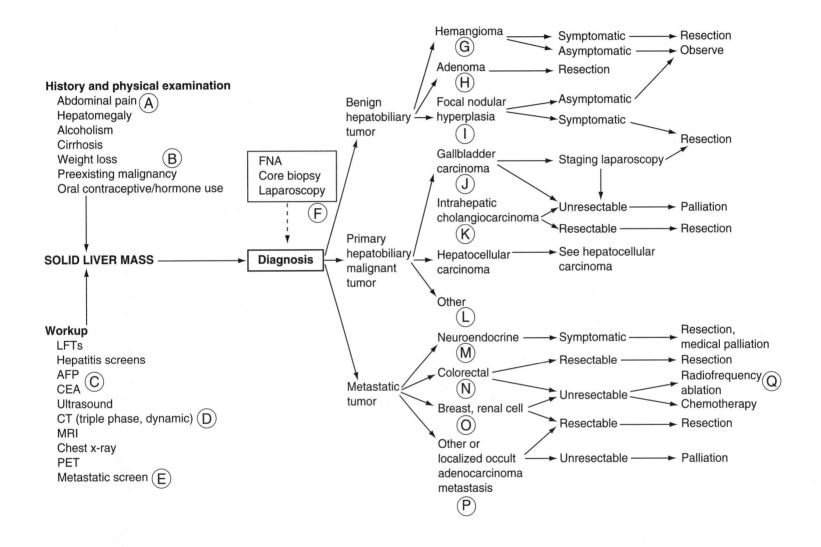

History and physical examination
Abdominal pain Ⓐ
Hepatomegaly
Alcoholism
Cirrhosis
Weight loss Ⓑ
Preexisting malignancy
Oral contraceptive/hormone use

Workup
LFTs
Hepatitis screens
AFP Ⓒ
CEA
Ultrasound
CT (triple phase, dynamic) Ⓓ
MRI
Chest x-ray
PET
Metastatic screen Ⓔ

SOLID LIVER MASS

FNA
Core biopsy
Laparoscopy
Ⓕ

Diagnosis

Benign hepatobiliary tumor

Primary hepatobiliary malignant tumor

Metastatic tumor

Hemangioma Ⓖ → Symptomatic → Resection
→ Asymptomatic → Observe

Adenoma Ⓗ → Resection

Focal nodular hyperplasia Ⓘ → Asymptomatic → Observe
→ Symptomatic → Resection

Gallbladder carcinoma Ⓙ → Staging laparoscopy → Resection
→ Unresectable → Palliation
→ Resectable → Resection

Intrahepatic cholangiocarcinoma Ⓚ

Hepatocellular carcinoma → See hepatocellular carcinoma

Other Ⓛ

Neuroendocrine Ⓜ → Symptomatic → Resection, medical palliation

Colorectal Ⓝ → Resectable → Resection
→ Unresectable → Radiofrequency ablation Ⓠ
→ Chemotherapy

Breast, renal cell Ⓞ → Resectable → Resection

Other or localized occult adenocarcinoma metastasis Ⓟ → Unresectable → Palliation

(P) A biopsy-proven adenocarcinoma metastasis from an occult primary can be resected when possible; however, this is rare. Chemotherapy should be considered, and several clinical trials are investigating combination therapy. Prognosis remains extremely poor.

(Q) Ablative therapies are being used more commonly, with goals of cure as well as palliation. Radiofrequency ablation (RFA) is now often used in patients who are deemed unresectable or who are poor candidates for resection. Many surgeons also use RFA as an adjunct to resection. This technology is continually evolving, and a survival advantage has yet to be proven. Cryosurgery has been used in the past, but is less often used now because it is associated with increased systemic complications such as pulmonary insufficiency and renal impairment.

REFERENCES

Benson III, AB: Hepatobiliary Cancer, Clinical Practice Guidelines in Oncology. Journal of the National Comprehensive Cancer Network 1:94–108, 2003.

Chari RS, Callery MP: Colorectal Cancer Metastatic to the Liver: Resection and Intraarterial Chemotherapy. In Cameron JL (ed): Current Surgical Therapy, 7th ed. St Louis: Mosby, 2001.

Chari RS, Carwenlaa, H, Meyers WC: Diagnostic Imaging in Liver Surgery. In Townsend CM (ed): Sabiston Textbook of Surgery, 16th ed. Philadelphia: WB Saunders, 2001.

Chen ZY, Qi QH, Dong ZL: Etiology and management of hemorrhage in spontaneous liver rupture: A report of 70 cases. World J Gastroenterol 8:1063–1066, 2002.

Choy PY Koe J, McCall J, et al: The role of radiofrequency ablation in the treatment of primary and metastatic tumours of the liver: Initial lessons learned. NZ Med J 115:1159, 2002.

Delbeke D, Martin WM, Sandler MP, et al: Evaluation of benign vs. malignant hepatic lesions with positron emission tomography. Arch Surg 133:510–515, 1998.

Hogan BA, Thornton FJ, Brennigan M, et al: Hepatic metastases from an unknown primary neoplasm (UPN): Survival, prognostic indicators and value of extensive investigations. Clin Radiol 57:1073–1077, 2002.

Kuvshinoff BW, Ota DM: Radiofrequency ablation of liver tumors: Influence of technique and tumor size. Surgery 132:605–611, 2002.

Meyers WC, Chari RS, Schaffer BK, et al: Neoplasms. In Townsend CM (ed): Sabiston Textbook of Surgery, 16th ed. Philadelphia: WB Saunders, 2001.

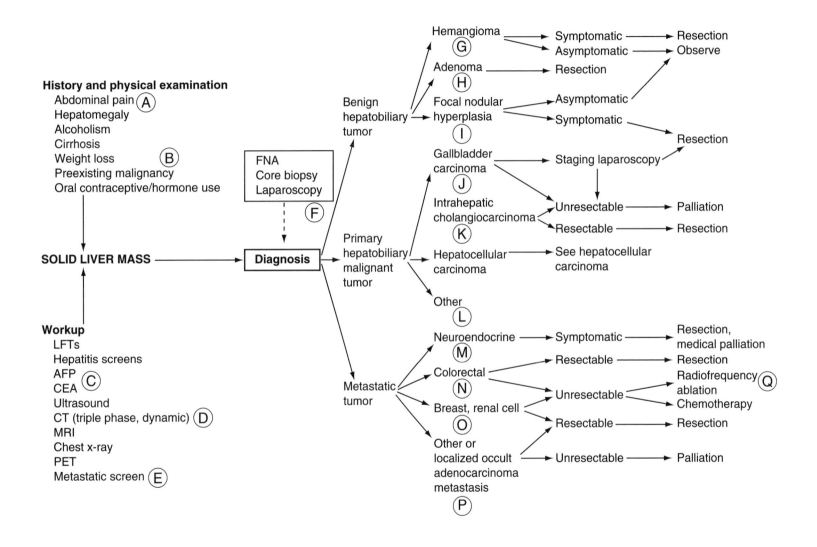

History and physical examination
Abdominal pain (A)
Hepatomegaly
Alcoholism
Cirrhosis
Weight loss   (B)
Preexisting malignancy
Oral contraceptive/hormone use

SOLID LIVER MASS

Workup
LFTs
Hepatitis screens
AFP   (C)
CEA
Ultrasound
CT (triple phase, dynamic) (D)
MRI
Chest x-ray
PET
Metastatic screen (E)

FNA
Core biopsy
Laparoscopy
(F)

Diagnosis

Benign hepatobiliary tumor

Primary hepatobiliary malignant tumor

Metastatic tumor

Hemangioma (G) → Symptomatic → Resection
→ Asymptomatic → Observe

Adenoma (H) → Resection

Focal nodular hyperplasia (I) → Asymptomatic
→ Symptomatic → Resection

Gallbladder carcinoma (J) → Staging laparoscopy → Resection
→ Unresectable → Palliation

Intrahepatic cholangiocarcinoma (K) → Unresectable → Palliation
→ Resectable → Resection

Hepatocellular carcinoma → See hepatocellular carcinoma

Other (L)

Neuroendocrine (M) → Symptomatic → Resection, medical palliation

Colorectal (N) → Resectable → Resection
→ Unresectable → Radiofrequency ablation (Q)
→ Chemotherapy

Breast, renal cell (O) → Resectable → Resection

Other or localized occult adenocarcinoma metastasis (P) → Unresectable → Palliation

Chapter 52 *Hepatocellular Carcinoma*

LISA A. RUTSTEIN, MD ● DAVID A. GELLER, MD

(A) Hepatocellular carcinoma (HCC) is one of the most common cancers in the world, with approximately 1 million cases diagnosed each year. Incidence in the United States increased by 70% between the mid-1970s and the mid-1990s.

(B) The incidence of HCC is highest in Mozambique, Zimbabwe, and in Southeast Asia, where the rate exceeds 30 cases per 100,000 population per year. High rates are also seen in Japan, Greece, and Africa. The disease is less common in northern Europe, Canada, and in the United States, although recent data indicate an increase in HCC in the United States.

(C) HCC, an epithelial tumor derived from hepatocytes, accounts for 80% of primary hepatic tumors. It affects men three times more commonly than women and is usually associated with underlying hepatic cirrhosis (70% of HCCs develop in cirrhotic livers). There is a strong association between hepatitis B (HBV) and HCC, especially in non-Western countries. In Western countries, cirrhosis associated with alcoholism and hepatitis C (HCV) infection shows the strongest association. The annual incidence of HCC in patients with cirrhosis is 3% to 5%. Up to 5 % of Child's class A patients are found to have small tumors, and this figure rises to 15% in patients with Child's B or C cirrhosis.

(D) Other significant risk factors for the development of cirrhosis and an increased risk of HCC include metabolic disorders such as tyrosinemia; α1-antitrypsin deficiency; Wilson's disease; hypercitrullinemia; porphyria cutanea tarda; and, most notably, primary and secondary hemochromatosis. Oral contraceptive use is associated with the development of hepatic adenoma, which can rarely undergo malignant change. In addition, aflatoxins, thorotrast (thorium dioxide), vinyl chloride monomer, arsenic, and prolonged use of anabolic steroids all have an association with the development of HCC.

(E) Hepatocellular carcinoma may present with abdominal symptoms, an elevated serum alpha-fetoprotein (AFP), or as an incidental finding on radiologic investigation.

(F) When symptomatic, presentation may include weight loss, upper abdominal pain, jaundice, ascites, or fever. In addition, patients may present with signs of chronic liver disease and stigmata of portal hypertension (e.g., varices, splenomegaly, gastrointestinal bleeding, or encephalopathy). Symptomatic presentation is more likely representative of unresectable disease.

(G) Ultrasonography is used in the screening of the cirrhotic patient with a raised alpha-fetoprotein level to detect masses within the liver parenchyma and to demonstrate associated vascular pathology including tumor thrombus or overt vessel invasion. As a primary imaging modality, transabdominal ultrasonography has a 70% to 80% sensitivity for the detection of HCC.

(H) Most HCCs appear as hypervascular enhancing masses during the arterial phase of a dual-phase helical computed tomography (CT) scan. Small HCCs (smaller than 2 cm) may enhance in a manner similar to hepatic parenchyma because of their predominantly portal venous supply. Dual-phase CT scanning with separate hepatic arterial and portal venous phase imaging has demonstrated a sensitivity of 93% to 96% in the detection of HCC, although this decreases to less than 90% in patients with lesions smaller than 3 cm in diameter. Magnetic resonance imaging, especially in association with dynamic bolus gadolinium contrast, shows the highest detection rate.

(I) AFP determination and transcutaneous ultrasonography are the most widely used screening tests for HCC. AFP is elevated in 80% to 90% of patients in Asia and in 60% to 70% of patients in the United States and Europe. There is no exact correlation between the level of AFP and the actual extent of HCC. Des-y-carboxy prothrombin (DCP) is another serologic assay for HCC. CEA is occasionally elevated by HCC.

(J) Angiography, in combination with dual-phase CT scan, increases the sensitivity of tumor detection and can be used to determine vascular invasion by tumor. As well, a characteristic vascular blush in a liver mass will confirm HCC.

(K) Stage I HCC is a solitary tumor of any size with no vascular invasion (T1NOMO). Stage II disease is a solitary tumor with vascular invasion or multiple tumors all less than 5 cm in diameter (T2NOMO). Both stage I and stage II patients may be resectable depending on liver status (cirrhosis) and the extent of tumor. Ideal resection candidates include noncirrhotic or Child's class A patients with a single lesion and no metastatic disease. Stage IIIA HCC includes one or more tumors greater than 5 cm with invasion of the portal and/or hepatic veins (T3NOMO). Stage IIIB is a tumor that invades organs other than the gallbladder or tumor perforation (T4NOMO). Stage IIIC HCC includes any tumor with nodal involvement (Any T, N1MO). Stage IV HCC is any tumor with associated metastatic disease (Any T, NM1). Stages III and IV disease are rarely resectable because of the extent of tumor and cirrhosis.

(L) The degree of cirrhosis determines the possibility of or extent of resection. In general, a normal liver patient can tolerate 75% resection; a Child's class A cirrhotic can undergo 50% resection; a Child's class B cirrhotic can undergo 25% resection; and a Child's class C cirrhotic cannot tolerate resection. Patients with minimal or no cirrhosis have a better prognosis following resection.

(M) Liver transplantation (LTX) is a good option for HCC because it removes the cancer and the underlying premalignant condition (cirrhosis). From early LTX experiences, it has been determined that certain characteristics of HCC are associated with better outcomes after LTX. Attempts to define the optimal upper limits of tumor size and number as predictors for outcome after LTX have yielded conflicting results.

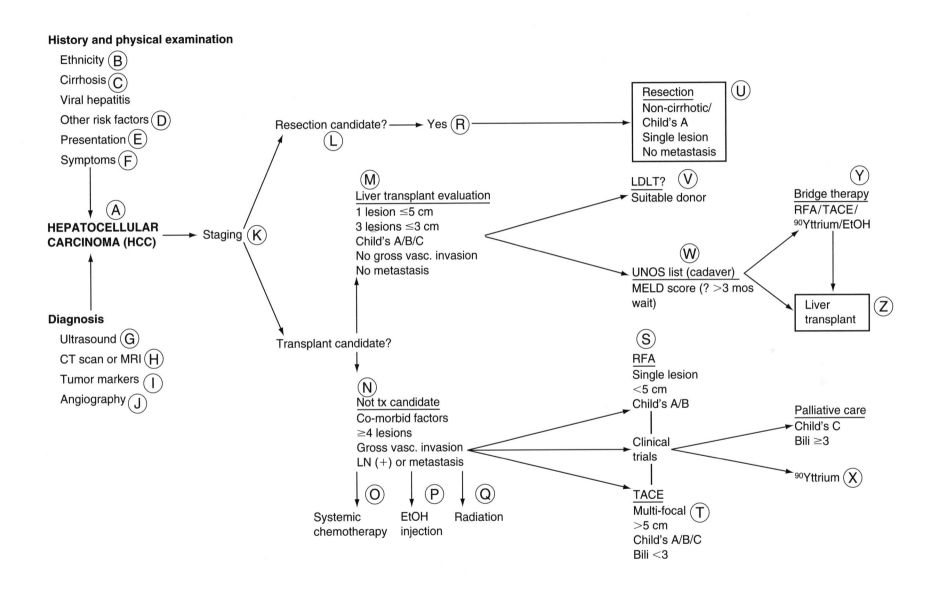

History and physical examination

Ethnicity (B)

Cirrhosis (C)

Viral hepatitis

Other risk factors (D)

Presentation (E)

Symptoms (F)

(A)

HEPATOCELLULAR CARCINOMA (HCC)

Diagnosis

Ultrasound (G)

CT scan or MRI (H)

Tumor markers (I)

Angiography (J)

Staging (K)

Resection candidate? → Yes (R)
(L)

Resection (U)
Non-cirrhotic/
Child's A
Single lesion
No metastasis

(M)
Liver transplant evaluation
1 lesion ≤5 cm
3 lesions ≤3 cm
Child's A/B/C
No gross vasc. invasion
No metastasis

LDLT? (V)
Suitable donor

UNOS list (cadaver) (W)
MELD score (? >3 mos wait)

Bridge therapy (Y)
RFA/TACE/
⁹⁰Yttrium/EtOH

Liver transplant (Z)

Transplant candidate?

(N)
Not tx candidate
Co-morbid factors
≥4 lesions
Gross vasc. invasion
LN (+) or metastasis

Systemic chemotherapy (O)

EtOH injection (P)

Radiation (Q)

(S)
RFA
Single lesion
<5 cm
Child's A/B

Clinical trials

TACE
Multi-focal (T)
>5 cm
Child's A/B/C
Bili <3

Palliative care
Child's C
Bili ≥3

⁹⁰Yttrium (X)

(N) Patients who are not considered transplant candidates include those with prohibitive comorbid factors, with 4 or more lesions, with gross vascular invasion and involved lymph nodes, or those with metastatic tumor burden. Options for treatment include radiofrequency ablation (RFA) via a percutaneous or laparoscopic approach, transarterial chemoembolization (TACE), or 90 Yttrium selective internal radiation therapy. Candidates for RFA include Child's class A or B patients with a solitary lesion smaller than 5 cm. Ongoing clinical trials using TACE or 90 Yttrium microspheres have involved Child's class A/B/C patients with multifocal disease, lesions larger than 5 cm, and a serum bilirubin lower than 3 mg/dl. Selective internal radiation therapy with 90 Yttrium microspheres involves injection of radiation microspheres into the hepatic artery; this has shown reasonable objective response rates with decreases in both serum tumor markers and in tumor burden on CT scan.

(O) Systemic chemotherapy has been largely abandoned in the management of HCC because of its limited effectiveness. The overall partial response rate to the most effective agent (Adriamycin) is 20% with a median survival of 16 weeks. In addition, systemic toxicity from this treatment is significant with the majority of patients reporting severe side effects.

(P) Injection of 99.5% ethanol into a HCC less than 5 cm in diameter by either a percutaneous or open operative approach leads to the ablation of tumor foci in many cases. Despite its low side effect profile and reported effectiveness, the recurrence rate at 5 years is greater than 80%. Multiple treatments are usually required because of the tumor's propensity for recurrence.

(Q) Radiation therapy as a primary modality has limited effectiveness because of tumor resistance and the risk of radiation-induced hepatitis. Radiation therapy can be used as part of a multimodality regimen.

(R) Routine preoperative evaluation includes serum AFP determination; liver function tests (i.e., ALT, AST, total bilirubin, protime, and PTT); dual-phase CT scan of the abdomen; and CT scan of the chest.

(S) RFA involves ultrasound-guided placement of an electrode into the center of a tumor by an open operative, laparoscopic, or percutaneous technique. The electrode is connected to a radiofrequency generator that heats the probe and results in coagulative necrosis of the tumor. RFA can be used as primary therapy in cirrhotic patients who are not candidates for resection or as bridging therapy in patients who are awaiting transplantation. At many centers in the United States, RFA has replaced cryotherapy because there is less morbidity associated with the ablation technique.

(T) A variety of embolization techniques have been undertaken for the treatment of HCC, including the use of polyvinyl chloride alcohol particles, gelatin particles, ivalon, Gelfoam, or Lipiodol, either alone or in combination with chemotherapeutic agents (e.g., Adriamycin, Mitomycin-C, or cisplatin). Embolization acts by causing ischemic necrosis of tumor. Combining chemotherapeutic agents with Lipiodol may enhance antitumor effect because of the affinity of the iodized oily agent for HCC. Chemoembolization can be used as a neoadjuvant therapy to downsize tumor burden before resection, as a palliative treatment in patients with unresectable lesions, or as a bridge therapy in patients awaiting transplantation. Many studies of chemoembolization demonstrate a borderline survival advantage but they are nonrandomized clinical series. One multicenter trial showed 62% of patients treated with chemoembolization were alive at 1 year, in comparision with 44% of patients treated symptomatically. Current clinical trials using transarterial chemoembolization (TACE) involve Child's class A/B/C patients with multifocal disease, tumors larger than 5 cm, and a bilirubin level lower than 3 mg/dl.

(U) The ideal candidate for resection is a noncirrhotic or Child's class A patient with a single lesion and no metastasis. Unfortunately, less than 20% of patients diagnosed with HCC fulfill the criteria for surgical resection. Overall, improved outcomes have been observed in cases of single and small tumors, absence of vascular invasion, absence of cirrhosis, negative node involvement, absence of metastases, negative resection margins, and fibrolamellar types. Surgical resection of HCC

has reported 1- and 5-year survival rates of 55% to 90% and 10% to 50%, respectively. Mortality rates in cirrhotic and noncirrhotic patients are 7% to 25% and less than 3%, respectively. Deaths beyond the immediate postoperative period are most commonly associated with tumor recurrence. It is well documented that the greatest risk factor for the development of a second HCC in the liver is a previous diagnosis of HCC. Data suggest that this risk is up to 40% at 2 years for patients with a single initial lesion.

(V) Living donor liver transplantation (LDLT) is also an alternative for patients with HCC in the setting of cirrhosis. LDLT was first offered in Asia where cadaver liver donation is rare, but LDLT has gained acceptance in the United States and is offered by many transplant centers.

(W) In February 2002, the Model for End-Stage Liver Disease (MELD) scoring system was implemented in the United States to allocate the scarce liver organ donors. The MELD system ranks patients with cirrhosis based on their risk of death. The MELD priority score (a 6 to 40 point scale) is calculated from a formula that takes into account serum total bilirubin, INR, and serum creatinine. Recognizing that early stage HCC patients have a limited period in which to receive a potentially curative liver transplant, additional MELD priority points are assigned to patients with stage I (24 points) and stage II (29 points) HCC. The United Network of Organ Sharing (UNOS) has adopted the criteria proposed by the group from Milan: stage I, solitary tumor smaller than 2 cm; stage II, solitary tumor smaller than 5 cm, or three or fewer lesions none of which is larger than 3 cm (the Milan Criteria). The traditional pathologic tumor-node-metastasis (TNM) classification does not seem to have sufficient prognostic power with respect to survival and risk for HCC recurrence after LTX. Modifications of both the TNM and the Milan criteria have been based on microvascular or macrovascular invasion, lobar distribution, tumor size, and lymph node involvement. These newly proposed criteria (UCSF Criteria and the Pittsburgh Modified TNM Criteria) seem to provide a more clear-cut discrimination with respect to posttransplant survival for each TNM tumor stage (I to IV).

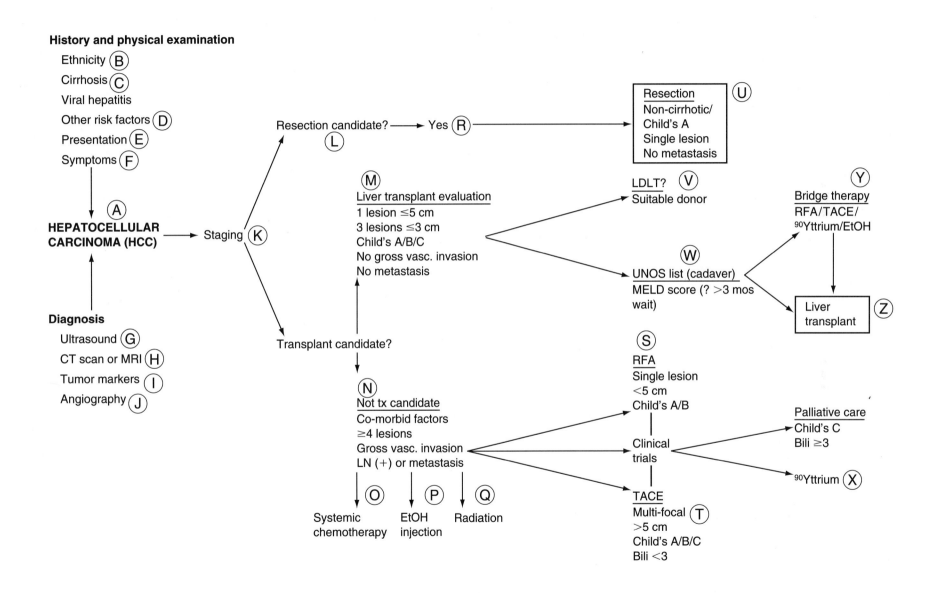

Ⓧ Internal radiation therapy can be administered in the form of 90 Yttrium microspheres, which are delivered via the hepatic artery. This form of radiation is better tolerated by nontumorous tissue than traditional external beam radiotherapy. Repeated treatments can be given to residual or recurrent tumor in the patient with nonresectable HCC. Objective response is measured by following serum AFP levels and serial CT findings.

Ⓨ Neoadjuvant therapy (or bridge therapy) including RFA, TACE, 90 Yttrium, or ETOH injection can be utilized once the patient is placed on the UNOS list with an initial MELD score in order to slow disease progression and compensate for the increased waiting time. These therapies have been used to help maintain eligibility for those transplant candidates with progressive disease.

Ⓩ Liver transplantation for HCC results in 1- and 5-year survival rates ranging from 42% to 71% and from 20% to 45%, respectively. Improved outcomes have been reported with incidentally discovered HCC and fibrolamellar variants. Despite this, prolonged waiting times and the lack of readily available organs have led to the progression of tumors to the extent that many potential recipients become noneligible candidates for transplantation.

REFERENCES

Adam R, Akpinar E, Johann M et al: Place of cryosurgery in the treatment of malignant liver tumors. Ann Surg 225:39–50, 1997.

Carr BI: Hepatic artery chemoembolization for advanced stage HCC: Experience of 650 patients. Hepatogastroenterology 49:79–86, 2002.

Cheng SJ, Freeman RB, Wong JB: Predicting the probability of progression-free survival in patients with small hepatocellular carcinoma. Liver Transplantation 8:323–328, 2002.

Chi-Leung L, Sheung-Tat F: Nonresectionable therapies for hepatocellular carcinoma. Am J Surg 173:358–365, 1997.

Cai-De L, Shu-You P, Xien-Chuan J et al: Pre-operative transcatheter arterial chemoembolization and prognosis of patients with hepatocellular carcinomas: Retrospective analysis of 120 cases. World J Surg 23:293–300, 1999.

Fong Y, Blumgart LH: American Cancer Society Clinical Atlas of Oncology: Hepatobiliary Cancer 43–74, 2001.

Fung J, Marsh W: The quandary over liver transplantation for hepatocellular carcinoma: The greater sin? Liver Transplantation 8:775–777, 2002.

Goodman M, Geller DA: Radiofrequency Ablation for Hepatocellular Carcinoma. In Carr B (ed): Hepatocellular Carcinoma. In press.

Harada T, Matsuo K, Inoue T et al: Is preoperative hepatic arterial chemoembolization safe and effective for hepatocellular carcinoma? Ann Surg 224:4–9, 1996.

Holbrook R, Koo K, Ryan J: Resection of malignant primary liver tumors. Am J Surg 171:453–455, 1996.

Iwatsuki S, Dvorchik I, Marsh JW et al: Liver transplantation for hepatocellular carcinoma: A proposal of a prognostic scoring system. J Am Coll Surg 191:389–394, 2000.

Lezoche E, Paganini A, Felliciotti F et al: Ultrasound-guided laparoscopic cryoablation of hepatic tumors: Preliminary report. World J Surg 22:829–836, 1998.

Marsh JW, Dvorchik I, Bonham CA et al: Is the pathologic TNM staging system for patients with hepatoma predictive of outcome? Cancer 88:538–543, 2000.

Molmenti EP, Klintmalm GB: Liver transplantation in association with hepatocellular carcinoma: An update of the international tumor registry. Liver Transplantation 8:736–748, 2002.

Nagasue N, Kohno H, Chang YC et al: Liver resection for hepatocellular carcinoma. Ann Surg 217:375–384, 1993.

Yamanaka N, Tanaka T, Oriyama T et al: Microwave coagulonecrotic therapy for hepatocellular carcinoma. World J Surg 20:1076–1108, 1996.

Yao FY, Ferrell L, Bass NM, et al: Liver transplantation for hepatocellular carcinoma: Expansion of the tumor size limits does not adversely impact survival. Hepatology 33:1394–1403, 2001.

Yao FY, Ferrell L, Bass NM, et al: Liver transplantation for hepatocellular carcinoma: Comparison of the proposed UCSF criteria with the Milan criteria and the Pittsburgh modified TNM criteria. Liver Transplantation 8:765–774, 2002.

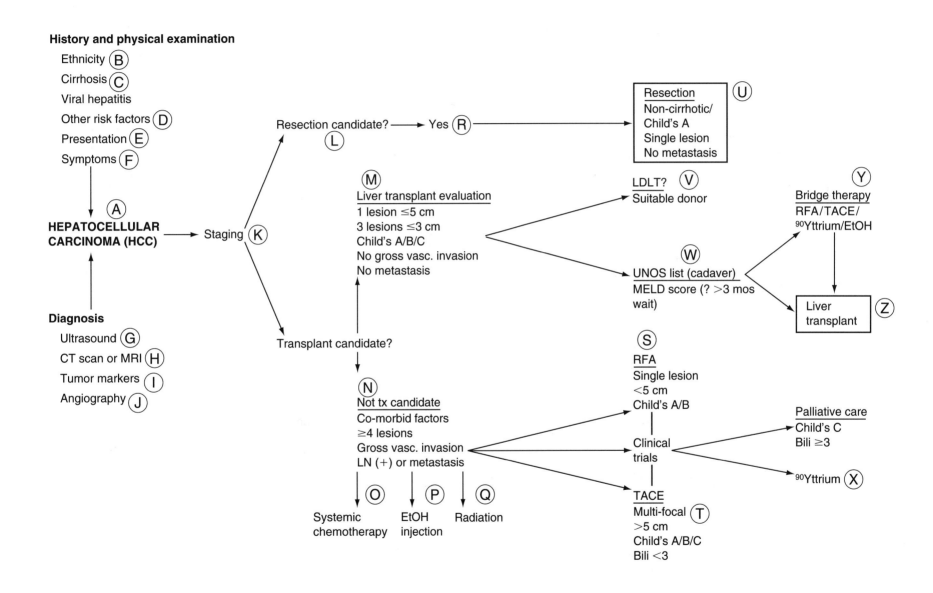

History and physical examination

Ethnicity (B)

Cirrhosis (C)

Viral hepatitis

Other risk factors (D)

Presentation (E)

Symptoms (F)

(A)

HEPATOCELLULAR CARCINOMA (HCC)

Diagnosis

Ultrasound (G)

CT scan or MRI (H)

Tumor markers (I)

Angiography (J)

Staging (K)

Resection candidate? (L) → Yes (R)

Resection (U)
Non-cirrhotic/
Child's A
Single lesion
No metastasis

(M)
Liver transplant evaluation
1 lesion ≤5 cm
3 lesions ≤3 cm
Child's A/B/C
No gross vasc. invasion
No metastasis

LDLT? (V)
Suitable donor

UNOS list (cadaver) (W)
MELD score (? >3 mos wait)

Bridge therapy (Y)
RFA/TACE/
⁹⁰Yttrium/EtOH

Liver transplant (Z)

Transplant candidate?

(N)
Not tx candidate
Co-morbid factors
≥4 lesions
Gross vasc. invasion
LN (+) or metastasis

(S)
RFA
Single lesion
<5 cm
Child's A/B

Clinical trials

TACE (T)
Multi-focal
>5 cm
Child's A/B/C
Bili <3

Palliative care
Child's C
Bili ≥3

⁹⁰Yttrium (X)

Systemic chemotherapy (O)

EtOH injection (P)

Radiation (Q)

Chapter 53 Hepatic Abscess

SCOTT W. HELTON, MD

(A) The best indication of an amebic or parasitic infection is a history of travel to an endemic area such as Mexico, Central America, or Southeast Asia. Hydatid disease occurs in sheep-raising countries. Tropical climate is associated with amebiasis.

(B) The most common cause of pyogenic liver abscess is biliary tract obstruction or cholangitis (35%) caused by gallstones or malignancy. In the past, the most common cause was portal pyemia caused by diverticulitis, inflammatory bowel disease, or perforated appendicitis; this now accounts for 20% of cases.

(C) Approximately 20% of hepatic abscesses are cryptogenic and associated with other morbid medical conditions.

(D) Increased risk associated with these syndromes.

(E) These are classic symptoms, but the presentation is often varied. A single abscess may present gradually and insidiously, whereas multiple abscesses are associated with more systemic symptoms.

(F) Clinically, the liver can be palpated and percussion over the ribs may aggravate the pain.

(G) Leukocytosis is present in most patients.

(H) Liver function tests are abnormal in most patients but the elevations are seldom marked. In recent years, the percentage of patients with abnormal liver function tests has decreased. This difference may reflect the increased incidence of abscess in patients with biliary stents. Alkaline phosphatase elevations tend to be higher when compared with other liver function tests.

(I) If hepatic abscess is detected, serologic tests should be performed to rule out active amebiasis or echinococcal infection. *Entamoeba histolytica*–specific antigen detection or PCR is preferred to confirm the diagnosis of amebiasis. Echinococcal liver abscess can be confirmed by means of an elevated indirect hemagglutination (IHA) titer or by an IgG enzyme–linked immunoabsorbent assay (ELISA).

(J) Blood cultures and/or bile cultures (obtained at ERCP) are important because they are positive in half of patients and can aid in directing antimicrobial therapy. Cultures from abscess cavities are commonly sterile because of prior antimicrobial therapy. Presence of *Streptococcus milleri* in the blood may be associated with a visceral abscess.

(K) Ultrasonography is the study of choice in patients with suspected biliary disease and in patients who must avoid intravenous contrast or radiation exposure. It has excellent sensitivity (80% to 90%) and can demonstrate lesions as small as 2 cm in liver substance. Most liver abscesses occur in the right lobe: 40% are 1.5- to 5-cm in diameter, 40% are 5- to 8-cm in diameter, and 20% are more than 8 cm in diameter.

(L) CT scanning is superior to ultrasound for evaluating the presence of air and abscesses as small as 0.5 cm in diameter, especially near the hemidiaphragm. Abdominal CT is the method of choice in the postoperative patient. CT imaging is the best guide for complex drainage procedures.

(M) ERCP is indicated when gallstones or biliary malignancy is the potential source of the abscess. Percutaneous transhepatic cholangiography/drainage is indicated when ERCP is nondiagnostic or unavailable.

(N) Infectious etiology is important in making management decisions. It is essential to differentiate hydatid cysts from amebic or pyogenic abscess because special precautions are required for the drainage of echinococcal cysts to prevent the risk of spillage and anaphylaxis. Less common infectious agents such as fungus and mycobacterium may also cause hepatic abscess. These are more likely to occur in patients that are immunosuppressed (e.g., because of malignancy, postorgan transplant, steroids, chronic diseases, or the elderly).

(O) Diagnostic percutaneous aspiration is critical in cases where the etiology is unclear or if the patient is acutely ill and requires emergent therapy. It should be performed after ruling out the possibility of a hydatid cyst through serologic studies. Aspiration may also be beneficial in left-sided abscesses and in extremely large abscesses (greater than 10 cm). Aspiration can be both diagnostic and therapeutic. Aspirated material should always be sent for culture.

(P) Amoebic abscesses are the most common liver abscess worldwide and constitute 10% of all abscesses. Infection with *Entamoeba histolytica* is prevalent in subtropical and tropical climates and in developing countries where sanitation and public health measures are poor. Immigration and travel between countries has increased the incidence of this disease in developed countries. The cystic form enters the human through oral ingestion of contaminated material. Trophocytes are released and multiply in the colon, especially the cecum. The trophocytes reach the liver through the portal vein, the lymphatics, or by direct extension through the colon wall into the peritoneum and then through the liver capsule. Amebic abscesses develop in ischemic necrotic areas caused by obstruction of the small venules by the trophocytes and their byproducts. Like pyogenic abscesses, they are more commonly found in the right lobe of the liver. Amebic abscess tends to be solitary. The clinical signs and symptoms of amebic liver abscess are similar to those of pyogenic abscesses. There are often no detectable parasites in the stool of patients with amebic liver abscess. Serologic testing for antibodies to *E. histolytica* is more useful. It is important to note that a positive titer can represent a previous infection rather than current illness; therefore imaging techniques are important in the diagnosis. In addition to US and CT, 99mTc nuclide hepatic scanning may be useful for differentiating an amebic liver abscess from a pyogenic abscess. Amebic abscesses do not contain leukocytes and

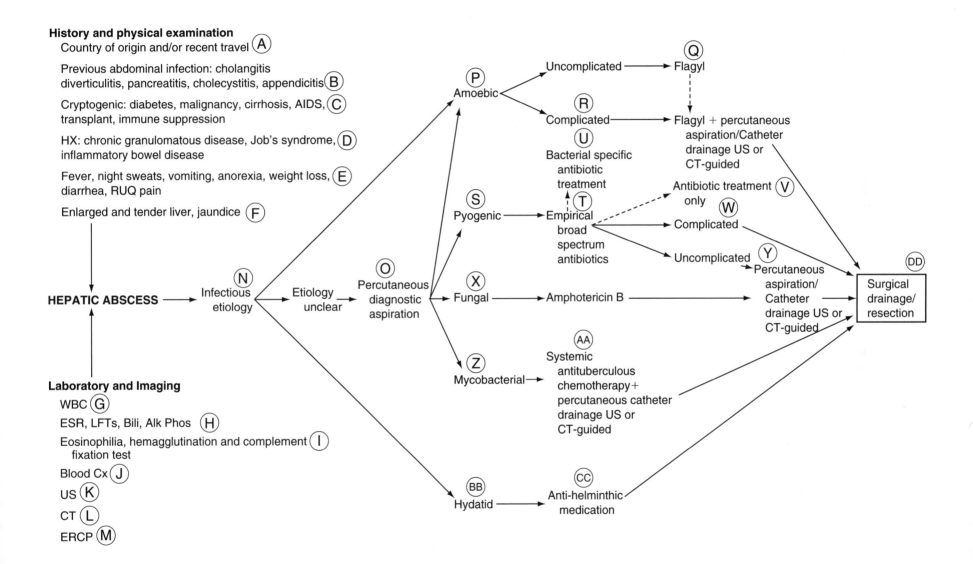

History and physical examination

Country of origin and/or recent travel (A)

Previous abdominal infection: cholangitis
diverticulitis, pancreatitis, cholecystitis, appendicitis (B)

Cryptogenic: diabetes, malignancy, cirrhosis, AIDS, (C)
transplant, immune suppression

HX: chronic granulomatous disease, Job's syndrome, (D)
inflammatory bowel disease

Fever, night sweats, vomiting, anorexia, weight loss, (E)
diarrhea, RUQ pain

Enlarged and tender liver, jaundice (F)

HEPATIC ABSCESS

Laboratory and Imaging

WBC (G)

ESR, LFTs, Bili, Alk Phos (H)

Eosinophilia, hemagglutination and complement (I)
fixation test

Blood Cx (J)

US (K)

CT (L)

ERCP (M)

(N) Infectious etiology

Etiology unclear

(O) Percutaneous diagnostic aspiration

(P) Amoebic

(S) Pyogenic

(X) Fungal

(Z) Mycobacterial

(BB) Hydatid

Uncomplicated ⟶ (Q) Flagyl

Complicated ⟶ (R) Flagyl + percutaneous aspiration/Catheter drainage US or CT-guided

(U) Bacterial specific antibiotic treatment

(T) Empirical broad spectrum antibiotics

(V) Antibiotic treatment only

(W) Complicated

Uncomplicated ⟶ (Y) Percutaneous aspiration/ Catheter drainage US or CT-guided

Amphotericin B

(AA) Systemic antituberculous chemotherapy+ percutaneous catheter drainage US or CT-guided

(CC) Anti-helminthic medication

(DD) Surgical drainage/ resection

appear as "cold" lesions, whereas pyogenic liver lesions contain leukocytes and may be visualized as "hot" lesions on the nuclide scan.

(Q) Metronidazole is the treatment of choice for uncomplicated amebic liver abscess. It enters the parasite by passive diffusion, then is converted into a reactive cytotoxic nitro radical by reduced ferridoxin or flavodoxin. It is effective against both systemic and intestinal manifestations, and clinical improvement usually occurs within 3 days. Patients failing this therapy should receive chloroquine therapy. After the patient has been treated, a luminal agent such as iodoquinol, paromomycin, or diloxanide furoate should be administered for treatment of the asymptomatic colonization state. Failure to use luminal agents will lead to relapse of infection in approximately 10% of patients.

(R) Patients who require percutaneous aspiration or catheter drainage are those with a high risk of abscess rupture, abscess cavity size greater than 5 cm, left lobe abscess (associated with higher mortality and higher frequency of peritoneal leak or rupture into the pericardium), and those that fail to respond clinically to drug therapy within 5 to 7 days.

(S) Pyogenic abscesses are the most common hepatic abscess in the United States; mortality is as high as 30%. The incidence has slowly increased from 13 to 20 per 100,000 hospital admissions. Aggressive operative and nonoperative approaches to the management of hepatobiliary and pancreatic neoplasms (e.g., hepatic artery embolization and biliary stenting) may be contributing to this trend. Most patients with pyogenic abscess present with fever and abdominal pain. With the exception of alkaline phosphatase and leukocyte count, most laboratory findings are normal. Most pyogenic abscesses are located in the right lobe of the liver. This is thought to be caused by the preferential blood supply of the superior mesenteric vein to the right lobe of the liver. Pyogenic liver abscesses tend to be multiple.

(T) Antibiotics should be started as soon as the diagnosis is suspected. Empirical antimicrobials should include coverage for anaerobes, gram-negative bacilli, and streptococcus species.

Monotherapy or multidrug therapy can be used depending on the severity and suspicion of the inciting bacteria. The typical regimen consists of an aminoglycoside, a penicillin (ampicillin), and metronidazole (to cover the possibility of an amebic abscess). In certain cases, a carbapenem can substitute for the penicillin and a fluoroquinolone can substitute for the aminoglycoside and penicillin.

(U) Blood culture and abscess aspiration cultures should be obtained to help guide antimicrobial therapy. Once microbiologic data are obtained, antibiotic therapy should be tailored to the organisms isolated and the antibiotic susceptibility profiles. Duration of antibiotic therapy will be dictated by the patient's clinical response and any follow-up imaging studies. Typically, treatment consists of parenteral antibiotic therapy for 3 weeks and another 4 to 6 weeks of oral antibiotics. In most cases abscesses completely resolve, but on occasion a residual cavity may persist, prolonging therapy. Patients should be followed up by CT scanning 1 to 2 months after cessation of therapy.

(V) Antibiotic treatment alone may have a role in selected patients. Indications for antibiotics alone may include high-risk patients who cannot tolerate procedures or those with multiple small liver abscesses.

(W) Complicated cases of pyogenic liver abscess require operative treatment. These include failed percutaneous drainage, very large and/or multiple loculated abscesses, patients with concurrent intra-abdominal disease, and impending rupture or rupture into pericardium or peritoneum.

(X) Fungal abscesses are less common than pyogenic or amebic liver abscesses. Fungus should be considered, particularly in patients that have solid-tissue or hematologic malignancies or are immunosuppressed (e.g., post-transplant, steroids, HIV-positive, or chemotherapy). The most common causative organism is Candida albicans. Others include aspergillus, cryptococcus, histoplasma, and mucormycosis. In many cases, both the liver and spleen are involved. Typically, the lesions are multiple and may appear as hypoechoic areas or lesions of low attenuation on ultrasound or CT, respectively. These lesions can be difficult

to distinguish from pyogenic liver abscesses. Percutaneous aspiration under ultrasound or CT guidance is indicated for definitive diagnosis. Amphotericin B will usually eradicate hepatic fungal infection.

(Y) The preferred treatment of hepatic abscess secondary to bacteria, fungus, or mycobacteria is ultrasound or CT-guided percutaneous drainage. This can consist of repeated percutaneous needle aspirations or continuous drainage with a catheter. If reaccumulation occurs after aspiration, continuous catheter drainage is recommended. Needle aspiration is less invasive, less expensive, avoids problems of catheter care, and multiple cavities can be aspirated. The success rate with aspiration has been reported to be 60% to 100%; however, the higher success rates were associated with up to four aspiration sessions per patient. A prospective randomized study found more effective treatment of liver abscesses with percutaneous catheter drainage (100%) when compared with needle aspiration (60% after up to two aspirations). The average time for total resolution of abscess was the same (15 weeks). Failure of needle aspiration to cure was associated with large abscesses and abscesses with thick, viscous pus.

(Z) Tuberculous liver abscess is rare and occurs most often in areas where tuberculosis is still prevalent. Tuberculosis in the liver usually presents in diffuse form (miliary) or as multiple caseating granulomas. Imaging studies can be diagnostic in these cases. Occasionally, a hepatic abscess thought to be pyogenic or amebic in etiology is discovered to be caused by mycobacteria. It is thought that the organisms reach the liver by hematogenous spread from tuberculous foci in the lungs or via the hepatic artery or through the portal vein from tuberculous foci in the gut. Most patients present with symptoms similar to pyogenic or amebic abscess. The diagnosis can be difficult when there is no evidence of extrahepatic tuberculosis. Tuberculous liver abscess occurs more often in patients being treated for extrahepatic tuberculosis who have acquired drug resistance or who are noncompliant with the medication regimen. The patient's history as well as percutaneous diagnostic

History and physical examination

Country of origin and/or recent travel 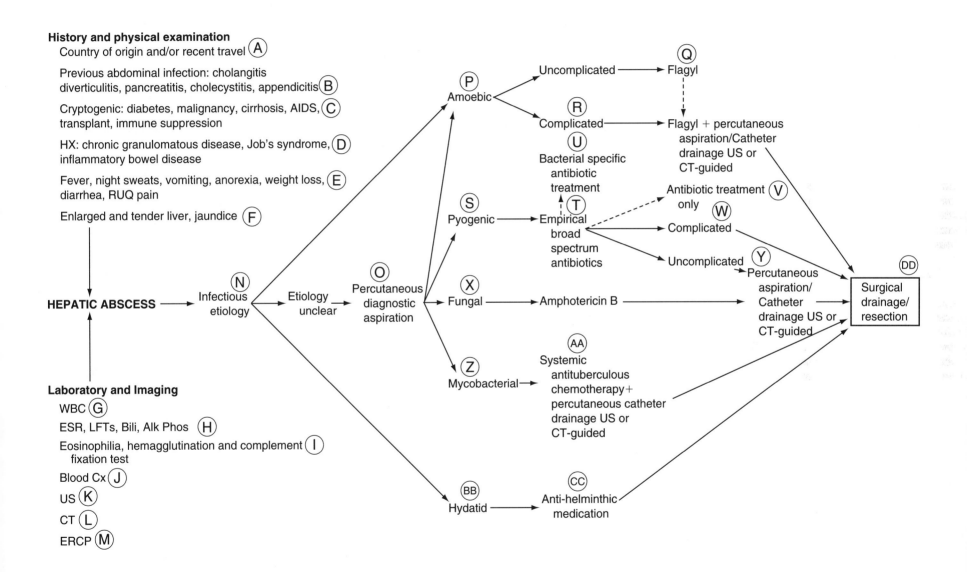(A)

Previous abdominal infection: cholangitis diverticulitis, pancreatitis, cholecystitis, appendicitis (B)

Cryptogenic: diabetes, malignancy, cirrhosis, AIDS, (C) transplant, immune suppression

HX: chronic granulomatous disease, Job's syndrome, (D) inflammatory bowel disease

Fever, night sweats, vomiting, anorexia, weight loss, (E) diarrhea, RUQ pain

Enlarged and tender liver, jaundice (F)

HEPATIC ABSCESS

Laboratory and Imaging

WBC (G)

ESR, LFTs, Bili, Alk Phos (H)

Eosinophilia, hemagglutination and complement (I) fixation test

Blood Cx (J)

US (K)

CT (L)

ERCP (M)

(N) Infectious etiology

Etiology unclear

(O) Percutaneous diagnostic aspiration

(P) Amoebic

Uncomplicated ⟶ (Q) Flagyl

Complicated ⟶ Flagyl + percutaneous aspiration/Catheter drainage US or CT-guided (R)

(U) Bacterial specific antibiotic treatment

(S) Pyogenic ⟶ Empirical broad spectrum antibiotics (T)

Antibiotic treatment only (V)

Complicated (W)

Uncomplicated (Y)

Percutaneous aspiration/ Catheter drainage US or CT-guided

(X) Fungal ⟶ Amphotericin B

(Z) Mycobacterial ⟶ (AA) Systemic antituberculous chemotherapy+ percutaneous catheter drainage US or CT-guided

(BB) Hydatid ⟶ (CC) Anti-helminthic medication

(DD) Surgical drainage/ resection

aspiration may serve as the only indicators for tuberculous abscess. The tuberculin test as well as other serologic examinations may be noncontributory.

(AA) Treatment consists of a multi-drug regimen such as rifampicin, isoniazid, pyrazinamide, and ethambutol, along with a drainage procedure. Most recommend using percutaneous catheter drainage. The abscess usually resolves after 2 to 3 weeks. There are also reports of combined treatment using catheter drainage with transcatheter infusion of antituberculous drugs into the cavity.

(BB) Hydatid cysts are caused by the dog tapeworm *Echinococcus granulosus*. The disease is endemic to sheep-raising countries. Infection occurs when ingestion of ova leads to invasion through intestinal wall and passage through the portal vein to the liver. Infected patients have symptoms similar to those with pyogenic or amebic abscesses. Rupture of the cyst into the peritoneum may result in urticaria, anaphylactic shock, eosinophilia, and implantation into the surrounding abdominal viscera. Percutaneous aspiration of cysts that could be echinococcal should not be performed for this reason. The diagnosis is confirmed using hemagglutination and complement-fixation tests.

(CC) All cysts require surgical removal and treatment with antihelminthic medications such as albendazole, flubendazole, and/or praziquantel. After surgical removal, antihelminthic drugs are continued for at least 2 weeks postoperatively to prevent recurrence. Drug therapy alone is reserved for those patients who are unable to undergo surgery.

(DD) Surgery is now reserved for hydatid disease and complicated pyogenic, amebic, fungal, and tuberculosis cases that cannot be treated by percutaneous techniques. Operations for hydatid disease include capitonnage, omentoplasty, cyst excision, cystoenterostomy, and laparoscopic deroofing. Surgical treatment of pyogenic, amebic, fungal, and tuberculosis abscess (performed open or laparoscopically) consists of either a drainage procedure or resection. Resection (wedge, segment, or lobe) is defined by the extent of the disease and the amount of destruction in the surrounding liver parenchyma.

REFERENCES

Akgun Y, Tacyildiz IH, Celik Y: Amebic liver abscess: Changing trends over 20 years (see comments). World J Surg 23:102–106, 1999.

Aktan AO, Yalin R: Preoperative albendazole treatment for liver hydatid disease decreases the viability of the cyst. Eur J Gastroenterol Hepatol 8:877–879, 1996.

Aktan AO, Yalin R, Yegen C et al: Surgical treatment of hepatic hydatid cysts. Acta Chirurgica Belgica 93:151–153, 1993.

Alvarez JA, Gonzalez JJ, Baldonedo RF et al: Single and multiple pyogenic liver abscesses: Etiology, clinical course, and outcome. Digestive Surgery 18:283–288, 2001.

Alvarez Perez JA, Gonzalez JJ, Baldonedo RF et al: Clinical course, treatment, and multivariate analysis of risk factors for pyogenic liver abscess. Am J Surg 181:177–186, 2001.

Andersson R, Forsberg L, Hederstrom E et al: Percutaneous management of pyogenic hepatic abscesses. HPB Surgery 2:185–188, 1990.

Balik AA, Basoglu M, Celebi F et al: Surgical treatment of hydatid disease of the liver: Review of 304 cases. Arch Surg 134:166–169, 1999.

Huang CJ, Pitt HA, Lipsett PA et al: Pyogenic hepatic abscess. Changing trends over 42 years. Ann Surg 223:600–607, 1996.

Hughes MA, Petri WA Jr: Amebic liver abscess. Inf Dis Clin N Am 14:565–582, 2000.

Johannsen EC, Sifri CD, Madoff LC: Pyogenic liver abscesses. Inf Dis Clin N Am 14:547–563, 2000.

Krige JE, Beckingham IJ: ABC of diseases of liver, pancreas, and biliary system. BMJ 322:537–540, 2001.

Marcus SG, Walsh TJ, Pizzo PA et al: Hepatic abscess in cancer patients: Characterization and management. Arch Surg 128:1358–1364, 1993.

Maxwell AJ, Mamtora H: Fungal liver abscesses in acute leukaemia: A report of two cases. Clin Radiol 39:197–201, 1988.

McDonald MI: Pyogenic liver abscess: Diagnosis, bacteriology and treatment. Eur J Clin Microbiol 3:506–509, 1984.

Petri A, Hohn J, Hodi Z et al: Pyogenic liver abscess: 20 years' experience. Comparison of results of treatment in two periods. Langenbecks Arch Surg 387:27–31, 2002.

Pitt HA: Surgical management of hepatic abscesses. World J Surg 14:498–504, 1990.

Rahmatulla RH, al-Mofleh IA, al-Rashed RS et al: Tuberculous liver abscess: A case report and review of literature. Eur J Gastroenterol Hepatol 13:437–440, 2001.

Rajak CL, Gupta S, Jain S et al: Percutaneous treatment of liver abscesses: Needle aspiration versus catheter drainage. AJR 170:1035–1039, 1998.

Rustgi AK, Richter JM: Pyogenic and amebic liver abscess. Med Clin N Am 73:847–858, 1989.

Sharma MP, Rai RR, Acharya SK et al: Needle aspiration of amoebic liver abscess. BMJ 299:1308–1309, 1989.

History and physical examination

Country of origin and/or recent travel Ⓐ

Previous abdominal infection: cholangitis diverticulitis, pancreatitis, cholecystitis, appendicitis Ⓑ

Cryptogenic: diabetes, malignancy, cirrhosis, AIDS, Ⓒ transplant, immune suppression

HX: chronic granulomatous disease, Job's syndrome, Ⓓ inflammatory bowel disease

Fever, night sweats, vomiting, anorexia, weight loss, Ⓔ diarrhea, RUQ pain

Enlarged and tender liver, jaundice Ⓕ

HEPATIC ABSCESS

Laboratory and Imaging

WBC Ⓖ

ESR, LFTs, Bili, Alk Phos Ⓗ

Eosinophilia, hemagglutination and complement Ⓘ fixation test

Blood Cx Ⓙ

US Ⓚ

CT Ⓛ

ERCP Ⓜ

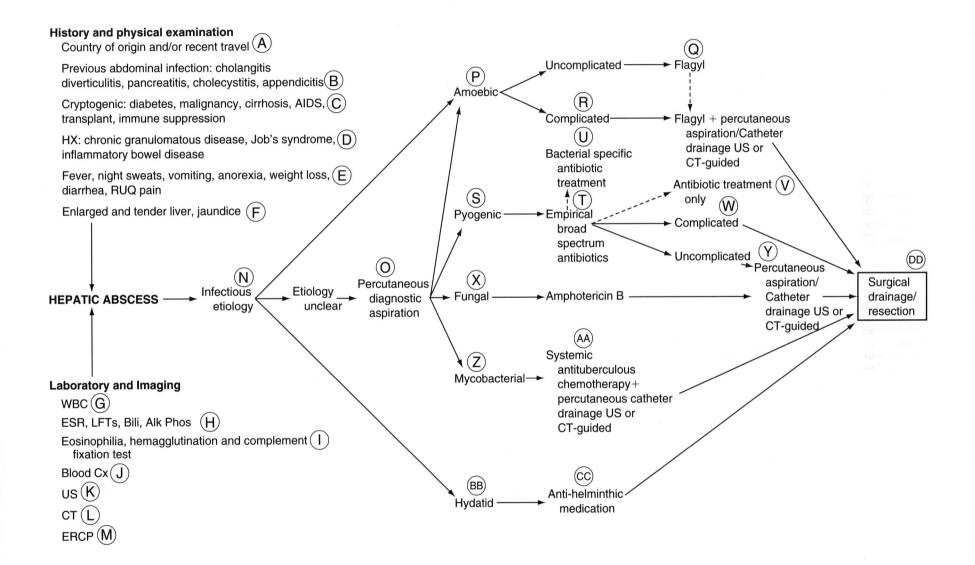

Chapter 54 **Acute Pancreatitis**

ALEXANDER S. ROSEMURGY, MD • SHARONA B. ROSS, MD

(A) Acute pancreatitis is a common disorder that varies markedly in severity and predictability. The diagnosis of acute pancreatitis may involve a constellation of symptoms and signs including epigastric abdominal pain, nausea and vomiting, and jaundice with hyperamylasemia and hyperlipidemia. Pancreatic enzymes elevations alone are not enough to make the diagnosis because there are extrapancreaticobiliary causes of hyperamylasemia and abdominal pain. For approximately 80% of patients, attacks are mild and resolve spontaneously with low mortality rates. Pancreatic necrosis develops to some degree in approximately 20% of patients. As a consequence, patients may experience systemic complications such as fluid sequestration; adult respiratory distress syndrome; hepatic failure; acute renal failure; hypotension; and death, with mortality rates as high as 40% in the most severe occurrences of acute pancreatitis.

There are multiple etiologies for acute pancreatitis. The most common causes are choledocholithiasis and alcohol, with relative frequencies in the United States of 40% and 30%, respectively.

(B) Serum amylase and lipase levels are used to confirm the diagnosis of acute pancreatitis, although their degree of elevation does not correlate with disease severity. Few patients with acute pancreatitis fail to demonstrate any elevation in amylase and/or lipase. Elevations in base deficit, hematocrit, creatinine, and blood urea nitrogen (BUN) reflect volume contraction. Serum trypsin level is the most accurate laboratory indicator for pancreatitis; however, a usable assay is not readily available. A rapid dipstick screening test for pancreatitis based on immunochromatographic measurement of urinary trypsinogen-2 was developed by Kemppainen and colleagues. A negative urinary trypsinogen-2 test result rules out acute pancreatitis with high probability, whereas a positive result identifies patients that should undergo further evaluation. Ranson's criteria, the APACHE II, and multiple organ system failure scales provide prognostic

information at the time of admission and, other than Ranson's criteria, may be repeated daily to monitor disease progression.

Ranson's criteria includes 11 signs that assess the severity of acute pancreatitis:

Criteria at admission	Criteria within first 48 hours
Age >55 years	HCT fall by >10%
White blood cell count >16,000/mm³	Fluid sequestration >6000 ml
LDH >350 IU/L	BUN rise >5 mg /dl
SGOT >250 μ/dl	Serum calcium <8 mg/dl
Blood glucose >200 mg/dl	PO₂ <60 mm Hg
	Base deficit >4

Patients with fewer than three signs generally experience mild pancreatitis, whereas those with more than three signs are at higher risk to suffer from severe pancreatitis and have increased mortality.

The APACHE II (acute physiology score and chronic health evaluation):

A. Physiologic Variables: Temperature (°C), Mean Arterial Pressure (mmHg), Pulse, Respirations, PaO₂, Arterial PH, Serum Na, Serum K, Serum Creatinine (mg/dl), HCT (%), White Blood Count, Glasgow Coma Score, and Serum HCO₃ (mmol/L)
B. Age Points
C. Chronic Health Points

The APACHE II score is equal to A+B+C. This system provides a mechanism to evaluate the disease process successively on a daily basis. A score below 9 predicts mild acute pancreatitis and better survival rates; scores above 13 indicate severe acute pancreatitis and higher likelihood of mortality.

(C) Mild to moderate acute pancreatitis (based on Ranson's criteria with fewer than 3 signs):

1. Intravenous hydration
2. No food by mouth (NPO): bowel rest
3. Pain control

Adjunctive treatments, which include inhibition of pancreatic secretion and antiproteases, do not improve the clinical course of the average patient. Nasogastric tube suction appears to have no benefit when used routinely; however, it should be considered for patients with vomiting or altered sensorium.

(D) For patients with self-limited mild to moderate gallstone pancreatitis, a laparoscopic cholecystectomy should be undertaken before discharge to prevent future episodes of acute pancreatitis (early [less than 4 days after onset] with mild disease or late [more than 14 days after onset] with more severe disease). An intraoperative cholangiogram during the cholecystectomy should be undertaken; if stones in the common bile duct are found, common bile duct exploration and stone extraction is indicated either through laparoscopic common bile duct exploration or postoperative endoscopic sphincterotomy with stone extraction.

(E) Severe acute pancreatitis (based on Ranson's criteria with more than 3 signs):

1. Intensive care admission
2. Intravenous hydration
3. No food by mouth (NPO): bowel rest
4. Nasogastric tube suction
5. Pain control
6. Nutritional support: total parenteral nutrition (TPN) with gradual transition into enteral feeding via feeding tube
7. Support body systems (oxygen, mechanical ventilation, dialysis)
8. Prophylactic antibiotics/antifungals: Prophylactic antibiotics are believed to reduce morbidity and mortality of severe acute pancreatitis, but benefit in acute mild to moderate pancreatitis is not well established. Imipenem is the drug of choice because of its superior concentration level in the pancreatic parenchyma and its ability to cover multiple pathogens.
9. Treatment of underlying cause of pancreatitis

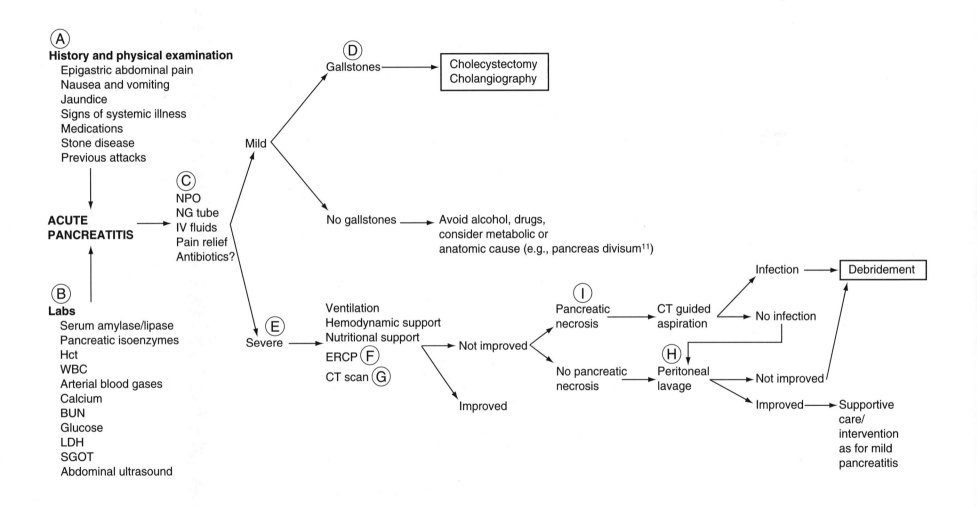

Ⓐ
History and physical examination
    Epigastric abdominal pain
    Nausea and vomiting
    Jaundice
    Signs of systemic illness
    Medications
    Stone disease
    Previous attacks

**ACUTE
PANCREATITIS**

Ⓑ
Labs
    Serum amylase/lipase
    Pancreatic isoenzymes
    Hct
    WBC
    Arterial blood gases
    Calcium
    BUN
    Glucose
    LDH
    SGOT
    Abdominal ultrasound

Ⓒ
NPO
NG tube
IV fluids
Pain relief
Antibiotics?

Mild

Ⓓ
Gallstones → Cholecystectomy / Cholangiography

No gallstones → Avoid alcohol, drugs, consider metabolic or anatomic cause (e.g., pancreas divisum[11])

Severe Ⓔ →
Ventilation
Hemodynamic support
Nutritional support
ERCP Ⓕ
CT scan Ⓖ

→ Not improved
    Ⓘ Pancreatic necrosis → CT guided aspiration → Infection → **Debridement**
                               → No infection
    No pancreatic necrosis → Ⓗ Peritoneal lavage → Not improved → **Debridement**
                                       → Improved → Supportive care/ intervention as for mild pancreatitis

→ Improved

(F) A small group of critically ill patients who fail to improve in the first 12 to 24 hours of treatment may benefit from an early approach to clearing the common bile duct. If ultrasonography confirmed the presence of gallstones, then ERCP, sphincterotomy, and stone extraction within 48 hours decreases mortality. Laparoscopic cholecystectomy is delayed until recovery from pancreatitis occurs, but is usually undertaken during the same hospitalization.

(G) Patients with severe pancreatitis should undergo dynamic oral and intravenous contrast-enhanced CT examination. Finding peripancreatic fluid collections, pseudocysts, or peripancreatic necrosis is not an absolute indication for operative treatment. Instead, in the absence of deterioration and sepsis, supportive care is in order. However, patients thought to be septic with hypoperfused areas (suggestive of necrosis) on CT scan should undergo CT-guided fine-needle aspiration (FNA) for Gram stain and culture to detect infection. If the FNA results show sterile necrosis, medical management needs to be maximized for the next 24 to 48 hours. However, if the patient's condition fails to improve, peritoneal lavage and/or operative debridement may be helpful. If infected pancreatic necrosis is identified, broad-spectrum intravenous antibiotics and antifungal therapy with operative debridement are recommended. The risk of death for patients with very severe peripancreatic necrosis can be reduced from 40% to 10% by aggressive operative treatment.

(H) Peritoneal lavage for patients with severe acute pancreatitis is an adjunctive therapy in some centers. It is used to aid in the elimination of toxic substances that may collect within the peritoneal cavity during this illness. However, a multi-center randomized controlled trial failed to show any benefit. Nonetheless, the authors continue to use peritoneal lavage in severely ill patients with extrapancreatic manifestations of acute pancreatitis.

(I) It has been thought that there is no role for percutaneous drainage of infected peripancreatic necrosis: the authors believe that this is true. However, with the use of very, very large drains and the application of transcatheter endoscopic debridement, "nonoperative" management is being reevaluated. Results with open and closed drainage after operative debridement are comparable. With very severe peripancreatic necrosis, there may be a role for debridement with marsupialization. Pancreatectomy is rarely, if ever, necessary in the treatment of severe pancreatitis.

REFERENCES

Andriulli A, Leandro G, Clemente R et al: Meta-analysis of somatostatin, octreotide, and gabexate mesilate in the therapy of acute pancreatitis. Aliment Pharmacol Ther 12:237–245, 1998.

Kemppainen EA, Hedstrom JI, Puolakkainen PA et al: Rapid measurement of urinary trypsinogen-2 as a screening test for acute pancreatitis. N Engl J Med 336:1788–1793, 1997.

Mayer AD, McMahon MJ, Corfield AP et al: Controlled clinical trial of peritoneal lavage for the treatment of severe acute pancreatitis. N Engl J Med 312:399–404, 1985.

Rosemurgy AS, Bloomston M: The Management of Pancreas Divisum. In Cameron J (ed): Current Surgical Therapy, 7th ed. St. Louis: Mosby, pp. 533–538.

Sarr MG, Sanfey H, Cameron JL: Prospective, randomized trial of nasogastric suction in patients with acute pancreatitis. Surgery 100:500–504, 1986.

Tang E, Stain SC, Tang G et al: Timing of laparoscopic surgery in gallstone pancreatitis. Arch Surg 130:496–499, 1995.

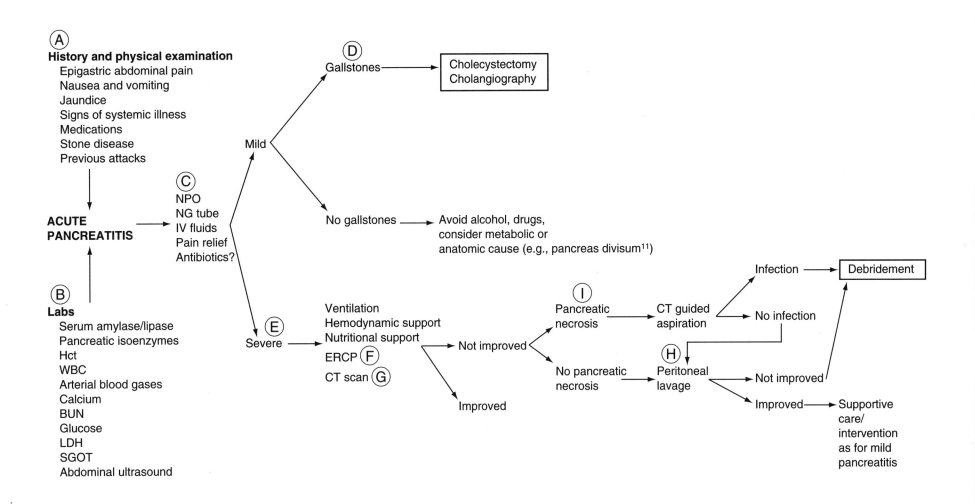

Ⓐ
History and physical examination
   Epigastric abdominal pain
   Nausea and vomiting
   Jaundice
   Signs of systemic illness
   Medications
   Stone disease
   Previous attacks

Ⓒ
   NPO
   NG tube
   IV fluids
   Pain relief
   Antibiotics?

ACUTE PANCREATITIS

Ⓑ
Labs
   Serum amylase/lipase
   Pancreatic isoenzymes
   Hct
   WBC
   Arterial blood gases
   Calcium
   BUN
   Glucose
   LDH
   SGOT
   Abdominal ultrasound

Mild

Ⓓ
Gallstones → Cholecystectomy / Cholangiography

No gallstones → Avoid alcohol, drugs, consider metabolic or anatomic cause (e.g., pancreas divisum[11])

Severe Ⓔ →
   Ventilation
   Hemodynamic support
   Nutritional support
   ERCP Ⓕ
   CT scan Ⓖ

Not improved

Improved

Ⓘ Pancreatic necrosis → CT guided aspiration → Infection → Debridement
                                              → No infection

No pancreatic necrosis → Ⓗ Peritoneal lavage → Not improved
                                             → Improved → Supportive care/ intervention as for mild pancreatitis

Chapter 55 *Chronic Pancreatitis*

HUNG HO, MD ● CHARLES F. FREY, MD

(A) Chronic pancreatitis often leads to persistent or recurrent abdominal pain, pancreatic exocrine and endocrine insufficiency, and malnutrition. Patients may present with anatomical complications of the disease such as biliary or duodenal obstruction, pseudoaneurysm formation, and splenic vein thrombosis.

(B) Chronic pancreatitis is an inflammatory process associated with a progressive replacement of the normal pancreatic tissue by fibrosis, often with pancreatic ductal stricturing and intraductile calcification. Management of chronic pancreatitis is mainly palliative. The ideal treatment for chronic pancreatitis should be able to exclude the existence of malignancy, provide long-lasting pain relief, and correct pancreatitis-related local complications. Operative treatment should be as simple and safe as possible and should preserve the remaining endocrine and exocrine functions of the pancreas.

(C) Diagnostic tests to objectively document the existence of chronic pancreatitis should be done, especially in the patient whose sole complaint is abdominal pain. Hyperamylasemia may be present during exacerbations of chronic pancreatitis. Clinical steatorrhea can be confirmed by fecal fat studies. The use of cholecystokinin or secretin stimulation tests to assess pancreatic exocrine function is time-consuming, and the results are abnormal only in advanced disease. Imaging studies to assess pancreatic structural abnormalities include endoscopic retrograde cholangiopancreaticography, helical dynamic CT scan, and magnetic resonance cholangiopancreatography (MRCP).

(D) Intractable abdominal pain associated with chronic pancreatitis can be severe and disabling enough to lead to narcotic addiction. Most patients would benefit from early surgical intervention before the problem with narcotic dependency arises. There is still controversy regarding the mechanisms contributing to pain in chronic pancreatitis, and hence the best method to treat pain. The original theory of pain caused by either pancreatic ductal hypertension or postprandial pancreatic hyperstimulation can only partially explain the complex pain associated with chronic pancreatitis. Recent studies have suggested that neuropathic changes (e.g., nerve and perineural destruction) and alteration in neurotransmitters may in fact account for the root of pain associated with chronic pancreatitis. On the other hand, ductal hypertension may induce a compartment-syndrome effect on the pancreatic parenchyma, leading to scarring and fibrosis and accounting for the neuropathic changes.

(E) Clinically significant obstruction of the common bile duct (CBD) occurs in about 10% to 20% of patients with chronic pancreatitis. In the absence of intractable abdominal pain, either a Roux-en-Y choledochojejunostomy or a choledochoduodenostomy can effectively deal with the problem. A retrocolic retrogastric loop gastrojejunostomy is the treatment of choice for duodenal obstruction from chronic pancreatitis without intractable abdominal pain. If pancreatic pain is present, then the Frey (LR-LPJ) or the Beger procedure may be employed not only to relieve pain but to completely decompress the common bile duct. Alternatively, a variation of the classic Whipple operation will achieve the same effect.

(F) Pseudoaneurysms in chronic pancreatitis most commonly involve the splenic artery, followed by the inferior and superior pancreaticoduodenal arteries and their branches. These are best treated by angiographic embolization. No further surgery is required for the pseudoaneurysms, and surgery is rarely required for the commonly associated pseudocysts. The patients can be observed to see if the pseudocysts resolve spontaneously after angiographic embolization of the pseudoaneurysms, because more than 60% of pseudocysts do resolve spontaneously and few of the remainder may be symptomatic. Resection of the involved portion of the pancreas or ligation of the involved artery is rarely indicated unless angiographic embolization is unsuccessful in stopping the bleeding. Left-sided portal hypertension from splenic vein thrombosis can be alleviated by angiographic embolization of the splenic artery. Following angiographic embolization of the splenic artery, splenectomy is not necessary unless there are associated bleeding gastric varices.

(G) Disruption of the pancreatic duct may lead to pancreatic ascites or fistula. The condition can be persistent if there is associated obstruction or stricture of the proximal pancreatic duct. A trial of total parental nutrition (TPN) is warranted because some of these fistulae will close spontaneously. The efficacy of somatostatin analog therapy has not been proven or accepted. When a pancreatic fistula fails to close after nonoperative trial, an internal drainage procedure should be performed with a Roux-en-Y jejunal limb anastomosed to the matured fistula tract on the surface of the pancreas.

(H) The risk of pancreatic cancer in patients with chronic pancreatitis is difficult to assess, but the standardized incidence ratio in various cohort studies ranged as high as 18.5 to 26.7 when compared with the number of expected cases in the normal population. Differentiation between an inflammatory mass and a malignant one can be extremely difficult even with the most advanced imaging test. In such cases, the use of endoscopic ultrasonography with fine-needle aspiration of a small mass (less than 2 cm in diameter) may be very useful. When in doubt, it is best to perform a Whipple procedure rather than any of the duodenum-preserving head resections in patients with an enlarged head of the pancreas. Discrete mass in the body or tail of the pancreas can be effectively dealt with by distal pancreatectomy, often with splenectomy.

(I) Medical treatment of chronic pancreatitis emphasizes the correction of malnutrition and reduction of pancreatic stimulation by providing pancreatic enzyme supplements to facilitate absorption of fat, protein, and other nutrients. Proteolytic enzymes may inhibit the release of cholecystokinin from the

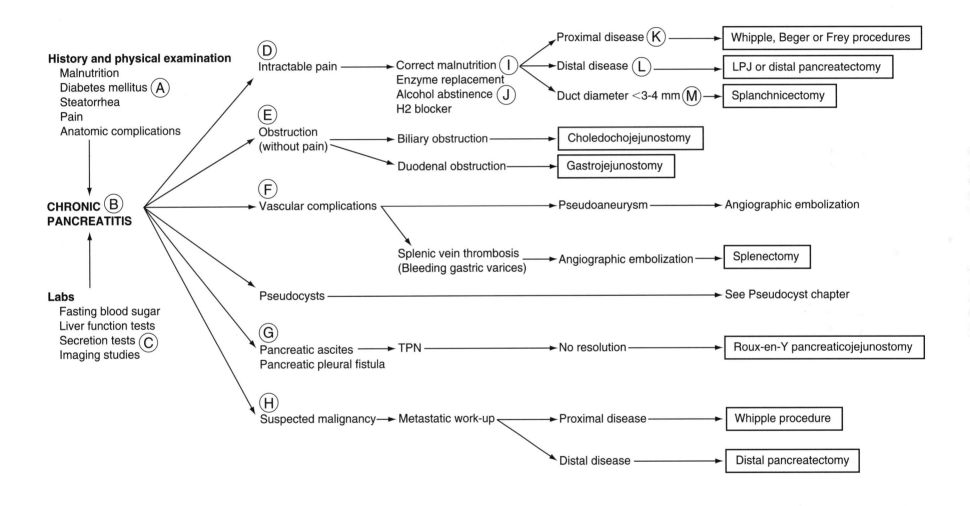

History and physical examination
Malnutrition
Diabetes mellitus (A)
Steatorrhea
Pain
Anatomic complications

CHRONIC (B)
PANCREATITIS

Labs
Fasting blood sugar
Liver function tests
Secretion tests (C)
Imaging studies

(D) Intractable pain → Correct malnutrition (I)
Enzyme replacement
Alcohol abstinence (J)
H2 blocker

Proximal disease (K) → Whipple, Beger or Frey procedures
Distal disease (L) → LPJ or distal pancreatectomy
Duct diameter <3-4 mm (M) → Splanchnicectomy

(E) Obstruction
(without pain)
→ Biliary obstruction → Choledochojejunostomy
→ Duodenal obstruction → Gastrojejunostomy

(F) Vascular complications
→ Pseudoaneurysm → Angiographic embolization
→ Splenic vein thrombosis (Bleeding gastric varices) → Angiographic embolization → Splenectomy

Pseudocysts → See Pseudocyst chapter

(G) Pancreatic ascites → TPN → No resolution → Roux-en-Y pancreaticojejunostomy
Pancreatic pleural fistula

(H) Suspected malignancy → Metastatic work-up
→ Proximal disease → Whipple procedure
→ Distal disease → Distal pancreatectomy

duodenum and therefore reduce cholecystokinin-induced stimulation of the fibrotic pancreas. Correction of malnutrition is essential before initiating surgical intervention for the structural abnormalities of the pancreas.

(J) Continued alcohol consumption accelerates further deterioration of pancreatic exocrine and endocrine function. It is important to involve the patient early in a program to maintain alcohol abstinence. It is equally important to realize that alcohol abstinence may slow down but does not halt further deterioration of pancreatic endocrine and exocrine function.

(K) Pancreatic resection for chronic pancreatitis is based on the assumption that complete removal of the diseased pancreatic tissue eliminates the pain regardless of the cause. For proximal disease, the various versions of the classic Whipple procedure were the standard operation for chronic pancreatitis for decades. However, these operations have been slowly replaced by versions of duodenum-preserving resection of the head of the pancreas such as the Beger or the Frey procedures. The poor quality of life associated with the effects of iatrogenically induced exocrine and endocrine insufficiency after total pancreatectomy or 85% to 95% distal pancreatectomy rarely warrants their use in chronic pancreatitis. Total pancreatectomy does not even ensure long-term pain relief, and it is associated with an approximately 20% failure rate.

(L) The Partington-Rochelle modification of the original Puestow longitudinal pancreaticojejunostomy (LPJ) may be effective when the diseased pancreatic duct involves only portions within the body or tail of the pancreas and when the head of the gland and its ducts are normal and are found to be soft on palpation at the time of the operation. Alternatively, distal pancreatectomy may be effective in patients with disease confined to the body or tail of the pancreas. When the head of the pancreas is thickened, it is essential that duodenum-preserving resection of the head of the pancreas (by either the Beger or Frey procedure) be performed to adequately drain the ducts of Wirsung and Santorini, the ducts within the uncinate process and their tributaries, as well as any retention cysts.

(M) In patients who have small-duct chronic pancreatitis (i.e., pancreatic duct smaller than 3 to 4 mm in diameter) without any structural lesion amenable to surgical intervention (e.g., stricture, pseudocyst, or retention cysts), bilateral thoracoscopic splanchnicectomy provides a minimally invasive approach to a very selective subgroup of these complex patients.

REFERENCES

Adams DB, Ford MC, Anderson MC: Outcome after pancreatico-jejunostomy for chronic pancreatitis. Ann Surg 219:481–489, 1994.

Beger HG, Schlosser W, Firiess HM et al: Duodenum-preserving head resection in chronic pancreatitis changes the natural course of the disease: A single-centre 26-year experience. Ann Surg 230:512–523, 1999.

Buchler MW, Friess H, Muller MW et al: Randomized trial of duodenum-preserving pancreatic head resection versus pylorus-preserving Whipple in chronic pancreatitis. Am J Surg 169:65–69, 1995.

Frey CF, Amikura K: Local resection of the head of the pancreas combined with longitudinal pancreaticojejunostomy in the management of patients with chronic pancreatitis. Ann Surg 220:492–507, 1994.

Howard TJ, Swofford JB, Wagner DL et al: Quality of life after bilateral thoracoscopic splanchnicectomy: Long-term evaluation in patients with chronic pancreatitis. J Gastrintest Surg 6:845–854, 2002.

Hutchins MS, Hart RS, Pacifico M et al: Long-term results of distal pancreatectomy for chronic pancreatitis in 90 patients. Ann Surg 236:612–618, 2002.

Izbicki JR, Bloeche C, Knoefel WT et al: Drainage versus resection in surgical therapy of chronic pancreatitis of the head of the pancreas: A randomized study. Chirurg 68:369–377, 1997.

Izbicki JR, Bloechle C, Broering DC et al: Extended drainage versus resection in surgery for chronic pancreatitis: A prospective randomized trial comparing the longitudinal pancreaticojejunostomy combined with local pancreatic head excision with the pylorus-preserving pancreaticoduodenectomy. Ann Surg 228:771–779, 1998.

Jordan PH, Pikoulis M: Operative treatment for chronic pancreatitis pain. J Am Coll Surg 192:498–509, 2001.

Klempa I, Spatny M, Menzel J et al: Pancreatic function and quality of life after resection of the head of the pancreas in chronic pancreatitis: A prospective, randomized, comparative study after duodenum-preserving resection of the head of the pancreas versus Whipple's operation. Chirurg 66:350–359, 1995.

Lowenfels AB, Maisonneuve P, Cavallini G et al: Pancreatitis and the risk of pancreatic cancer. N Engl J Med 328:143–147, 1993.

Malka D, Hammel P, Maire F et al: Risk of pancreatic adenocarcinoma in chronic pancreatitis. Gut 51:849–852, 2002.

Markowitz JS, Rattner DW, Warshaw AL: Failure of symptomatic relief after pancreaticojejunal decompression for chronic pancreatitis: Strategies for salvage. Arch Surg 129:374–379, 1994.

Nealon WH, Townsend CM Jr, Thompson JC: Operative drainage of the pancreatic duct delays functional impairment in patients with chronic pancreatitis: A prospective analysis. Ann Surg 208:321–329, 1988.

Talamini G, Falconi M, Bassi C et al: Incidence of cancer in the course of chronic pancreatitis. Am J Gastroenterol 94:1253–1260, 1999.

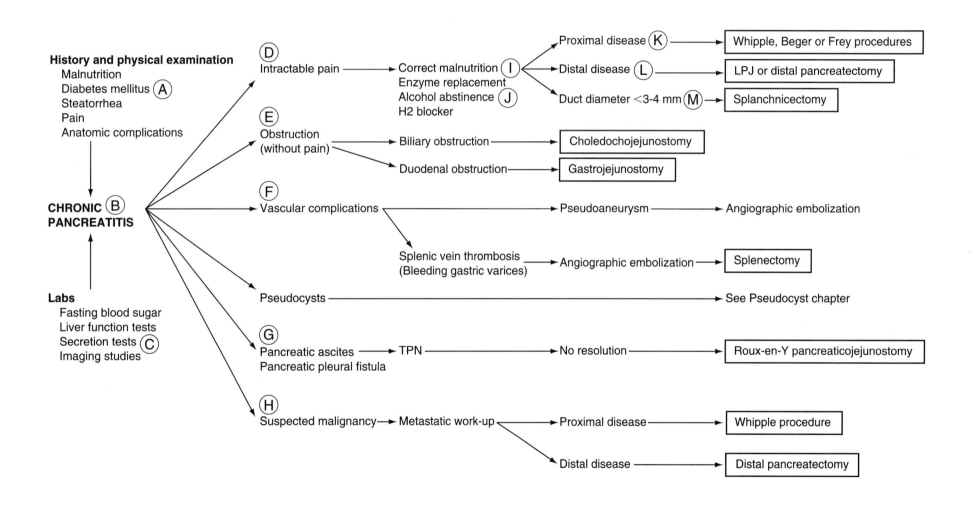

History and physical examination
  Malnutrition
  Diabetes mellitus Ⓐ
  Steatorrhea
  Pain
  Anatomic complications

CHRONIC Ⓑ
PANCREATITIS

Labs
  Fasting blood sugar
  Liver function tests
  Secretion tests Ⓒ
  Imaging studies

Ⓓ Intractable pain

Correct malnutrition Ⓘ
Enzyme replacement
Alcohol abstinence Ⓙ
H2 blocker

Proximal disease Ⓚ → Whipple, Beger or Frey procedures

Distal disease Ⓛ → LPJ or distal pancreatectomy

Duct diameter <3-4 mm Ⓜ → Splanchnicectomy

Ⓔ Obstruction (without pain)

Biliary obstruction → Choledochojejunostomy

Duodenal obstruction → Gastrojejunostomy

Ⓕ Vascular complications

Pseudoaneurysm → Angiographic embolization

Splenic vein thrombosis (Bleeding gastric varices) → Angiographic embolization → Splenectomy

Pseudocysts → See Pseudocyst chapter

Ⓖ Pancreatic ascites → TPN → No resolution → Roux-en-Y pancreaticojejunostomy
Pancreatic pleural fistula

Ⓗ Suspected malignancy → Metastatic work-up

Proximal disease → Whipple procedure

Distal disease → Distal pancreatectomy

Chapter 56 Pancreatic Pseudocysts

MATTHEW M. HUTTER, MD • DAVID W. RATTNER, MD

(A) The diagnosis of a pancreatic pseudocyst is suspected in the patient with acute pancreatitis or pancreatic trauma whose symptoms do not resolve within 10 to 14 days. Persistent pain, nausea, vomiting, and early satiety are common complaints.

(B) Pancreatic pseudocysts are fluid collections that develop from the inflammatory process created by enzyme-rich pancreatic juices that have leaked from disrupted pancreatic ducts into surrounding tissues. Duct disruption can occur secondary to pancreatitis (either acute or chronic) or trauma. The pseudocyst wall is composed of fibrous tissue from the peritoneum, retroperitoneum, and/or the serosa of adjacent viscera. The absence of an epithelial lining differentiates pseudocysts from cystic neoplasms and congenital pancreatic cysts. The development of a mature pseudocyst follows a fairly predictable progression from inflammatory mass to an acute fluid collection and, ultimately, to the development of an encapsulated collection of amylase-rich fluid with a fibrous wall. This process takes about 4 to 6 weeks. More than 50% of acute fluid collections resolve on their own and never become mature pseudocysts, so intervention of any type should be delayed for 6 weeks from the onset of illness unless there is reason to be concerned about sepsis.

(C) Serum amylase levels are elevated 50% of the time. A CT scan is the preferred way to make the diagnosis; it also provides important anatomic detail that can help guide management.

(D) If the patient has a history of chronic pancreatitis, it is important to determine if this is an acute exacerbation of a chronic condition, which would merit an observational period to determine if it resolves; or a chronic problem, which could be acted on right away. Most patients with known chronic pancreatitis are in the latter category.

(E) The natural history of pancreatic pseudocysts in asymptomatic patients has recently been redefined. Historically, recommendations were to operate on all pseudocysts that were present for more than 6 weeks. More recent studies have shown high rates of resolution (57% to 60%) and low rates of complications (3% to 9%) with expectant management in asymptomatic patients. Therefore asymptomatic patients with pancreatic pseudocysts should be managed nonoperatively and followed as outpatients with serial CT scans. Drainage is indicated only for those patients who develop symptoms or complications, or for those whose pseudocysts are enlarging. There are no strict size criteria for the pseudocyst itself that make drainage a requirement.

(F) The symptomatic patient who has a cyst that has not resolved by 6 weeks warrants drainage. Symptoms can persist because of obstruction of the GI and/or biliary tracts from this space-occupying mass, or because of the inflammatory process that led to its creation.

(G) Jaundice results from biliary obstruction either because of compression of the bile duct by the pseudocyst or from fibrosis in the head of the pancreas. Hence biliary obstruction may not resolve with drainage of the pseudocyst. A cholangiogram following cyst decompression should be performed to assess the caliber of the distal common duct. When narrowing of the distal common duct persists following cyst decompression, consideration should be given to biliary enteric bypass (choledochoduodenostomy or choledochojejunostomy).

(H) Rupture of the pseudocyst can cause pain from chemical peritonitis as the enzyme-rich fluid is released into the peritoneum. Pancreatic fistula or pancreatic ascites can also result.

(I) Hemorrhage can result from erosion into nearby vessels by elastase and other enzymes in the fluid. Bleeding can occur into the cyst itself, into the retroperitoneum, or into the duodenum if there is communication to the cyst via the pancreatic duct. Angiography and embolization can often localize and stop life-threatening bleeding. Operative drainage and possible resection may be necessary to drain infection and prevent recurrent bleeding.

(J) A history of an antecedent, inciting event is important in determining both the diagnosis and subsequent management of cystic pancreatic lesions. Cystic lesions in or near the pancreas without a history of either pancreatitis or trauma must be viewed as cystic neoplasms until proven otherwise. CT findings of septations within the cyst, or multiple cysts, especially in middle-aged woman, are worrisome for cystic neoplasm. Cyst fluid sampling revealing mucin excludes an inflammatory pseudocyst. The presence of mucin mandates that the cyst be approached as a cystic neoplasm. Other markers (e.g., CEA, CA 19-9) are less reliable in confirming or refuting the diagnosis of a cystic neoplasm. Cyst wall biopsy at time of operation is mandatory to assess for the presence or absence of an epithelial lining. Unfortunately, the epithelial lining may be denuded over large areas in neoplastic cysts, so clinical judgment is often the final arbiter in the decision to resect (for cystic neoplasm) or drain (for pseudocyst) a cystic lesion.

(K) Infection should be suspected if there is a fever and/or a high white blood cell count, especially in patients who have been previously instrumented either by percutaneous aspiration or ERCP. In patients with necrotizing pancreatitis, however, there is no laboratory test or clinical parameter that can differentiate infected from sterile necrosis. Therefore fine-needle aspiration for Gram stain and culture may be necessary in unstable patients. Pseudocysts containing fluid that is grossly purulent or containing large amounts of necrotic tissue should not be anastomosed to another segment of the GI tract. In this setting, operative debridement, irrigation, and external drainage is the procedure of choice. Often fluid analysis reveals the presence of microorganisms microscopically, but as long as the fluid is thin and not grossly purulent, internal drainage with an enteric anastomosis is likely to provide successful decompression.

(L) ERCP is helpful primarily in patients with chronic pancreatitis. ERCP identifies the subset

History and physical examination
Pancreatitis—acute or chronic
Trauma
Alcoholism   (A)
Biliary colic
Abdominal pain
Jaundice
Abdominal mass

Labs
Amylase, lipase
LFTs
WBC count   (C)
Abdominal CT with IV contrast
   (ultrasound)

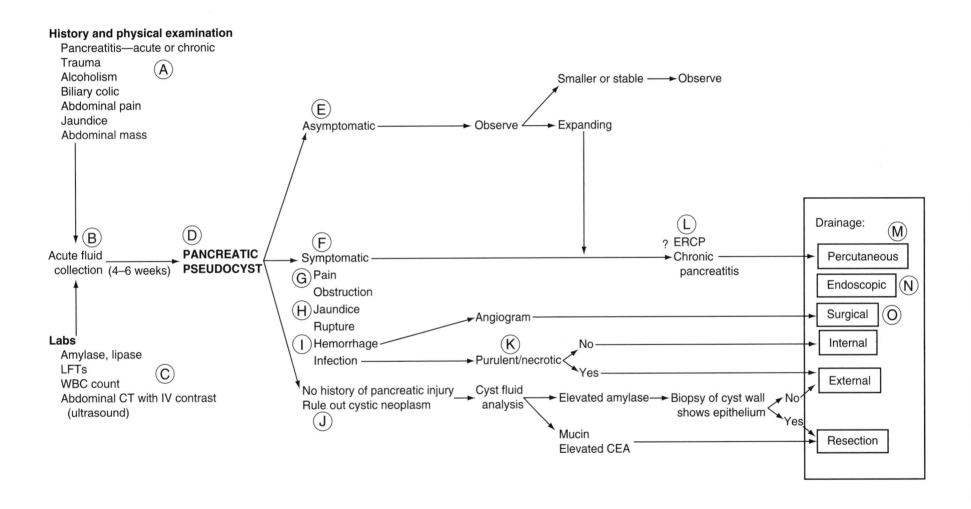

of patients with both pseudocysts and dilated or obstructed ducts. These findings can change surgical management in 25% of patients. Patients with chronic pancreatitis also have a relatively high incidence of bile duct strictures that can be addressed at the time of surgery. ERCP itself carries its own risks, including pancreatitis and infection. ERCP should therefore be done within 24 to 48 hours of the scheduled drainage procedure so that if the pseudocyst is seeded with bacteria, it has little time to develop into a clinically significant infection.

(M) Percutaneous needle aspiration can assist with diagnosis, but percutaneous drainage is not commonly used as definitive therapy because of the greater than 70% recurrence rate. Percutaneous drainage catheters can be placed with either CT or US guidance. Although many claim that percutaneous drainage is effective and safe, recent retrospective comparisons of percutaneous drainage versus surgery have shown high rates of failure and septic complications, as well as unacceptably long drainage times with catheter drainage.

(N) Endoscopic drainage includes transpapillary stenting and transgastric and transduodenal cystenterostomies. Results to date have been encouraging, but these techniques require significant expertise that is not available in all communities. New technology such as combined video-echoscopes may make this modality even safer. Aggressive care of stents placed following endoscopic cystenterostomies is essential to achieve a successful long-term result.

(O) Surgical treatment of pseudocysts includes internal drainage, external drainage, and resection. Internal drainage is the preferred method of drainage, either via cystgastrostomy, cystduodenostomy, or Roux-en-Y cystjejunostomy. The choice of procedure depends on the anatomic location and size of the pseudocyst. Principles that should be followed include: (1) biopsy of the cyst wall to rule out neoplasm, especially in patients with atypical presentations; (2) debridement of all necrotic debris from the pseudocyst cavity; (3) an operative plan to adequately dependently drain the cavity; and (4) a strategy that addresses any underlying ductal abnormalities. External drainage should be used for immature pseudocysts whose walls will not hold sutures, and for infected pseudocysts with grossly purulent or necrotic intracystic debris. Resection should be considered if malignancy cannot be ruled out and for pseudocysts in the pancreatic tail involving the splenic hilum. Laparoscopic cystgastrostomy and Roux-en-Y cystjejunostomy are less invasive options and should be considered by surgeons possessing advanced laparoscopic skills.

REFERENCES

Bradley EL III, Clements JL Jr, Gonzalez AC: The natural history of pancreatic pseudocysts: A unified concept of management. Am J Surg 137:135–141, 1979.

Hutter MM, Mulvihill SJ: Laparoscopic Management of Pancreatic Pseudocysts. In Zucker K (ed): Surgical Laparoscopy, 2nd ed, New York, McGraw-Hill, 1997.

Nealon WH, Walser E: Main pancreatic ductal anatomy can direct choice of modality for treating pancreatic pseudocysts (surgery versus percutaneous drainage). Ann Surg 235:751–758, 2002.

Pitchumoni CS, Agarwal N: Pancreatic pseudocysts: When and how should drainage be performed? Gastro Clin N Amer 28:615–639, 1999.

Vitas GJ, Sarr MG: Selected management of pancreatic pseudocysts: Operative versus expectant management. Surgery 111:123–130, 1992.

Warhaw AL, Fernandez-del Castillo C, Rattner DW: Pancreatic Cysts, Pseudocysts and Fistulas. In Zinner M (ed): Maingot's Abdominal Operations, 10th ed, Philadelphia, Lippincott Williams & Wilkins, 2001.

Yeo CJ, Bastidas JA, Lynch-Nyhan A et al: The natural history of pancreatic pseudocysts documented by computed tomography. Surg Gynecol Obstet 170:411–417, 1990.

History and physical examination
Pancreatitis—acute or chronic
Trauma
Alcoholism   Ⓐ
Biliary colic
Abdominal pain
Jaundice
Abdominal mass

Labs
Amylase, lipase
LFTs
WBC count   Ⓒ
Abdominal CT with IV contrast
  (ultrasound)

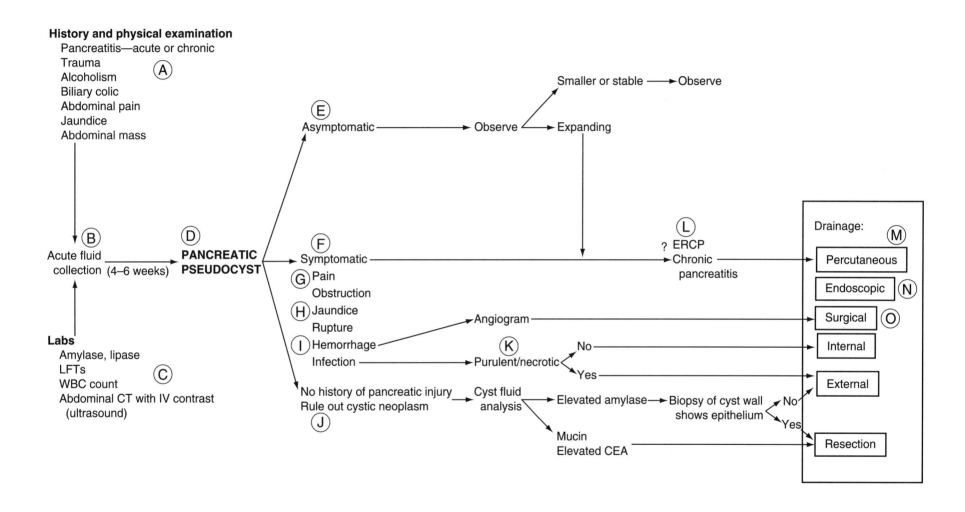

Chapter 57 *Periampullary Carcinoma*

KEITH D. LILLEMOE, MD • JOHN L. CAMERON, MD

(A) The early presentation of periampullary carcinoma often includes vague and nonspecific symptoms. The development of painless obstructive jaundice usually leads to the diagnosis. Abdominal or back pain and weight loss may be seen but usually represent a more advanced stage. Smoking is the only established environmental risk factor for pancreatic cancer. New-onset diabetes may be seen in patients with pancreatic cancer, but diabetes has not consistently been shown to be a risk factor, nor has chronic pancreatitis or alcohol. A family history of pancreatic cancer in two or more first-degree relatives is associated with an increased risk.

(B) Elevation of CA-19-9, a tumor-associated antigen, to a level above 100 U/ml is 90% accurate in diagnosing pancreatic cancer. CA-19-9 is also useful for prognosis and monitoring during the course of treatment.

(C) Spiral (helical) computed tomography (CT) has overall accuracy of more than 90% in the diagnosis of periampullary carcinoma. CT provides essential information for the diagnosis of both obstructive jaundice and a pancreatic mass. Furthermore, spiral CT accurately stages periampullary cancer by identifying hepatic or peritoneal metastases or major visceral vessel invasion. The quality of these studies has eliminated the need for routine visceral angiography. Transcutaneous ultrasound provides less information than CT; however, endoscopic ultrasound may be helpful to further stage periampullary cancers by detecting adenopathy or major vessel involvement. Recently, enthusiasm for magnetic resonance cholangiography/pancreatography (MRCP) has developed owing to the ability of this technique to clearly demonstrate the tumor mass and to define the biliary and pancreatic ducts and the peripancreatic vessels with a single examination.

(D) A tissue diagnosis can be obtained by either CT-guided percutaneous biopsy or by endoscopic ultrasound directed fine-needle aspirate. A histologic diagnosis is not generally required in potentially resectable lesions, but is useful in patients to be treated with neoadjuvant therapy or in patients considered unresectable in order to direct palliative therapy.

(E) Nonoperative palliation of obstructive jaundice can be performed by endoscopic or percutaneous techniques. Endoscopic stenting is successful in more than 90% of patients and is the procedure of choice in most cases. Metallic expandable stents (Wallstents) appear to remain patent longer than polyethylene stents.

(F) Cholangiography, either by the endoscopic (ERCP) or percutaneous (PTC) route, may be indicated for jaundiced patients suspected of having periampullary carcinoma. Although preoperative biliary stenting has not been shown to be of value in randomized trials, stenting is valuable in patients in whom delay in surgical management is expected or in those with malnutrition, sepsis, or coexisting medical conditions.

(G) The actual site of origin of a periampullary malignancy can be difficult to determine by clinical findings and radiographic imaging. Ampullary and duodenal cancers may be seen endoscopically and biopsy can be performed. Organs of origin of resectable periampullary tumors have the following distribution: pancreas, 40% to 60%; distal bile duct, 10%; ampulla of Vater, 20% to 40%; and duodenum, 10%. Because pancreatic carcinoma is more often unresectable, the overall likelihood of a periampullary tumor being pancreatic in origin is 90%.

(H) Staging laparoscopy before full abdominal exploration is favored in a number of centers.

Several series have reported detection of unsuspected liver or peritoneal metastases in up to 20% of patients. Laparoscopic US can also be performed to assess local invasion of major visceral vessels.

(I) The results of chemotherapy for disseminated pancreatic carcinomas are disappointing. Prospective trials indicate that the agent gemcitabine can improve both survival and, importantly, disease-related symptoms. Other, newer agents are under investigation.

(J) A number of neoadjuvant protocols employ both preoperative radiation therapy and chemotherapy. Most preliminary reports show no significant increase in perioperative morbidity and mortality. No significant survival advantage has been demonstrated over standard postoperative adjuvant therapy.

(K) In high-volume centers, pancreaticoduodenectomy is performed with perioperative mortality rates of less than 3%. Perioperative morbidity remains high (35%), although most complications are not life threatening. Interest has been raised in more radical resection, including extensive lymph node dissection for pancreatic cancer. Although results from Japanese groups show favorable survival with more radical resection when compared with historical controls, prospective, randomized trials performed in Western centers have not confirmed a survival benefit.

(L) Both randomized and nonrandomized series have been performed to address the role of postoperative chemotherapy and radiation following adjuvant pancreaticoduodenectomy for pancreatic carcinoma. The results have been conflicting, although most groups still favor combination therapy for most patients.

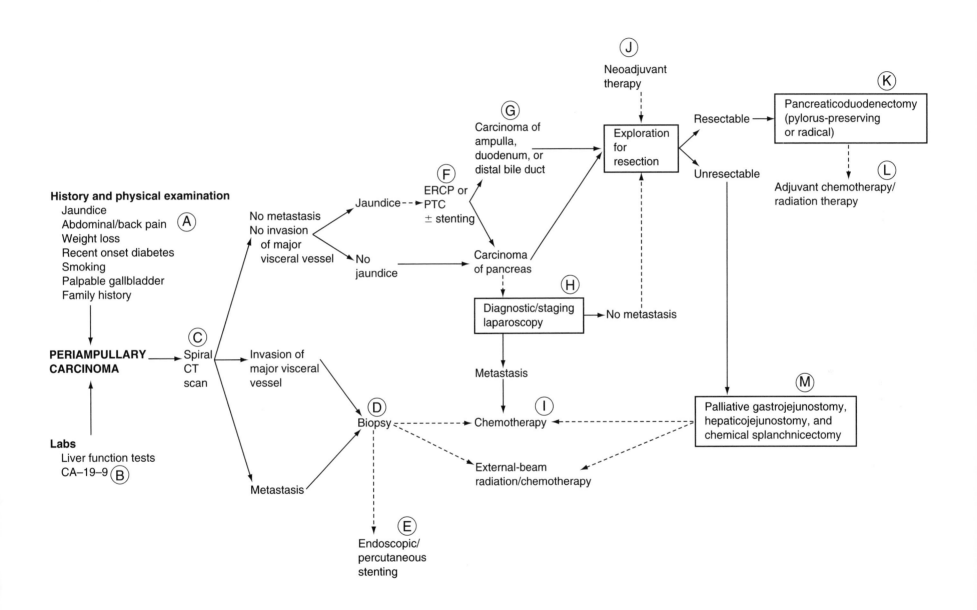

(M) If at the time of laparotomy, unresectable disease is diagnosed, appropriate palliative surgical procedures should be performed. A biliary drainage procedure (hepaticojejunostomy), a gastrojejunostomy, and chemical splanchnicectomy should palliate symptoms of obstructive jaundice, gastric outlet obstruction, and pain. The routine use of gastrojejunostomy and chemical splanchnicectomy is supported by prospective randomized trials.

REFERENCES

Fernandez-del Castillo C, Rattner DW, Warshaw AL: Standards for pancreatic resection in the 1990s. Arch Surg 130: 295–300, 1995.

Gastrointestinal Tumor Study Group: Further evidence of effective adjuvant combined radiation and chemotherapy following curative resection of pancreatic cancer. Cancer 59: 2006–2010, 1987.

Jimenez RE, Washaw AL, Ratner DW et al: Impact of laparoscopic staging in the treatment of pancreatic cancer. Arch Surg 135:409–414, 2000.

Lillemoe KD: Current management of pancreatic carcinoma. Ann Surg 221:133–148, 1995.

Lillemoe KD, Cameron JL, Hardacre JM et al: Is prophylactic gastrojejunostomy indicated for unresectable periampullary cancer? Ann Surg 230:322–330, 1999.

Neoptolemos JP, Dunn JA, Stocken DD et al: Adjuvant chemoradiotherapy and chemotherapy in resectable pancreatic cancer: A randomized controlled trial. Lancet 358:1576–1585, 2001.

Sohn TA, Lillemoe KD, Cameron JL et al: Surgical palliation of unresectable periampullary carcinoma in the 1990s. J Am Coll Surg 188:658–669, 1999.

Watanapa P, Williamson RCN: Surgical palliation for pancreatic cancer: Developments during the past two decades. Br J Surg 79:8–20, 1992.

Yeo CJ, Cameron JL, Sohn TA et al: 650 consecutive pancreaticoduodenectomies in the 1990s: Pathology, complications, outcomes. Ann Surg 226:248–260, 1997.

Yeo CJ, Cameron JL, Lillemoe KL et al: Pancreaticoduodenectomy for cancer of the head of the pancreas in 201 patients. Ann Surg 221:721–733, 1995.

Yeo CJ, Cameron JL, Lillemoe KD et al: Pancreaticoduodenectomy with or without extended retroperitoneal lymphadenectomy for periampullary adenocarcinoma: Evaluation of survival, morbidity, and mortality. Ann Surg 236:355–368, 2002.

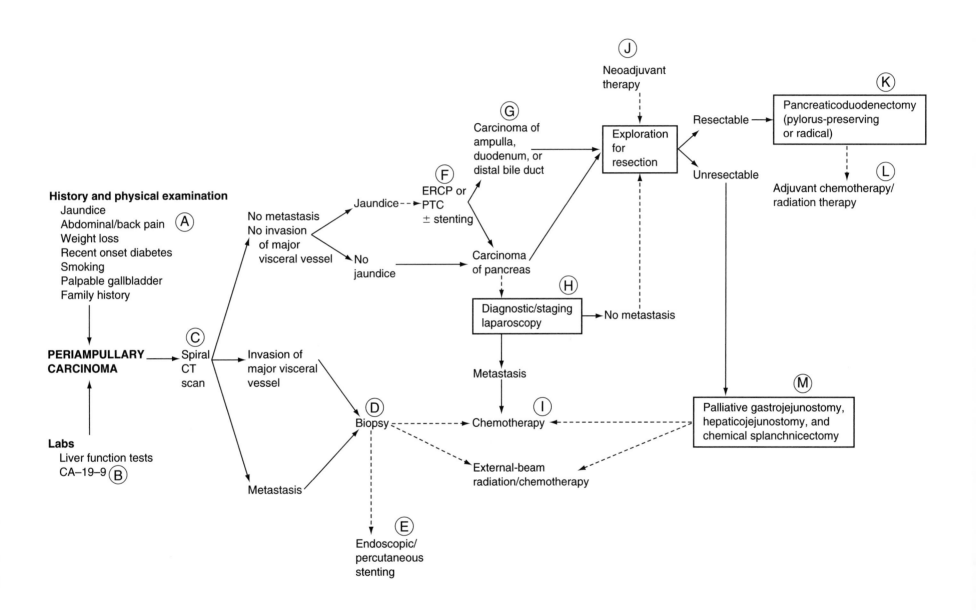

History and physical examination
Jaundice
Abdominal/back pain (A)
Weight loss
Recent onset diabetes
Smoking
Palpable gallbladder
Family history

PERIAMPULLARY CARCINOMA → (C) Spiral CT scan

Labs
Liver function tests
CA–19–9 (B)

No metastasis
No invasion of major visceral vessel

Jaundice

No jaundice

Invasion of major visceral vessel

Metastasis

(D) Biopsy

(E) Endoscopic/percutaneous stenting

(F) ERCP or PTC ± stenting

(G) Carcinoma of ampulla, duodenum, or distal bile duct

Carcinoma of pancreas

(H) Diagnostic/staging laparoscopy → No metastasis

Metastasis

(I) Chemotherapy

External-beam radiation/chemotherapy

(J) Neoadjuvant therapy

Exploration for resection

Resectable

Unresectable

(K) Pancreaticoduodenectomy (pylorus-preserving or radical)

(L) Adjuvant chemotherapy/radiation therapy

(M) Palliative gastrojejunostomy, hepaticojejunostomy, and chemical splanchnicectomy

Chapter 58 *Small Bowel Obstruction*

KATHERINE A. BARSNESS, MD • ROBERT C. MCINTYRE, JR., MD

(A) The presenting symptoms of a small bowel obstruction (SBO) are abdominal pain, distention, obstipation, nausea, and vomiting. The history commonly includes a prior abdominal operation or a new, painful mass in the groin or abdominal wall. The examination should evaluate for signs of peritonitis, abdominal mass, focal tenderness, or the presence of an incarcerated hernia.

(B) No single laboratory test confirms bowel ischemia or necrosis. Leukocytosis, acidosis, and electrolyte abnormalities are often present.

(C) Plain radiographs should include an upright view of the chest and upright and supine views of the abdomen. Free air is best seen on the upright chest x-ray. Distended loops of small bowel with air-fluid levels suggest mechanical small bowel obstruction, but this picture can also be caused by paralytic ileus. When the diagnosis is uncertain based on examination and plain radiographs, computed tomography (CT) can aid in the diagnosis of small bowel obstruction with a sensitivity of 78% to100% for high-grade obstructions. A CT scan may also provide additional information when the etiology of the obstruction is unclear.

(D) The metabolic effects of small bowel obstruction are caused by decreased fluid intake, vomiting, and a shift of fluid from the vascular and extracellular spaces into the lumen of the proximal bowel (third spacing). Immediate treatment is resuscitation with intravenous fluids and replacement of depleted electrolytes. The effectiveness of resuscitation is gauged by hemodynamic parameters and urine output. A nasogastric tube (NGT) should be placed to decompress the stomach and proximal small bowel and to reduce the risk of aspiration of gastric contents. The NGT also prevents swallowed air from increasing the distention of the proximal bowel.

(E) Emergent surgical indications may include fever, shock, acidosis, leukocytosis, and peritonitis. Any or all of these signs and symptoms may indicate ongoing bowel ischemia and/or necrosis.

If bowel ischemia is in question, a laparotomy is warranted. Additionally, any patient with SBO initially treated with conservative therapy who develops any of these signs or symptoms should also be considered for immediate laparotomy.

(F) If reduction of a groin hernia relieves the signs and symptoms of SBO, the patient is observed, and then a herniorrhaphy is performed on an elective basis. A nonreducible hernia is a surgical emergency.

(G) Adhesive obstructions are the most common type of SBO. Many of these obstructions will resolve with bowel rest and decompression. In the absence of clinical improvement, additional radiographic studies may be indicated. Any patient with worsening signs or symptoms should undergo immediate laparotomy and lysis of adhesions (LOA).

(H) The operative procedure for an incarcerated groin hernia depends largely on the operating surgeon's preference. A standard anterior approach is adequate treatment, with a laparotomy added to the procedure only in cases of bowel necrosis. Alternatively, a laparoscopic repair using the transabdominal preperitoneal (TAPP) approach allows for evaluation of bowel viability as well as repair of the hernia defect via a single procedure. Finally, a preperitoneal approach allows for repair of the hernia defect as well as evaluation of the bowel for viability. Further, in cases of questioned viability, bowel resections can be done through the preperitoneal exposure, thereby abrogating the need for a midline laparotomy.

(I) Less than 10% of all SBOs occur as a result of a distal obstruction. The most common colonic obstruction is colon cancer. In cases of suspected large bowel tumors, information obtained from a preoperative colonoscopy or barium enema can aid in the operative management of the tumor. Additionally, a decompressing stent may be placed during colonoscopy, allowing for a full bowel prep before the definitive operation.

(J) Gallstone ileus is obstruction of the small bowel caused by an intraluminal gallstone.

Treatment is enterotomy and removal of the stone. Swallowed objects or bezoars can also cause bowel obstruction and require removal via enterotomy.

(K) Intussusception of the small bowel is uncommon in adults. The lead point for an intussusception is a tumor in most patients, although adhesive bands or inflammatory lymph nodes may also be causative. Simple reduction or lysis of adhesions may be the only treatment necessary. Patients with tumors require resection of the mass after reduction of the intussusception.

(L) A volvulus is a rotation of a loop of bowel at least 180 degrees around its mesenteric axis. A cecal volvulus can present as an SBO and usually requires a laparotomy for treatment. Resection of the redundant colon reduces the rate of recurrence as compared with detorsion/fixation alone.

(M) Crohn's disease can present with intestinal obstruction either during an acute inflammatory episode or, more commonly, from chronic stricture formation. Acute inflammatory obstructions usually resolve with bowel rest.

(N) An ileus is a functional obstruction secondary to decreased motility of the small intestine, usually associated with an underlying condition. Despite the lack of a true obstruction, these patients are also volume/electrolyte depleted and uncomfortable from abdominal distention. Treatment should therefore address the volume status and electrolytes of the patient and may include an NGT until the underlying etiology for decreased motility can be addressed. Additionally, all medications that cause decreased motility (e.g., narcotics and anticholinergics) should be decreased in dose or withheld until resolution of the ileus.

(O) If a patient fails to make progress within 24 to 48 hours of observation, a gastrograffin study of the small bowel can aid in differentiating between a partial and a complete obstruction. Failure of gastrograffin to reach the colon within 24 hours of ingestion suggests a complete obstruction, and this patient will benefit from immediate laparotomy

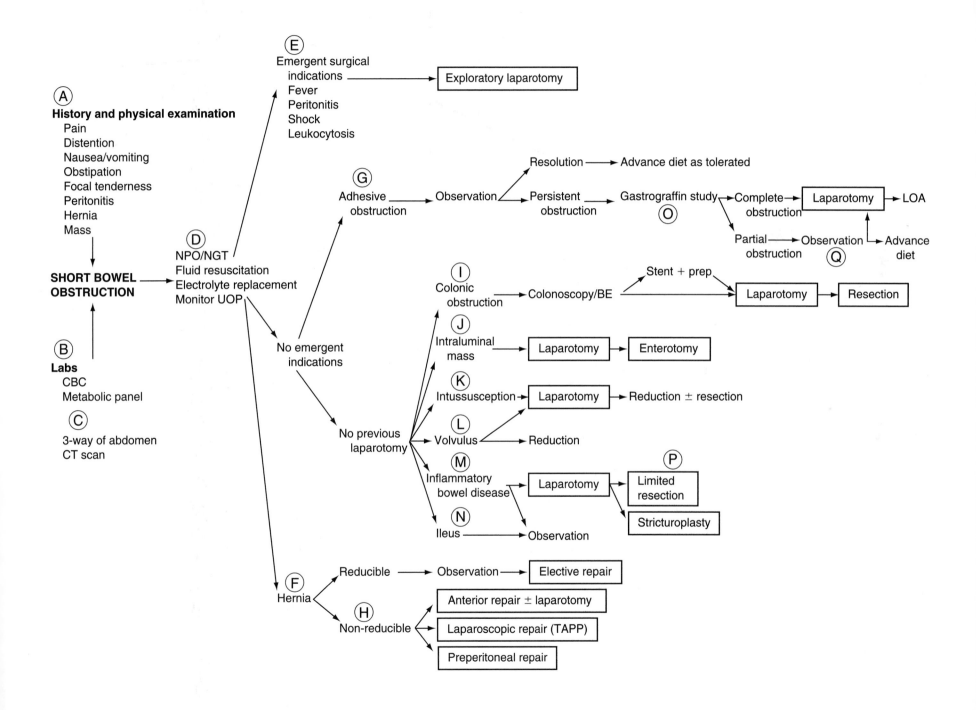

(A)
History and physical examination
 Pain
 Distention
 Nausea/vomiting
 Obstipation
 Focal tenderness
 Peritonitis
 Hernia
 Mass

SHORT BOWEL OBSTRUCTION

(B)
Labs
 CBC
 Metabolic panel

(C)
3-way of abdomen
CT scan

(D)
NPO/NGT
Fluid resuscitation
Electrolyte replacement
Monitor UOP

(E)
Emergent surgical indications
Fever
Peritonitis
Shock
Leukocytosis

Exploratory laparotomy

No emergent indications

(G)
Adhesive obstruction → Observation
Resolution → Advance diet as tolerated
Persistent obstruction → Gastrograffin study (O)
Complete obstruction → Laparotomy → LOA
Partial obstruction → Observation (Q) → Advance diet

No previous laparotomy

(I)
Colonic obstruction → Colonoscopy/BE → Stent + prep → Laparotomy → Resection

(J)
Intraluminal mass → Laparotomy → Enterotomy

(K)
Intussusception → Laparotomy → Reduction ± resection

(L)
Volvulus → Reduction

(M)
Inflammatory bowel disease → Laparotomy → Limited resection (P) / Stricturoplasty

(N)
Ileus → Observation

(F)
Hernia
 Reducible → Observation → Elective repair
 (H) Non-reducible → Anterior repair ± laparotomy / Laparoscopic repair (TAPP) / Preperitoneal repair

and LOA. However, if gastrograffin passes into the colon within 24 hours of ingestion, up to 75% of these patients will have resolution of their SBO with observation alone.

Ⓟ A laparotomy is often required for obstruction from chronic stricture formation in Crohn's disease. Because frequent obstructive episodes are the rule rather than the exception in this chronic inflammatory disease, operations that preserve small bowel length (e.g., stricturoplasty or limited resections) are preferred.

Ⓠ Further observation for a partial obstruction can extend for another 24 to 48 hours with few adverse sequelae. If there is still failure to improve, the patient should undergo a laparotomy for LOA.

REFERENCES

Begos DG, Sandor A, Modlin IM: The diagnosis and management of adult intussusception. Am J Surg 173:88–94, 1997.

Choi HK, Chu KW, Law WL: Therapeutic value of gastrograffin in adhesive small bowel obstruction after unsuccessful conservative treatment: A prospective randomized trial. Ann Surg 236:1–6, 2002.

Dietz DW, Laureti S, Strong SA et al: Safety and long-term efficacy of strictureplasty in 314 patients with obstructing small bowel Crohn's disease. J Am Coll Surg 192:330–337, 337–338, 2001.

Fevang BT, Jensen D, Svanes K et al: Early operation or conservative management of patients with small bowel obstruction? Eur J Surg 168:475–481, 2002.

Maglinte DD, Heitkamp DE, Howard TJ et al: Current concepts in imaging of small bowel obstruction. Radiol Clin North Am 41:263–283, 2003.

Shih SC, Jeng KS, Lin SC et al: Adhesive small bowel obstruction: How long can patients tolerate conservative treatment? World J Gastroenterol 9:603–605, 2003.

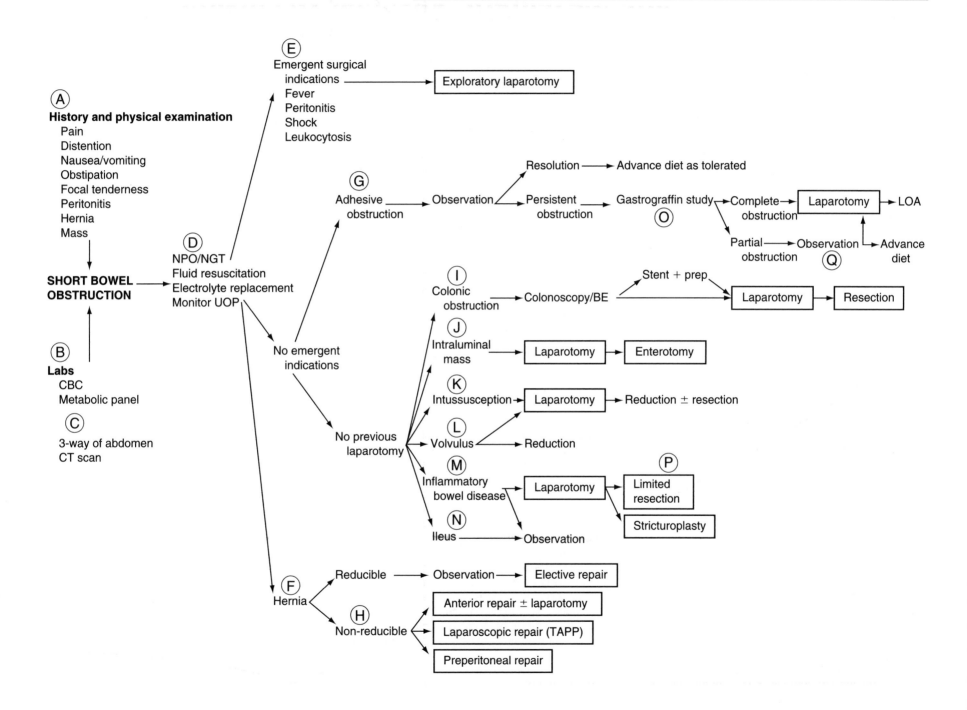

Chapter 59 *Acute Mesenteric Vascular Occlusion*

WILLIAM H. PEARCE, MD • NANCY SCHINDLER, MD

(A) Characteristically, patients present with severe abdominal pain of abrupt onset that is out of proportion to physical findings and immediate bowel evacuation. The classic triad of abdominal pain, fever, and heme-positive stools is present in only one third of patients. A history of prior abdominal pain with weight loss is indicative of an acute arterial thrombosis. Patients with acute mesenteric thrombosis may present with vague, nonspecific abdominal pain.

(B) Acute mesenteric ischemia (AMI) is uncommon (1 in 100,000 hospital admissions). Because of this and the often nonspecific symptoms, diagnosis is often delayed and the mortality rate is high. Recent series have not shown significant improvements in mortality rates despite medical advancements. Prompt diagnosis is critical to survival, and therefore the index of suspicion needs to be high and the threshold for diagnostic tests low.

(C) Acute mesenteric vascular occlusion may result from arterial embolism, thrombotic occlusion of an existing stenosis, nonocclusive ischemia secondary to shock, mesenteric venous occlusion, or hypercoagulable states. Risk factors therefore include age, associated atherosclerotic disease, arrhythmias, recent myocardial infarction, cardiogenic shock with pressor support or intra-aortic balloon, and known hypercoagulable states. Mesenteric ischemia occurs more often in females than in males.

(D) Unfortunately, no simple noninvasive test is reliable for diagnosing intestinal ischemia. Acidosis develops in only 50% of patients and it is generally a late sign signifying transmural bowel infarction. Hyperamylasemia, hemoconcentration, and elevations of creatinine phosphokinase and lactic dehydrogenase are associated with intestinal ischemia but are neither sensitive nor specific. Leukocytosis is common and is usually greater than 15,000/µl.

(E) Electrocardiography (ECG) may be helpful in identifying arrhythmias or a recent myocardial infarction. Echocardiography (TEE) may identify a proximal source of embolus such as a significant ventricular wall motion abnormality, valvular heart disease, or intra-arterial or ventricular thrombus.

(F) Plain abdominal x-rays are nonspecific and not sensitive. Findings suggestive of AMI include thickening of bowel wall, pneumatosis, and portal vein air. Because of the ready availability of CT scan, plain x-rays of the abdomen are rarely performed. CT or CTA will show aortic calcification at the origins of the visceral vessels and contrast within the visceral arteries.

(G) When mesenteric ischemia is suspected, clotting profiles should be performed to identify any underlying hypercoaguable state. These tests should include a complete blood count; platelet count; prothrombin time; partial thromboplastin time; protein C; protein S; antithrombin III; activated protein C resistance; and genetic tests for mutation of the Factor V Leyden, prothrombin 20210, and MHTHR genes. Hematologic testing should be performed prior to anticoagulation.

(H) Resuscitation of the patient is important to improve perfusion of still viable gut. A Swan-Ganz catheter may be helpful to optimize cardiac output and treat underlying cardiac disease. This should not delay angiography or laparotomy.

(I) Biplanar mesenteric angiography is the diagnostic test of choice for suspected mesenteric ischemia. The origins of the mesenteric vessels are visualized on the lateral projection. In patients with nonocclusive ischemia, angiography may play a therapeutic role as well. Placement of a selective catheter for intra-arterial injection of papaverine or other vasodilator may improve ischemia. Magnetic resonance arteriography is an excellent tool for the evaluation of chronic mesenteric ischemia. Its use in the diagnosis of acute mesenteric vascular occlusion is limited by time needed to perform and interpret images.

(J) When a diagnosis of mesenteric ischemia is made, the patient is prepared for laparotomy with access to the greater saphenous vein. A vein bypass graft is preferred over prosthetic graft when bowel necrosis has occurred. Self-retaining retractors are very helpful in obtaining adequate exposure, especially of the supraceliac aorta.

(K) On occasion, a patient may be explored for a diagnosis other than AMI and be found to have necrotic bowel. The root of the mesentery should be examined for the presence of a pulse. Absence of any pulse in the small bowel mesentery is consistent with thrombotic occlusion of the superior mesenteric artery (SMA) at its origin. Similarly, the pattern of bowel necrosis may suggest the etiology. Bowel ischemia from the ligament of Treitz to the mid-transverse colon is characteristic of a thrombotic occlusion. With embolic occlusions, the proximal branches of the SMA are spared and provide collateral bloodflow to the proximal jejunum.

(L) Patients with nonocclusive ischemia are usually seen after complicated coronary artery bypass surgery with long pump times and cardiogenic shock. Every attempt should be made before laparotomy to resuscitate the patient and reestablish adequate cardiac output. Intra-arterial papaverine into the SMA may be beneficial in relieving the vasoconstriction. When peritoneal signs develop, exploration is necessary.

(M) Venous thrombosis is becoming a more common cause of abdominal pain and intestinal ischemia. CT and MRI have greatly enhanced our ability to diagnose mesenteric venous thrombosis. Selective SMA angiography is rarely required. Approximately 80% of these patients have an underlying hypercoagulable state and 44% have a history of deep venous thrombosis. These patients should be treated with long-term anticoagulation.

(N) Embolic occlusion of the mesenteric vessels follows ventricular dysfunction or arrhythmia. Intravenous heparin is given when the diagnosis is made. Chances of survival are significantly improved when the operation is performed within

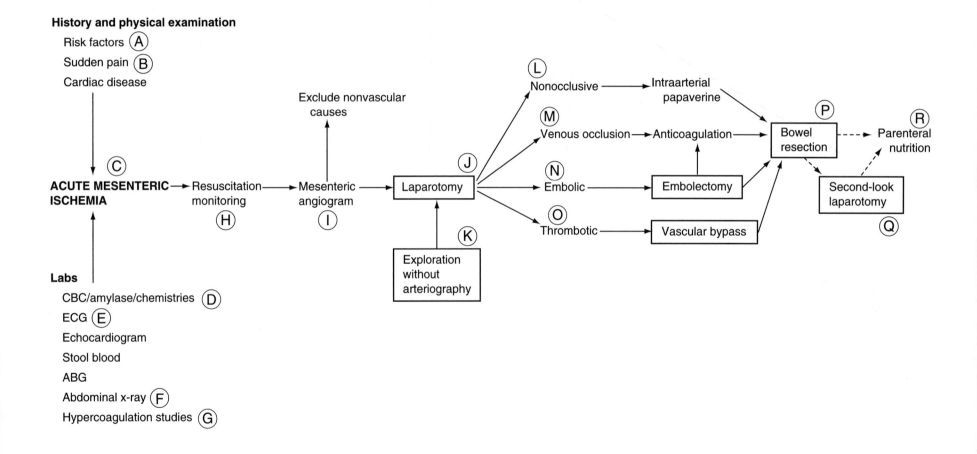

History and physical examination

Risk factors (A)

Sudden pain (B)

Cardiac disease

Exclude nonvascular causes

(C)

ACUTE MESENTERIC → Resuscitation → Mesenteric → Laparotomy
ISCHEMIA monitoring angiogram

(H) (I) (J)

Exploration without arteriography (K)

(L) Nonocclusive → Intraarterial papaverine

(M) Venous occlusion → Anticoagulation

(N) Embolic → Embolectomy

(O) Thrombotic → Vascular bypass

(P) Bowel resection

(R) Parenteral nutrition

Second-look laparotomy (Q)

Labs

CBC/amylase/chemistries (D)

ECG (E)

Echocardiogram

Stool blood

ABG

Abdominal x-ray (F)

Hypercoagulation studies (G)

8 hours of the initial symptoms. Long-term anti-coagulation is necessary to prevent recurrent embolization. Embolectomy may be performed through a transverse arteriotomy if the vessel appears normal and of adequate size. If the vessel is diseased or small, a longitudinal arteriotomy with patch is preferred.

Ⓞ Multiple visceral artery occlusion is present in patients with thrombotic occlusion. Initially, revascularization of the bowel is performed with a venous graft to the SMA. Restoration of bloodflow minimizes the amount of bowel that must be resected. Single-vessel revascularization is usually performed. The infrarenal aorta is often too diseased to serve as an inflow vessel. Options for inflow may include the supraceliac aorta or the iliac arteries. In rare patients intra-arterial thrombolysis may be considered; however, because the metabolic demands of the gut are high, operative exploration and embolectomy should be performed when there is any delay in obtaining the angiogram or in infusing thrombolytics. Limited reports of angioplasty and stenting of acute mesenteric vascular occlusions are available. Any attempts at percutaneous treatment should be limited to patients without peritoneal signs.

Ⓟ After revascularization, viability of the bowel is assessed with Doppler ultrasound or fluorescein injection. Necrotic bowel is resected. A second-look operation is performed when there are areas of questionable bowel viability.

Ⓠ Once the decision has been made to perform a second-look operation, clinical improvement should not alter the decision.

Ⓡ For young patients, removal of the entire small bowel may be indicated. The patient may then be maintained on hyperalimentation or considered for a small bowel transplant. In the very elderly with significant comorbidities, quality of life and long-term survival may influence the decision to resect necrotic bowel and to resuscitate the patient.

REFERENCES

Bjorck M, Acosta S, Lindberg F et al: Revascularization of the superior mesenteric artery after acute thromboembolic occlusion. Brit J Surg 89:923–927, 2002.

Endean ED, Barnes SL, Kwolek CJ et al: Surgical management of thrombotic acute intestinal ischemia. Ann Surg 233:801–808, 2001.

Morasch MD, Ebaugh JL, Chiou AC et al: Mesenteric venous thrombosis: A changing clinical entity. J Vasc Surg 34:680–684, 2001.

Vosshenrich R, Fischer U: Contrast-enhanced MR angiography of abdominal vessels: Is there still a role for angiography? Eur Radiol 12:218–230, 2002.

Yamaguchi T, Saeki M, Iwasaki Y et al: Local thrombolytic therapy for superior mesenteric artery embolism: Complications and long-term clinical follow-up. Radiation Med 17:27–33, 1999.

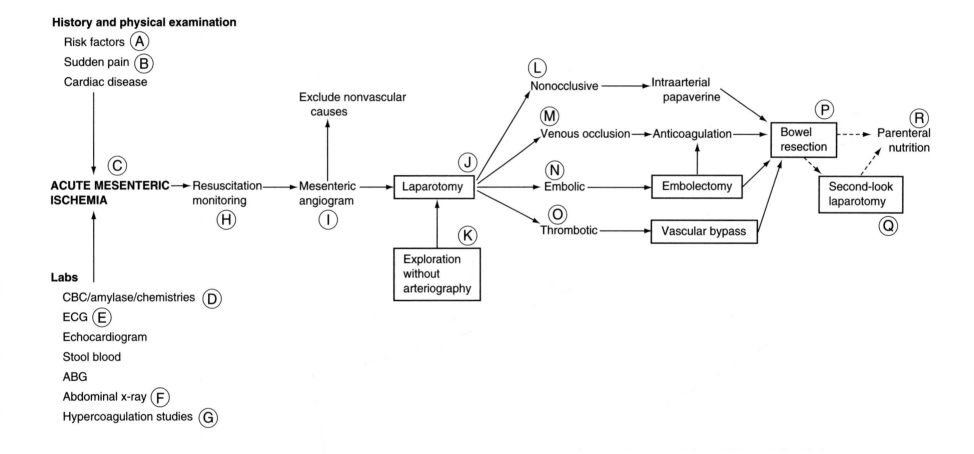

History and physical examination

Risk factors (A)

Sudden pain (B)

Cardiac disease

ACUTE MESENTERIC ISCHEMIA (C)

Labs

CBC/amylase/chemistries (D)

ECG (E)

Echocardiogram

Stool blood

ABG

Abdominal x-ray (F)

Hypercoagulation studies (G)

Resuscitation monitoring (H)

Mesenteric angiogram (I)

Exclude nonvascular causes

Laparotomy (J)

Exploration without arteriography (K)

Nonocclusive (L) → Intraarterial papaverine

Venous occlusion (M) → Anticoagulation

Embolic (N) → Embolectomy

Thrombotic (O) → Vascular bypass

Bowel resection (P)

Second-look laparotomy (Q)

Parenteral nutrition (R)

Chapter 60 **Short Bowel Syndrome**

JON S. THOMPSON, MD

(A) The Short Bowel Syndrome (SBS) is characterized by malnutrition, weight loss, dehydration, diarrhea, and electrolyte abnormalities. This clinical syndrome and its associated complications are related primarily to the length of the remaining functioning intestine. However, the site of resection, underlying intestinal disease, presence or absence of the ileocecal valve, functional status of the remaining digestive organs, and adaptive capacity of intestinal remnant are important factors as well. Patients left with less than 60 cm of small intestine are almost uniformly dependent on parenteral nutrition (PN) long-term. Those with greater than 120 cm of intestine can usually be rehabilitated to enteral nutrition (EN). Those with 60 to 120 cm of intestine will usually require PN for up to a year but will often be rehabilitated to EN, depending on the other factors mentioned above.

(B) SBS occurs when resection of the intestine results in absorptive capacity that does not meet the needs of the patient. This generally occurs when less than 120 cm of small bowel is remaining in the adult. Conditions that lead to SBS include mesenteric vascular disease, Crohn's disease, malignancy and/or radiation therapy, and a variety of benign causes including trauma and intestinal obstruction. Seventy-five percent of incidences result from single massive intestinal resection, and 25% result from multiple sequential resections.

(C) The early management of patients with the SBS is often that of the care of a critically ill surgical patient. Maintaining fluid electrolyte balance and initiation of nutritional support are important. Sepsis is often present.

(D) During the initial phase, nutrition support usually requires PN, particularly until the patient's condition stabilizes. Initiation of enteral therapy as soon as feasible will be important during this period. Approximately 70% of patients will survive massive intestinal resection.

(E) Adaptation of the remaining intestinal remnant occurs over a period of months following resection. Luminal contents (e.g., pancreaticobiliary secretions and nutrients and hormonal factors) appear to be important in this process. The initial dietary management should include frequent small feedings, although continuous therapy may be useful in very short remnants. Hyperosmolar solution should be avoided early on. Initially a high-carbohydrate, high-protein diet is appropriate to maximize absorption. Provision of nutrients in their simplest form, so that digestion is not a limiting factor, is also useful. A low-oxalate (i.e., no cola, tea, or spinach), low-fat, lactose-free diet is recommended. Separating the ingestion of solids and liquids may decrease the frequency of bowel movements.

(F) Patients with SBS are at risk for several complications. Metabolic complications are present, particularly in patients requiring PN. These include metabolic acidosis and alkalosis, hypocalcemia, hyper- and hypoglycemia, and D-lactic acidosis. Specific nutrient deficiencies may also occur depending on absorption and replacement therapy. Bacterial overgrowth may exacerbate diarrhea and impair absorption and may contribute to D-lactic acidosis. Cholelithiasis occurs in at least one third of patients. Prophylactic cholecystectomy should be considered in patients with SBS. Gastric hypersecretion occurs transiently during the first several months after resection and should be managed with H_2-blockers or proton pump inhibitors. Kidney stones, which develop in one third of patients, usually are calcium oxalate stones. This occurs primarily in patients with remaining colon where the free oxalate is absorbed. Diarrhea can be treated generally with agents such as loperamide, codeine, or lomotil. Octreotide is useful in selected patients. Using cholestyramine to bind bile acids may also be helpful. Treating gastric hypersecretion and bacterial overgrowth, as mentioned above, is also important.

(G) Patients who successfully transition to total EN will require long-term monitoring and care to prevent complications. Patients who do not successfully transition to EN require further efforts at intestinal rehabilitation. The initial step is to optimize dietary intake. This is done to maximize absorption from the intestinal remnant. However, the diet can also be modified, and other treatment introduced, to maximize the intestinal adaptive response. Provision of fat and dietary fiber may be important in this regard. Other therapies, including glutamine and growth factors such as growth hormone or glucagon-like peptide, continue to be investigated but their efficacy is unclear. Surgical therapy may also be helpful. Intestinal obstruction should be sought as a cause of bacterial overgrowth and stasis. Intestinal continuity should be restored whenever feasible to recruit downstream intestine. However, this may be result in worsening diarrhea and perianal complications that may limit the diet. Generally, the overall remnant should be at least 90 cm to prevent these complications.

(H) Patients who cannot be successfully rehabilitated during a 1- to 2-year period after their resections are considered to have irreversible intestinal failure. These patients are anticipated to be permanently dependent on PN. The 5-year survival for this therapy is approximately 85%. Complications of long-term PN include line sepsis, thrombosis with difficulty maintaining vascular access, and PN-related liver failure. Hepatic failure occurs in approximately one third of patients on long-term PN. This can be minimized by maximizing delivery of nutrients via the enteral route.

(I) Selected patients who have intestinal failure may become candidates for nontransplant operations to improve intestinal function. Patients who have a dilated intestinal remnant may be considered for intestinal tapering and lengthening to improve their motility and intestinal absorption and to lengthen the intestinal remnant. This has been more commonly performed in children. The success rate of this approach is approximately 75%. Patients who have a moderate intestinal remnant and rapid transit with significant diarrhea and electrolyte problems may be candidates for procedures

History and physical examination (A)
Weight loss
Diarrhea
Steatorrhea
Malnutrition
Ostomy
Perianal disease

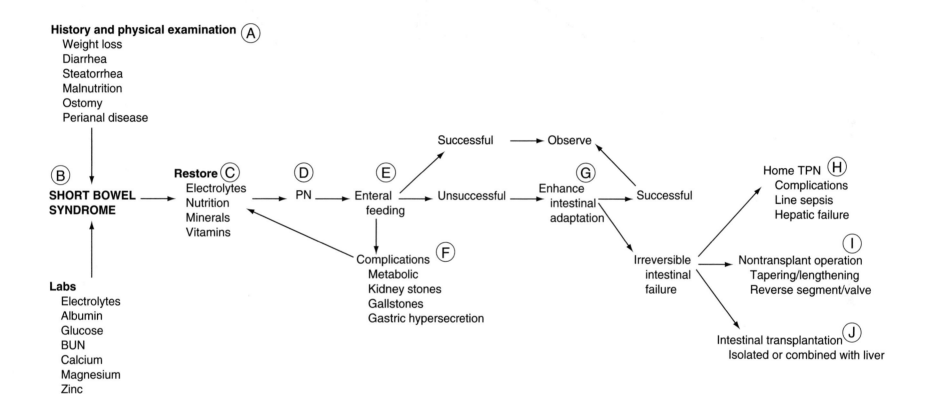

(B)

SHORT BOWEL SYNDROME

Restore (C)
Electrolytes
Nutrition
Minerals
Vitamins

(D) PN

(E) Enteral feeding

Successful ⟶ Observe

Unsuccessful

Complications (F)
Metabolic
Kidney stones
Gallstones
Gastric hypersecretion

(G) Enhance intestinal adaptation

Successful

Irreversible intestinal failure

Labs
Electrolytes
Albumin
Glucose
BUN
Calcium
Magnesium
Zinc
LFT

Home TPN (H)
Complications
Line sepsis
Hepatic failure

(I)
Nontransplant operation
Tapering/lengthening
Reverse segment/valve

Intestinal transplantation (J)
Isolated or combined with liver

such as reversed intestinal segment, artificial valve, or colon interposition. The success rate of these procedures designed to slow motility is only 50%.

Ⓙ   Patients with irreversible intestinal failure who develop complications of long-term PN are candidates for intestinal transplantation. Isolated intestinal transplantation is acceptable for patients who have recurrent sepsis and difficulty with vascular access but reversible liver disease. Patients with irreversible liver disease will require combined liver-intestinal transplantation. These procedures are successful in 75% of patients at 1 year and 50% of patients at 5 years.

REFERENCES

Abu-Elmagd K, Reyes J, Todo S et al: Clinical intestinal transplantation: New perspectives and immunologic considerations. J Am Coll Surg 186:512–527, 1998.

Chan S, McCowen KC, Bistran BR et al: Incidence, prognosis, and etiology of end stage liver disease in patients receiving home total parenteral nutrition. Surgery 126:28–34, 1999.

Jeppesen PB, Hartmann B, Thulesen J: GLP-2 improves nutrient absorption and nutritional status in short bowel patients with no colon. Gastroenterology 120:806–815, 2001.

Messing B, Crenn P, Beau P et al: Long-term survival and parenteral nutrition dependence in adult patients with the short bowel syndrome. Gastroenterology 117:1043–1050, 1999.

Thompson JS, Langnas AN, Pinch LW et al: Surgical approach to the short bowel syndrome. Ann Surg 222:600–607, 1995.

Thompson JS, Langnas AN: Surgical approaches to improving intestinal function in the short bowel syndrome. Arch Surg 134:706–711, 1999.

Thompson JS: The role of prophylactic cholecystectomy in the short bowel syndrome. Arch Surg 131:556–560, 1996.

Thompson JS: Surgical approach to the short bowel syndrome: Procedures to slow intestinal transit. Eur J Ped Surg 9:263–266, 1999.

Vanderhoof JA, Langnas AN: Short bowel syndrome in children and adults. Gastroenterology 113:1767–1778, 1997.

Wilmore DW, Byrne TA, Persinger RL: Short bowel syndrome: New therapeutic approaches. Curr Prob Surg 34:309–444, 1997.

History and physical examination (A)
Weight loss
Diarrhea
Steatorrhea
Malnutrition
Ostomy
Perianal disease

(B)

SHORT BOWEL SYNDROME

Labs
Electrolytes
Albumin
Glucose
BUN
Calcium
Magnesium
Zinc
LFT

Restore (C)
Electrolytes
Nutrition
Minerals
Vitamins

(D)
PN

(E)
Enteral feeding

Successful → Observe

Unsuccessful

Complications (F)
Metabolic
Kidney stones
Gallstones
Gastric hypersecretion

(G)
Enhance intestinal adaptation

Successful

Irreversible intestinal failure

Home TPN (H)
Complications
Line sepsis
Hepatic failure

(I)
Nontransplant operation
Tapering/lengthening
Reverse segment/valve

Intestinal transplantation (J)
Isolated or combined with liver

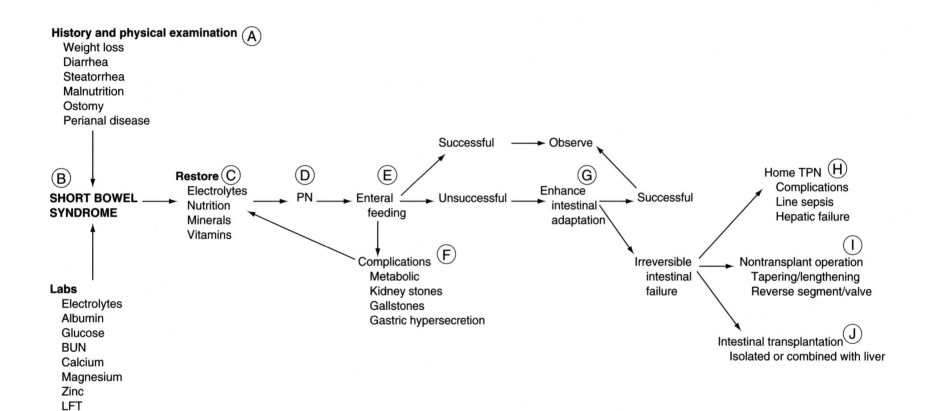

Chapter 61 *Enterocutaneous Fistula*

JOSEF E. FISCHER, MD

(A) Enterocutaneous fistula continues to carry a 20% mortality rate, although in some studies mortality has been as low as 6%. Satisfactory results require both judgment and meticulous care. Death is usually caused by sepsis, now that malnutrition and electrolyte imbalance are preventable. Adequate nutrition of patients with established sepsis remains difficult to achieve because of the lack of satisfactory utilization of either carbohydrate or fat calories and because proteolysis continues unabated.

(B) A sinogram of every sinus tract (No. 5 pediatric feeding tube), using water-soluble contrast media, delineates the source and extent of the tract and associated abscesses. Barium studies rarely are required and, if performed, often do not reveal fistulas. The same is true of CT scans.

(C) Bowel function and healing are impaired by abnormal colloid oncotic pressure caused by low serum albumin levels. Liberal albumin administration may restore albumin to 3.3 g/dl, a level at which healing is promoted and bowel function is more normal.

(D) Needle aspiration of an obvious pointing abscess can be followed by a Hypaque sinogram to delineate the extent of the abscess and its origin from the bowel before drainage.

(E) A subclavian cannula is inserted for total parenteral nutrition. Patients should be hydrated with crystalloid to ensure safe cannulation of large veins.

(F) Antibiotics are required when a patient is frankly septic. An average of eight or nine antibiotics are ultimately required during the total course of therapy for a patient with a fistula.

(G) An abscess adjacent to the fistula keeps the tract open.

(H) Fistulas arising from irrevocably damaged bowel do not heal.

(I) Nasogastric suction does not decrease fistula output and may produce reflux esophagitis and subsequent stricture.

(J) Enteral nutrition should be begun with immunoactive enteral formulas. It is usually wise to maintain parenteral nutrition for 5 to 10 days after starting enteral feedings because it takes 5 days to achieve adequate enteral nutrition and the gut at rest does not resume effective absorption immediately. About 4 feet of normal gut is needed for enteral nutrition.

(K) Mortality after an operation to repair a fistula should be 2% or less. A complication rate of 12% or less is expected.

(L) If the fistula has not closed after 4 to 5 weeks without sepsis, an operation is usually necessary. Preoperative nutritional status can be evaluated by measuring short–half-life proteins (e.g., transferrin, retinol-binding protein, and thyroxine-binding prealbumin). When transferrin increases spontaneously, hepatic protein synthesis is adequate. Principles of operative management include incision through healthy skin, relief of all distal obstruction, excision of marginally competent bowel, reanastomosis of all small intestinal blind loops, gastrostomy, feeding jejunostomy, and postoperative parenteral nutrition until enteral nutrition is resumed.

(M) Histamine H_2-antagonists or proton-pump inhibitors may decrease drainage from enterocutaneous fistulas. Somatostatin or the octreotide analog has not proven helpful in closing enterocutaneous fistulas. Somatostatin or an analog may be helpful in closing pancreatic fistulas, however. In several large series using contemporary treatment, a spontaneous closure rate of 33% to 45% was reported. Spontaneous closure may be followed by return of a fistula if there is diseased bowel such as in inflammatory bowel disease or distal obstruction.

REFERENCES

Aguirre A, Fischer JE, Welch CE: The role of surgery and hyperalimentation in therapy of gastrointestinal-cutaneous fistulae. Ann Surg 180:393–400, 1974.

Edmunds LH, Williams GM, Welch CE: External fistulas arising from the gastrointestinal tract. Ann Surg 152:445–471, 1960.

Fischer JE: The management of high-output intestinal fistulas. Adv Surg 9:139–179, 1975.

Fischer JE: The pathophysiology of enterocutaneous fistulas. World J Surg 7:446–450, 1983.

Kuvshinoff BW, Brodish RJ, McFadden DW et al: Serum transferrin as a prognostic indicator of spontaneous closure and mortality in gastrointestinal cutaneous fistulas. Ann Surg 217:615–623, 1993.

McPhayden VB Jr, Dudrick SJ: Management for gastrointestinal fistulas with parenteral hyperalimentation. Surgery 74:100–105, 1973.

Reber MA, Robert C, Way LW et al: Management of external gastrointestinal fistulas. Ann Surg 188:460–467, 1978.

Soeters PB, Ebeid AM, Fischer JE: Review of 404 patients with gastrointestinal fistulas: Impact of parenteral nutrition. Ann Surg 190:189–202, 1979.

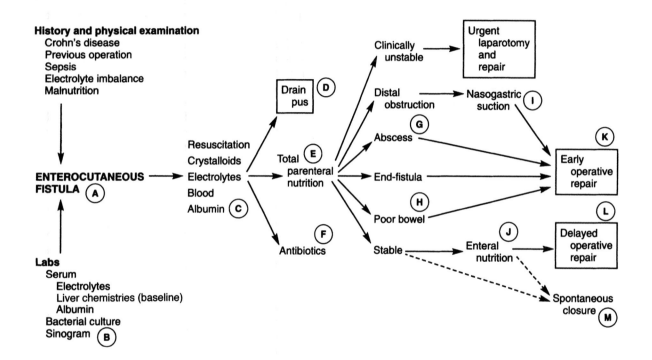

History and physical examination
Crohn's disease
Previous operation
Sepsis
Electrolyte imbalance
Malnutrition

ENTEROCUTANEOUS FISTULA (A)

Labs
Serum
  Electrolytes
  Liver chemistries (baseline)
  Albumin
Bacterial culture
Sinogram (B)

Resuscitation
Crystalloids
Electrolytes
Blood
Albumin (C)

Drain pus (D)

Total parenteral nutrition (E)

Antibiotics (F)

Clinically unstable

Distal obstruction

Abscess (G)

End-fistula

Poor bowel (H)

Stable

Urgent laparotomy and repair

Nasogastric suction (I)

Enteral nutrition (J)

Early operative repair (K)

Delayed operative repair (L)

Spontaneous closure (M)

Chapter 62 *Gastrointestinal Lymphoma*

CHRISTINA A. FINLAYSON, MD

(A) Epigastric pain is the most common presenting symptom for GI lymphoma. Weight loss is the most common systemic sign. Melena from mucosal ulceration is present if the stomach or ileoceal region is involved, but massive gastrointestinal hemorrhage is unusual. Perforation is rare. Night sweats, fevers, and peripheral adenopathy are unusual in primary GI lymphoma and signify more advanced disease.

(B) The incidence of small bowel lymphoma is increasing as the number of people who are immunosuppressed, either from disease or medication, increases.

(C) Because gastric lymphoma is a submucosal lesion, it may be undetectable on upper GI contrast (UGI) series. When a lesion is seen, it may appear as a mass, as diffuse infiltration of the stomach, or as an ulcer in the mucosa. Often, small bowel lymphoma is not appreciated on UGI.

(D) Endoscopy can visualize a gastric or colonic lesion directly and provide diagnosis via biopsy; it is rarely useful for diagnosing small bowel lymphoma.

(E) Chronic blood loss can occur if the lesion ulcerates through the mucosa. This can be detected by stool guaiac testing. The degree of blood loss should be assessed.

(F) Small bowel lymphoma is usually diagnosed at laparotomy (80%). Gastric and colonic lymphoma is more likely to be correctly identified preoperatively. When lymphoma is encountered during laparotomy, it is incumbent on the surgeon to take the following measures:
1. Establish a tissue diagnosis
2. Accurately stage the extent of disease with thorough examination of all viscera, mesentery, and nodal tissue and with biopsy of any abnormal-looking sites
3. Treat any current complications of the tumor

4. If possible, completely resect the primary tumor and any localized regional disease (laparotomy is not indicated for staging purposes alone)

(G) Most gastric and colonic lymphomas can be diagnosed by endoscopic biopsy. Multiple biopsies that are deep to the mucosa are required for adequate tissue sampling. Endoscopic ultrasound (US) can accurately gauge the depth of invasion of gastric lymphoma and, in many patients, can predict involvement of perigastric lymph nodes.

(H) Computed tomography (CT) can evaluate the local extent of disease and enlargement of retroperitoneal or mediastinal lymph nodes. For small bowel lymphoma, it is often the only positive radiologic study if the diagnosis is made preoperatively. Evaluation of the chest by x-ray or CT may demonstrate parenchymal disease, pleural effusion, or mediastinal or hilar adenopathy.

(I) Waldeyer's ring is commonly a site of distant involvement and, if it is involved, the tumor stage would be upgraded.

(J) Involvement of the bone marrow with lymphoma indicates disseminated disease (stage IV).

(K) Bone scan is indicated if the patient has bone pain or an elevated alkaline phosphatase value.

(L) Most low-grade MALT lymphomas are associated with *Helicobacter pylori* infection. Eradication of *H. pylori* with antibiotic treatment can result in significant and sometimes complete regression. Surgery is reserved for an incomplete response.

(M) Stage I_E disease is confined to one extranodal (i.e., stomach, small bowel or colon) site. Stage II_E is disease in one extranodal site with local or regional (abdominal) lymph node involvement.

(N) Stage III is one extranodal site and lymph node involvement on both sides of the diaphragm (stage III_E), or splenic involvement (III_S),

or both (III_{ES}). Stage IV is diffuse or disseminated disease.

(O) The appropriate treatment for GI lymphoma is controversial. Historically, complete surgical excision has been the mainstay of treatment. In small bowel lymphoma, stage I_E and II_E, this produced 5-year survival rates of 50% and 25%, respectively. The addition of chemotherapy has improved survival for this group of patients to 75% to 85%. Patients whose tumors are completely resected tend to do better than those with incomplete resection. Radiation therapy has also been used for local treatment of the primary tumor and involved lymph nodes, and good results have been reported, particularly when combined with chemotherapy.

(P) Advanced-stage disease, if diagnosed preoperatively, is usually treated with chemotherapy followed by surgery or radiation therapy as needed. Although with surgery alone there were no long-term survivors of stage III and IV GI lymphoma, a combined-modality approach has achieved 10% to 25% 5-year survival rates.

REFERENCES

Crump M, Gospodarowicz M, Shepherd FA: Lymphoma of the gastrointestinal tract. Semin Oncol 26:324–337, 1999.

Longo DL, DeVita VT, Jaffe ES, et al: Lymphocytic Lymphomas. In DeVita VT, Hellman S, Rosenberg SA (eds): Cancer: Principles and Practice of Oncology, 6th ed. Philadelphia: Lippincott, Williams & Wilkins, 2001.

Kida M: Endoscopic tumor diagnosis and treatment. Endoscopy 34:860–870, 2002.

Koch P, del Valle F, Berdel WE et al: Primary gastrointestinal non-Hodgkin's lymphoma: I. Anatomic and histologic distribution, clinical features, and survival data of 371 patients registered in the German Multicenter Study GIT NHL 01/92. JCO 19:3861–3873, 2001.

Schechter NR, Yahalom J: Low-grade MALT lymphoma of the stomach: A review of treatment options. Int J Rad Onc Bio Phy 46:1093–1103, 2000.

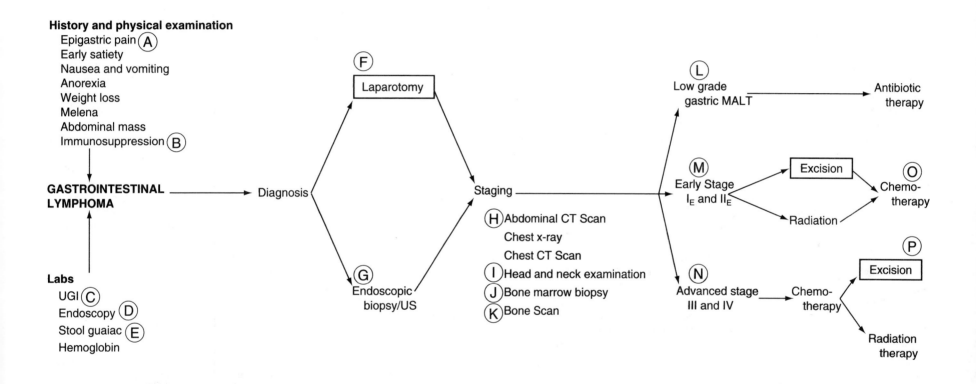

History and physical examination
Epigastric pain (A)
Early satiety
Nausea and vomiting
Anorexia
Weight loss
Melena
Abdominal mass
Immunosuppression (B)

GASTROINTESTINAL LYMPHOMA

Labs
UGI (C)
Endoscopy (D)
Stool guaiac (E)
Hemoglobin

Diagnosis

(F)
Laparotomy

(G)
Endoscopic biopsy/US

Staging

(H) Abdominal CT Scan
Chest x-ray
Chest CT Scan
(I) Head and neck examination
(J) Bone marrow biopsy
(K) Bone Scan

(L)
Low grade gastric MALT ——→ Antibiotic therapy

(M)
Early Stage I$_E$ and II$_E$
Excision
Radiation
(O) Chemo-therapy

(N)
Advanced stage III and IV ——→ Chemo-therapy
(P) Excision
Radiation therapy

Chapter 63 *Crohn's Disease of the Small Bowel*

TRACY L. HULL, MD

(A) Patients with small bowel Crohn's disease may present with abdominal pain, diarrhea, fever, weight loss, fatigue, anal pain, or an abdominal mass. If lesions are present that bleed, either overtly or occultly, anemia may be present.

(B) The etiology of Crohn's disease is unknown. It can affect the GI tract anywhere from the mouth to the anus. The ileocolic region is most often affected. Neither medical nor surgical treatment is curative. The aim of management is to maintain quality of life and to foster the longevity of the bowel, not simply to deal with the current problem.

(C) Upper and lower intestinal contrast x-rays outline the location of disease. Colonoscopy allows visualization of the disease process and the opportunity to do biopsies. Patients with duodenal disease can have biopsies done via an esophagogastroduodenoscopy (EGD). In patients without obstruction, capsule video endoscopy may help locate disease that is difficult to see on contrast studies. This test may be useful for occult bleeding and when looking for ulcers in the small bowel. Experience is being gained with MRI to locate and evaluate disease.

(D) Medical treatment should be started in patients with nonacute problems. The aim is to alleviate symptoms, restore nutrition, and provide emotional support. Steroids are usually the mainstay of initial treatment. Antibiotics such as metronidazole are commonly used. Azathioprine and 6-mercaptopurine are used for steroid-sparing effects, although such effects can take up to 6 months to appear. These drugs are used if a patient cannot be weaned from steroids or has had multiple small bowel resections. Oral 5-ASA compounds (but not sulfasalazine) are also used to treat small bowel Crohn's disease. Intravenous infliximab has gained support for induction of remission and maintenance treatment of inflammatory disease.

(E) Acute ileitis can mimic an acute flare-up of Crohn's disease. The bowel is spongy, edematous, and violaceous. The lumen is not narrowed, and the cecum is normal. Should appendectomy be done, fistulization from the appendiceal stump or diseased ileum is rare, in contrast with appendectomy associated with Crohn's ileitis.

(F) Vagotomy and gastrojejunostomy are used when medical treatment of gastroduodenal Crohn's disease fails. Revision rates in some studies approach 70% at 10 years. When feasible, strictureplasty can be done with better long-term outcomes in some cases.

(G) Resection of diseased small bowel is favored over bypass procedures in almost all patients with intractable disease or obstruction. In the few instances when resection is too hazardous, and bypass of ileum to the side of the transverse colon is done, the bypassed segment is resected at a second stage. Midline incisions are favored to preserve the right and left lower quadrants for stoma sites, which may be needed later in the patient's lifetime. Patients should have physiologic deficits such as anemia and electrolyte imbalances corrected before surgery. At 10 years after surgery, 30% of patients with distal ileal disease need more than one operation and 5% need more than three for recurrent disease.

(H) It is optimal to drain abscesses before abdominal surgery in stable patients. This avoids free contamination of pus in the abdominal cavity at surgery. Drainage can be done with CT guidance by the radiologists and a drain can be placed. If persistent sepsis or a fistula develops, surgery is done.

(I) When resection is done, wide resection margins (2 to 3 cm) are not needed and microscopic margins need not be checked. Patients presenting for elective first operations for ileocecectomy may be ideal candidates for laparoscopic assisted surgery. Open surgery is usually selected for those who have had multiple operations or enterostomies that preclude safe, time-efficient laparoscopy.

(J) Strictureplasty is used instead of resection to treat all feasible strictures. It is usually not considered with active sepsis, fistula, or when transverse closure of the enterotomy is vulnerable to leakage. This procedure allows for small bowel preservation. Short strictures (less than 10 cm) are treated with Heinke-Mikulicz type of construction. Longer strictures are corrected with Finney type reconstruction. Strictureplasty can be combined with resection of small intestine. Rates of complications such as abdominal sepsis (6%) and reoperation for new strictures (28% at a median of 7 years follow-up) compare favorably with resection.

(K) The decision to perform an anastomosis or to divert the intestine after resection is based on the patient's condition with respect to residual sepsis, malnutrition, and other factors that affect dehiscence. Preoperative total parenteral nutrition in a debilitated patient may decrease the risk of primary anastomotic dehiscence. Preoperative stoma marking should be done if there is a possibility that a stoma may be needed.

REFERENCES

Delaney CP, Fazio VW: Crohn's disease of the small bowel. Surg Clin N Am 81:137–158, 2001.

Dietz DW, Fazio VW, Laureti S et al: Strictureplasty in diffuse Crohn's jejunoileitis. Dis Colon Rectum 45:764–770, 2002.

Hoffmann JC, Zeitz M: Treatment of Crohn's disease. Hepato-Gastroenterology 47:90–100, 2000.

Milsom JW, Hammerhofer KA, Bohnm B et al: Prospective, randomized trial comparing laparoscopic vs. conventional surgery for refractory ileocolic Crohn's disease. Dis Colon Rectum 44:1–9, 2001.

Reiber A, Nussle K, Reinshagen M et al: MRI of the abdomen with positive oral contrast agents for diagnosis of inflammatory bowel disease. Abdominal Imaging 27:394–399, 2002.

Strong SA: Surgical treatment of inflammatory bowel disease. Curr Opin Gastroenterol 18:441–446, 2002.

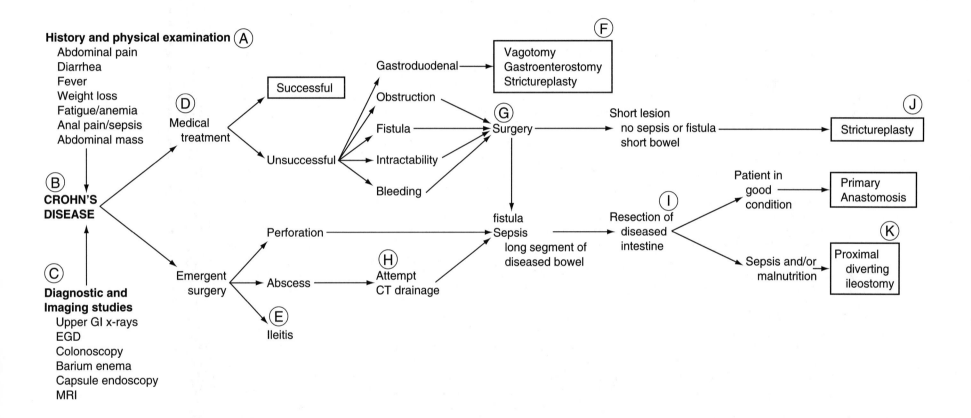

History and physical examination (A)
Abdominal pain
Diarrhea
Fever
Weight loss
Fatigue/anemia
Anal pain/sepsis
Abdominal mass

(B)
**CROHN'S
DISEASE**

(C)
**Diagnostic and
Imaging studies**
Upper GI x-rays
EGD
Colonoscopy
Barium enema
Capsule endoscopy
MRI

(D)
Medical
treatment

Successful

Unsuccessful

Emergent
surgery

Perforation

Abscess

(E)
Ileitis

(H)
Attempt
CT drainage

Gastroduodenal

Obstruction

Fistula

Intractability

Bleeding

(F)
Vagotomy
Gastroenterostomy
Strictureplasty

(G)
Surgery

fistula
Sepsis
long segment of
diseased bowel

Short lesion
no sepsis or fistula
short bowel

(J)
Strictureplasty

(I)
Resection of
diseased
intestine

Patient in
good
condition

Primary
Anastomosis

Sepsis and/or
malnutrition

(K)
Proximal
diverting
ileostomy

Chapter 64 *Acute Right Lower Quadrant Pain*

C. CLAY COTHREN, MD • JULIE K. HEIMBACH, MD

(A) In the majority of patients, history and physical examination point to the etiology of acute right lower quadrant (RLQ) pain. Appendicitis, the most common etiology of RLQ pain, is characterized by vague umbilical discomfort that intensifies and localizes to McBurney's point. In contrast, gynecologic sources tend to originate in the RLQ and are often sudden in onset, such as in the case of a ruptured ovarian cyst or ovarian torsion. Associated symptoms may help differentiate the etiology; nausea and vomiting following the onset of pain suggests appendicitis, whereas emesis before the onset of pain is more consistent with gastroenteritis. Diarrhea, while nonspecific, is more suggestive of inflammatory bowel disease (IBD) or regional/infectious enteritis. Vaginal complaints point to a gynecologic etiology, whereas dysuria is consistent with cystitis or pyelonephritis. Hematuria suggests renal or ureteral stones. Physical examination should rule out such sources as an incarcerated hernia, epididymitis or testicular pathology, musculoskeletal complaints, or a rectus sheath hematoma.

(B) Laboratory studies should routinely include white blood cell (WBC) count, urinalysis, and βHCG in women. Leukocytosis with a left shift is indicative of inflammatory conditions; if a patient has a normal WBC count, the incidence of significant intra-abdominal pathology is lower, and a trial of observation may be warranted.

(C) Imaging is often helpful in equivocal cases (e.g., patients without a classic history, suggestive examination, or suggestive lab results), in female patients, and in patients at either extreme of age. Pelvic ultrasound is the first-line test in patients with suspected gynecologic pathology, whereas appendicitis, diverticulitis, and IBD are best visualized by CT scan with contrast.

(D) Thorough evaluation may not reveal an obvious cause of the patient's RLQ pain. Patients with a normal WBC count and negative imaging who are able to tolerate a diet may be considered for outpatient management with repeat evaluation in 24 hours. Alternatively, patients may be admitted for close observation, serial examinations, and repeat lab studies.

(E) Patients with appendicitis should receive appropriate preoperative fluid resuscitation and intravenous antibiotic coverage for polymicrobial infection (e.g., cefotetan).

(F) In cases of nonperforated appendicitis, open or laparoscopic appendectomy are advocated techniques. Laparoscopy is often preferred if the diagnosis is in question, if there is concern for pelvic pathology, and in obese patients.

(G) Patients with a CT scan diagnosis of perforated appendicitis with associated abscess may be considered for percutaneous drainage if technically feasible. Subsequent need for standard "interval appendectomy" 6 weeks following resolution is controversial and often debated in the literature.

(H) Common gynecologic etiologies include a tubo-ovarian abscess, pelvic inflammatory disease, a ruptured ovarian cyst, ovarian torsion, and ectopic pregnancy. Pelvic examination and imaging are critical to appropriate diagnosis.

(I) Mesenteric adenitis or infectious ileitis are often diagnoses of exclusion but may be suggested by CT scan findings of a thickened ileum. Conservative therapy is warranted.

Meckel's diverticulitis may be noted on CT scan but is often discovered at the time of operation when a normal-appearing appendix is identified, resulting in further exploration. The morphology of the diverticulum determines diverticulectomy versus segmental resection.

Ideally, IBD is detected before surgery unless the initial presentation is perforation or obstruction necessitating intervention. Medical therapy includes steroids and sulfasalazine. Appendectomy is performed if the appendix/base of the cecum is not involved with disease.

Diverticulitis may be cecal or sigmoid in origin (a redundant sigmoid colon may easily be located in the RLQ); treatment is identical regardless. Medical therapy consists of bowel rest, IV hydration, and broad-spectrum antibiotics until the patient's examination improves and the WBC returns to normal. If complicated by free perforation or obstruction, operative therapy is necessary, typically with segmental resection and fecal diversion. If an isolated abscess is present, percutaneous drainage and IV antibiotics may be an alternative.

Cecal cancer requires a right hemicolectomy and intraoperative evaluation for metastatic disease.

A psoas abscess can often be drained percutaneously and treated with culture-directed antibiotics. Search for an underlying cause (e.g., IVDA, primary renal or intestinal pathology, and osteomyelitis) is important.

REFERENCES

Berg DF, Bahadursingh AM, Kaminski DL et al: Acute surgical emergencies in inflammatory bowel disease. Am J Surg 184:45–51, 2002.

Fa-Si-Oen PR, Roumen RM, Croiset van Uchelen FA: Complications and management of Meckel's diverticulum–a review. Eur J Surg 165:674–678, 1999.

Ferzoco LB, Raptopoulos V, Silen W: Acute diverticulitis. N Engl J Med 338:1521–1526, 1998.

Groebli Y, Bertin D, Morel P: Meckel's diverticulum in adults: Retrospective analysis of 119 cases and historical review. Eur J Surg 167:518–524, 2001.

Kurtz RJ, Heimann TM: Comparison of open and laparoscopic treatment of acute appendicitis. Am J Surg 182:211–214, 2001.

Lipscomb GH, Stovall TG, Ling FW: Nonsurgical treatment of ectopic pregnancy. N Engl J Med 343:1325–1329, 2000.

Liu S, Siewert B, Raptopoulos V et al: Factors associated with conversion to laparotomy in patients undergoing laparoscopic appendectomy. J Am Coll Surg 194:298–305, 2002.

Nagel TC, Sebastian J, Malo JW: Oophoropexy to prevent sequential or recurrent torsion. J Am Assoc Gynecol Laparosc 4:495–498, 1997.

Pittman-Waller VA, Nyers JG, Stewart RM et al: Appendicitis: Why so complicated? Analysis of 5755 consecutive appendectomies. Am Surg 66:548–554, 2000.

Rao PM, Rhea JT, Novelline RA et al: Effect of computed tomography of the appendix on treatment of patients and use of hospital resources. N Engl J Med 338:141–146, 1998.

Ross J: Pelvic inflammatory disease. BMJ 322:658–659, 2001.

Wilson EB, Cole JC, Nipper ML et al: Computed tomography and ultrasonography in the diagnosis of appendicitis: When are they indicated? Arch Surg 136:670–674, 2001.

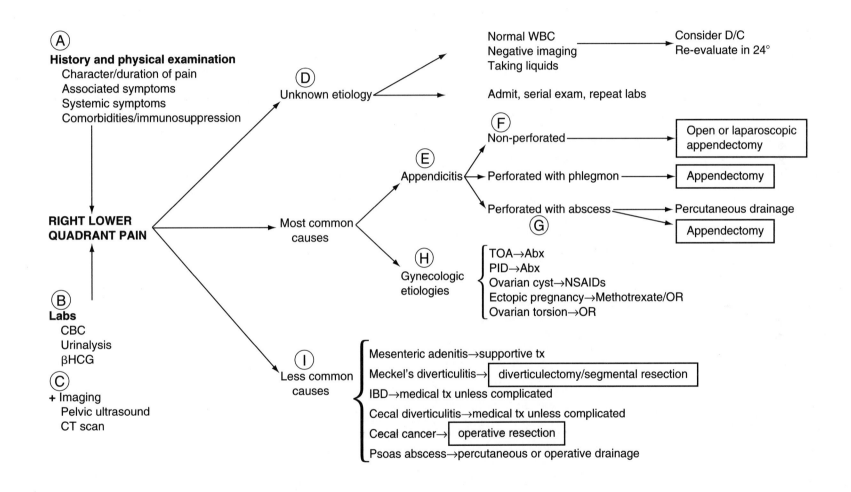

A

History and physical examination
Character/duration of pain
Associated symptoms
Systemic symptoms
Comorbidities/immunosuppression

RIGHT LOWER QUADRANT PAIN

B
Labs
CBC
Urinalysis
βHCG

C
+ Imaging
Pelvic ultrasound
CT scan

D Unknown etiology

Normal WBC
Negative imaging
Taking liquids
→ Consider D/C
Re-evaluate in 24°

Admit, serial exam, repeat labs

Most common causes

E Appendicitis

F Non-perforated → Open or laparoscopic appendectomy

Perforated with phlegmon → Appendectomy

Perforated with abscess → Percutaneous drainage
G → Appendectomy

H Gynecologic etiologies
{
TOA→Abx
PID→Abx
Ovarian cyst→NSAIDs
Ectopic pregnancy→Methotrexate/OR
Ovarian torsion→OR
}

I Less common causes
{
Mesenteric adenitis→supportive tx
Meckel's diverticulitis→ diverticulectomy/segmental resection
IBD→medical tx unless complicated
Cecal diverticulitis→medical tx unless complicated
Cecal cancer→ operative resection
Psoas abscess→percutaneous or operative drainage
}

Chapter 65 *Volvulus*

MARK D. WALSH JR., MD • ROBERT C. MCINTYRE JR., MD

(A) Volvulus of either the small or large intestine causes abdominal pain, distention, nausea with or without vomiting, and constipation/obstipation in most patients. Sigmoid volvulus often affects older male individuals institutionalized with neuropsychiatric disorders. Cecal volvulus is most common in middle-aged persons who have increased cecal mobility as a result of anomalous fixation of the cecum. Approximately 10% of patients with cecal volvulus have cecal bascule, an anterior cephalad folding of the cecum.

(B) Volvulus, a twisting of the bowel around its mesenteric axis, causes less than 10% of all bowel obstructions. In the colon, sigmoid volvulus is the most common (50% to 80%), followed by cecal volvulus (10% to 40%). Some series have reported almost equal incidences of cecal and sigmoid volvulus. Small bowel volvulus in children is often the result of congenital malrotation.

(C) In most instances, abdominal x-rays differentiate between the types of volvulus. A dilated loop of colon in the right upper quadrant with an "omega" or "bent inner tube" configuration suggests sigmoid volvulus. A dilated loop of colon with central density in the left upper quadrant or "coffee bean" configuration is a clue to cecal volvulus. Pseudo-obstruction of the colon (Ogilvie's syndrome) and acute gastric dilatation can be mistaken for volvulus on radiographs. Plain films are diagnostic in 60% to 70% of cases. CT scan is accurate and may suggest ischemic changes of the bowel.

(D) The addition of a barium enema is usually the only additional test required when the diagnosis is in question. Barium enema should not be performed in patients who have evidence of gangrenous bowel (e.g., fever, tachycardia, or hypotension); peritonitis; pneumatosis intestinalis; or pneumoperitoneum.

(E) Operation for small bowel obstruction caused by volvulus is undertaken after adequate resuscitation. Resection of bowel with end-to-end anastomosis is required more often than simple lysis of adhesions.

(F) Fluoroscopic placement of a rectal tube or endoscopy is usually effective for decompression. Proctosigmoidoscopy provides satisfactory decompression of sigmoid volvulus in 80% to 90% of patients. The sigmoid twist is usually encountered by 25 cm. The mucosa should be carefully examined for viability while withdrawing the scope following decompression. If gangrenous mucosa is noted before decompression, the procedure should be aborted and the patient should be operatively managed.

(G) After decompression, elective resection of the sigmoid colon is recommended for good risk patients because the risk of recurrent volvulus is about 60%.

(H) If proctosigmoidoscopy fails to decompress the sigmoid colon, or if peritoneal signs develop, the patient should be operated on urgently. Depending on the degree of risk, either an end sigmoid colostomy with a Hartmann's pouch or a sigmoid resection with a primary anastomosis is performed. An alternative surgical option is laparoscopically assisted sigmoid colectomy after colonoscopic decompression. "Extraperitonealization" of the sigmoid colon after decompression is an option to prevent recurrence.

(I) In unstable or high-risk patients with viable bowel, detorsion and cecopexy should be performed. Cecostomy, although associated with higher morbidity than cecopexy, has a lower incidence of recurrence and may be performed without a formal laparotomy. Resection is necessary in the presence of cecal necrosis, and detorsion should not be attempted because of increased rates of sepsis and higher mortality.

(J) In young, healthy persons, right colectomy should be done to prevent recurrence. The mortality rate for right colectomy is less than 2%, and the complication rate is about 5%.

(K) Patients with sigmoid volvulus often have complications. The mortality rate for the first episode is 5% to 15% because of associated comorbidities. A gangrenous colon is associated with an increased mortality in the range of 10% to 25%.

REFERENCES

Ballantyne GH, Brandner MD, Beart RW et al: Volvulus of the colon: Incidence and mortality. Ann Surg 202:83–92, 1985.

Chung RS: Colectomy for sigmoid volvulus. Dis Colon Rectum 40:363–365, 1997.

Chung YF, Eu KW, Nyam DC et al: Minimizing recurrence after sigmoid volvulus. Br J Surg 86:231–233, 1999.

Friedman JD, Odland MD, Burbrick MP: Experience with colonic volvulus. Dis Colon Rectum 32:409–416, 1989.

Frizelle FA, Wolff BG: Colonic volvulus. Adv Surg 29:131–139, 1996.

Grossmann EM, Longo WE, Stratton MD et al: Sigmoid volvulus in Department of Veterans Affairs medical centers. Dis Colon Rectum 43:414–418, 2000.

Khanna AK, Misra MK, Kumar K: Extraperitonealization for sigmoid volvulus: A reappraisal. Aust NZ J Surg 112:512–517, 1995.

Kuzu MA: Emergent resection for acute sigmoid volvulus: Results of 106 cases. Dis Colon Rectum 45:1085–1090, 2002.

Madiba TE, Thomson SR: The management of cecal volvulus. Dis Colon Rectum 45:264–267, 2002.

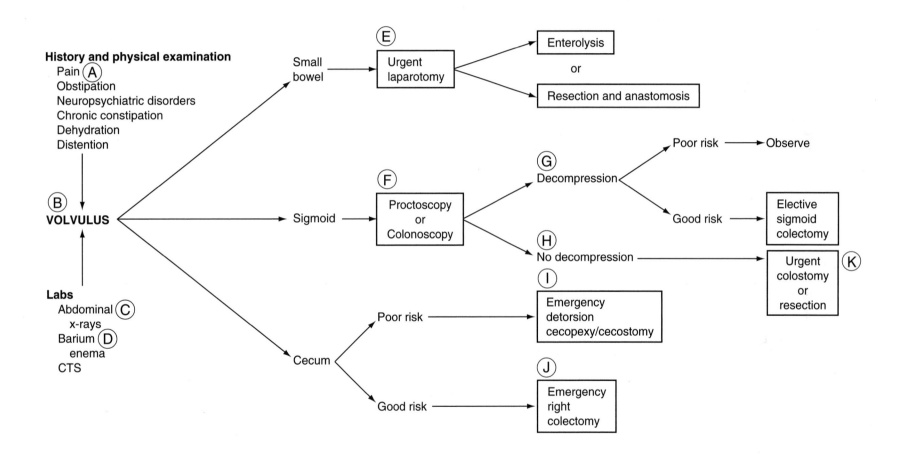

History and physical examination
Pain Ⓐ
Obstipation
Neuropsychiatric disorders
Chronic constipation
Dehydration
Distention

Ⓑ
VOLVULUS

Labs
Abdominal Ⓒ
  x-rays
Barium Ⓓ
  enema
CTS

Small
bowel

Ⓔ
Urgent
laparotomy

Enterolysis

or

Resection and anastomosis

Sigmoid

Ⓕ
Proctoscopy
or
Colonoscopy

Ⓖ
Decompression

Poor risk → Observe

Good risk →

Elective
sigmoid
colectomy

Ⓗ
No decompression

Ⓚ
Urgent
colostomy
or
resection

Cecum

Poor risk

Ⓘ
Emergency
detorsion
cecopexy/cecostomy

Good risk

Ⓙ
Emergency
right
colectomy

Chapter 66 *Diverticulitis*

MIKE KUO LIANG, MD • ANTHONY LAPORTA, MD

(A) Clinical diverticulitis presents most commonly with left lower abdominal pain, tenderness, and involuntary guarding (greater than 90%); with fever (greater than 60%); and with nonspecific gastrointestinal and urinary symptoms. Many patients state that they feel they would get better if they could have a bowel movement.

(B) Colonic diverticula are outpouchings from the colon wall categorized as true diverticula (containing all wall layers) or false diverticula (containing only the mucosal layer). Diverticulitis is the inflammation and perforation of a diverticulum. Often the perforation is microscopic. Diverticulosis is routinely used to describe a false diverticulum, most commonly on the left side of the colon. Diverticula develop because of multiple factors that include an inherent weakness in the colon wall where the vasa recta penetrate the colon along the border of the taneia coli, elastosis, a low-fiber diet, and hard stools. True diverticula of the colon are usually in the cecum.

Colonic diverticulosis occurs in 5% of individuals 50 years of age; it progressively increases such that it occurs in 80% of individuals 80 years of age. Ninety percent of diverticula occur in the sigmoid colon. Symptomatic diverticulitis develops in 20% of people with diverticula.

(C) Patients commonly (more than 70%) have an elevated WBC and abnormal urinalysis.

An upright chest x-ray should be obtained to evaluate for free air and pulmonary infiltrates; these are abnormal in 30% of patients with acute diverticulitis.

A CT scan should be obtained when the diagnosis is unclear, the severity is indeterminant, or for failure to improve with medical therapy. The CT scan has a sensitivity and specificity greater than 90% and can detect the degree of inflammation.

Ultrasound (US) can be a useful diagnostic tool but is user-dependent and variable in its accuracy. A water-soluble contrast enema is also an available diagnostic tool if CT scan is unavailable. Barium enema and endoscopy should be avoided in the acute period of diverticulitis because of the risk of perforation.

(D) Mild diverticulitis can be treated on an outpatient basis with broad-spectrum oral antibiotic coverage. Diabetic and immunosuppressed patients should not be treated as outpatients. Subsequent endoscopic or contrast evaluation to rule out malignancy is recommended once the acute inflammation has resolved. A high-fiber diet is recommended to reduce future attacks.

(E) Moderate or severe diverticulitis should be treated on an inpatient basis with broad-spectrum antibiotics, bowel rest, and analgesia. Fever, white count, peritoneal signs, and knowledge of the patient's immune status help determine the severity of the problem.

(F) Obstruction of the colon can occur with inflammation. It is difficult to differentiate from carcinoma even with negative biopsies. Resection is mandatory; however, if the obstruction resolves with conservative measures, surgery can be delayed after a bowel preparation.

(G) Fistulas can occur from the colon to the bladder (65%), vagina (25%), small bowel, or skin. These can be repaired electively with resection of the fistulized bowel and repair of the adjacent organ.

(H) Of patients presenting with their first bout of diverticulitis, 15% will require surgery and 85% will resolve with medical therapy. Of those respondent to conservative treatment, 33% will resolve with no future symptoms, 33% will continue to have vague abdominal complaints, and 33% will have a second attack.

(I) Of patients presenting with a second bout of diverticulitis, 60% will be complicated and 60% will have a third attack if left untreated. It is recommended to have an elective sigmoid resection after the second attack.

Patients under the age of 50 years have a higher recurrence rate and more severe disease process. It is recommended to consider an elective sigmoid resection after the first attack for patients 50 years or younger.

(J) Small pericolic abscesses can be treated with antibiotic therapy alone; however, large abscesses require drainage. CT-guided drainage has become the treatment of choice for most abscesses. Collections not amenable to percutaneous drainage may require surgical intervention. Elective vs. emergent surgery is then determined by the patient's response to the antibiotics and drainage.

(K) For the patient undergoing emergent surgery because of perforation, abscess, or obstruction, the treatment of choice is a two-stage Hartmann's procedure (sigmoidectomy, end colostomy, and closed rectal stump) followed by a colostomy closure in the future. The use of on-table lavage with primary anastomosis, primary anastomosis with protective loop ileostomy or transverse loop colostomy, or primary anastomosis alone have all been advocated in select cases. For patients who are either unstable or unable to tolerate a full resection, a diverting ileostomy or transverse colostomy alone should be performed. Some 20% of patients fail to have their colostomy reversed for various reasons.

(L) For patients undergoing an elective resection, a sigmoidectomy with primary anastomosis following a bowel preparation is the recommended procedure. The distal margin is to the rectum where the taneia coli diverge, and the proximal margin is to soft, pliable bowel. Either laparoscopic or hand-assisted laparoscopic colon resection are options.

Patients with fistulas can undergo a bowel resection including the colonic fistula with primary anastomosis and repair of the fistulized organ.

REFERENCES

Ambrosetti P, Jenny A, Becker C et al: Acute left colonic diverticulitis—compared performance of computed tomography and water-soluble contrast enema: Prospective evaluation of 420 patients. Disease of the Colon and Rectum 43:1363–1367, 2000.

Belmonte C, Klas JV, Perez JJ et al: The Hartmann procedure: First choice or last resort in diverticular disease? Arch Surg 131:612–615, 1996.

Blair N, Germann E: Surgical management of acute sigmoid diverticulitis. Am J Surg 183:525–528, 2002.

Bouillot J, Berthou J, Champault G et al: Elective laparoscopic colonic resection for diverticular disease. Surg Endoscop 16:1320–1323, 2002.

Chautems R, Ambrosetti P, Ludwig A et al: Long-term follow-up after first acute episode of sigmoid diverticulitis: Is surgery mandatory? A prospective study of 118 patients. Dis Colon Rectum 45:962–966, 2002.

Kohler L, Sauerland S, Neugebauer E: Diagnosis and treatment of diverticular disease: Results of a consensus development conference. Surg Endoscop 13:430–436, 1999.

Schechter S, Eisenstat TE, Oliver GC et al: Computerized tomographic scan guided drainage of intra-abdominal abscesses: Preoperative and postoperative modalities in colon and rectal surgery. Dis Colon Rectum 37:984–988, 1994.

Stollman N, Raskin J: Practice guidelines: Diagnosis and management of diverticular disease of the colon in adults. Am J Gastroenterol 94:3110–3121, 1999.

Wong W, Wexner S: Practice parameters for the treatment of sigmoid diverticulitis: Supporting documentation. Dis Colon Rectum 43:290–297, 2000.

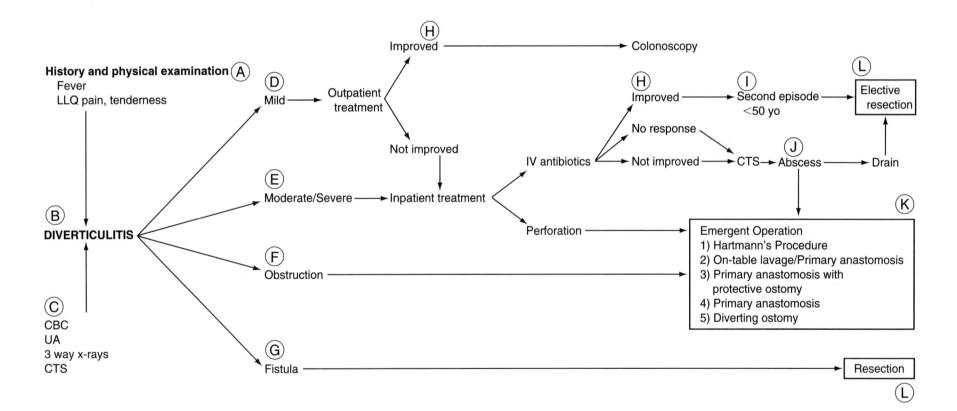

Chapter 67 Lower Gastrointestinal Bleeding

THOMAS N. ROBINSON, MD • SONIA RAMAMOORTHY, MD

(A) Lower gastrointestinal (GI) bleeding is defined as bleeding that originates distal to the ligament of Trietz. Blood per rectum, however, can originate from anywhere along the GI tract. It is estimated that approximately 24% of all intestinal bleeds are from a lower GI source. Spontaneous resolution can occur in up to in 85% of lower GI bleeds; however, up to 25% of patients will have recurrent bleeding. Massive lower GI bleeding (more than 3 units of transfused blood) has a reported mortality as high as 21%. The most common etiologies of major lower GI bleeding include diverticulosis (30%), vascular ectasia (10% to 20%), inflammatory bowel disease (9%), polyps (9%), malignancy (8%), and anorectal disease (10%). Minor lower GI bleeding (i.e., blood that is only seen with defecation, intermittently, or seen coming from the surface of the anus) is often caused by anorectal pathology.

(B) Clinical information can assist in the differential diagnosis of a lower GI bleed. Painless bleeding is suggestive of diverticulosis, angiodysplasia, hemorrhoids, or neoplasm. Abdominal pain with bleeding suggests ischemic bowel, inflammatory bowel disease, or other forms of colitis. Rectal pain with bleeding suggests an anorectal process such as anal fissure or proctitis.

(C) Massive lower GI bleeding is a life-threatening condition. The tenets of management of any GI bleed include the following: (1) resuscitation; (2) localization; and (3) treatment. Minimum requirements for initial resuscitation include two large-bore IVs, obtaining blood for transfusion, and diagnosing the presence of a coagulopathy. The acuity of the hemorrhage dictates the aggressiveness of the resuscitative measures. Expedient measures to start localizing the source of a lower GI bleed include digital rectal examination, anoscopy, and sigmoidoscopy. Nasogastric intubation for gastric lavage with return of bile is essential to exclude an upper GI source of hemorrhage. Some 10% of patients initially thought to have a lower GI source of hemorrhage are ultimately found to have an upper GI source.

(D) Colonoscopy is the test of choice for localization of lower GI bleeding; it provides both diagnostic and therapeutic potential. The diagnostic accuracy of colonoscopy ranges from 69% to 80% and may be improved by a rapid oral colonic purging. Endoscopic therapy for a localized bleed includes electrocautery, photocoagulation, and injection of vasoconstrictors/sclerotherapy. The optimal use of colonoscopy is for patients in whom the rate of bleeding does not obscure the ability to visualize the colonic mucosa or for patients in whom the rate of bleeding is insufficient to detect. Angiography and radiolabeled red blood cell scanning are used to localize bleeding that cannot be assessed by colonoscopy.

(E) Angiography has the potential for both diagnostic and therapeutic intervention. Angiography detects bleeding rates as low as 1 to 1.5 cc/min. The ability of angiography to localize a lower GI bleed ranges from 40% to 78%. Once the location of the bleed is identified, and with the angiocatheter still in place, methylene blue can be instilled to facilitate intraoperative localization of the bleed. Therapeutic interventions include angiographic coil/gelfoam embolization and vasopressin infusion. Successful halting of the bleed occurs in 60% to 100% of patients, although rebleeding may occur in up to one half of patients. The recommended use of angiography is in acutely bleeding patients in whom the rate of bleeding prohibits colonoscopy from identifying the source.

(F) Radiolabeled red blood cell scanning provides for diagnosis and localization of the bleed but does not offer any therapeutic benefit. The advantage of tagged radionuclide scanning is the ability to identify lower GI bleeding at rates as low as 0.5 ml/min. The sensitivity of this test is variable, with reports ranging from 42% to 97%. Optimal usage of radiolabeled red blood cell scanning provides localization in a non–life-threatening bleed as a prelude to either angiography or surgery.

(G) Surgery provides definitive treatment of a localized lower GI bleed. Indications for an operation include hemorrhage of more than 6 to 8 units of blood in 24 hours, hemodynamic instability despite resuscitative efforts, or significant rebleeding within a short time. If hemodynamic stability allows, localization studies should be performed before an operation to direct a segmental resection. In a hemodynamically unstable patient, or in a bleeding patient in whom no bleeding site is located at surgery, a subtotal colectomy is the procedure of choice.

REFERENCES

Billingham RP: The conundrum of lower gastrointestinal bleeding. Surg Clin N Am 77:241–252, 1997.

Cappell MS, Friedel D: The role of sigmoidoscopy and colonoscopy in the diagnosis and management of lower gastrointestinal disorders: Endoscopic findings, therapy, and complications. Med Clin N Am 86:1253–1288, 2002.

Eisen GM, Dominitz JA, Faigel DO et al: An annotated algorithmic approach to acute lower gastrointestinal bleeding. Gastrointest Endosc 53:859–863, 2001.

Vernava AM III, Moore BA, Longo WE et al: Lower gastrointestinal bleeding. Dis Colon Rectum 40:846–858, 1997.

Zuckerman GR, Prakash C: Acute lower intestinal bleeding: Clinical presentation and diagnosis. Gastrointest Endosc 48:606–617, 1999.

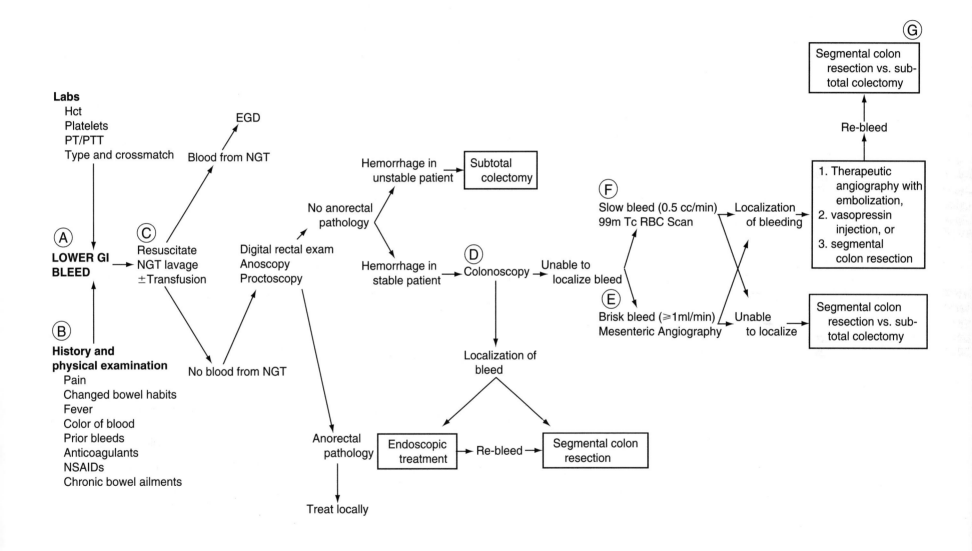

Labs
Hct
Platelets
PT/PTT
Type and crossmatch

EGD

Blood from NGT

Ⓐ

LOWER GI BLEED

Ⓒ
Resuscitate
NGT lavage
±Transfusion

Digital rectal exam
Anoscopy
Proctoscopy

No anorectal pathology

Hemorrhage in unstable patient → Subtotal colectomy

Hemorrhage in stable patient

Ⓓ
Colonoscopy

Unable to localize bleed

Ⓕ
Slow bleed (0.5 cc/min)
99m Tc RBC Scan

Localization of bleeding

Ⓖ
Segmental colon resection vs. sub-total colectomy

Re-bleed

1. Therapeutic angiography with embolization,
2. vasopressin injection, or
3. segmental colon resection

Ⓔ
Brisk bleed (≥1ml/min)
Mesenteric Angiography

Unable to localize

Segmental colon resection vs. sub-total colectomy

Ⓑ
History and physical examination
Pain
Changed bowel habits
Fever
Color of blood
Prior bleeds
Anticoagulants
NSAIDs
Chronic bowel ailments

No blood from NGT

Anorectal pathology

Localization of bleed

Endoscopic treatment → Re-bleed → Segmental colon resection

Treat locally

Chapter 68 *Ulcerative Colitis*

GLENN T. AULT, MD, MSEd • ROBERT W. BEART, JR., MD

(A) Ulcerative colitis usually presents with diarrhea, abdominal pain, and fever. Arthritis, uveitis, pyoderma, and hepatitis are sometimes systemic manifestations.

(B) Sigmoidoscopy is the first step in diagnosis. The rectal mucosa appears edematous and friable with continuous involvement of the colon beginning at the anus. An abdominal x-ray shows colonic dilatation (toxic megacolon) in 3% to 5% of patients with negative stool cultures.

(C) Massive hemorrhage is a rare complication of acute ulcerative colitis. If transfusion of more than 3000 ml of whole blood is required within 24 hours, emergency colectomy is necessary. The rectum should be carefully examined preoperatively and removed only when necessary to control bleeding.

(D) Perforation of the colon occurs in only 3% of patients but causes more deaths than any other complication. The perforation is most often in the sigmoid colon or splenic flexure. Perforation usually occurs in patients with toxic megacolon. The perforation may be associated with an abscess, but because this is a diffuse process, CT-guided drainage is not appropriate in this setting.

(E) Symptoms of toxicity are treated by nasogastric (NG) suction, IV corticosteroids, cyclosporine, antibiotics, and total parenteral nutrition (TPN). Potassium and blood transfusion are often needed. If toxic colitis (with or without megacolon) does not improve within 48 hours, emergency abdominal colectomy with Brooke ileostomy is performed. Emergency colectomy has a 3% to 6% mortality rate when performed less than 5 days after admission.

(F) Chronic ulcerative colitis can be intermittent or persistent. When medical therapy with steroids and 6-mercaptopurine and nutritional support fail to bring improvement within 6 months, the entire colon is removed. Signs of medical intractability are uncontrolled diarrhea, chronic debilitation and arrested development in children, and fibrosis with stricture.

(G) Extracolonic disease rarely is an indication for colectomy. Ankylosing spondylitis and liver disease do not consistently respond to resection.

(H) Abdominal colectomy is the most appropriate procedure today. Lesser procedures such as the Turnbull blowhole procedure are less appropriate. The colon is very fragile and great care must be taken during colectomy.

(I) Patients followed for more than 7 years should undergo annual colonoscopy and multiple biopsies to search for epithelial dysplasia. Severe dysplasia on several biopsies is associated with cancer of the colon in half of such patients. Patients with severe or moderate dysplasia require colectomy, but mild dysplasia is followed by close surveillance.

(J) The usual elective operation for medically intractable ulcerative colitis is total proctocolectomy with a Brooke ileostomy, continent ileostomy, ileorectal anastomosis, or ileoanal anastomosis. Some patients benefit from nutritional repletion before elective operation to ensure an operative mortality under 3%.

REFERENCES

Almogy G, Sachar DB, Bodian CA et al: Surgery for ulcerative colitis in elderly persons—Changes in indications for surgery and outcome over time. Arch Surg 136:1396–1400, 2001.

Beart RW Jr: Pouchitis. Br J Surg 82:566–567, 1995.

Cohen RD, Woseth DM, Thisted RA et al: A meta-analysis and overview of the literature on treatment options for left-sided ulcerative colitis and ulcerative proctitis. Am J Gastroenterol 95:1263–1276, 2000.

Eaden JA: The risk of colorectal cancer in ulcerative colitis: A meta-analysis. Gut 48:526–535, 2001.

Gorfine SR, Bauer JJ, Harris MT et al: Dysplasia complicating chronic ulcerative colitis—Is immediate colectomy warranted? Dis Colon Rectum 43:1575–1581, 2000.

Heuschen UA, Hinz U, Allemeyer EH et al: One- or two-stage procedure for restorative proctocolectomy: Rationale for a surgical strategy in ulcerative colitis. Ann Surg 234:788–794, 2001.

McIntyre PB, Pemberton HJ, Wolff BG et al: Comparing functional results 1 year and 10 years after ileal pouch-anal anastomosis for chronic ulcerative colitis. Dis Colon Rectum 37:303–307, 1994.

Podosky DK: Inflammatory bowel disease. N Engl J Med 347(6):417–429, 2002.

Sachar DB: Inflammatory bowel disease: Recent advances in pharmacotherapy. Gastrointestinal Dis Today 6:9–15, 1997.

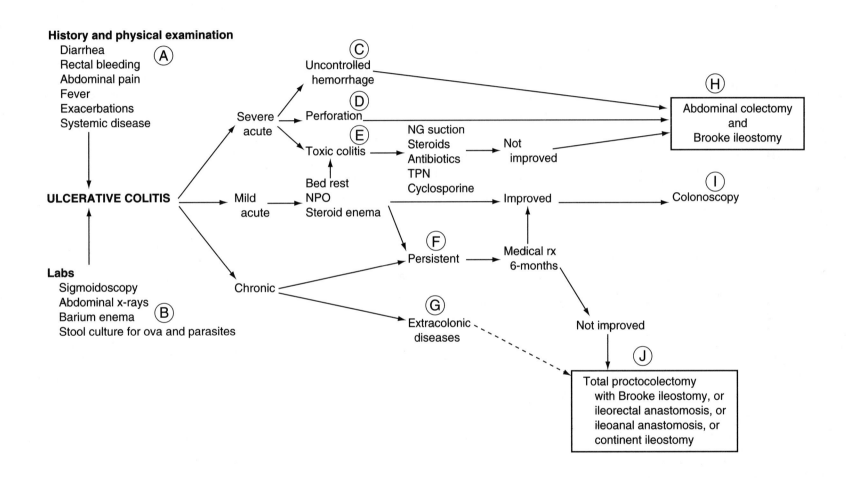

History and physical examination
- Diarrhea (A)
- Rectal bleeding
- Abdominal pain
- Fever
- Exacerbations
- Systemic disease

ULCERATIVE COLITIS

Labs
- Sigmoidoscopy
- Abdominal x-rays
- Barium enema (B)
- Stool culture for ova and parasites

Severe acute

(C) Uncontrolled hemorrhage

(D) Perforation

(E) Toxic colitis

Bed rest
NPO
Steroid enema

Mild acute

NG suction
Steroids
Antibiotics
TPN
Cyclosporine

Not improved

(H) Abdominal colectomy and Brooke ileostomy

Improved

(I) Colonoscopy

Chronic

(F) Persistent

Medical rx 6-months

Not improved

(G) Extracolonic diseases

(J) Total proctocolectomy with Brooke ileostomy, or ileorectal anastomosis, or ileoanal anastomosis, or continent ileostomy

Chapter 69 *Carcinoma of the Colon*

MARTIN D. MCCARTER, MD

(A) Risk factors include family history of colon cancer, inflammatory bowel disease, adenomatous polyps, and multiple polyp syndromes (e.g., FAP, Gardner's syndrome, and Peutz-Jegher's syndrome).

(B) The majority of colon cancers cases (65% to 85%) result from sporadic mutations; 10% to 25% are considered hereditary; 5% meet the criteria for hereditary nonpolyposis colorectal cancer (HNPCC, also known as Lynch syndrome); 0.5% meet the criteria for familial adenomatous polyposis (FAP); and approximately 0.1% result from rare polyposis syndromes. Consideration for genetic screening should be given to patients with a strong family history, young age of onset (age less than 30 years), and multiple (more than 100) polyps. The current (Amsterdam II) criteria for HNPCC can be remembered as 3,2,1 (3 relatives with HNPCC-associated cancers such as colorectal, endometrium, small bowel, genitourinary; over 2 successive generations; with 1 primary relative under 50 years of age at diagnosis).

(C) Colon cancer is the third most common cancer in the United States (148,300 new cases per year) and the third most common cause of death (56,600 per year) in both men and women. An individual's lifetime risk of developing colorectal cancer in the United States is 6%.

(D) Screening for colon cancer should begin by age 50 years or earlier for those at higher risk. Acceptable screening options include those in Table 69-1.

TABLE 69.1
Screening Options

Yearly fecal occult blood testing (FOBT) plus flexible
  sigmoidoscopy every 5 years*
Flexible sigmoidoscopy every 5 years
Yearly fecal occult blood testing
Colonoscopy every 10 years
Double-contrast barium enema every 5 years

*The combination of FOBT and flexible endoscopy is preferred over
  either modality alone.

(E) Rectal bleeding or the presence of occult fecal blood requires diagnostic evaluation. Endoscopic biopsy of the lesion and its histologic confirmation is the cornerstone of diagnosis and should not be delayed. The entire colon and rectum must be evaluated.

(F) Capsule endoscopy and virtual colonoscopy (with specialized CT scan and software) are still being evaluated and are considered experimental. The utility of these modalities may be limited in that they both require mechanical bowel preparation and any abnormalities detected would likely need endoscopic biopsy.

(G) Polyps may be found on a stalk (pedunculated) or may be broad-based (sessile) and may span the range from benign to adenomatous to cancerous. Three types of adenomatous polyps are recognized histologically: tubular adenoma, tubulovillous adenoma, and villous adenoma. Colon resection is recommended for cancerous polyps with positive polypectomy margins or with invasive cancer to Haggit level 4 (submucosal below the stalk).

(H) Staging and symptoms direct clinical management. Chest x-ray and CT scan of the abdomen and pelvis are helpful in planning potential therapy and extent of surgery. A baseline serum CEA measurement is helpful because it may serve as a marker for recurrence or therapy if the tumor secretes the antigen. Endorectal ultrasound has no role in colon cancer but is most accurate for rectal cancers. More advanced lesions (T3 or N1) will likely benefit from preoperative (neoadjuvant) chemoradiation therapy. This is summarized in Table 69-2.

(I) Mechanical and antibiotic bowel preparation may reduce perioperative infections.

(J) For patients with more than 100 polyps, FAP is likely and total proctocolectomy with ileal J-pouch is advised during the early teenage years if possible. If 10 to 100 polyps are found with relative rectal sparing, then total colectomy with ileal-rectal anastomosis is recommended.

TABLE 69.2
TNM Staging System

Stage	Depth	Nodes	Metastasis	Dukes
0	Tis	N0	M0	
I	T1 or T2	N0	M0	A
II	T3 or T4	N0	M0	B
III	Any T	N1 or N2	M0	C
IV	Any T	Any N	MI	

Tis=confined by basement membrane; T1=invades submucosa;
T2=invades muscularis propria; T3=invades through muscularis
into subserosa or pericolic tissue; T4=invasion into adjacent
organs or perforation; N1=metastasis to 1-3 regional nodes;
N2=metastasis to 4 or more nodes.

(K) The current standard remains open resection until the long-term data from large prospective randomized trials are available. Quality of life data published at 2 years showed minimal if any benefit to the laparoscopic approach. The initial scare about potential for port site recurrences is overrated. The adequacy and completeness of surgical resection are likely the most important surgical factors.

(L) The application of the sentinel lymph node concept and technique to colon cancer is currently undergoing study. It is somewhat operator dependent, but is successful in 70% to 90% of cases. The identification of a sentinel lymph node may alter the surgical resection (estimated at 5% to 10% of the time) and/or the staging. The significance of immunohistochemically detected microscopic metastasis (as compared with standard hemotoxylin and eosin staining) remains unclear.

(M) Treatment for most colon cancers includes a segmental resection to encompass the major vascular supply and lymphatic drainage to the affected segment with a minimum 5-cm margin on either side of the tumor. For accurate staging, a minimum of 12 lymph nodes must be examined.

(N) Liver metastases are identified in up to 30% of patients at the time of diagnosis. Of those with isolated colorectal cancer metastasis to the

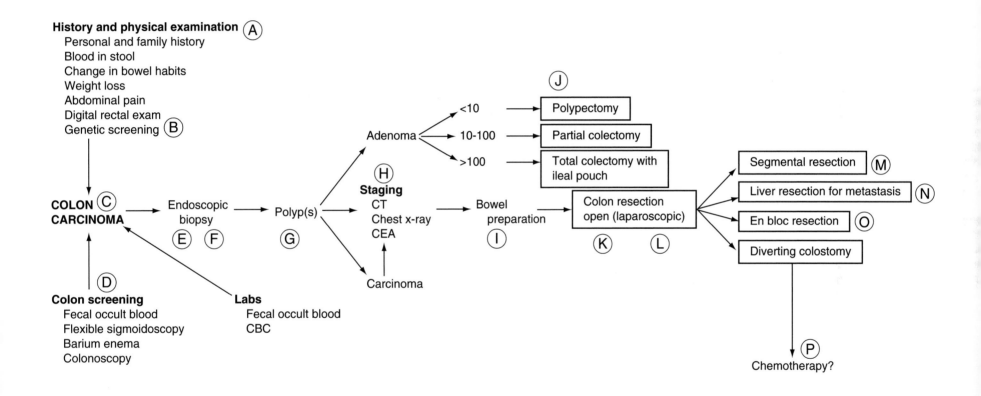

History and physical examination (A)
Personal and family history
Blood in stool
Change in bowel habits
Weight loss
Abdominal pain
Digital rectal exam
Genetic screening (B)

COLON (C)
CARCINOMA

Endoscopic
biopsy

(E) (F)

Polyp(s)

(G)

Adenoma

(H)
Staging
CT
Chest x-ray
CEA

Carcinoma

(J)

<10 → Polypectomy

10-100 → Partial colectomy

>100 → Total colectomy with
ileal pouch

Bowel
preparation

(I)

Colon resection
open (laparoscopic)

(K) (L)

Segmental resection (M)

Liver resection for metastasis (N)

En bloc resection (O)

Diverting colostomy

(P)
Chemotherapy?

(D)
Colon screening
Fecal occult blood
Flexible sigmoidoscopy
Barium enema
Colonoscopy

Labs
Fecal occult blood
CBC

liver, approximately one third (or 5% to 10% of all metastatic colorectal cancer patients) are candidates for liver resection. Average survival for untreated colorectal metastasis is 6 to 12 months and can be significantly improved (24 to 60 months) for selected patients with aggressive systemic chemotherapy combined with hepatic directed therapy.

(O) In the absence of metastatic disease, en bloc resection of adjacent organs should be considered when feasible and safe to do so. Despite stage IV disease, 25% to 50% of such patients may enjoy long-term survival.

(P) Adjuvant chemotherapy for colon cancer is generally recommended for patients with stage III (node positive) or IV (locally invasive/metastatic) disease. 5-Fluorouracil plus leucovorin is considered the standard for adjuvant therapy. Newer combination regimens (with 5-Fluorouracil plus CPT-11 or oxaliplatin) have shown considerable improvements in survival for patients with metastatic colorectal cancer. Radiation therapy for colon cancer is utilized only when there is contained perforation to the sidewall of the abdomen or when adjacent organs (e.g., bladder or uterus) are involved.

REFERENCES

American Cancer Society: Cancer Facts and Figures 2002. Atlanta: American Cancer Society, 2002.

Cohen AM, Minsky BD, Schilsky RL: Cancer of the Colon. In DeVita VT Jr., Hellman S, Rosenberg SA (eds): Cancer: Principles and Practice of Oncology. Philadelphia: Lippincott-Raven, 1997.

Corman ML: Colon and Rectal Surgery. Philadelphia: Lippincott-Raven, 1998.

Guillem JG, Smith AJ, Calle JP et al: Gastrointestinal polyposis syndromes. Curr Probl Surg 36:217–323, 1999.

Haggit RC, Glotzbach RE, Soffer EE et al: Prognostic factors in colorectal carcinomas arising in adenomas: Implications for lesions removed by endoscopic polypectomy. Gastroenterol 89:328–336, 1985.

McCarter MD, Fong Y: Metastatic liver tumors. Semin Surg Oncol 19:177–188, 2000.

Nelson H, Petrelli N, Carlin A et al: Guidelines 2000 for colon and rectal cancer surgery. J Natl Cancer Inst 93:583–596, 2001.

Paramo JC, Summerall J, Poppiti R et al: Validation of sentinel node mapping in patients with colon cancer. Ann Surg Oncol 9:550–554, 2002.

Van Cutsem E, Dicato M, Wils J et al: Adjuvant treatment of colorectal cancer (current expert opinion derived from the Third International Conference: Perspectives in Colorectal Cancer, Dublin, 2001). Eur J Cancer 38:1429–1436, 2002.

Vasen HF, Watson P, Mecklin JP et al: New clinical criteria for hereditary nonpolyposis colorectal cancer (HNPCC, Lynch syndrome) proposed by the International Collaborative Group on HNPCC. Gastroenterol 116:1453–1456, 1999.

Weeks JC, Nelson H, Gelber S et al: Short-term quality-of-life outcomes following laparoscopic-assisted colectomy vs. open colectomy for colon cancer: A randomized trial. JAMA 287:321–328, 2002.

Winawer SJ, Fletcher RH, Miller L et al: Colorectal cancer screening: Clinical guidelines and rationale. Gastroenterol 112:594–642, 1997.

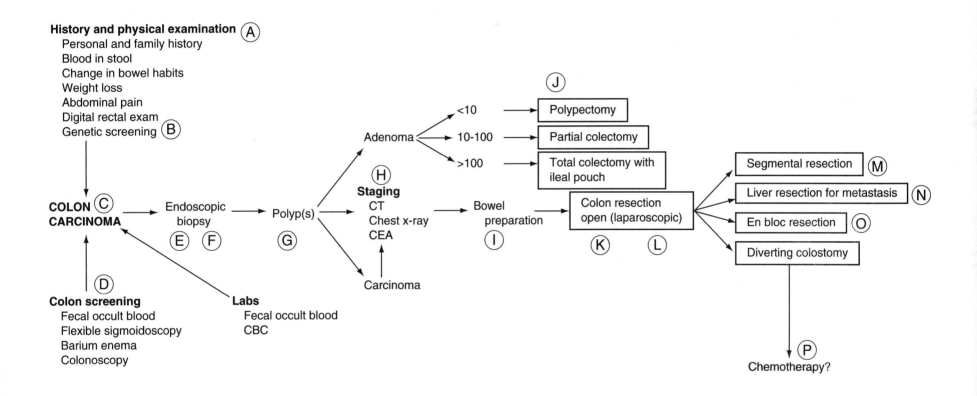

History and physical examination (A)
  Personal and family history
  Blood in stool
  Change in bowel habits
  Weight loss
  Abdominal pain
  Digital rectal exam
  Genetic screening (B)

COLON (C)
CARCINOMA

(D)
Colon screening
  Fecal occult blood
  Flexible sigmoidoscopy
  Barium enema
  Colonoscopy

Endoscopic
biopsy
(E) (F)

Polyp(s)
(G)

Labs
  Fecal occult blood
  CBC

Adenoma
  <10
  10-100
  >100

(H)
Staging
  CT
  Chest x-ray
  CEA

Carcinoma

(J)
Polypectomy

Partial colectomy

Total colectomy with
ileal pouch

Bowel
preparation
(I)

Colon resection
open (laparoscopic)
(K)   (L)

Segmental resection (M)

Liver resection for metastasis (N)

En bloc resection (O)

Diverting colostomy

(P)
Chemotherapy?

Chapter 70 *Carcinoma of the Rectum or Anus*

ERIC T. KIMCHI, MD ● MITCHELL C. POSNER, MD

(A) History and physical examination yield the diagnosis in more than 80% of patients with rectal or anal carcinoma. Pain is frequent in anal carcinoma and absent in rectal carcinoma unless the patient has an advanced lesion with tenesmus or perineural involvement causing back pain.

(B) Digital examination of the rectum is important to evaluate the mobility and size of the lesion and to palpate for pararectal nodes. Inguinal regions must also be examined for possible nodal metastases. If inguinal nodes are enlarged, biopsy (possibly fine-needle aspiration) is done.

(C) Hematest stool examination for occult blood is a cost-effective means of detecting colorectal neoplasms. Cancers detected by occult blood testing usually have a more favorable prognosis than those detected by symptoms.

(D) Some 5% of patients with biopsy-proven carcinoma develop synchronous or metachronous colon cancer and 30% have polyps. Examination of the entire colorectum is mandatory. Barium enema is cost-effective but has a 5% to 10% false-negative rate.

(E) Endorectal ultrasound (EUS) accurately identifies the extent of penetration of cancer into the rectal wall in 87% of patients. It is less accurate (74%) in determining the status of pararectal lymph nodes. In addition, EUS allows for guided sampling of pararectal nodes with fine-needle aspiration, which may aid in management decisions. Magnetic resonance imaging (MRI) with an endorectal coil has an accuracy of 84% in evaluating the penetration of cancer into the rectal wall. Its accuracy is also decreased (82%) in determining nodal status. Approximately 10% of patients are overstaged and 5% are understaged with either of these two modalities. Combined with physical examination by the surgeon, these tests determine the feasibility of local excision and sphincter preservation.

(F) Computed tomography (CT) of the abdomen and pelvis is useful because it defines the extent of extramural spread of T3 rectal cancer, evaluates the liver for the presence of metastases, and may detect lymph node metastases greater than 0.5 cm. MRI of the abdomen and pelvis will provide slightly better accuracy but at a substantially higher cost.

(G) Preoperative serum carcinoembryonic antigen is an important prognosticator because a level of 5 mg/ml or greater is associated with the subsequent appearance of distant metastasis in 46% to 85% of patients. CEA elevation should prompt a thorough evaluation of the liver and lungs, the most common sites of metastasis from rectal carcinoma.

(H) Colonoscopy has the advantage of permitting a tissue diagnosis. Rigid proctosigmoidoscopy or flexible sigmoidoscopy must be done by the surgeon to evaluate resectability of carcinoma or villous adenoma. Biopsy of anal and rectal cancer is pivotal to the diagnosis and treatment. Small in situ or noninvasive lesions can be safely excised locally (with negative margins) and given no further therapy. Invasive squamous carcinomas can be cured by chemoradiotherapy and usually do not require excision. Adenocarcinoma of the rectum arises above the dentate line, where a biopsy does not cause pain. Regional or general anesthesia is needed for excision, however, because submucosal or deeper dissection is painful.

(I) Carcinoma of the anus should be treated with chemoradiotherapy by the Nigro regimen. Patients who are incontinent or who fail chemoradiotherapy should undergo abdominoperineal resection (APR). Salvage chemoradiotherapy (5-fluorouracil and cisplatin) may avoid colostomy in certain patients in whom initial chemoradiation fails. For patients with enlarged metastatic inguinal nodes (15%) inguinal node dissection is palliative, but they should still receive chemoradiotherapy.

(J) Superficial adenocarcinomas (T1 and T2 lesions that involve but do not penetrate through the muscularis propria) may be considered for local excision if they are 10 cm or less above the dentate line; are mobile; are less than 3 cm in diameter; are well differentiated; and have no evidence of lymphatic, venous, or perineural invasion. Local excision can be performed transanally or, less commonly, through a transsacral approach. Lesions greater than 4 cm in diameter and 5 cm or less from the anal verge may require APR. Lesions 4 cm in diameter and more than 5 cm from the anal verge usually are removed by low anterior resection without permanent colostomy. T1 lesions locally excised with negative margins need no other therapy. The risk of recurrence of T2 lesions, 20% to 30% following local excision, warrants the addition of chemotherapy and radiotherapy after surgery. Lesions of 3- to 4-cm diameter are amenable to local excision depending on the site (e.g., proximity to sphincters).

(K) A deep-penetrating rectal adenocarcinoma (T3 lesion that invades the full thickness of the rectal wall) should not be locally excised. APR is done for lesions less than 5 cm from the anal verge; anterior resection is reserved for lesions more than 5 cm from the verge. All patients should receive adjuvant chemotherapy and radiotherapy, especially when lymph node metastases are present. For patients considered candidates for low anterior resection, preoperative chemoradiotherapy is considered to be the preferred approach by most surgeons because it may provide better functional results than postoperative (adjuvant) therapy. The local recurrence rate for T3 N0 or T3 N1 rectal cancer is approximately 25% after radical surgery alone and 12% after radical surgery and adjuvant chemoradiotherapy. Unfortunately, 20% to 40% of patients develop systemic disease.

(L) Cancer that is fixed to the pelvis, invades pelvic organs, or is greater than 5 cm in diameter may benefit from preoperative radiotherapy (with or without chemotherapy) to improve resectability. Patients can then undergo anterior resection or APR. Approximately 60% of fixed rectal cancers can be resected after radiotherapy.

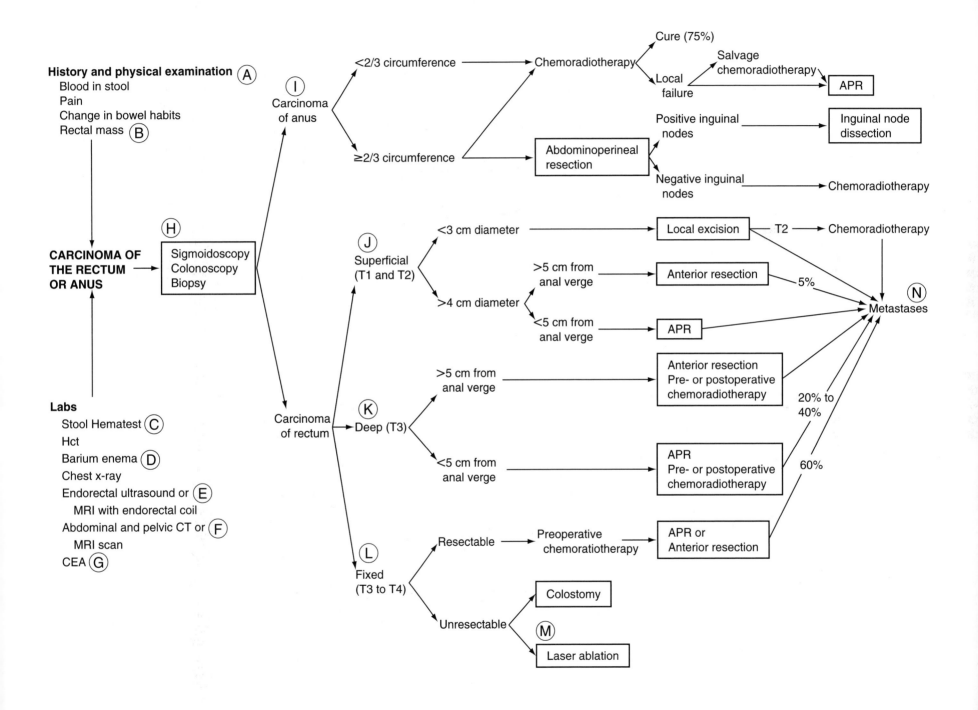

History and physical examination (A)
   Blood in stool
   Pain
   Change in bowel habits
   Rectal mass (B)

**CARCINOMA OF
THE RECTUM
OR ANUS**

(H) Sigmoidoscopy
Colonoscopy
Biopsy

Labs
   Stool Hematest (C)
   Hct
   Barium enema (D)
   Chest x-ray
   Endorectal ultrasound or (E)
     MRI with endorectal coil
   Abdominal and pelvic CT or (F)
     MRI scan
   CEA (G)

(I) Carcinoma of anus

<2/3 circumference → Chemoradiotherapy → Cure (75%)
   → Local failure → Salvage chemoradiotherapy → APR

≥2/3 circumference → Abdominoperineal resection
   → Positive inguinal nodes → Inguinal node dissection
   → Negative inguinal nodes → Chemoradiotherapy

Carcinoma of rectum

(J) Superficial (T1 and T2)
   <3 cm diameter → Local excision — T2 → Chemoradiotherapy
   >4 cm diameter
     >5 cm from anal verge → Anterior resection
     <5 cm from anal verge → APR

(K) Deep (T3)
   >5 cm from anal verge → Anterior resection / Pre- or postoperative chemoradiotherapy
   <5 cm from anal verge → APR / Pre- or postoperative chemoradiotherapy

(L) Fixed (T3 to T4)
   Resectable → Preoperative chemoratiotherapy → APR or Anterior resection
   Unresectable → Colostomy
   (M) → Laser ablation

(N) Metastases
   5%
   20% to 40%
   60%

(M) Patients whose cancers are unresectable and who have obstruction or impending obstruction need a diverting colostomy. Alternatively, endoscopic laser ablation of the rectal cancer may avoid a diverting colostomy. It can also be useful in patients with carcinoma who are receiving preoperative chemoradiotherapy.

(N) Systemic metastases are usually multiple and amenable only to systemic therapy. Occasional patients have three or fewer liver or lung metastases. Resection of these lesions with negative margins is associated with 20% to 42% 5-year survival. Resection of four or more lesions does not improve survival. Treatment with 5-fluorouracil, leucovorin, and irinotecan (CPT-11) can prolong survival of patients who have metastatic disease and good performance status (e.g., are out of bed more than 50% of the time). An average of approximately 6 months survival is added in patients who otherwise have a 9-month median survival. This advantage must be balanced against the 1% mortality and up to a 66% morbidity associated with chemotherapy.

REFERENCES

American Society of Clinical Oncology: Clinical practice guidelines for the use of tumor markers in breast and colorectal cancer. J Clin Oncol 14(10):2843–2877, 1996.

Bleday R, Steele G Jr.: Current protocols and outcomes of local therapy for rectal cancer. Surg Oncol Clin N Am 9(4):751–758, 2000.

Flam M, John M, Pajak TF et al: Role of mitomycin in combination with fluorouracil and radiotherapy, and of salvage chemoradiation in the definitive nonsurgical treatment of epidermoid carcinoma of the anal canal: Results of a phase III randomized intergroup study. J Clin Oncol 14(9):2527– 2539, 1996.

Harewood GC, Wiersema MJ, Nelson H et al: A prospective, blinded assessment of the impact of preoperative staging on the management of rectal cancer. Gastroenterol 123:24–32, 2002.

Hollomorgen CF, Meagher AP, Wolff BG et al: The long-term effect of adjuvant postoperative chemoradiotherapy for rectal cancer or bowel function. Ann Surg 220(5):676–682, 1994.

Jass JR, Atkin WS, Cuzick J et al: The grading of rectal cancer: Historical perspectives and a multivariate analysis. J Cancer Res Clin Oncol 113:586–592, 1987.

Kwok H, Bissett IP, Hill GL: Preoperative staging of rectal cancer. Int J Colorectal Dis 15:9–20, 2000.

Nigro NA, Vaitkevicius VK, Buroker T et al: Combined therapy for cancer of the anal canal. Dis Colon Rectum 24:73–74, 1981.

Parks JPS, Thompson AG: Per-anal endorectal operative techniques. In Rob C II, Smith R, Dudley HAF (eds): Operative Surgery. London: Butterworth, 1977.

Saltz LB, Cox JV, Blanke C et al: Irinotecan plus fluorouracil and leucovorin for metastatic colorectal cancer. Irinotecan Study Group. N Engl J Med 28:905–914, 2000.

Visser BC, Varma MG, Welton ML: Local therapy for rectal cancer. Surg Oncol 10:61–69, 2001.

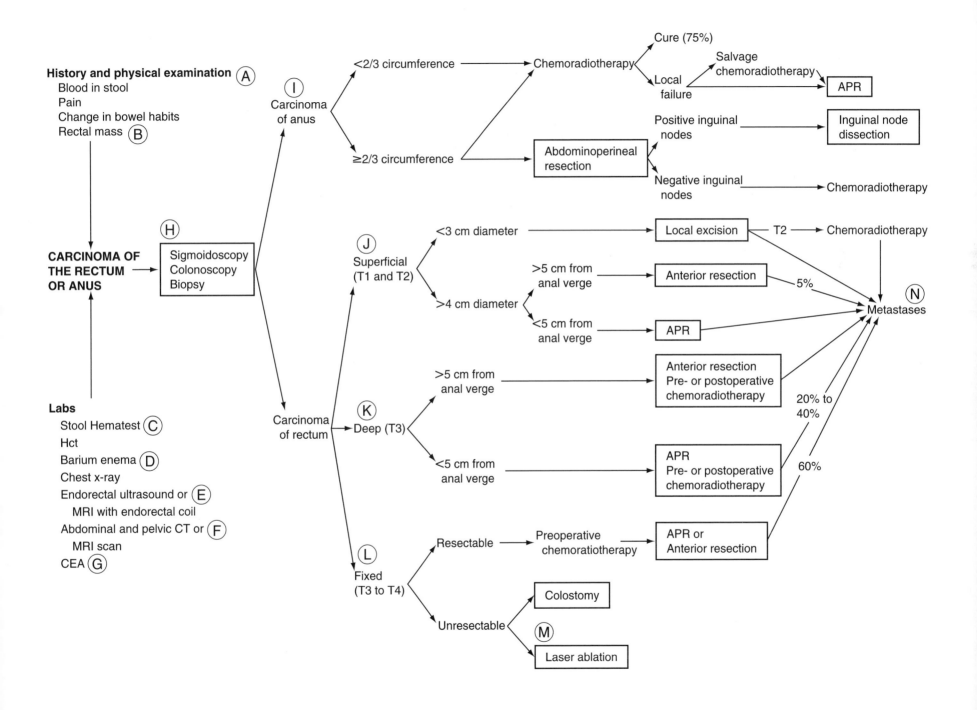

History and physical examination (A)
  Blood in stool
  Pain
  Change in bowel habits
  Rectal mass (B)

CARCINOMA OF
THE RECTUM
OR ANUS

Labs
  Stool Hematest (C)
  Hct
  Barium enema (D)
  Chest x-ray
  Endorectal ultrasound or (E)
    MRI with endorectal coil
  Abdominal and pelvic CT or (F)
    MRI scan
  CEA (G)

(H)
Sigmoidoscopy
Colonoscopy
Biopsy

(I)
Carcinoma
of anus

  <2/3 circumference → Chemoradiotherapy
    → Cure (75%)
    → Local failure → Salvage chemoradiotherapy → APR

  ≥2/3 circumference → Abdominoperineal resection
    → Positive inguinal nodes → Inguinal node dissection
    → Negative inguinal nodes → Chemoradiotherapy

Carcinoma
of rectum

(J)
Superficial
(T1 and T2)
  <3 cm diameter → Local excision → T2 → Chemoradiotherapy
  >4 cm diameter
    >5 cm from anal verge → Anterior resection
    <5 cm from anal verge → APR

(K)
Deep (T3)
  >5 cm from anal verge → Anterior resection / Pre- or postoperative chemoradiotherapy
  <5 cm from anal verge → APR / Pre- or postoperative chemoradiotherapy

(L)
Fixed
(T3 to T4)
  Resectable → Preoperative chemoratiotherapy → APR or Anterior resection
  Unresectable → Colostomy
               → Laser ablation (M)

(N)
Metastases
  5%
  20% to 40%
  60%

Chapter 71 **Anorectal Abscess/Fistula**

ROBERT E.H. KHOO, MD

(A) A patient with an anal abscess complains of severe, constant, throbbing anal or perianal pain. Unlike the pain of a fissure, which increases on defecation, abscess pain is constant but increases with straining or coughing. There may be a mass and fever. On examination, there may be signs of inflammation (e.g., swelling, tenderness, heat, or erythema), but occasionally little may be detected. The patient may not tolerate digital examination.

(B) An anal abscess usually arises from an infected anal gland. Abscess and fistula are part of a two-stage process. The acute initial phase is the abscess, and the chronic phase is the fistula.

(C) Anoscopy and sigmoidoscopy are not indicated in this acute setting because the findings would not alter management. The white blood cell (WBC) count may be elevated.

(D) Intersphincteric abscess presents with few external signs of anal sepsis. This condition can be difficult to distinguish from anal fissure. When it is suspected, the only way to make the diagnosis is to examine the patient under regional or general anesthesia. This abscess is treated by dividing the internal sphincter fibers overlying the abscess.

(E) Most horseshoe abscesses arise from the deep postanal space, but some arise from the deep anterior anal space. Incision and drainage should be done under general anesthesia. The lateral extensions are widely drained. There may be no sign of inflammation over a postanal space abscess. The deep postanal space is drained by dividing the overlying internal sphincter and the lower portion of the external sphincter. The incidence of fistula decreases when drainage is performed properly.

(F) Supralevator abscess can be an upward extension of an intersphincteric abscess; an upward extension of an ischiorectal abscess; or a result of intraperitoneal disease such as perforated diverticulitis, appendicitis, or Crohn's. Its origin should be determined before a route of drainage is chosen.

(G) Treatment of an anal abscess is immediate drainage. Antibiotics are not primary treatment, but they can be used as an adjunct in patients who are septic or immunosuppressed, or in those with valvular heart disease or a prosthetic heart valve. A common mistake is to wait for the abscess to "mature" and point to the skin surface: waiting invites trouble. Drainage can usually be done under local anesthesia in the office. Drainage in the operating room is more expensive and is necessary only if office drainage fails. Use of a drain is optional. If an abscess ruptures spontaneously, the patient should still be examined to ensure that drainage is adequate. Culture of the pus may predict fistula formation (enteric organisms), but doing a culture will not change the treatment. Fistulotomy at the time of abscess drainage should be avoided because of the following: (1) half of patients will not develop a fistula; (2) a false passage can be created; (3) this procedure requires an operating room, which increases costs; and (4) the risk of incontinence is increased. The internal opening cannot be identified in 65% of patients at the time of abscess drainage. If an abscess has recurred several times, it is reasonable to look for an internal fistula opening in the operating room and to perform fistulotomy while draining the abscess.

(H) After drainage, there is a 50% chance of developing an anal fistula (chronic phase). The manifestations are recurrent abscesses or persistent drainage resulting in skin excoriation and pruritus. A fistula will not resolve with medical therapy alone: antibiotics will not heal it. Surgery is always necessary. The patient should be questioned for critical history clues to associated GI disease (e.g., inflammatory bowel disease [IBD] or cancer) or systemic disease (e.g., HIV). Investigations with sigmoidoscopy or even total colon examination (colonoscopy or barium enema x-ray) may be indicated. Tests such as fistulography, endoanal ultrasound (US), or MRI are not done unless the fistula is recurrent or the internal opening is difficult to find.

(I) A fistula involving more than 30% of the sphincter fibers or any anterior fistula in women should not be subjected to fistulotomy because incontinence may result. (The puborectalis muscle is not present anteriorly.)

(J) Occasionally, the internal opening cannot be identified. The surgeon must avoid making a false passage with vigorous probing. Injecting the outside opening with hydrogen peroxide may help to identify an internal opening. Goodsall's rule is a guide to the internal opening location. When the external opening lies anterior to the transverse anal line, the track runs in a direct radial line to the internal opening in the anal canal. When the external opening is posterior to the transverse line, the tract curves backward to the posterior anal midline. An anterior external opening more than 3 cm from the anal verge will have a track that curves back to the posterior midline. If the opening still cannot be found, the fistula tract can be cored out and the internal sphincter overlying the presumptive infected anal gland can be divided. This technique preserves the external sphincter. If a fistula recurs and the internal opening is not clearly visualized, endoanal US can be used after injection of the fistula tract with hydrogen peroxide. Fistulography may also help. The colon may need to be investigated to rule out underlying disease. Rarely is the internal opening seen on barium enema.

(K) Lay-open fistulotomy should be avoided in IBD except for the most superficial fistulas because the subsequent fistulotomy wound will heal slower and the risk of incontinence is increased. The mainstay of treatment is the prevention of abscess. This is best done with a draining seton (soft vessel loop or loosely tied suture) that will keep the fistula tract ends open and draining. If the rectum is relatively disease free, an advancement flap or fibrin glue may be tried, but the success rate is only 60%. Infliximab, a monoclonal antibody to tumor necrosis factor alpha can be given intravenously to Crohn's disease patients and will heal half of all fistulas. Metronidazole can also be tried for these cases. Proctectomy is rarely indicated

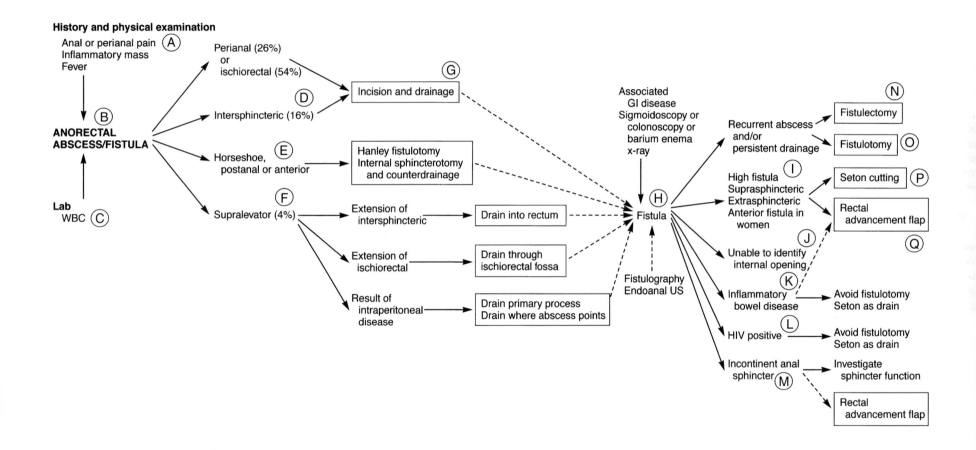

History and physical examination

Anal or perianal pain (A)
Inflammatory mass
Fever

Lab (C)
WBC

(B)
ANORECTAL ABSCESS/FISTULA

Perianal (26%)
or
ischiorectal (54%)

(D)
Intersphincteric (16%)

(E)
Horseshoe,
postanal or anterior

(F)
Supralevator (4%)

Extension of
intersphincteric

Extension of
ischiorectal

Result of
intraperitoneal
disease

(G)
Incision and drainage

Hanley fistulotomy
Internal sphincterotomy
and counterdrainage

Drain into rectum

Drain through
ischiorectal fossa

Drain primary process
Drain where abscess points

Associated
GI disease
Sigmoidoscopy or
colonoscopy or
barium enema
x-ray

(H)
Fistula

Fistulography
Endoanal US

Recurrent abscess
and/or
persistent drainage

(I)
High fistula
Suprasphincteric
Extrasphincteric
Anterior fistula in
women

Unable to identify
internal opening

(J)

(K)
Inflammatory
bowel disease

(L)
HIV positive

Incontinent anal
sphincter (M)

(N)
Fistulectomy

Fistulotomy (O)

Seton cutting (P)

Rectal
advancement flap

(Q)

Avoid fistulotomy
Seton as drain

Avoid fistulotomy
Seton as drain

Investigate
sphincter function

Rectal
advancement flap

but may be considered for intractable cases with uncontrolled sepsis.

(L) Becaause of possible poor wound healing, HIV-positive patients should be treated as IBD patients are. Avoid surgery in HIV-positive patients with asymptomatic fistula.

(M) If the patient is incontinent because of previous sphincter injury or age, standard lay-open fistulotomy should be avoided. Ideally, the sphincter is evaluated with manometry before surgery. A good option is flap advancement, possibly with sphincter repair or use of a draining seton. Fecal diversion is a consideration for persistent incontinence.

(N) Fistulectomy is often unnecessary: the resulting larger wound takes longer to heal and there is a greater risk of muscle separation and incontinence.

(O) Surgery for a fistula that develops after drainage of a perianal or ischiorectal abscess can usually be done as an outpatient procedure with local anesthesia. Most fistulas are intersphincteric (70%) or transphincteric (23%). Fistulotomy and marsupialization produces a smaller wound that heals within 6 weeks.

(P) A cutting seton is a nonabsorbable suture placed through the tract. It stimulates fibrosis and cuts through the encircled muscle gradually.

Later, the fistulotomy can be completed by dividing the remaining muscle. A seton can also be tightened gradually over weeks to eventually cut through the muscle. Using a seton in this way decreases but does not eliminate the risk of fecal incontinence (4% major and more than 50% minor).

(Q) Incontinence can be avoided by excising or curetting the fistula tract, advancing a flap of rectal mucosa and internal sphincter, and suturing it to the anal canal distal to the original internal opening. To avoid incontinence, suprasphincteric (5%) or extrasphincteric (2%) fistulas are best treated with this flap advancement technique. Another technique is injecting fibrin glue to fill the tract. Although recurrence rate is higher than for laying the tract open, the procedure can be repeated if it fails without greatly increasing the risk of incontinence. Using fibrin glue avoids the pain and prolonged healing of fistulotomy wounds.

REFERENCES

American Society of Colon and Rectal Surgeons Standards Task Force: Practice parameters for treatment of fistula-in-ano. Dis Colon Rectum 39:1361–1372, 1996.

Cintron JR, Park JJ, Orsay CP et al: Repair of fistulas-in-ano using fibrin adhesive: Long-term follow-up. Dis Colon Rectum 43:944–950, 2000.

Deen KI, Williams JG, Hutchinson R et al: Fistulas-in-ano: Endoanal ultrasonographic assessment assists decision making for surgery. Gut 35:391–394, 1994.

Fazio VW: Complex anal fistulae. Gastroenterol Clin N Am 16:93–114, 1987.

Garcia-Aguilar J, Belmonte C, Wong WD et al: Anal fistula surgery: Factors associated with recurrence and incontinence. Dis Colon Rectum 39:723–729, 1996.

Gordon PH: Anorectal Abscesses and Fistula-In-Ano. Gordon PH, Nivatvongs S (eds.). In Principles and Practice of Surgery for the Colon, Rectum, and Anus, 2nd ed. St Louis: Quality Medical Publishing, 241–286, 1999.

Hämäläinen KJ, Sainio AP: Cutting seton for anal fistulas: High risk of minor control defects. Dis Colon Rectum 40:1443–1447, 1997.

Ho YH, Tan M, Chui CH et al: Randomized controlled trial of primary fistulotomy with drainage alone for perianal abscess. Dis Colon Rectum 40:1435–1438, 1997.

Kodner IJ, Mazor A, Shemesh EI et al: Endorectal advancement flap repair of rectovaginal and other complicated anorectal fistulas. Surg 114:682–690, 1993.

McKee RF, Keenan RA: Perianal Crohn's disease: Is it all bad news? Dis Colon Rectum 39:136–142, 1996.

Parks AG, Gordon PH, Hardcastle JD: A classification of fistula-in-ano. Br J Surg 63:1–12, 1976.

Present DH, Rutgeerts P, Targan S et al: Infliximab for the treatment of fistulas in patients with Crohn's disease. N Engl J Med 340(18):1398–1405, 1999.

Ramanujam PS, Prasad ML, Abcarian H et al: Perianal abscesses and fistulas: A study of 1023 patients. Dis Colon Rectum 27:593–597, 1984.

History and physical examination

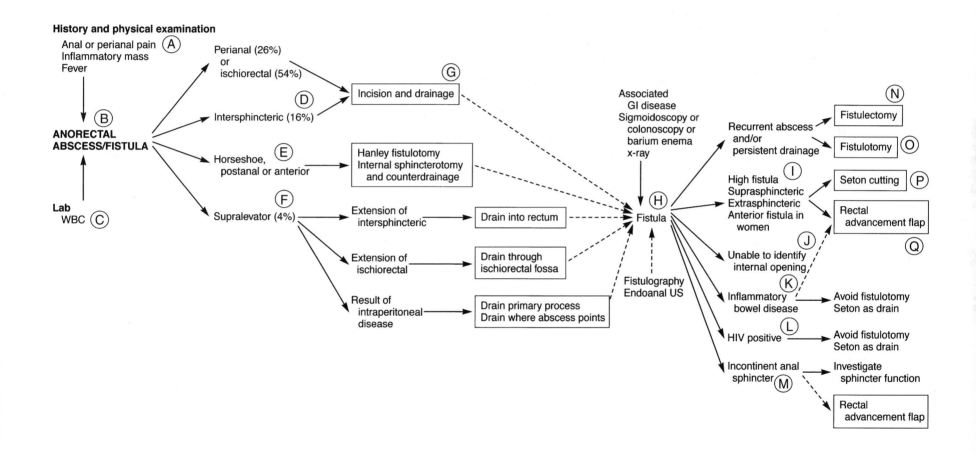

Chapter 72 *Hemorrhoids*

ROBERT E.H. KHOO, MD

(A) Hemorrhoids are vascular cushions normally found lining the anal canal. They are made up of arteries, arterioles, veins, venules, and connective tissue. The presence of hemorrhoids does not imply disease. The prevalence of symptomatic hemorrhoids is 4.4%; of these, a third require medical attention. Because hemorrhoids are not varicose veins, their prevalence is not increased in patients with portal hypertension. Straining associated with constipation or diarrhea causes engorgement of these vascular cushions. Stool trauma causes painless, often profuse, bright red bleeding. If straining persists, the connective tissue supports weaken, allowing the hemorrhoids to prolapse out of the anus. Hemorrhoids are found at three constant sites: left lateral, right posterior, and right anterior.

(B) Patients complaining of hemorrhoids must be examined for other anorectal lesions with inspection, digital rectal examination, anoscopy, and sigmoidoscopy. Further investigations of the colon are indicated for unexplained GI symptoms, anemia, or family history of colon polyps or cancer. The surgeon should never attribute rectal bleeding solely to hemorrhoids without first doing a thorough investigation.

(C) External hemorrhoids lie below the dentate line and are usually asymptomatic. They present as a skin tag or acute external thrombosis. External skin tags can be irritated by changes in diet or poor perianal hygiene but excision is not usually indicated.

(D) Internal hemorrhoids are located above the dentate line and are classified according to degree of prolapse by history. Because they lie in this insensitive zone, many treatment modalities can be done painlessly as office procedures.

(E) With acute external hemorrhoid thrombosis, a painful blue lump arises. Occasionally, the skin over the thrombus can become necrotic and rupture, leading to bleeding. When the external thrombus resolves, the sequela is an external skin tag.

(F) First-degree hemorrhoids present with bleeding only; second-degree hemorrhoids present with bleeding and spontaneously reducing prolapse.

(G) Third-degree hemorrhoids present with prolapse that requires manual reduction, and fourth-degree hemorrhoids are irreducible. When the prolapsed mucosa lies outside the anal canal, patients may complain of a mucous discharge.

(H) Occasionally, with fourth-degree internal hemorrhoid prolapse, spasm of the anal sphincter leads to vascular compromise, acute thrombosis, and severe pain. Conservative therapy requires hospitalization for bedrest and analgesics and a later admission for elective excision. The preferred treatment is immediate formal hemorrhoidectomy, which spares the patient an additional hospital stay and gives instant relief. The feared complication of anal stenosis can be avoided by carefully excising no more anoderm than is necessary during surgery.

(I) Most hemorrhoid symptoms that intensify during pregnancy and delivery later resolve. Thrombosed acute external hemorrhoids can be excised under local anesthesia. Formal hemorrhoidectomy is indicated for significant and persistent prolapse or strangulation.

(J) Diarrhea secondary to inflammatory bowel disease (e.g., ulcerative colitis or Crohn's disease) aggravates hemorrhoids. Control of proximal bowel disease and diarrhea and local perianal care is the initial treatment. Hemorrhoidectomy can be performed for patients with ulcerative colitis but should be avoided in Crohn's disease patients because of the increased risk of incontinence and poor wound healing.

(K) HIV-positive patients with hemorrhoids should be treated similarly to Crohn's disease patients, and surgery should be avoided.

(L) The preferred treatment for an acute external hemorrhoid thrombosis is excision in the office within the first 4 days. After this acute period, excision is rarely indicated because the pain is already decreasing and resolution is under way. Incision and evacuation of the blood clot is associated with a higher recurrence rate and results in a skin tag. Complete excision of the clot and the feeding vessels is the preferred treatment.

(M) Initial treatment of first- and second-degree hemorrhoids is a high-fiber diet and bulking agents and increased fluid intake to minimize straining at stool. Steroid ointments and suppositories are of little value.

(N) Nonsurgical treatment of third- and fourth-degree hemorrhoids is less than 50% successful. Surgery is 95% successful but is painful and results in up to 2 weeks off work. Surgery can be done under local anesthesia with sedation. Formal admission is rarely indicated, but an overnight stay may be necessary. Complications (e.g., hemorrhage, infection, and stenosis) occur in about 1% to 2% of patients. Urinary retention occurs in 5% to 10%. Variations of excisional hemorrhoidectomy using laser, harmonic scalpel, and Ligasure ligature have not succeeded in decreasing pain of surgery because all these procedures involve excision of sensitive anoderm. A new technique, stapled hemorrhoidectomy, excises loose rectal mucosa above the hemorrhoids circumferentially. This interrupts the blood supply to the hemorrhoids and restores the weakened suspensory ligaments, reducing the hemorrhoids back to their correct anatomic position inside the anal canal. Because this excision of mucosa is done above the dentate line, the pain of surgery is significantly less. Stapled hemorrhoidectomy appears to be as effective and safe as conventional surgery. Manual dilation of the anus as a primary treatment for hemorrhoids is rarely

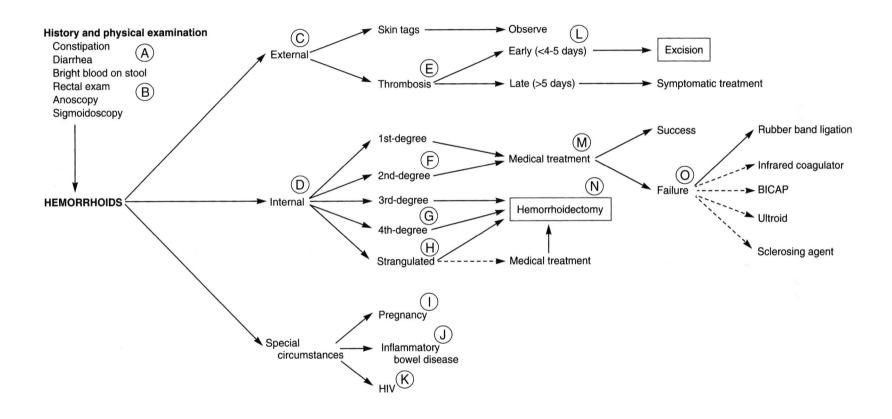

History and physical examination
Constipation Ⓐ
Diarrhea
Bright blood on stool
Rectal exam Ⓑ
Anoscopy
Sigmoidoscopy

HEMORRHOIDS

Ⓒ External

Skin tags ──────▶ Observe Ⓛ

Thrombosis Ⓔ

Early (<4-5 days) ──────▶ Excision

Late (>5 days) ──────▶ Symptomatic treatment

Ⓓ Internal

1st-degree Ⓕ
2nd-degree

3rd-degree Ⓖ
4th-degree

Strangulated Ⓗ

Medical treatment Ⓜ

Hemorrhoidectomy Ⓝ

Medical treatment

Success

Failure Ⓞ

Rubber band ligation

Infrared coagulator

BICAP

Ultroid

Sclerosing agent

Special circumstances

Pregnancy Ⓘ

Inflammatory bowel disease Ⓙ

HIV Ⓚ

practiced in the United States because of the risk of incontinence and persistent prolapse. Cryosurgery is not as effective as surgery, and it produces prolonged and profuse wound drainage. The depth of the wound destruction with the cryoprobe cannot be controlled precisely.

O Medical therapy for first- and second-degree hemorrhoids fails in 20% of cases; other treatment modalities can then be tried. Rubber band ligation is the most efficacious and cost-effective treatment (90% success). Infrared coagulation is less effective for prolapsing hemorrhoids (60% to 85% success) because more treatment visits are needed than for rubber banding. Bipolar coagulation (BICAP) is another expensive therapy whose success rate is similar to that for infrared coagulation.

Ultroid (direct current) application is expensive and time consuming. It is painful, and its efficacy is variable. Sclerotherapy causes scarring and fixation, but complications such as sloughing, infection, and thrombosis can occur. It is less effective then rubber banding.

REFERENCES

American Society of Colon and Rectal Surgery Standards Task Force: Practice parameters for the treatment of hemorrhoids. Dis Colon Rectum 36:1118–1120, 1993.

Gordon PH, Nivatvongs S: Hemorrhoids. In Principles and Practice of Surgery for the Colon, Rectum, and Anus, 2nd ed. St. Louis: Quality Medical Publishing, 1999.

Ho YH, Cheong WK, Tsang C et al: Stapled hemorrhoidectomy: Cost and effectiveness: Randomized, controlled trial including incontinence scoring, anorectal manometry, and endoanal ultrasound assessments at up to 3 months. Dis Colon Rectum 43:1666–1675, 2000.

Johanson JF, Rimm A: Optimal nonsurgical treatment of hemorrhoids: A comparative analysis of infrared coagulation, rubber band ligation, and injection sclerotherapy. Am J Gastroenterol 87:1601–1606, 1992.

Johanson JF, Sonnenberg A: The prevalence of hemorrhoids and chronic constipation: An epidemiologic study. Gastroenterol 98:380–386, 1990.

Loder PB, Kamm MA, Nicholls RJ et al: Haemorrhoids: Pathology, pathophysiology, and aetiology. Br J Surg 81:946–954, 1994.

MacRae HM, McLeod RS: Comparison of hemorrhoidal treatment modalities: A meta-analysis. Dis Colon Rectum 38:687–694, 1995.

Mazier WP, Wolkomir AF: Hemorrhoids. Semin Colon Rectal Surg 1:197–206, 1990.

Wexner SD: The quest for painless surgical treatment of hemorrhoids continues. J Am Coll Surg 193:174–178, 2001.

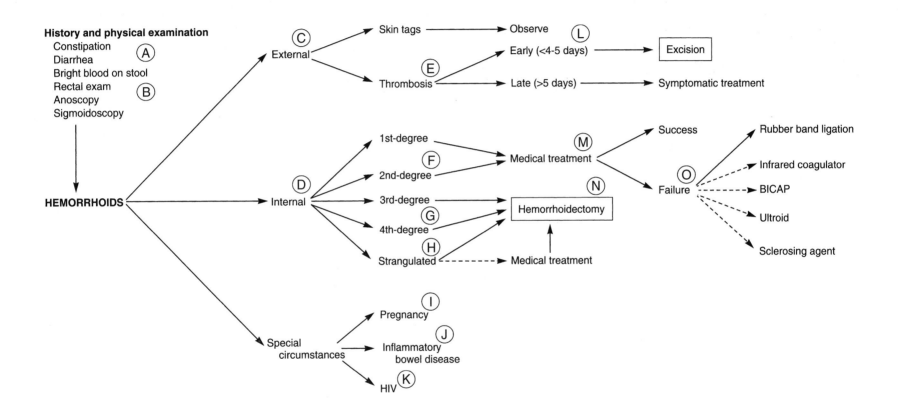

History and physical examination
Constipation   Ⓐ
Diarrhea
Bright blood on stool
Rectal exam   Ⓑ
Anoscopy
Sigmoidoscopy

HEMORRHOIDS

External   Ⓒ

Skin tags → Observe   Ⓛ

Thrombosis   Ⓔ

Early (<4-5 days) → Excision

Late (>5 days) → Symptomatic treatment

Internal   Ⓓ

1st-degree
2nd-degree   Ⓕ → Medical treatment   Ⓜ

3rd-degree
4th-degree   Ⓖ → Hemorrhoidectomy   Ⓝ

Strangulated   Ⓗ - - → Medical treatment

Success

Failure   Ⓞ

Rubber band ligation
Infrared coagulator
BICAP
Ultroid
Sclerosing agent

Special circumstances

Pregnancy   Ⓘ

Inflammatory bowel disease   Ⓙ

HIV   Ⓚ

Chapter 73 Pilonidal Disease

ROBERT E.H. KHOO, MD

(A) Pilonidal disease of the sacrococcygeal region affects young adults after puberty and is rare after age 40 years. There is a 4:1 male predominance. Originally, pilonidal disease was thought to be congenital, but now most agree that it is an acquired lesion produced by the burrowing of hairs into the natal cleft. The differential diagnosis includes anal fistula, hidradenitis suppurativa, and presacral tumor/cyst.

(B) Acute pilonidal disease (abscess) presents with pain, swelling, and erythema of the overlying skin.

(C) Chronic pilonidal disease is manifested as a chronic discharging sinus with one or more openings in the skin. This chronic infection can occasionally become an acute abscess. There are many treatment options, but the ideal treatment should achieve cure with minimal risk of recurrence, with brief hospitalization, and with little morbidity. Minimal surgery is as effective as radical excision, yet the cost to the patient in terms of pain and time lost from work is less.

(D) An acute pilonidal abscess should be drained without delay. This can be done under local anesthesia in the office. Antibiotics are not the primary treatment, but they may be used as an adjunct to drainage for patients with systemic sepsis, prosthetic implants, heart valve disease, immunosuppression, or diabetes.

(E) After drainage of a pilonidal abscess, 85% of patients develop chronic pilonidal disease.

(F) Incising the skin and laying open the sinus tracts and curettage with or without marsupialization of the wound edges is a simple yet effective treatment for chronic pilonidal disease. The wound is smaller than with excision so there is less pain and faster healing. This procedure can be done in an outpatient setting using local anesthesia.

The recurrence rate is no greater than with other techniques. Treatment of recurrence has a very high success rate. Recurrence is prevented by meticulous shaving or plucking of hairs around the wound and keeping the edges apart with cotton dressings while it heals from the base. Frequent follow-up visits to remove granulation tissue from the wound base with a small curette or silver nitrate is mandatory until healing is complete. If this is not done, the wound edges may heal together, causing bridging and a recurrent sinus.

(G) Excision of the pilonidal sinus produces a much larger wound, more pain, and longer healing time, all of which result in greater costs for the patient. General anesthesia is necessary for complete excision of extensive pilonidal disease. Recurrence rates with complete excision are higher than with simple laying open of the tracts followed by meticulous postoperative skin care.

(H) Excision with closure can be done with primary suture or skin flap coverage. Asymmetric closure or rotation flaps provide better results than does midline closure. These extensive procedures often require spinal or general anesthesia and hospitalization. To allow healing, restriction of activity may be necessary. When successful, this technique results in fast wound healing, but the recurrence rate is not decreased compared with simply laying the sinus tract open.

(I) The Bascom technique involves an incision lateral to the midline to curette infected granulation tissue from the sinus plus excision of all holes in the midline. The surgery can be done as an outpatient procedure with local anesthesia. Time lost from work is minimal (1 to 4 days) and the recurrence rate low. Success depends on how meticulously this technique is performed.

(J) The pilonidal sinus can be obliterated with phenol, but the success rate is not high.

(K) An unhealed midline natal cleft wound may be the result of overaggressive surgical treatment. The initial treatment of an unhealed wound is outpatient curettage or application of silver nitrate to the base and meticulous wound care (i.e., shaving, then packing the wound to keep the edges apart). Rosenberg describes reverse bandaging of the buttocks to flatten out the natal cleft, which allows the wound to heal. Should these initial conservative treatments fail, the cleft closure technique of Bascom can be done as an outpatient procedure and is 85% successful. Other methods of closure with skin flaps have variable success rates and are more technically demanding.

REFERENCES

Allen-Mersh TG: Pilonidal sinus: Finding the right track for treatment. Br J Surg 77:123–132, 1990.

Bascom JU: Recurrent Pilonidal Disease. In Wexner SD, Vernava AM (eds): Clinical Decision Making in Colorectal Surgery. New York: Igaku-Shoin, 1995.

Bascom J, Bascom T: Failed pilonidal surgery: New paradigm and new operation leading to cures. Arch Surg 137:1146–1150, 2002.

da Silva JH: Pilonidal cyst: Cause and treatment. Dis Colon Rectum 43:1146–1156, 2000.

Nivatvongs S: Pilonidal Disease. In Gordon PH, Nivatvongs S (eds.) Principles and Practice of Surgery for the Colon, Rectum and Anus, 2nd ed. St. Louis: Quality Medical Publishing, 287–301, 1999.

Petersen S, Koch R, Stelzner S et al: Primary closure techniques in chronic pilonidal sinus: A survey of the results of different surgical approaches. Dis Colon Rectum 45:1458–1467, 2002.

Rosenberg I: Reverse bandaging for the cure of the reluctant pilonidal wound. Dis Colon Rectum 20:290–291, 1977.

Schneider IH, Thaler K, Kockerling TF: Treatment of pilonidal sinuses by phenol injection. Int J Colorectal Dis 9:200–202, 1994.

Solla JA, Rothenberger DA: Chronic pilonidal disease: An assessment of 150 cases. Dis Colon Rectum 33:758–761, 1990.

Weinstein MA, Rubin RJ, Salvati EP: The dilemma of pilonidal disease: Pilonidal cystotomy, reappraisal of an old technique. Dis Colon Rectum 20:287–289, 1977.

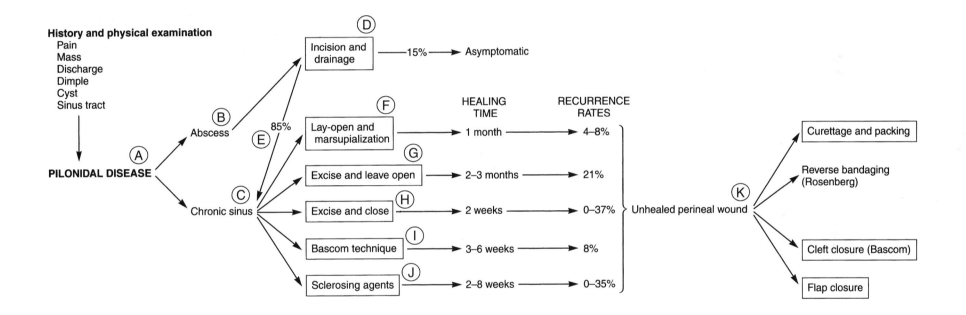

History and physical examination
Pain
Mass
Discharge
Dimple
Cyst
Sinus tract

PILONIDAL DISEASE

Ⓐ

Ⓑ Abscess

Ⓒ Chronic sinus

Ⓓ Incision and drainage — 15% → Asymptomatic

Ⓔ 85%

HEALING TIME   RECURRENCE RATES

Ⓕ Lay-open and marsupialization → 1 month → 4–8%

Ⓖ Excise and leave open → 2–3 months → 21%

Ⓗ Excise and close → 2 weeks → 0–37%

Ⓘ Bascom technique → 3–6 weeks → 8%

Ⓙ Sclerosing agents → 2–8 weeks → 0–35%

Ⓚ Unhealed perineal wound

Curettage and packing

Reverse bandaging (Rosenberg)

Cleft closure (Bascom)

Flap closure

Chapter 74 *Anal Fissure*

TONIA M. YOUNG-FADOK, MD, MS

(A) Anal fissure is a disruption of the sensate ano-derm lining the distal anal canal. This very common condition may occur following a large, hard bowel movement; or, conversely, may be associated with a bout of diarrhea. Most fissures are acute, heal within several days, and never come to medical attention. Increased resting anal pressure, attributed to spasm of the internal sphincter, may result in chronic anal fissure. The condition is commonly attributed to hemorrhoids by both patients and primary care physicians. The hallmark symptom is pain during and after defecation. The pain may last minutes with acute fissures or hours in the chronic setting, leading to avoidance of defecation. Rectal bleeding is common, typically consisting of small quantities of red blood noted on the toilet tissue.

(B) The typical patient is a young adult, and both sexes are equally affected. The history suggests the diagnosis, which is confirmed by physical examination. The key for a successful examination is slow, gentle distraction of the perianal skin by opposing traction with the thumbs. The vast majority of fissures will be in the posterior midline (25% of women have anterior fissures compared with 8% of men, and 3% of patients have both anterior and posterior fissures). A sentinel skin tag at the anal verge is an additional clue. Once the fissure is seen, instrumentation should be avoided because any attempt at digital examination or endoscopy is painful and not well tolerated. Further tests, such as colonoscopy to evaluate bleeding, should be deferred until the symptoms have resolved. When the diagnosis is in doubt, examination under anesthesia will rule out an occult perianal abscess.

(C) An acute anal fissure has been present for less than 1 month and has the appearance of a simple tear of the distal anoderm. Acute fissures usually heal with standard conservative measures.

(D) A chronic anal fissure may show heaping of the fissure edges, granulation tissue, and exposed fibers of the internal anal sphincter (IAS) muscle. A sentinel skin tag is often present at the distal end of the fissure, and a hypertrophied anal papilla may be seen at the proximal point.

(E) Fissures that are off the midline, are multiple or painless, and those that fail to heal require further evaluation. These should be examined under anesthesia with biopsies and cultures because this presentation may exist with Crohn's disease, anal carcinoma, lymphoma, HIV or AIDS, tuberculosis, syphilis, or melanoma.

(F) Most acute fissures heal with no intervention or respond to increased oral fluid intake, fiber supplementation, stool softeners, sitz baths, and topical analgesics. Sitz baths plus bran supplementation, or use of 2% hydrocortisone, result in healing of approximately 85% of acute fissures.

(G) Pharmacologic intervention is aimed at reduction of sphincter tone without the permanent dysfunction that can result from surgical approaches.

(H) Lateral internal sphincterotomy (LIS) is associated with healing rates of 95% to 100%. It is appropriate to proceed directly to LIS if pain is severe or intolerable or if prior conservative therapy has failed. Lateral sphincterotomy is performed to avoid the potential "keyhole deformity" associated with midline sphincterotomy—a groove that allows loss of flatus or liquid stool. Reported rates of incontinence vary widely from 0% to 38%, probably reflecting greater extent of IAS division in older studies plus subtle yet clinically unimportant changes that may be detected on questionnaires. Recent studies recommend that the extent of the sphincterotomy should correspond to the length of the fissure. Anal dilation is condemned: almost no studies are standardized and there is a high risk of causing incontinence.

(I) Although many acute fissures heal spontaneously, some become chronic. Ambulatory manometry has demonstrated sustained resting hypertonia with rare episodes of spontaneous IAS relaxation. Cadaveric studies show a reduction of vascularity in the normal posterior midline of the anal canal in 85% of individuals. Anodermal perfusion is dependent on arterioles that cross the IAS, so high anal pressures may reduce perfusion pressure to the posterior midline and prevent healing.

(J) Nitric oxide is the primary nonadrenergic, noncholinergic neurotransmitter in the IAS and results in IAS relaxation. Exogenous nitrates release nitric oxide: topical 0.2% glyceryl trinitrate or nitroglycerin (GTN) results in decreased anal pressure. Randomized trials show healing rates of 50% to 70%, but recurrence rates of 25% to 33%. Headache is the most common side effect in one-half to two-thirds of patients. In randomized trials GTN resulted in healing in only 30% to 60% compared with over 90% of patients using botulinum or undergoing LIS.

(K) Increased cellular calcium levels mediate contraction of the IAS, so calcium channel blockers (CCB) reduce IAS tone. Nifedipine gel (0.2%) and diltiazem gel (2%) result in healing of 65% to 95% of chronic anal fissures in randomized trials. Results of topical therapy with calcium channel blockers are similar to topical nitrates but without the side effect of headaches.

(L) Botulinum toxin (BT) prevents nerve impulses by inhibiting acetylcholine release from presynaptic nerve terminals. Randomized trials show healing in 75% to 96% of patients. In a randomized trial, BT resulted in healing in 96% versus 60% in the GTN group. Most studies have used 10 to 20 units of BT injected in aliquots into the internal sphincter.

(M) Randomized trials of GTN, CCB, and BT have suggested further healing in patients who have been given an additional trial of therapy. Further pharmacologic therapy may thus be justified if patients have mild to moderate symptoms only and wish to avoid operative intervention.

(N) LIS is the procedure of choice in patients who have elevated sphincter tone, have failed a trial of pharmacologic therapy, and who understand

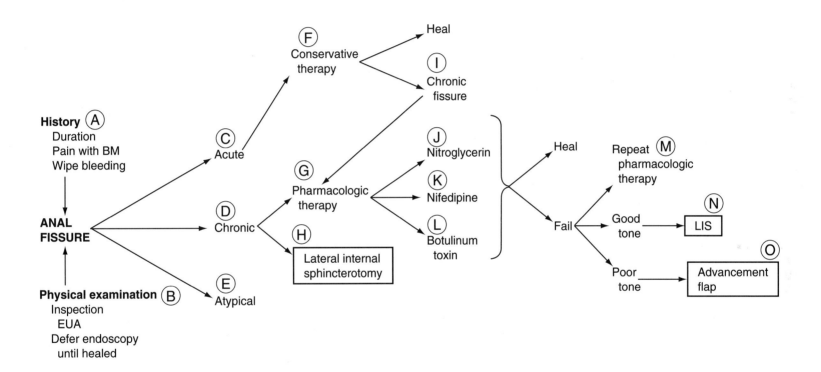

the potential albeit small risk of altered continence after LIS.

Ⓞ In those with fissures in conjunction with low sphincter tone (e.g., elderly patients and postpartum women), LIS is not recommended for failure of medical therapy. In these cases an anal or rectal advancement flap can aid healing.

REFERENCES

Carapeti EA, Kamm MA, Phillips RK: Topical diltiazem and bethanechol decrease anal sphincter pressure and heal anal fissures without side effects. Dis Colon Rectum 43:1359–1362, 2000.

Farouk R, Duthie GS, MacGregor AB et al: Sustained internal sphincter hypertonia in patients with chronic anal fissure. Dis Colon Rectum 37:424–429, 1994.

Hananel N, Gordon PH: Re-examination of clinical manifestations and response to therapy of fissure-in-ano. Dis Colon Rectum 40:229–233, 1997.

Hawley PR: The treatment of chronic fissure-in-ano: A trial of methods. Br J Surg 56:915–918, 1969.

Hyman NH, Cataldo PA: Nitroglycerin ointment for anal fissures: Effective treatment or just a headache? Dis Colon Rectum 42:383–385, 1999.

Jensen SL: Treatment of first episodes of acute anal fissure: Prospective randomized study of lignocaine ointment versus hydrocortisone ointment or warm sitz baths plus bran. Br M J (Clin Res Ed) 292:1167–1169, 1986.

Klosterhalfen B, Vogel P, Rixen H et al: Topography of the inferior rectal artery: A possible cause of chronic, primary anal fissure. Dis Colon Rectum 32:43–52, 1989.

Littlejohn DR, Newstead GL: Tailored lateral internal sphincterotomy for anal fissure. Dis Colon Rectum 40:1439–1442, 1997.

Richard CS, Gregoire R, Plewes EA et al: Internal sphincterotomy is superior to topical nitroglycerin in the treatment of chronic anal fissure: Results of a randomized, controlled trial by the Canadian Colorectal Surgical Trials Group. Dis Colon Rectum 43:1048–1057; discussion 1057–1058, 2000.

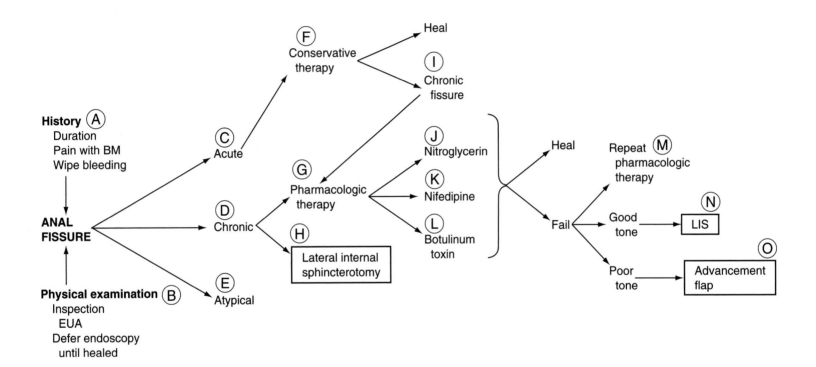

Chapter 75 *Hernia*

ALEXANDER P. NAGLE, MD • KENRIC M. MURAYAMA, MD

(A) The history of a patient with hernia often includes an intermittent bulge and/or a dull sensation in the groin. The symptoms are often worse with heavy lifting, straining, or exercise. A history of heavy lifting is important, both in planning of postoperative disability and in considering long-term recurrence rates. The history should also include questions about chronic coughing, straining to defecate, and difficulties with urination. These symptoms may reveal an underlying pathology (e.g., BPH or prostate, colon, or lung cancer). Preoperative urinary dysfunction also indicates an increased risk for postoperative urinary retention. The examination consists of observing the groin area for evidence of a bulge while the patient coughs. This is repeated with the examiner's index finger invaginated into the external ring: palpation of a bulge or a significant pressure impulse denotes a hernia. If the hernia is incarcerated, the physical examination should note any signs of strangulation (e.g., fever, tenderness, and erythema).

(B) 97% of groin hernias are inguinal and 3% are femoral. The male-to-female ratio is 9:1. The most common type of inguinal hernia is an indirect hernia in both sexes. Femoral hernias are more common in women. Inguinal hernias are bilateral in 20% of cases. The lifetime risk of developing an inguinal hernia is about 10%. Groin hernias have a pronounced adverse economic impact, including the cost of the operation and hospital stay plus the incapacity and lost working hours.

(C) Ultrasound may be helpful for patients who report symptoms but do not have a palpable defect. Ultrasound of the inguinal area with the patient in the supine and upright positions, and with the patient attempting the Valsalva maneuver, has a reported diagnostic sensitivity and specificity of greater than 90%; however, ultrasound is highly operator dependent.

(D) In general, all reducible inguinal hernias should be repaired electively because of the risk of incarceration.

(E) If the patient has an incarcerated inguinal hernia, and strangulation is not suspected, it is appropriate to attempt reduction by using sedation, Trendelenburg's positioning, and gentle sustained pressure over the groin mass. Vigorous repetitive attempts at reducing an incarcerated hernia are ill-advised and may produce "reduction en masse," wherein the entire hernia sac and its contents are reduced so that even though the external bulge is gone the incarceration within the sac remains. If there are any indications of strangulation (e.g., fever, erythema, pain, leukocytosis, bowel obstruction, or peritonitis), reduction should not be attempted.

(F) A strangulated hernia implies that the vascular supply to the contents of the hernia is compromised. A strangulated inguinal hernia is a surgical emergency. The patient should be prepared with IV hydration, a nasogastric tube, correction of electrolytes, and IV antibiotics.

(G) Most elective inguinal hernia repairs can be done on an outpatient basis. Recurrence rates for groin hernias range from 1% to 10%. With the many techniques available, treatment should be individualized. Excellent results with very low recurrence rates have been reported for both open and laparoscopic techniques. There has been a trend towards using prothetic mesh because of the tension-free nature of the repair. Although there is controversy regarding laparoscopic repair for unilateral, newly diagnosed hernias, it seems ideally suited for recurrent and/or bilateral hernias. Recurrent hernias repaired without mesh have a higher rate of recurrence and therefore are best managed utilizing mesh via either an open or a laparoscopic approach.

(H) When operating for an incarcerated or possible strangulated hernia, most surgeons would use the standard anterior inguinal incision. The hernia sac is dissected and then opened under direct vision. It is important to control the base of the hernia sac in order to prevent dropping the contents into the abdominal cavity before adequate inspection. If necessary, it may be possible to do a bowel resection and anastomosis through the inguinal incision. There should be a low threshold to convert to a midline incision if the bowel cannot be adequately inspected. If the bowel is ischemic or if a bowel resection is performed, mesh should not be used because of the high risk of infection. If the defect is too large to close primarily, then a piece of absorbable or biologic (e.g., small intestine submucosa) mesh may be used to repair the hernia defect. An alternative technique is an open preperitoneal (posterior) approach. This has the advantage of being able to convert to a laparotomy without a separate incision.

(I) Laparoscopic inguinal herniorrphapy has the following potential advantages: (1) less postoperative pain; (2) reduced recovery time; (3) easier repair of a recurrent hernia because the repair is performed in a tissue plane that has not been dissected previously; (4) the ability to treat bilateral hernias; (5) the performance of a simultaneous diagnostic laparoscopy; and (6) improved cosmesis. The earlier return to full activity is an important socioeconomic factor because the decrease in the time away from work could potentially offset higher operative costs. The laparoscopic repair might have a lower recurrence rate because of the mechanical advantage gained by placing the mesh on the inside of the adominal wall musculature. The main arguments against laparoscopic inguinal hernia are as follows: (1) conventional inguinal hernia repair is an effective operation performed as an outpatient procedure with low morbidity and mortality; (2) it requires general anesthesia; (3) it is more expensive; and (4) it requires mesh. Some abdominal incisions or treatments (e.g., prostatectomy, prostate XRT) preclude adequate or safe laparoscopic dissection. The type of laparoscopic approach—either TAPP (transabdominal preperitoneal) or TEP (totally extraperitoneal)—depends mainly on the surgeon's preference and level of experience.

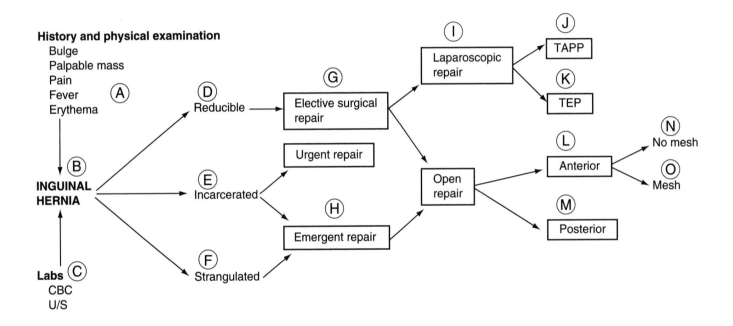

History and physical examination
Bulge
Palpable mass
Pain   Ⓐ
Fever
Erythema

Ⓑ
INGUINAL HERNIA

Labs Ⓒ
CBC
U/S

Ⓓ Reducible

Ⓔ Incarcerated

Ⓕ Strangulated

Ⓖ Elective surgical repair

Urgent repair

Ⓗ Emergent repair

Ⓘ Laparoscopic repair

Open repair

Ⓙ TAPP

Ⓚ TEP

Ⓛ Anterior

Ⓜ Posterior

Ⓝ No mesh

Ⓞ Mesh

(J) The TAPP approach involves a transperitoneal approach to the inguinal region. The peritoneum is incised and a peritoneal flap is created. Once the preperitoneal space is entered, the dissection and conduct of the operation is similar to the TEP. After the mesh is placed, it is then covered by the peritoneal flap. The disadvantage of a TAPP is that it requires entrance into the peritoneal cavity and exposes the patient to potential intra-abdominal injury and late adhesion formation.

(K) The TEP repair stays completely extraperitoneal. A specialized balloon is passed along the posterior rectus sheath down to the pubis symphysis. The balloon is then used to dissect the preperitoneal space, exposing the entire myopectineal orifice. The cord is skeletonized, the hernia sac is reduced, and mesh is used to cover the defect. Medially the mesh is tacked to Cooper's ligament. Laterally the mesh is tacked to the lateral aspect of the transversus abdominis aponeurosis and to the ileopubic tract. Tacks should not be placed below the lateral iliopubic tract in order to avoid injury to the genitofemerol and the lateral femoral cutaneous nerves. The other anatomical landmark of great importance is the "triangle of doom." This triangle is bordered laterally by the spermatic vessels and medially by the vas deferens; located within this triangle are the external iliac artery and vein and the femoral nerve.

(L) The open anterior approach is still the gold standard against which other techniques must be measured. Most hernias can be treated at a low cost by using local anesthesia in an outpatient setting. Excellent results with very low recurrence rates have been reported for both primary repairs (without mesh) and for repairs utilizing mesh. The advantage of a mesh repair is that it provides a tension-free repair. In cases of a large defect, attenuated tissue, or recurrence, a mesh repair is favorable. Although there has been a trend toward an increased use of mesh, there is a slight risk of mesh erosion and infection, which much be considered.

(M) The open preperitoneal (posterior) approach has been advocated by Nyhus and Stoppa. For unilateral hernias, it utilizes a horizontal skin incision in the right or left lower quadrant above the traditional incision used for an anterior repair. For bilateral hernias, a subumbilical midline or Pfannenstiel incision is used. The preperitoneal space is created and the entire myopectineal orifice is exposed. Direct, indirect, and femoral hernias can all be repaired via this approach. Modifications utilizing prosthetic material have become more popular, particularly for recurrent or bilateral hernias. The Stoppa technique uses a giant prosthetic mesh that extends far beyond the myopectineal orifice and envelops the visceral sac. In cases of recurrent or re-recurrent hernia this approach avoids dissection in scar tissue.

(N) Excellent results have been reported for hernia repaired primarily (without mesh). The technique involves opening the external oblique and freeing the spermatic cord. The hernia sac is dissected and usually ligated. Common repairs include the Bassini, the McVay, and the Shouldice. The Bassini repair and its modifications are accomplished by suturing the conjoined tendon of the transversus abdominis and the internal oblique muscles to Poupart's ligament. The McVay repair pulls the floor of the inguinal canal laterally and attaches it to Cooper's ligament under the inguinal ligament. The Shouldice repair utilizes a multilayer, imbricated repair of the inguinal canal floor with running sutures.

(O) Many surgeons routinely use mesh in an effort to reduce tension and recurrence. The mesh incites the formation of scar tissue to further increase tensile strength beyond that provided by the mesh alone. The Lichenstein repair utilizes a segment of prosthetic mesh sutured medially to the pubic tubercle, inferiorly to Poupart's ligament, and superiorly to the conjoined tendon. Laterally the mesh is split, wrapped around the spermatic cord, and the tails sutured together. The use of the mesh "plug" as described by Rutkow has gained popularity because it is relatively simple, fast, and requires only minimal dissection. The mesh plug is placed in the internal ring or onto the inguinal floor and secured with interrupted sutures. A second piece of mesh is placed on the inguinal canal from the pubic tubercle to above the internal ring. The onlay mesh may or may not be secured with sutures. The onlay mesh is intended to strengthen the direct space in an indirect repair and the area of the internal ring in a direct repair. The onlay piece of mesh is meant to serve as a form of prophylaxis against future herniation by creating further tissue ingrowth.

REFERENCES

Felix EL, Michas Caa, Gonzalez MH: Laparoscopic hernioplasty: TAPP vs TEP. Surg Endosc 9:984–989, 1995.

Fitzgibbons RJ Jr., Camps J, Cornet DA et al: Laparoscopic inguinal herniorrhaphy: Result of a multicenter trail. Ann Surg 221:3–13, 1995.

Phillips EH, Arregui M, Carroll BJ et al: Incidence of complications following laparoscopic hernioplasty. Surg Endosc 9:16–21, 1995.

Stoppa RE: The Preperitoneal Approach and Prosthetic Repair of Groin Hernias. In Nyhus LM, Condon RE (eds): Hernia, 4th ed. Philadelphia: JB Lippincott, 1995.

Lichtenstein IL, Shulman AG, Amid PK, et al: The tension-free hernioplasty. Am J Surg 157:188–193, 1989.

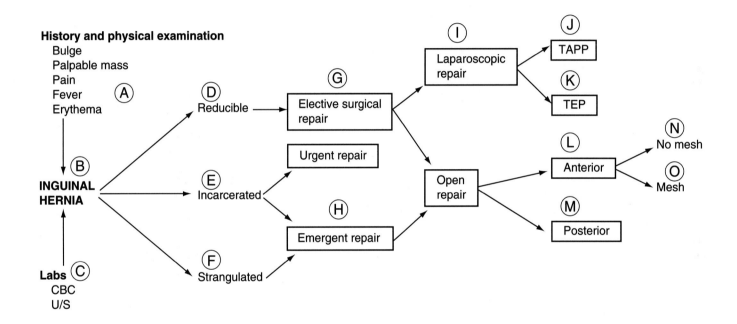

History and physical examination
Bulge
Palpable mass
Pain   Ⓐ
Fever
Erythema

Ⓑ
**INGUINAL
HERNIA**

Labs Ⓒ
CBC
U/S

Ⓓ
Reducible

Ⓔ
Incarcerated

Ⓕ
Strangulated

Ⓖ
Elective surgical
repair

Urgent repair

Ⓗ
Emergent repair

Ⓘ
Laparoscopic
repair

Open
repair

Ⓙ
TAPP

Ⓚ
TEP

Ⓛ
Anterior

Ⓜ
Posterior

Ⓝ
No mesh

Ⓞ
Mesh

Chapter 76 Cancer of Unknown Primary

CHRISTOPHE L. NGUYEN, MD • CARLTON C. BARNETT, JR., MD

(A) A complete history and physical examination is essential for patients with metastatic cancer of unknown primary. Related symptoms may be of relatively recent onset (less than 3 months) with rapid progression of disease. All nodal basins including those of the head and neck, as well as the supraclavicular, axillary, and inguinal region should be carefully examined for lymphadenopathy.

(B) In most patients, the origin of metastases is never identified. Only 25% of cases of unknown primary are identified during the patient's lifetime. At autopsy, the primary site will be identified in only 70% of cases.

(C) Tissue biopsy is a crucial step in the work-up of patients with cancer of unknown primary. FNA is recommended initially, although core biopsy, excisional biopsy, or incisional biopsy may be useful when larger tissue specimens are required. The histologic subtype of the metastases can be identified by light microscopy. Electron microscopy can help differentiate squamous cell carcinoma from adenocarcinoma. Immunohistochemistry may also delineate tumor origin. This histologic information is critical in determining the subsequent work-up and treatment.

(D) Chemotherapy remains the standard treatment for most lymphomas. Although patients with Hodgkin's disease may require staging laparotomy, surgery is generally not indicated in non-Hodgkin's lymphoma because of tumor distribution and spread. Laparotomy to obtain tissue may be required to direct more appropriate chemotherapy.

(E) Approximately 5% of patients with melanoma present with metastatic disease to the lymph nodes from an unknown primary tumor. Historically, patients with metastatic melanoma and unknown primary tumors were thought to have a worse prognosis. Recent studies suggest that the survival rates of these patients are comparable to those of patients with known primary tumors. The nodal basin of patients with unknown primary tumors should be approached by radical lymphadenectomy followed by adjuvant immunotherapy.

(F) Biopsies of cervical lymphadenopathy often demonstrate metastatic squamous cell cancer. The most common site of metastasis in these patients is the jugulodigastric (level II upper internal jugular chain nodes), followed by the midjugular (zone III and IV) nodes.

(G) Based on a large series, the expected 5-year survival for patients with metastatic squamous cell cancer following combined therapy is from 32% to 55%, and overall rate of control of neck disease is 75% to 85%. Outcome for patients with metastatic adenocarcinoma is less favorable. Rate of local recurrence is nearly 100%, and the 5-year survival rate is 0% to 10%.

(H) There are three general approaches to the treatment of women with breast adenocarcinoma metastatic to the axilla. Immediate mastectomy has been the traditional therapy for these patients; it has 10-year survival rates of 79%. Axillary dissection with observation of the breast is another option, although local recurrence is 25% to 75% in these patients. The third approach is breast conservation therapy, which results in survival rates comparable to traditional therapy.

(I) Women with peritoneal carcinomatosis should be approached in a similar manner to those with known advanced ovarian cancer. Surgical cytoreduction followed by platinum-based chemotherapy results in median survival rates of 16 months to 2 years.

(J) Overall response of metastatic cancer from an unknown primary tumor to chemotherapy remains poor with expected 5-year survival rates between 5% and 10% in unselected groups of patients. However, recent studies suggest that cisplatin-based regimens and combination treatments of paclitaxel, carboplatin, and etoposide may improve such responses.

(K) Overall survival for patients with liver metastases and unknown primary remains poor with median survival of 7 months. Palliative hepatic resection may provide relief for symptoms of compression. Percutaneous or standard radiofrequency ablation may provide symptomatic relief, particularly for hormonally active metastases. In general, supportive care is most appropriate, although recent reviews suggest symptomatic benefit from palliative chemotherapy.

REFERENCES

Abbruzzese JL, Lenzi R, Raber MN: Carcinoma of Unknown Primary. In Abeloff MD, Armitage JD, Lichter AS (eds): Clinical Oncology, 2nd ed. New York: Churchill Livingstone, 2000.

Ayoub JP, Hess KR, Abbruzzese MC et al: Unknown primary tumors metastatic to liver. J Clin Oncol 16:2105–2112, 1998.

Chorost MI, McKinley B, Tsachoi M et al: The management of the unknown primary. J Am Col Surg 193:666–677, 2001.

Feig BW, Berger DH, Fuhrman GM: The M.D. Anderson Surgical Oncology Handbook, 3rd ed. Philadelphia: Lippincott Williams & Wilkins, 2003.

Greco FA, Burris HA, Erland JB et al: Carcinoma of unknown primary site: Long-term follow-up after treatment with paclitaxel, carboplatin, and etoposide. Cancer 89:2655–2660, 2000.

Rades D, Kuhnel G, Wildfang I et al: Localised disease in cancer of unknown primary (CUP): The value of positron emission tomography (PET) for individual therapeutic management. Ann Oncol 12:1605–1609, 2001.

Wolff AC, Lange JR, Davidson NE: Occult Primary Cancer with Axillary Nodal Metastases. In Singletary SE, Robb GL (eds): Adjuvant Therapy of Breast Disease. Hamilton: BC Decker, 2000.

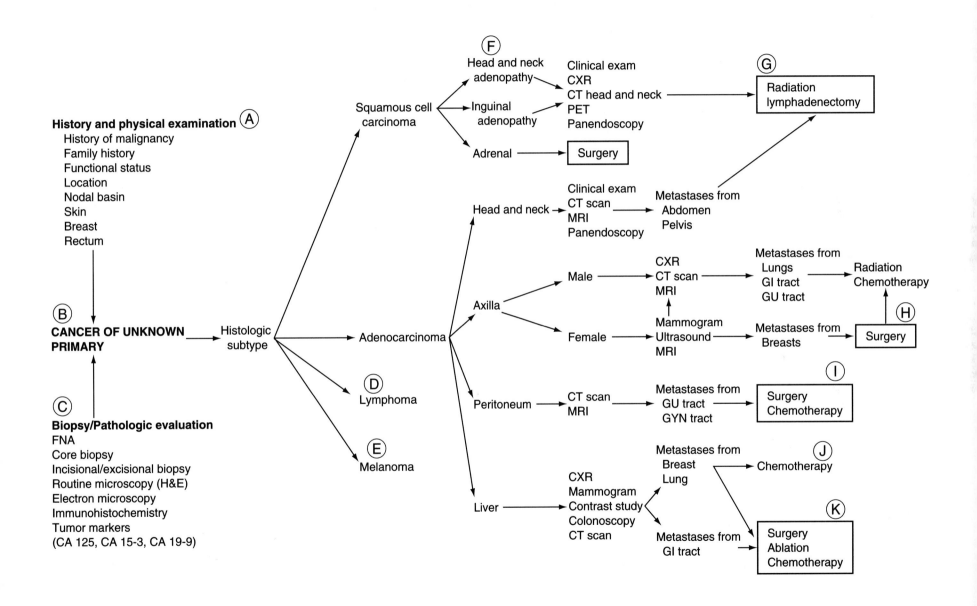

History and physical examination (A)
History of malignancy
Family history
Functional status
Location
Nodal basin
Skin
Breast
Rectum

(B)
CANCER OF UNKNOWN PRIMARY

(C)
Biopsy/Pathologic evaluation
FNA
Core biopsy
Incisional/excisional biopsy
Routine microscopy (H&E)
Electron microscopy
Immunohistochemistry
Tumor markers
(CA 125, CA 15-3, CA 19-9)

Histologic subtype

Squamous cell carcinoma

(F)
Head and neck adenopathy
Inguinal adenopathy

Clinical exam
CXR
CT head and neck
PET
Panendoscopy

(G)
Radiation lymphadenectomy

Adrenal → Surgery

Adenocarcinoma

Head and neck →
Clinical exam
CT scan
MRI
Panendoscopy
→ Metastases from
Abdomen
Pelvis

Axilla

Male →
CXR
CT scan
MRI
→ Metastases from
Lungs
GI tract
GU tract
→ Radiation
Chemotherapy

Female →
Mammogram
Ultrasound
MRI
→ Metastases from
Breasts
→
(H)
Surgery

Peritoneum →
CT scan
MRI
→ Metastases from
GU tract
GYN tract
→
(I)
Surgery
Chemotherapy

Liver →
CXR
Mammogram
Contrast study
Colonoscopy
CT scan

Metastases from
Breast
Lung
→
(J)
Chemotherapy

Metastases from
GI tract
→
(K)
Surgery
Ablation
Chemotherapy

(D)
Lymphoma

(E)
Melanoma

BREAST AND SOFT NIPPLE

Chapter 77 Nipple Discharge

V. SUZANNE KLIMBERG, MD

(A) Nipple discharge is most often (more than 99%) benign. The history specific to nipple discharge and associated ductal abnormalities has to do with the nature of the discharge, including spontaneity; unilaterality; single versus multiple ducts; color of the discharge (e.g., milky, cheesy, purulent, serous, green, black, or bloody); signs or history of infection; endocrine disorders; and pregnancy or drugs (e.g., caffeine, smoking, hormones, marijuana, or cimetidine or similar drugs). Any good history should include those factors that may increase the patient's risk of breast cancer and calculate that risk using the Gail or Clause model.

(B) Bilateral, nonspontaneous, nonbloody discharge from multiple ducts is benign. The examiner should apply pressure in a clockwise fashion around the areolar in an attempt to identify a specific site, mass, or duct that produces discharge.

(C) Gross examination and guaiac of the nipple discharge can reveal macroscopic or microscopic blood. Gram stain can be performed if there is a suspicion of infection. Examination under the office microscope will confirm fat in benign milky discharge. Cytological examination of the nipple fluid has a false negative rate for cancer of approximately 50%. In any patient with potential endocrine abnormality prolactin, thyroid and/or pregnancy tests should be performed.

Mammography is a must in any patient older than 40 years to rule out associated underlying pathology. A negative mammogram should be ignored.

(D) Milky or clear discharge can be present for years, especially after pregnancy. In a small percentage of patients a milky discharge may represent prolactinemia secondary to a prolactinoma of the pituitary.

(E) Unilateral, spontaneous discharge requires further evaluation. It can be caused by fibrocystic changes; intraductal papilloma; duct ectasia; nipple adenoma; pregnancy; postlactation; infection; chronic mastitis or subareolar abscess; and, less commonly (less than 1%), by breast cancer.

(F) Some intraductal lesions, including cancer, produce no detectable blood. Ductography, cytology of nipple aspiration, or ductal lavage or ductoscopy may help detect such disease.

(G) Grossly bloody or hemoccult-positive unilateral discharge requires further evaluation or treatment. The most common causes are intraductal papilloma (45%), duct ectasia (36%), carcinoma (8%), infection (8%), and other (3%). Bilateral spontaneous bloody discharge can be seen in pregnancy.

(H) An elevated prolactin level, confirmed by repeat testing, is an indication for pituitary imaging to diagnose a prolactinoma.

(I) Galactography or ductogram, ultrasound, and aspiration cytology are useful only when positive but have a high rate of false-negative results. Ductography is abnormal almost 80% of the time and therefore is of limited usefulness. Ductal lavage to increase cell retrieval, in combination with cytology and ductal endoscopy, is an emerging technique that may prove useful in the future. Ductal lavage has its best use, at this time, in the high-risk patient. Ductal endoscopy, although promising for visual and cytological diagnosis, does not yet have the ability for minimally invasive resection.

(J) Colored, clear, or milky discharge either unilaterally or bilaterally often resolves with cessation of smoking and/or caffeine.

(K) In spontaneous unilateral nipple discharge (bloody or not), ductal excision is the only reliable procedure in establishing a diagnosis as well as in controlling the discharge. A palpable mass or blood-filled duct may guide excision (microdochectomy). The bloody duct should be excised as far proximal as possible because most cancers are located proximally. Other surgical aids may include a probe or dye placed in the abnormal duct to guide excision.

(L) If no such mass or duct can be identified, then nipple core biopsy (taking all the ductal structures under the nipple-areolar complex) is mandated.

REFERENCES

Das DK, Al-Ayadhy B, Ajrawi MT et al: Cytodiagnosis of nipple discharge: A study of 602 samples from 484 cases. Diag Cytopathol 25:25–37, 2001.

Hou MF, Huang TJ, Liu GC: The diagnostic value of galactography in patients with nipple discharge. Clin Imaging 25:75–81, 2001.

Khan SA, Baird C, Staradub VL et al: Ductal lavage and ductoscopy: The opportunities and the limitations. Clin Breast Cancer 3:185–191, 2002.

King TA, Carter KM, Bolton JS et al: A simple approach to nipple discharge. Am Surg 66:960–966, 2000.

Mokbel K, Elkak AE: The evolving role of mammary ductoscopy. Curr Med Res Opin 18:30–32, 2002.

Sakorafas GH: Nipple discharge: Current diagnostic and therapeutic approaches. Cancer Treat Rev 27:275–282, 2001.

Vaidyanathan L, Barnard K, Elnicki DM: Benign breast disease: When to treat, when to reassure, when to refer. Cleve Clin J Med 69:425–432, 2002.

Vargas HI, Romero L, Chlebowski RT: Management of bloody nipple discharge. Curr Treat Options Oncol 3:157–161, 2002.

Williams RS, Brook D, Monypenny IJ et al: The relevance of reported symptoms in a breast screening programme. Clin Radiol 57:725–729, 2002.

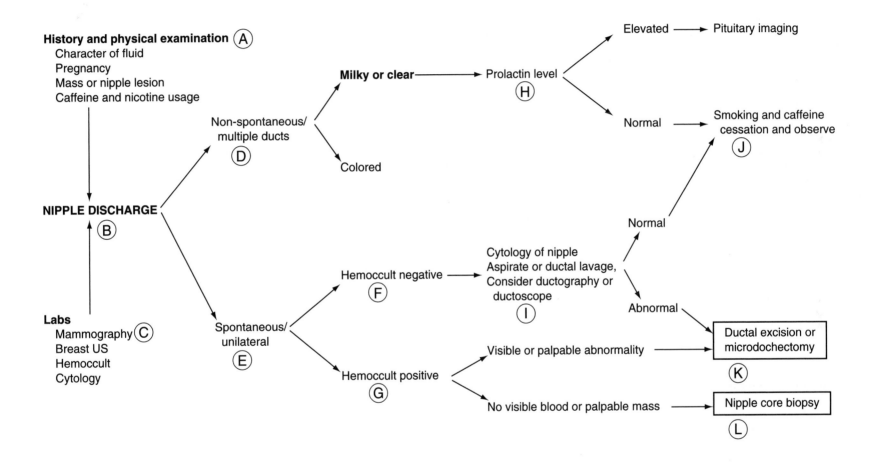

History and physical examination Ⓐ
    Character of fluid
    Pregnancy
    Mass or nipple lesion
    Caffeine and nicotine usage

NIPPLE DISCHARGE Ⓑ

Labs
    Mammography Ⓒ
    Breast US
    Hemoccult
    Cytology

Non-spontaneous/multiple ducts Ⓓ

Milky or clear

Colored

Prolactin level Ⓗ

Elevated ⟶ Pituitary imaging

Normal ⟶ Smoking and caffeine cessation and observe Ⓙ

Spontaneous/unilateral Ⓔ

Hemoccult negative Ⓕ

Hemoccult positive Ⓖ

Cytology of nipple
Aspirate or ductal lavage,
Consider ductography or
ductoscope Ⓘ

Normal

Abnormal

Visible or palpable abnormality

No visible blood or palpable mass

Ductal excision or microdochectomy Ⓚ

Nipple core biopsy Ⓛ

Chapter 78 **Gynecomastia**

CHRISTINA A. FINLAYSON, MD

(A) There are three common peaks in age distribution for the development of a mass in the male breast. It is very common for both male and female newborns to have breast enlargement. There is a second pubertal peak between ages 10 and 16 years in boys. Pubertal breast enlargement usually regresses spontaneously but may persist for 2 to 3 years. Some 30% of middle-aged men may develop gynecomastia, and that incidence increases to 60% by age 70 years.

(B) Gynecomastia often presents as a painful breast mass. It may be unilateral or bilateral.

(C) It is characterized as a rubbery, round, or oval mass located directly behind the areola although it may be large enough to extend outside the margins of the areola. Breast cancer is more often not painful and presents as a unilateral, hard mass usually located eccentric to the nipple or areola.

(D) Men with nipple discharge are more likely to have breast cancer than gynecomastia.

(E) Enlarged axillary lymph nodes raise concerns about breast cancer.

(F) Mammography is most useful to discriminate between pseudogynecomastia (fatty breast) and a solid mass (gynecomastia, breast cancer). Gynecomastia may have a characteristic pattern on mammography that provides a diagnosis.

(G) Ultrasound is most useful to discriminate between cystic and solid lesions. True male breast masses are virtually never cystic. Ultrasound has limited utility in evaluating a male breast mass.

(H) A mass located eccentric from the areola, particularly if it is hard to the touch, is worrisome for malignancy. Breast cancer, as well as sarcoma or soft-tissue metastatic disease, can present

in this location. Other conditions to consider are lipoma, neurofibroma, and epidermal inclusion cyst.

(I) A rubbery mass located directly behind and concentric with the areola is usually gynecomastia.

(J) Pseudogynecomastia, or diffuse fatty enlargement of the male breast area, is a cosmetic problem.

(K) Biopsy of a mass located eccentric from the areola can be done by fine-needle aspiration (FNA), core biopsy, or excisional biopsy.

(L) Gynecomastia, although a benign phenomenon, can be a presenting symptom for a more worrisome underlying disease. A very careful and extensive history, physical examination, and review of systems are required. Elucidation of drug use (e.g., prescription medications, marijuana, alcohol, and anabolic steroids); symptoms of pituitary, thyroid, hepatic, renal or adrenal disease; changes in libido and sexual functioning; and the presence of testicular masses all need to be pursued.

(M) If a careful history and physical examination does not reveal an underlying cause of gynecomastia, a biochemical profile should be performed, particularly if the patient falls outside the usual age distribution for gynecomastia. Laboratory evaluation begins with a B-hCG, luteinizing hormone (LH), estradiol, and testosterone levels. Elevated B-hCG points toward a testicular tumor. Elevated estradiol is concerning for a Leydig, Sertoli, or adrenal tumor. Increased LH and testosterone points to hyperthyroidism or androgen resistance. Decreased LH and testosterone is concerning for a prolactin-secreting pituitary tumor. If all studies are normal, idiopathic gynecomastia is the diagnosis.

(N) Most men with gynecomastia do not require treatment. If an underlying condition is identified, steps can be taken to modify medications or treat disease. Mild pain medication such as acetaminophen or NSAIDs can provide symptomatic relief. Most discomfort resolves although it may take 12 to 24 months.

(O) Tamoxifen can decrease size and discomfort for painful gynecomastia. Side effects of tamoxifen are relatively mild. Danazol is can also be helpful but side effects are more severe and often limit treatment.

(P) Surgical removal of gynecomastia can remove the mass, but the cosmetic result is often unsatisfying with a scar as well as flattening of the nipple-areolar complex. Lack of sensation of the nipple-areolar complex can occur. Plastic surgical removal combined with liposuction provides the best cosmetic outcome.

(Q) Fatty enlargement of the breast is a cosmetic problem that can be nicely improved with plastic surgery including liposuction.

REFERENCES

Braunstein GD: Gynecomastia. In Harris JR, Lippman ME, Morrow M et al (eds): Diseases of the Breast. Philadelphia: Lippincott-Raven, 1996.

Daniels TR, Layer GT: Gynaecomastia. Eur J Surg 167: 885–892, 2001.

Gunhan-Bilgen I, Bozkaya H, Ustun EE et al: Male breast disease: Clinical, mammographic, and ultrasonographic features. Eur J Radiol 43:246–255, 2002.

Mathur R, Braunstein GD: Gynecomastia: Pathomechanisms and treatment strategies. Horm Res 48:95–102, 1997.

Rohrich RJ, Ha RY, Kenkel JM et al: Classification and management of gynecomastia: Defining the role of ultrasound-assisted liposuction. Plast Reconstr Surg 111:909–925, 2003.

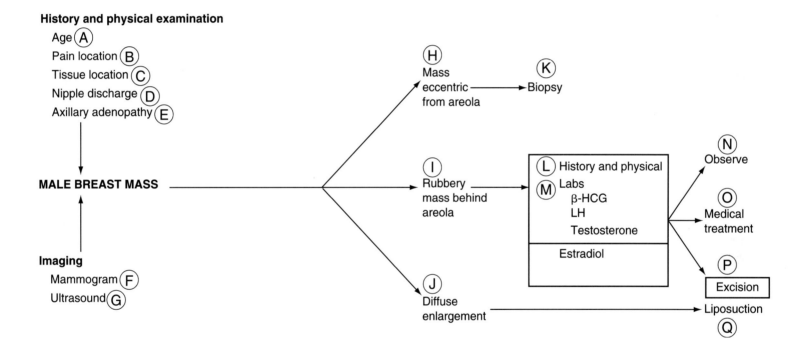

History and physical examination
Age Ⓐ
Pain location Ⓑ
Tissue location Ⓒ
Nipple discharge Ⓓ
Axillary adenopathy Ⓔ

MALE BREAST MASS

Imaging
Mammogram Ⓕ
Ultrasound Ⓖ

Ⓗ
Mass eccentric ──► Biopsy
from areola

Ⓚ

Ⓘ
Rubbery mass behind areola

Ⓙ
Diffuse enlargement

Ⓛ History and physical
Ⓜ Labs
β-HCG
LH
Testosterone

Estradiol

Ⓝ
Observe

Ⓞ
Medical treatment

Ⓟ
Excision

Liposuction
Ⓠ

Chapter 79 *Dominant Breast Mass*

MARY A. HOOKS, MD

(A) Important considerations regarding a new breast mass include the duration and change since initial detection. For premenopausal women, this includes changes associated with menstrual cycle including associated pain and change in size. Associated symptoms include changes of the skin or nipple areolar complex, nipple discharge, pain, and tenderness.

(B) Breast cancer risk factors should be included in the history of all women presenting with a dominant breast mass. These include age, family history (especially first-degree relatives), previous personal history of breast cancer or certain types of benign pathology (e.g., atypical hyperplasia or lobular carcinoma in situ), and hormonal factors (e.g., age at menarche and menopause, parity, use of exogenous hormones). Seventy-five per cent of women diagnosed with breast cancer have advanced age as the only risk factor. The absence of other risk factors should not limit the work-up of a dominant mass.

(C) A dominant palpable breast mass is most often detected by the patient, reinforcing the need to instruct and encourage patients to perform monthly breast self-exam.

(D) Clinical breast examination (CBE) is extremely important in breast cancer screening and in evaluating a patient who presents with a new breast mass. Between 15% and 20% of breast masses are not detected with screening mammography, emphasizing the importance of CBE. Patients should be examined in upright and in supine positions. Pattern of search should include the area bordered by the clavicle superiorly, the lateral border of sternum medially, the inframammary fold inferiorly, and the latissimus dorsi muscle laterally. The vertical strip method has been shown to be most sensitive. Pads of the fingers should be used because they are much more sensitive than the fingertips; varying pressure provides assessment of tissue at differing depths in the breast, and the hand should not be removed from the breast during the examination.

(E) Ultrasonography is most useful in characterizing masses that are well circumscribed. In particular, it is best at distinguishing cystic lesions from solid ones. It is also the most useful imaging procedure in younger women, who have denser breasts. Ultrasound can also be used to perform image-guided biopsies or cyst aspiration. In the case of cyst aspiration, the complete collapse of the cyst can be visualized. For solid masses, ultrasound guidance provides targeted sampling of the concerning lesion.

(F) Mammography is the gold standard imaging technique. For women with a palpable mass, a diagnostic mammogram will include magnification views of the area containing the palpable mass. This is especially helpful in characterizing the mass and identifying associated calcifications and/or architectural distortion. In the presence of a palpable mass, the mammogram will also evaluate the remaining breast tissue. In some cases this may reveal multifocal disease or separate foci of calcifications. Imaging should be performed before biopsy to avoid distortion caused by hematoma formation following biopsy. Fine-needle aspiration (25- or 27-gauge needle) may safely be performed before biopsy in a woman with a previous history of cystic masses and clinical findings consistent with a simple cyst.

(G) Magnetic resonance imaging is not considered part of the routine work-up of a dominant palpable mass. It may be useful in the diagnostic work-up of patients who present with axillary lymphadenopathy and have a normal clinical breast examination and mammogram and who may possess an occult primary tumor. It may also be useful in patients with implants or a history of other breast surgery, including women with a previous personal history of breast cancer.

(H) Simple cysts can be aspirated if symptomatic or if followed clinically. When aspirated, a simple cyst should yield clear fluid and the mass should completely disappear. If/when a cyst recurs, surgical excision is advisable.

(I) Complex cysts and solid masses require definitive diagnosis.

(J) If aspiration yields blood or the mass does not completely resolve, fluid should be submitted for cytology and the mass should be surgically excised.

(K) Needle biopsy results provide important information for definitive surgical treatment planning and are usually encouraged. A diagnosis of carcinoma with needle biopsy allows fewer steps in the definitive surgical treatment.

(L) Core needle biopsy is well tolerated and provides architectural information unavailable with cytology alone. It has a high sensitivity (90%) and specificity (98% to 100%) and is easily performed in a clinic setting. The large needle requires use of local anesthesia and a small skin incision. There is a higher risk of bruising or hematoma formation compared with fine-needle aspiration.

(M) Fine-needle aspiration (FNA) is highly dependent on the skill of the person performing the procedure and of the cytopathologist analyzing the specimen. Local anesthesia is usually not required because of the small size of the needle. The use of FNA has decreased significantly since implementation of larger core needles, which yield more information.

(N) Surgical excision is the definitive diagnostic procedure and in most cases is itself therapeutic with regard to the breast lesion itself.

(O) There are many types of benign breast masses, and the plan for definitive treatment and/or follow up depends on specific pathology.

(P) Fibroadenomas may be either followed clinically or surgically excised. If the mass meets criteria of the "triple test" (i.e., clinical examination, imaging criteria, and needle biopsy), then the mass can be followed clinically. If stable following short-term follow-up (3 to 4 months) or surgical excision, the patient can return to routine screening.

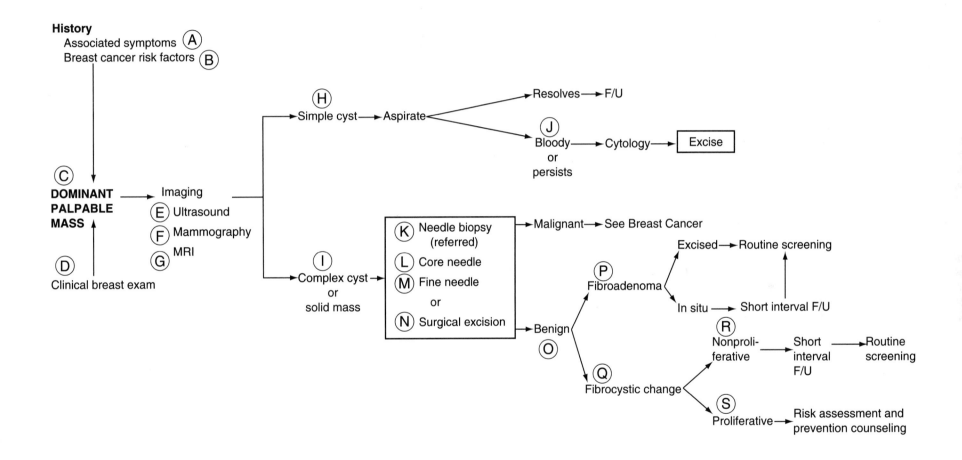

History
Associated symptoms (A)
Breast cancer risk factors (B)

(H)
Simple cyst → Aspirate → Resolves → F/U
(J)
Bloody → Cytology → Excise
or
persists

(C)
**DOMINANT
PALPABLE
MASS**

Imaging
(E) Ultrasound
(F) Mammography
(G) MRI

(D)
Clinical breast exam

(I)
Complex cyst
or
solid mass

(K) Needle biopsy (referred) → Malignant → See Breast Cancer
(L) Core needle
(M) Fine needle
or
(N) Surgical excision

→ Benign
(O)

(P)
Fibroadenoma → Excised → Routine screening
→ In situ → Short interval F/U

(Q)
Fibrocystic change
(R)
Nonproliferative → Short interval F/U → Routine screening
(S)
Proliferative → Risk assessment and prevention counseling

Q Fibrocystic change includes a variety of breast pathology. In the presence of a dominant palpable mass and needle biopsy results consistent with fibrocystic change, surgical excision should be performed.

R Nonproliferative fibrocystic change does not increase the risk of breast cancer, and these patients should continue with routine breast cancer screening to include monthly breast self-examination, annual clinical breast examination, and annual mammography.

S Proliferative fibrocystic change includes hyperplasia, which increases breast cancer risk minimally. The presence of atypia increases breast cancer risk four to five times over the general public, and lobular carcinoma in situ increases risk to 15% to 30% at 15 years following diagnosis. Patients with atypia and LCIS should be counseled regarding breast cancer risk and advised of preventive measures such as the use of tamoxifen or prophylactic surgery.

REFERENCES

August DA, Advisory Council for Surgery: Breast Disease Curriculum, American College of Surgeons, 1996.

Fisher B, Costantino J, Wickerham DL et al: Tamoxifen for prevention of breast cancer: Report of the National Surgical Adjuvant Breast and Bowel Project P-1 Study. J Natl Cancer Inst 90:1871–1888, 1998.

Freund KM: Rationale and technique of clinical breast examination. Medscape Women's Health, 5:E2, 2000.

Harris JR, Lippmann ME, Morrow M et al: Diseases of the Breast, 2nd ed. Philadelphia: Lippincott Williams & Wilkins, 1999.

Norton LW: Solitary Breast Mass. In Norton LW, Steele G, Eiseman B (eds): Surgical Decision Making, 3rd ed. Philadelphia: WB Saunders, 1993.

Pruthi S: Detection and evaluation of a palpable mass. Mayo Clin Proc 76:641–647, 2001.

Shannon J, Douglas-Jones AG, Dallimore NS: Conversion to core biopsy in preoperative diagnosis of breast lesions: Is it justified by results? J Clin Pathol 54:762–765, 2001.

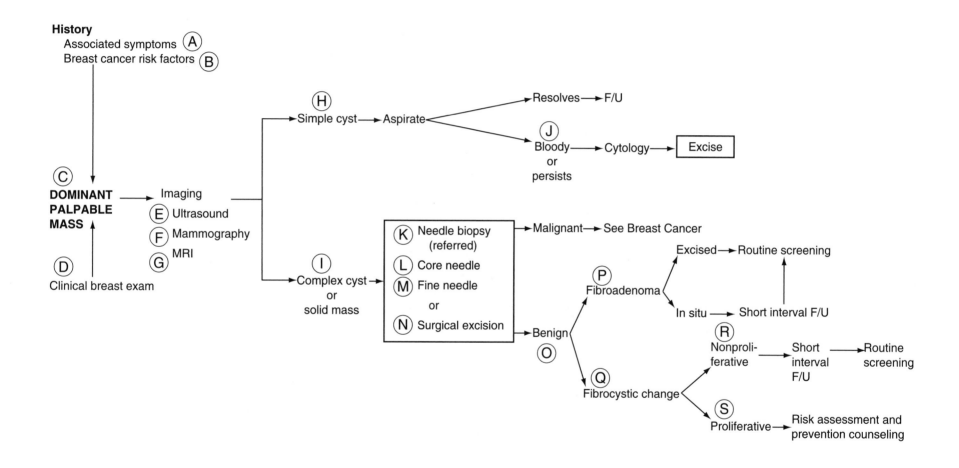

History
Associated symptoms (A)
Breast cancer risk factors (B)

(C)
DOMINANT PALPABLE MASS

(D)
Clinical breast exam

Imaging
(E) Ultrasound
(F) Mammography
(G) MRI

(H) Simple cyst → Aspirate

Resolves → F/U

(J) Bloody or persists → Cytology → Excise

(I) Complex cyst or solid mass

(K) Needle biopsy (referred)
(L) Core needle
(M) Fine needle
or
(N) Surgical excision

Malignant → See Breast Cancer

Benign
(O)

(P) Fibroadenoma

Excised → Routine screening

In situ → Short interval F/U

(Q) Fibrocystic change

(R) Nonproliferative → Short interval F/U → Routine screening

(S) Proliferative → Risk assessment and prevention counseling

Chapter 80 *Occult Breast Lesions*

JYOTI ARYA, MD • C. CLAY COTHREN, MD

(A) Important past medical history such as prior breast disease (e.g., fibrocystic change, proliferative breast lesions, or cancer); biopsy; trauma; or infection is needed. Previous biopsies, trauma, and infection may cause scarring that is visualized as architectural distortion or even a mass. Fat necrosis, which can occur after trauma, may mimic a malignancy. History of a proliferative breast lesion (e.g., atypical ductal hyperplasia or lobular carcinoma in situ) places the patient at increased risk for breast cancer and may alter the decision to follow vs. biopsy the patient.

(B) An occult breast lesion is an abnormality noted on an imaging study that has no physical manifestation (e.g., palpable mass, nipple discharge, or skin changes). The vast majority of occult lesions are noted on screening mammography. An acceptable screening mammography program will identify 5% to 10% of mammograms as abnormal. Radiologists use the Breast Imaging Reporting and Data System (BI-RADS) guidelines to evaluate mammograms, ultrasounds, and breast MRI images. Radiologists need the patient's pertinent medical history, breast cancer risk assessment, and physical examination information in order to best interpret the images.

(C) MRI occult lesions can be more challenging. If a lesion is identified on MRI, the patient's prior mammograms should be carefully re-evaluated. If no retrospective corresponding lesion is noted, additional focused mammograms and a focused breast ultrasound should be obtained. If the MRI-identified lesion can be seen with conventional imaging and is indeterminate or suspicious, it should be biopsied using standard techniques. If no mammographic or ultrasound abnormality is found, but the lesion is suspicious, a MRI-guided biopsy is technically possible but often limited to a few specialized breast imaging centers. Breast MRI is still an evolving imaging modality, and if standard biopsy or MRI-guided biopsy techniques are not available, it is reasonable to closely follow these patients.

(D) The common mammographic abnormalities warranting evaluation are architectural distortion, asymmetry, a mass, or calcifications. The first step in evaluating a mammographic abnormality is additional mammographic views (e.g., spot compression, oblique images, and magnification). This is particularly important for areas of architectural distortion or asymmetry. If on the additional views the architectural distortion dissipates, follow-up recommendation is a repeat mammogram in 6 months. If there is a suggestion of a mass on the additional views, an ultrasound may be helpful. If the distortion persists, it should undergo biopsy. Asymmetric areas that remain concerning after additional views should have a biopsy.

(E) Masses noted on mammography should always have an ultrasound to further characterize the lesion. Ultrasound is helpful in differentiating between solid vs. cystic masses and benign vs. suspicious masses. Simple cysts require no additional follow-up and complex cysts should be re-examined in 6 months. Highly suspicious, complex cysts should be biopsied. Ultrasound-guided fine-needle aspiration can be used to biopsy/aspirate a benign-appearing cyst if follow-up is questionable or if the patient requests. Benign solid masses should have either 6-month follow-up or undergo FNA biopsy depending upon the clinical situation. All indeterminate or suspicious solid masses should be biopsied. The biopsy can be performed under ultrasound guidance or stereotactically, although ultrasound is usually preferable in order to minimize radiation exposure and to maximize patient comfort.

(F) Calcifications are a common mammographic abnormality; if large they are considered benign. Microcalcifications are evaluated based upon their morphology; distribution within the breast; and associated abnormalities, such as a mass. The radiologist will assign a category and give follow-up recommendations. Categories I-II (benign) need only routine follow-up. Category III (likely benign)

calcifications can be biopsied if the risk of breast cancer is high and clinical suspicion is present, or a 6-month follow-up examination is reasonable. Category IV-V (suspicious or highly suspicious) calcifications should always be biopsied.

(G) The biopsy technique is determined by what is available in the community. Core needle biopsies are preferable over needle localized surgical biopsy. The success rate and accuracy of needle biopsies is comparable to operative biopsies; however, needle biopsies typically are less morbid, less expensive, and may reduce the number of operative procedures required for patients diagnosed with a malignancy. If a stereotactic needle biopsy is not available, then a needle-guided surgical biopsy should be performed if the imaging and clinical suspicion is high.

(H) The accuracy of needle core biopsy is influenced by the gauge of the needle, the technique, and the number of core samples. A needle 14 g or larger, with vacuum assistance, provides a high-quality tissue sample and a large number of cores with minimal complications. Smaller gauge needles are available but often result in tissue distortion and difficulty in pathologic interpretation. Ten to 15 cores or complete removal of the lesion is possible with a vacuum-assisted device and has a low false negative rate. Ultrasound-guided needle biopsies typically remove 4 or 5 core tissue samples. If the lesion is completely removed by the core biopsy, a mammographic clip should be placed in order to guide a future surgical biopsy if necessary. Core biopsies for microcalcifications should have specimen mammography to confirm the presence of the calcifications, and the pathologist should also be able to identify calcifications in the specimen.

(I) The ABBI system (advanced breast biopsy instrumentation) is also available for mammographic lesions. The ABBI requires a small incision but provides a large tissue sample and has a low false negative rate. Unfortunately, the ABBI is not

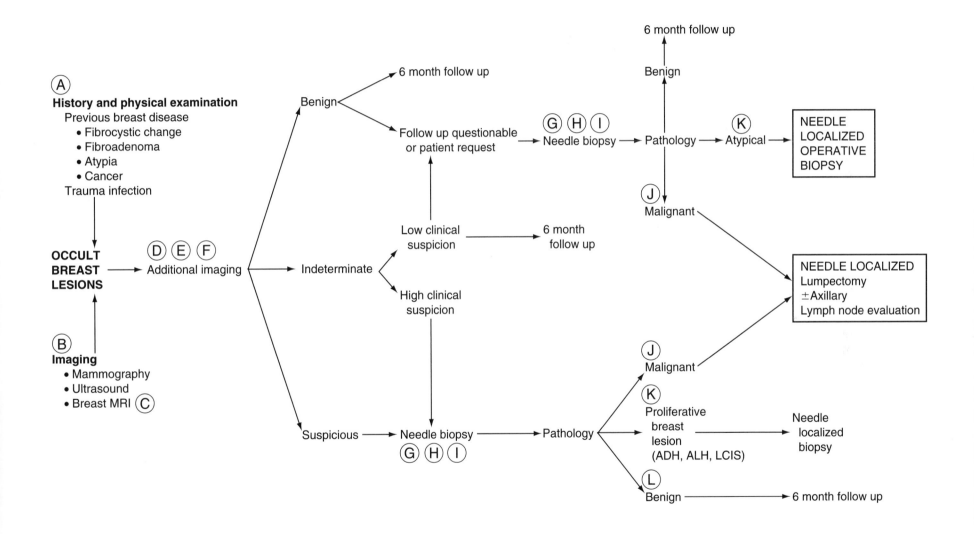

approved for the treatment of carcinoma; therefore a follow-up surgical excision is necessary.

(J) Once a pathologic diagnosis of a malignant lesion is made, a discussion with the patient can occur and the appropriate operative treatment rendered. For mammographically detectable cancers, a lumpectomy with axillary lymph node analysis followed by radiation therapy is often appropriate management.

(K) An operative biopsy should be performed if the pathology demonstrates atypical ductal hyperplasia, atypical lobular hyperplasia, radial scar, lobular carcinoma in situ, a papillary lesion, phyllodes tumor, or pseudoangiomatous stromal hyperplasia. The highest risk of an associated carcinoma is with atypical ductal hyperplasia, and 10% to 25% of patients will be upstaged to DCIS or invasive carcinoma upon surgical biopsy.

(L) Pathology found on needle biopsy should be concordant with what is suspected based upon the mammographic, ultrasound, or MRI image as well as the clinical suspicion. If the pathology is benign, but the images are concerning and the clinical index of suspicion is high, the patient should be rebiopsied or undergo a needle localized operative biopsy.

REFERENCES

Liberman L, Menell JH: Breast imaging reporting and data system (BI-RADS). Radiol Clin N Am 40:409–430, 2002.

Meyer JE, Smith DN, Lester SC et al: Large-core needle biopsy of nonpalpable breast lesions. JAMA 281:1638–1641, 1999.

Morris EA, Liberman L, Ballor DJ et al: MRI of occult breast carcinoma in a high-risk population. Am J Roentgenology 181:619–626, 2003.

Reynolds HE: Core needle biopsy of challenging benign breast conditions: A comprehensive literature review. Am J Roentgenology 174:1245–1250, 2000.

Seoudi H, Mortier J, Basile R et al: Stereotactic core needle biopsy of nonpalpable breast lesions. Arch Surg 133:366–372, 1998.

Stuart SJ: Benign breast disease and breast cancer risk: Morphology and beyond. Am J Surg Pathol 27:836–841, 2003.

Winchester DJ: Upstaging of atypical ductal hyperplasia after vacuum-assisted 11-gauge stereotactic core needle biopsy. Arch Surg 138:619–623, 2003.

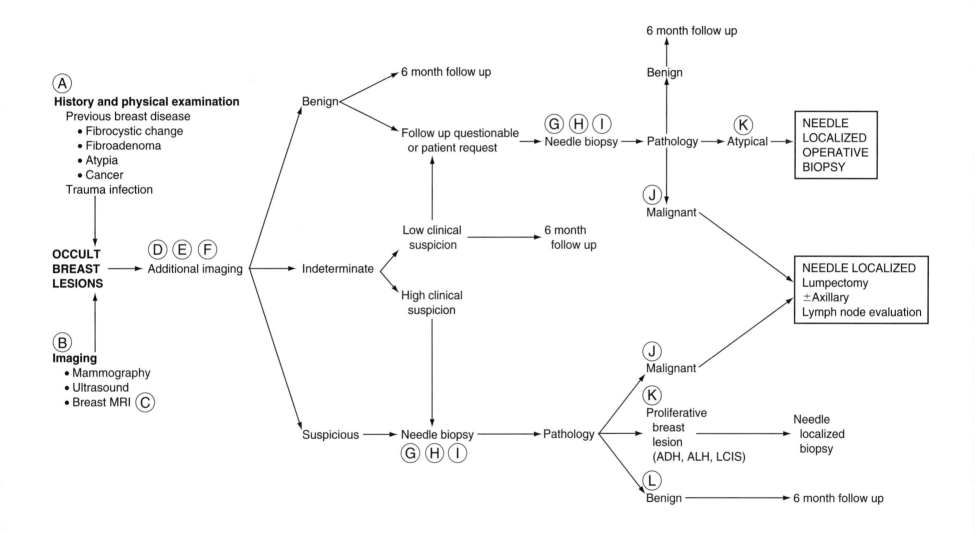

Ⓐ
History and physical examination
Previous breast disease
• Fibrocystic change
• Fibroadenoma
• Atypia
• Cancer
Trauma infection

OCCULT BREAST LESIONS

Ⓑ
Imaging
• Mammography
• Ultrasound
• Breast MRI Ⓒ

Ⓓ Ⓔ Ⓕ
Additional imaging

Benign
6 month follow up
Follow up questionable or patient request

Indeterminate
Low clinical suspicion → 6 month follow up
High clinical suspicion

Suspicious → Needle biopsy
Ⓖ Ⓗ Ⓘ
→ Pathology

Ⓖ Ⓗ Ⓘ
Needle biopsy → Pathology → Atypical Ⓚ

Benign → 6 month follow up

Ⓙ
Malignant

NEEDLE LOCALIZED OPERATIVE BIOPSY

NEEDLE LOCALIZED
Lumpectomy
±Axillary
Lymph node evaluation

Ⓙ
Malignant

Ⓚ
Proliferative breast lesion (ADH, ALH, LCIS) → Needle localized biopsy

Ⓛ
Benign → 6 month follow up

Chapter 81 *Early Breast Carcinoma*

CHRISTINA A. FINLAYSON, MD

(A) Age is the most important risk factor for the development of breast cancer. Postmenopausal women have a rate of developing breast cancer 17 times higher than that of premenopausal women.

(B) Risk factors for breast cancer development include a family history of breast or ovarian cancer, particularly in first-degree relatives. Previous breast biopsies, particularly if the pathology was atypical ductal, or lobular hyperplasia or lobular carcinoma in situ, increase the risk of the future development of breast cancer. Lesser risk factors are early menarche, late menopause, nulliparity, or personal history of previous breast or ovarian cancer of the uterus or ovary. Known mutation of the BRCA I or II genes increases the risk of developing breast cancer substantially, although various mutations have different degrees of penetrance.

(C) Early breast cancer (i.e., T1–2, N0–1, M0) is a disease that can often be treated by breast conservation. Some 80% of breast cancers detected by either mammography or physical examination are early-stage disease.

(D) Screening mammography should begin at age 40 years and be performed annually thereafter. Cancer detected by mammography has an earlier stage with better prognosis than do tumors identified on physical examination. If a cancer presents as a palpable mass, diagnostic mammography evaluates the remainder of the ipsilateral breast as well as the contralateral breast for occult, synchronous lesions that can impact recommendations for therapy.

(E) Ultrasound is useful for further evaluation of mammographic and palpable lesions. It can discriminate cystic vs. solid masses. Ultrasound can be used to direct core biopsy for solid masses.

(F) Minimum staging studies include a chest x-ray, CBC, platelets, and liver function tests. Asymptomatic patients with stage I tumors that are less than 2 cm and with negative lymph nodes are very unlikely to have true positive findings on more extensive studies. Stage II and higher patients may warrant further investigation with CT scan of the chest, abdomen, and pelvis, and a bone scan. PET scanning has not been established as a cost-effective staging tool.

(G) There are a number of genetic and biochemical studies that can be performed on tumor samples. Currently, only estrogen receptor (ER), progesterone receptor (PR), and Her-2-neu amplification provide information that might impact treatment recommendations.

(H) Ductal carcinoma in situ (DCIS, or intraductal carcinoma) is a heterogeneous tumor of varying histology and grade. The primary characteristic of in situ disease is malignant-appearing cells that are confined within the basement membrane of the ductal epithelium. There is no invasion into surrounding breast tissue. Treatment focuses on local control because survival is excellent (greater than 98%).

(I) Early stage invasive breast cancer is defined as stage I and IIA. This includes tumors smaller than 5 cm and axillary lymph nodes that, if they contain metastatic disease, are not matted. There is also no sign of tumor spread to other regional lymph node basins or distant sites.

(J) DCIS can be localized to one area of the breast or it can be widely scattered throughout the breast. If more than one site of disease is present, multifocal disease is localized in one quadrant, whereas multicentric disease is scattered throughout two or more quadrants. Breast conservation can be performed if negative margins of resection can be obtained while preserving breast appearance. If this is not possible, total mastectomy is required. Immediate reconstruction is available for interested women.

(K) Stages I and IIA invasive carcinomas respond to breast conservation or mastectomy with similar survival rates. Successful breast conservation requires removal of the tumor with a margin of normal breast surrounding the lesion, and residual breast tissue is sufficient to provide an acceptable cosmetic outcome. In addition, there should be no contraindications to postoperative radiation therapy. These contraindications include previous radiation therapy to the area and collagen vascular disease.

(L) Total mastectomy is often required for patients with large tumors, particularly if the breast is small; and for patients with multifocal or multicentric disease, or who have contraindications for radiation therapy. Twenty percent of women who have the option of breast conservation will choose mastectomy. Total mastectomy involves removal of the nipple/areolar complex, breast tissue from the clavicle to the inframammary fold, and the fascia of the pectoralis major muscle. If immediate reconstruction is undertaken, a skin-sparing mastectomy can preserve the skin envelope and improve cosmetic outcome without compromising oncologic outcome.

(M) Prospective, randomized studies of DCIS treatment have demonstrated decreased risk of local recurrence if adjuvant radiation is provided after lumpectomy. There is retrospective, uncontrolled data that suggest small, low-grade DCIS excised with negative margins may be treated by surgery alone. Current ongoing clinical trials are being conducted to further clarify the need for radiation in very good prognosis DCIS.

(N) Sentinel lymph node biopsy (SNBx) for invasive breast cancer is used to identify the more than 70% of women who have node-negative disease. If the sentinel lymph node is negative, the remainder of the axillary lymph nodes do not need to be removed. Surgical management of the axillary lymph nodes is currently undergoing significant investigation and change in clinical practice patterns. Axillary lymph node dissection (Ax Dx) is currently recommended if the sentinel lymph node is positive.

(O) The addition of tamoxifen after breast conservation treatment for DCIS decreases the incidence of local recurrence as well as new disease in the contralateral breast.

(P) Chemotherapy can improve relative survival rates by approximately 30%. Women with poor prognosis tumors (e.g., large tumors, node-positive tumors, or ER-negative tumors) have the greatest

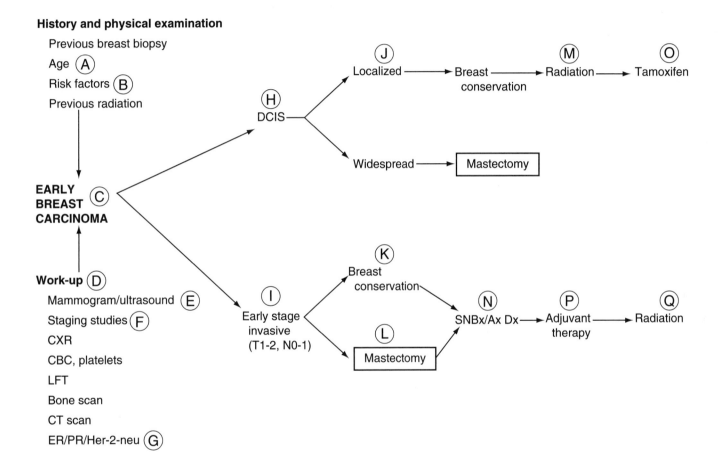

History and physical examination

Previous breast biopsy

Age (A)

Risk factors (B)

Previous radiation

EARLY BREAST CARCINOMA (C)

Work-up (D)

Mammogram/ultrasound (E)

Staging studies (F)

CXR

CBC, platelets

LFT

Bone scan

CT scan

ER/PR/Her-2-neu (G)

(H) DCIS

(J) Localized → Breast conservation → (M) Radiation → (O) Tamoxifen

Widespread → Mastectomy

(I) Early stage invasive (T1-2, N0-1)

(K) Breast conservation

(L) Mastectomy

(N) SNBx/Ax Dx → (P) Adjuvant therapy → (Q) Radiation

absolute benefit from chemotherapy. Women with small, node-negative, good prognosis tumors will have less absolute benefit from chemotherapy because their risk of recurrence is already small. General recommendations for chemotherapy currently include all women with node-positive disease and most women with tumors over 1 cm. Hormonal therapy with tamoxifen or an aromatase-inhibitor can be used alone or in combination with chemotherapy for women who have tumors that are ER positive, particularly if they are postmenopausal.

Q Breast conservation surgery for invasive disease is followed by local radiation therapy to the breast to decrease the incidence of local recurrence. Whole-breast radiation to 5500 cGy has been standard and involves a course of 25 to 30 treatments over a 5- to 6-week period. Brachytherapy radiation is now being used to shorten the treatment time to 1 week or less. Mastectomy is followed by radiation therapy when the tumor is larger than 5 cm, the pectoral muscle has been invaded by tumor, or when four or more axillary lymph nodes contain metastatic disease. There is accruing evidence that radiation therapy for all node-positive patients treated with mastectomy may improve local control and survival.

REFERENCES

Breast Cancer: NCCN Oncology Practice Guidelines. Accessible at: www.nccn.org

Coleman RE: Current and future status of adjuvant therapy for breast cancer. Cancer 97:880–886, 2003.

de Mascarel I, Bonichon F, MacGrogan G et al: Application of the Van Nuys prognostic index in a retrospective series of 367 ductal carcinomas in situ of the breast examined by serial macroscopic sectioning: Practical considerations. Breast Cancer Res Treat 61:151–159, 2000.

Fisher B, Anderson S, Bryant J et al: Twenty-year follow-up of a randomized trial comparing total mastectomy, lumpectomy, and lumpectomy plus irradiation for the treatment of invasive breast cancer. N Engl J Med 347:1233–1241, 2002.

Mokbel K: Towards optimal management of ductal carcinoma in situ of the breast. Eur J Surg Oncol 29:191–197, 2003.

Schwartz GF, Giuliano AE, Veronesi U: Proceedings of the consensus conference on the role of sentinel lymph node biopsy in carcinoma of the breast, April 19-22, 2001, Philadelphia, Pennsylvania. Cancer 94:2542–2551, 2002.

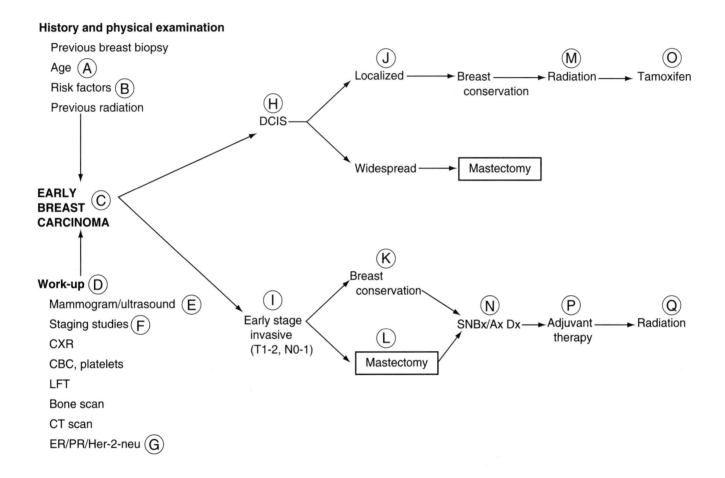

History and physical examination

Previous breast biopsy

Age (A)

Risk factors (B)

Previous radiation

(H)
DCIS

EARLY BREAST CARCINOMA (C)

Work-up (D)

Mammogram/ultrasound (E)

Staging studies (F)

CXR

CBC, platelets

LFT

Bone scan

CT scan

ER/PR/Her-2-neu (G)

(J)
Localized → Breast conservation → (M) Radiation → (O) Tamoxifen

Widespread → Mastectomy

(I)
Early stage invasive (T1-2, N0-1)

(K)
Breast conservation

(L)
Mastectomy

(N)
SNBx/Ax Dx → (P) Adjuvant therapy → (Q) Radiation

Chapter 82 *Advanced Breast Carcinoma*

DOUGLAS E. MERKEL, MD • DAVID P. WINCHESTER, MD

(A) Clinical staging for patients with bulky or advanced disease should include chest x-ray; bone scan; and, if liver enzymes are elevated, computed tomography (CT) of the liver. Although routine bone scan and CT are not indicated in the evaluation of asymptomatic patients with early breast cancer, distant metastases are more often associated with locally advanced disease.

(B) According to the staging system of the American Joint Committee on Cancer, T0 tumors are in situ, T1 tumors are 2.0 cm or less in greatest dimension, T2 tumors are more than 2.0 cm but 5.0 cm or less in greatest dimension, T3 tumors are more than 5.0 cm in greatest dimension, and T4 lesions are any size and have direct extension to the skin or chest wall. Stage T4 includes inflammatory carcinoma. N1 represents metastases to moveable ipsilateral axillary nodes or microscopic involvement of the internal mammary nodes, detected by sentinel lymph node dissection using lymphoscintigraphy but not by imaging studies or clinical examination. N2 represents metastases in ipsilateral axillary lymph nodes (fixed or matted) or in clinically apparent* ipsilateral internal mammary nodes in the absence of clinically evident axillary lymph node metastases. N3a represents metastases in ipsilateral infraclavicular lymph node(s), N3b represents metastases in ipsilateral internal mammary lymph node(s) and axillary lymph node(s), and N3c represents metastasis in ipsilateral supraclavicular lymph node(s).

(C) The algorithm for stage IV or systemic disease presumes that the breast was treated previously and the disease controlled. Locally directed therapy for metastases in addition to systemic therapy is indicated under special circumstances. For example, it is unusual for systemic therapy to

control pleural effusion. Tube thoracostomy and a sclerosing agent may be required. Recurrent effusion can be treated by repeat sclerosis, thoracentesis, parietal pleurectomy, or pleural-peritoneal shunting. Similarly, prophylactic stabilization of bony lesions in high-risk, weight-bearing areas may be indicated in addition to stabilization of fractures.

(D) Core needle biopsy for definitive histological diagnosis and determination of estrogen receptor, progesterone receptor, and HER-2 status is preferred over aspiration cytology or open biopsy.

(E) Mastectomy is the preferred approach for patients with T3 tumors who decline chemotherapy or for whom it is contraindicated.

(F) Neoadjuvant chemotherapy and conventional postoperative adjuvant treatment produce equivalent control of distant micrometastases and equivalent survival rates. Chemotherapy regimens including doxorubicin and docetaxel produce objective responses in a majority of patients. Those with complete responses will have an excellent prognosis, and partial responders may become candidates for lumpectomy.

(G) Neoadjuvant chemotherapy for clinically unresectable breast cancer is given for at least three cycles, or to the point of maximum response. Regimens containing doxorubicin or taxanes are usually employed.

(H) Systemic adjuvant therapy is given to all patients with resected advanced breast cancer. Chemotherapy is indicated for all node-positive or receptor-negative patients, and hormonal therapy is indicated for all receptor-positive patients. Hormonal therapy could consist of ovarian ablation and/or tamoxifen for premenopausal women, and tamoxifen or anastrozole for postmenopausal women.

(I) Laparoscopic oophorectomy or ovarian suppression with gonadotropin-releasing hormone agonists is first-line therapy for this group of patients.

Chemotherapy is added only for patients with more rapidly progressive visceral disease.

(J) The aromatase inhibitors anastrozole and letrozole are more active than tamoxifen and should be considered as first-line systemic therapy. Chemotherapy should be considered only for rapidly progressive visceral metastases.

(K) Adjuvant radiotherapy after mastectomy may improve survival, particularly for women with 4 or more involved axillary lymph nodes, and may also be considered for high-risk premenopausal patients with 1 to 3 involved nodes.

(L) Lumpectomy should be considered for patients with T3 tumors who respond to neoadjuvant chemotherapy. Overall survival is identical, but local recurrence is more common than for patients with T1-T2 tumors.

(M) The optimal sequence for administering systemic adjuvant therapy and radiotherapy following successful cytoreduction and resection of stage III disease has not been determined. The relative risk for local or distant sites of first relapse should determine the order in which these modalities are administered.

---

*Clinically apparent is defined as detected by imaging studies (excluding lymphoscintigraphy) or by clinical examination or pathologically grossly visible.

REFERENCES

Adjuvant therapy for breast cancer. NIH Consens Statement 17(4):1–23, 2000.

Baum M, Budzar AU, Cuzick J.: Anastrozole alone or in combination with tamoxifen versus tamoxifen alone for adjuvant treatment of postmenopausal women with early breast cancer: First results of the ATAC randomised trial. Lancet 359:2131–2139, 2002.

Attia-Sobol J, Ferriere J-P, Cure H et al: Treatment results, survival, and prognostic factors in 109 inflammatory breast cancers. Eur J Cancer 29A:1081–1088, 1993.

Bonadonna G, Veronesi U, Brambilla C et al: Primary chemotherapy to avoid mastectomy in tumors with diameters of 3 centimeters or more. J Natl Cancer Inst 82: 1539–1545, 1990.

De Lena M, Zucali R, Viganotti G et al: Combined chemotherapy-radiotherapy approach in locally advanced (T3-b-4) breast cancer. Cancer Chemother Pharmacol 1:53–59, 1978.

Fisher ER, Wang J, Bryant J et al: Pathobiology of preoperative chemotherapy. Cancer 95:681–695, 2002.

Hery M, Namer M, Moro M et al: Conservative treatment (chemotherapy/radiotherapy) of locally advanced breast cancer. Cancer 57:1744–1749, 1986.

Hortobagyi GN, Ames FC, Buzdar AV et al: Management of stage III primary breast carcinoma with primary chemotherapy, surgery, and radiation therapy. Cancer 62:2507–2516, 1988.

Olson JE, Neuberg D, Pandya KJ: The role of radiotherapy in the management of operable locally advanced breast carcinoma. Cancer 79:1138–1149, 1997.

Perlo FFM, Lesnick GJ, Korzun A et al: Combination chemotherapy with mastectomy or radiotherapy for stage III breast carcinoma: A Cancer and Leukemia Group B study. J Clin Oncol 6:261–269, 1988.

Schwartz GF, Birchansky CA, Komarnicky LT et al: Induction chemotherapy followed by breast conservation for locally advanced carcinoma of the breast. Cancer 73:362–369, 1994.

Touboul E, Buffat L, Lefranc J-P: Possibility of conservative local treatment after combined chemotherapy and preoperative irradiation for locally advanced noninflammatory breast cancer. Int J Radiat Oncol Biol Phys 34:1019–1028, 1996.

Veronisi U, Bonadonna G, Zurrida S et al: Conservation surgery after primary chemotherapy in large carcinomas of the breast. Ann Surg 222:612–618, 1995.

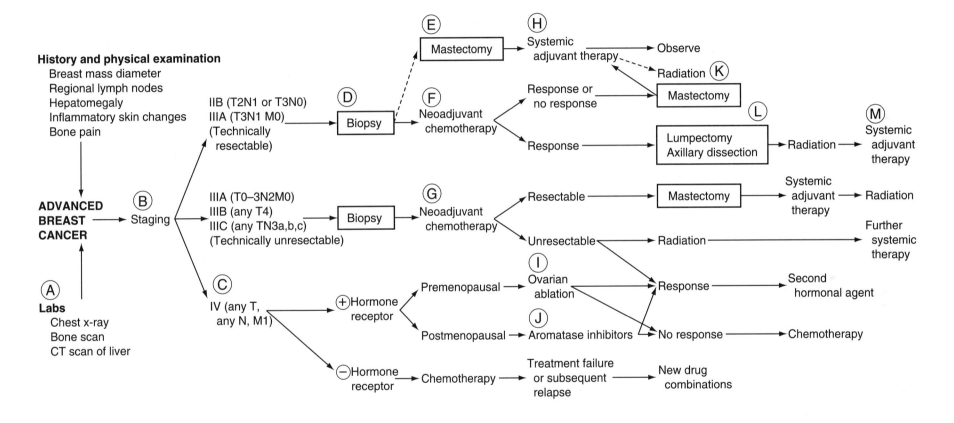

Chapter 83 *Recurrent Breast Carcinoma*

MAUREEN CHUNG, MD, PHD • BLAKE CADY, MD

(A) Recurrent breast cancer can be divided into local (breast), regional (axilla), and systemic recurrences. Local and regional recurrences are an indication of the biology of the disease and do not alter survival. Systemic recurrences have a significant impact on outcome and are a major determinant of survival.

Patients who develop a local (breast) recurrence within the first 3 years after initial diagnosis are more likely to have a recurrence of the original cancer. Patients who recur within the breast more than 5 years after initial diagnosis are more likely to have developed a new primary. Local recurrence after mastectomy is more ominous than that after breast conservation.

(B) All lesions thought to be breast cancer recurrences should be biopsied utilizing fine-needle aspiration (FNA), core needle biopsy (CNB), or open surgical biopsy. An exception might be the presence of multiple bone metastases in a typical pattern, where biopsy may be more difficult and painful. Estrogen and progesterone receptor proteins should be measured on the recurrent lesion even if this has been done previously because hormone receptor status may differ from the primary tumor status in 25% to 35% of patients.

(C) The primary determinants of treatment of locally recurrent breast carcinoma are the nature of the previous treatments, the site and extent of disease recurrence, and the interval from primary diagnosis to recurrent disease. Local recurrence, particularly after mastectomy, is an indication of the poor biology of the disease and patients should be considered for a metastatic evaluation. The most likely sites of distant disease are the bone, lungs, and liver, and the appropriate imaging studies should be ordered.

(D) Patients who develop distant metastases before or concurrent with local-regional failure should be offered chemotherapy or hormone therapy. They are observed for evidence of advancing local disease or symptoms. Patients with a complete or major response are considered for aggressive local therapy such as chest wall resection. Neither chemotherapy nor hormonal therapy given for local recurrence increases local control or disease-free survival.

(E) Local-regional recurrence after previous mastectomy is associated with a grave prognosis (5- and 10-year disease-free survival rates of 30% and 7%, respectively). Thirty-three percent of patients with local-regional recurrence of breast cancer have concurrent distant metastasis. Complete staging, consisting of chest x-ray, chest CT, bone scan, and liver function tests, should be done. Chest CT may show additional lesions in up to 50% of patients evaluated for local-regional recurrence, including disease in internal mammary nodes, sternal erosion, axillary nodes, and bone metastases.

If LFTs are abnormal, scans of the liver by ultrasound, CT, or magnetic resonance imaging are indicated. Survival patterns vary considerably depending on a number of factors, including size, organ involvement, the number of organs involved, and the disease-free interval. Important palliation usually can be provided with further treatment, and patients may have extended survival.

(F) Data from randomized trials in the United States and Europe indicate that local recurrence after lumpectomy and radiation ranges between 8% to 14% at 20 years of follow-up. Distant metastatic disease that develops before local recurrence in the retained breast is uncommon. Concurrent distant metastases are found in only 5% to 25% of patients; therefore complete staging is not always necessary. Exceptions are symptomatic patients and those whose bone scan or LFT is abnormal.

(G) The local recurrence rate is higher after lumpectomy without radiation than with radiation. Data from the randomized trials indicate that local recurrence may approach 40%, even with radiation therapy, if the cancer was large (Tl_c, T_2) and margins were inadequate. Even if the primary cancer is small (Tl_a, Tl_b), the local recurrence rate is 10% to 15% if the tumor-free margin is less than 1 cm. Local recurrence is low if the primary cancer is small, of low grade, and there is a tumor-free margin of 1 cm or greater.

(H) Total-field radiation should be used for local or regional nodal recurrent breast cancer rather than radiation limited to the specific site of recurrence. Patients previously treated with radiation may require chemotherapy or hormonal treatment. Complete excision of the recurrence may not be necessary because the response of the palpable or measurable lesion is often the best indicator of successful systemic therapy. Many times, chemotherapy produces complete regression with initial drug treatment. Most lesions recur at the site of original disease. The previously dissected axilla should not be radiated unless recurrence is confirmed by biopsy of suspicious nodes.

(I) Patients who recur in the axilla after previous sentinel lymphadenectomy (regional recurrence) should have an axillary node dissection. These patients may be rendered disease free by nodal dissection. Depending on the number of lymph nodes involved, they may be evaluated for adjuvant chemotherapy or hormonal therapy.

(J) Usual treatment for local breast recurrence after lumpectomy and radiation is mastectomy. Conservative re-excision with preservation of the breast may be feasible in one third of patients with small (less than 2 cm), mobile lesions without skin or extensive lymph node involvement or for patients with in situ cancer recurrence. Overall survival rates after local recurrence following lumpectomy and radiation have been reported to be between 45% to 70% at 5 years. These overall survival rates are dependent upon initial tumor size, nodal status, and time interval to recurrence. Breast reconstruction is an option after mastectomy, and

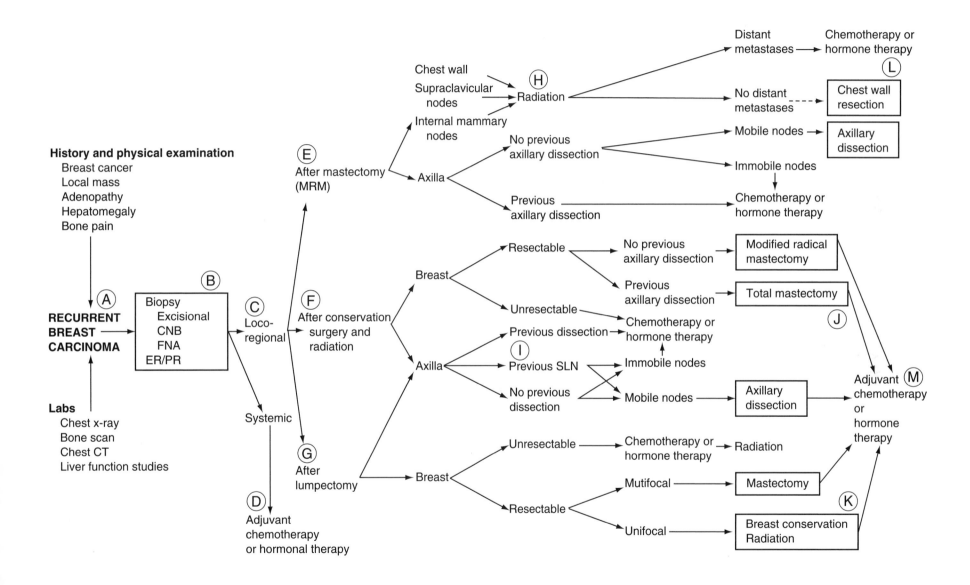

History and physical examination
Breast cancer
Local mass
Adenopathy
Hepatomegaly
Bone pain

RECURRENT BREAST CARCINOMA

Labs
Chest x-ray
Bone scan
Chest CT
Liver function studies

(A)

(B) Biopsy
Excisional
CNB
FNA
ER/PR

(C) Loco-regional

(D) Adjuvant chemotherapy or hormonal therapy

Systemic

(E) After mastectomy (MRM)

Chest wall
Supraclavicular nodes
Internal mammary nodes

(H) Radiation

Distant metastases → Chemotherapy or hormone therapy

No distant metastases

(L) Chest wall resection

Axilla

No previous axillary dissection

Mobile nodes → Axillary dissection

Immobile nodes

Previous axillary dissection → Chemotherapy or hormone therapy

(F) After conservation surgery and radiation

Breast

Resectable

No previous axillary dissection → Modified radical mastectomy

Previous axillary dissection → Total mastectomy

Unresectable → Chemotherapy or hormone therapy

Axilla

Previous dissection → Chemotherapy or hormone therapy

(I) Previous SLN → Immobile nodes

No previous dissection → Mobile nodes → Axillary dissection

(J)

(M) Adjuvant chemotherapy or hormone therapy

(G) After lumpectomy

Breast

Unresectable → Chemotherapy or hormone therapy → Radiation

Resectable

Mutifocal → Mastectomy

Unifocal → Breast conservation Radiation

(K)

this is best done with a rectus abdominis myocutaneous flap in patients who previously had radiation.

(K) Patients who recur in the breast after wide local incision without radiation are more likely to be amenable to breast conservation (up to two-thirds of patients). If the recurrent disease can be excised with a tumor-free margin, whole breast radiation should be used. Patients who recur with multifocal cancer after a lumpectomy should have a mastectomy. If the lymph nodes have not been evaluated at the time of lumpectomy, they should be evaluated with a sentinel lymphadenectomy or axillary node dissection to determine nodal status.

(L) Some patients benefit from chest wall resection for advanced or persistent local chest wall recurrence. Even those with large, isolated recurrences may have prolonged survival after resection. Local control is possible for most patients. The presence of distant metastases is not, in itself, a contraindication to local resection, but the procedure should generally be reserved for those expected to survive at least a year or for those with fungating, ulcerated, infected, or bleeding masses.

(M) The usefulness of adjuvant chemotherapy or hormone therapy after excision of local-regional recurrence has not been evaluated; however, such treatment seems reasonable because local recurrence is an indication of a more aggressive biology of disease and patients have an increased risk of distant metastases. The role of adjuvant systemic treatment for patients who have previously been treated at the time of the primary is also not clear. The use of new cytotoxic treatments may be reasonable.

REFERENCES

Aberizk WJ, Silver B, Henderson IC et al: The use of radiotherapy for treatment of isolated local regional recurrence of breast cancer after mastectomy. Cancer 158:1214–1218, 1986.

Ames FC, Balch CM: Management of local and regional recurrence after mastectomy or breast conserving treatment. Surg Clin North Am 70:1115–1124, 1990.

Bedwinek JM, Lee J, Fineberg B et al: Prognostic indicators in patients with isolated local-regional recurrence of breast cancer. Cancer 47:2232–2235, 1981.

Bedwinek JM, Monroe D, Fineberg B: Local regional treatment of patients with simultaneous local regional recurrence and distant metastases following mastectomy. Am J Clin Oncol 6:295–300, 1983.

Chung M, Steinhoff M, Cady B: Clinical axillary recurrence in breast cancer patients after a negative sentinel node biopsy. Am J Surg 184:310–313, 2002.

Fisher B, Anderson S, Bryant J et al: Twenty-year follow-up of a randomized trial comparing total mastectomy, lumpectomy, and lumpectomy plus irradiation for the treatment of invasive breast cancer. N Engl J Med 347:1233–1241, 2002.

Fisher B, Bryant J, Dignam JJ et al: Tamoxifen, radiation therapy, or both for prevention of ipsilateral breast tumor recurrence after lumpectomy in women with invasive breast cancers of one centimeter or less. J Clin Oncol 20:4141–4149, 2002.

Kurtz JM, Amalric R, Brandone H et al: Results of salvage surgery for mammary recurrence following breast-conserving therapy. Ann Surg 207:347–351, 1987.

Lindfors KK, Meyer JE, Busse PM et al: CT evaluation of local and regional breast recurrence. AJR 145:833–837, 1985.

Mirza NQ, Vlastos G, Meric F et al: Predictors of loco regional recurrence among patients with early-stage breast cancer treated with breast-conserving therapy. Ann Surg Oncol 9:256–265, 2002.

Newman LA, Hunt KK, Buchholz T et al: Presentation, management and outcome of axillary recurrence from breast cancer. Am J Surg 180: 252–256, 2000.

Osteen RT, Smith BL: Results of conservative surgery and radiation for breast cancer. Surg Clin North Am 70:1005–1021, 1990.

Recht A, Hayes DF: Specific Sites of Metastatic Disease and Emergencies: Local Recurrence. In Harris JR, Helman S, Henderson IC et al (eds): Breast Diseases, 2nd ed. Philadelphia: JB Lippincott, 1991.

Veronesi U, Caseinelli N, Mariani L et al: Twenty-year follow-up of a randomized study comparing breast-conserving surgery with radical mastectomy for early breast cancer. N Engl J Med 347:1227–1232, 2002.

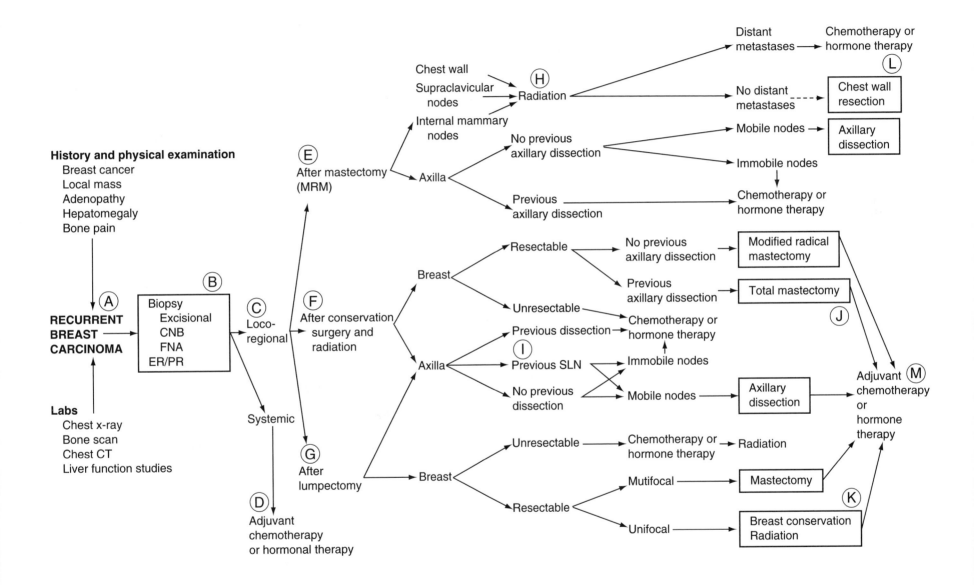

History and physical examination
Breast cancer
Local mass
Adenopathy
Hepatomegaly
Bone pain

Labs
Chest x-ray
Bone scan
Chest CT
Liver function studies

(A) **RECURRENT BREAST CARCINOMA**

(B) Biopsy
Excisional
CNB
FNA
ER/PR

(C) Loco-regional

(E) After mastectomy (MRM)

Chest wall
Supraclavicular nodes
Internal mammary nodes
(H) Radiation

Distant metastases → Chemotherapy or hormone therapy

No distant metastases ---- (L) Chest wall resection

Axilla

No previous axillary dissection → Mobile nodes → Axillary dissection

Immobile nodes

Previous axillary dissection → Chemotherapy or hormone therapy

(F) After conservation surgery and radiation

Breast
Resectable → No previous axillary dissection → Modified radical mastectomy

Previous axillary dissection → Total mastectomy (J)

Unresectable → Chemotherapy or hormone therapy

Axilla
Previous dissection → Chemotherapy or hormone therapy
(I) Previous SLN → Immobile nodes
No previous dissection → Mobile nodes → Axillary dissection

(G) After lumpectomy

Breast
Unresectable → Chemotherapy or hormone therapy → Radiation

Resectable
Mutifocal → Mastectomy
Unifocal → Breast conservation Radiation (K)

(M) Adjuvant chemotherapy or hormone therapy

Systemic

(D) Adjuvant chemotherapy or hormonal therapy

Chapter 84 Retroperitoneal Mass

FRITZ C. EILBER, MD • MURRAY F. BRENNAN, MD

(A) The initial presentation of patients with a retroperitoneal mass tends to be relatively nonspecific unless the patient has a functional adrenal lesion or a history of a primary malignancy in another location. Common presenting symptoms include a mass, abdominal or back pain, gastrointestinal complaints, and weight loss. Physical examination can vary widely from a normal physical examination to an obvious abdominal or flank mass.

(B) Retroperitoneal masses predominately originate from the mesenchymal soft tissues of the retroperitoneum. Other sites of origin, in decreasing order of frequency, include para-aortic lymph nodes, kidney and adrenal gland, visceral/splanchnic nerves and sympathetic chain, and aorta. The majority of retroperitoneal masses are malignant and the most commonly encountered malignant diagnoses are soft tissue sarcoma (55%), lymphoma (24%), and renal or adrenal tumors (4%). Benign lesions such as adrenocortical adenomas, schwannomas, paragangliomas, benign renal tumors, and other uncommon neoplasms are also found in the retroperitoneum.

(C) Computed tomography (CT) remains the best modality to identify and characterize retroperitoneal masses. The widespread use of abdominal CT to evaluate patients with minimal or no symptoms has made the incidental discovery of masses in the retroperitoneum much more common.

(D) Soft tissue sarcomas are the most common primary retroperitoneal tumors and are usually discovered in the fifth and sixth decades of life. Because of their nonspecific symptoms and physical findings, the majority (71%) of retroperitoneal sarcomas are greater than 10 cm at diagnosis. Histologically, retroperitoneal sarcomas are predominately liposarcomas (42% to 63%) and leiomyosarcomas (19% to 27%). Additional histologic subtypes include malignant fibrous histiocytoma, fibrosarcoma, hemangiopericytoma, and malignant peripheral nerve sheath tumors. Approximately two-thirds of retroperitoneal sarcomas are high grade. CT is critical for diagnosis, staging, and operative planning. Except in low-grade liposarcomas, local involvement of adjacent organs is common, and metastatic spread is primarily to the liver with pulmonary metastases occurring rarely. Treatment is en bloc resection and requires resection of contiguous organs such as the kidney, adrenal, pancreas, spleen, and/or colon in up to 75% of the cases. Eighty percent of primary retroperitoneal sarcomas can be completely resected with an aggressive surgical approach. Unresectability is predominately caused by major vascular involvement, peritoneal implants, and metastatic disease. High histologic grade, unresectable primary tumor, positive gross margin, and stage at presentation are all strongly associated with tumor mortality.

(E) Adrenal masses are discovered incidentally in up to 5% of patients undergoing CT for other indications. Nonfunctioning adenomas account for up to 90% of adrenal lesions, with biochemically active tumors being much less common. Biochemically active tumors, regardless of size, should be removed. These functional tumors (producing hypercortisolism, pheochromocytoma, virilizing or feminizing syndrome, and hyperaldosteronism) can be identified by measuring urine for 24-hour free cortisol, catecholamines, metanephrines, 17-hydroxysteroids, and 17-ketosteroids; and measuring blood for aldosterone-to-renin ratio. Adrenocortical carcinomas are very rare with an annual incidence of approximately 0.5 to 2 cases per million. The probability that an incidentally discovered adrenal mass is malignant is directly related to size. The mean size of adrenal carcinomas at presentation ranges from 12 to 16 cm, with greater than 95% being larger than 6 cm. Although the exact size that necessitates removal of an adrenal "incidentaloma" is controversial, lesions greater than 4 cm should be considered for removal. Both biochemically active and inactive adrenal lesions can be safely removed either laparoscopically or by traditional open techniques. The adrenal gland is a common site for metastases, particularly from lung, breast, and melanoma. CT-guided fine-needle aspiration (FNA) is useful for diagnosing metastasis; however, it should only be done after the possibility of a pheochromocytoma has been excluded.

(F) Because of the variety of histologic types in secondary retroperitoneal tumors, it is necessary to obtain a tissue diagnosis before beginning treatment. CT-guided FNA and core needle biopsies are usually successful in obtaining tissue. Laparoscopic biopsy is an accurate and less morbid alternative to open biopsy after image-guided techniques fail.

(G) Patients with a history of cancer and elevated levels of lactic dehydrogenase (LDH), alpha-fetoprotein (AFP), or β-human chorionic gonadotropin (β-hCG) should be considered for core biopsy. Success of CT-guided core biopsy in making the diagnosis of lymphoma is 87% compared with 70% for FNA. Failure to obtain a tissue diagnosis with these techniques warrants laparoscopic biopsy. In selective situations, resection of isolated metastases is warranted.

(H) Retroperitoneal metastases occur in 10% to 25% of patients with testicular malignancies. Residual embryonic tissue presenting as a primary retroperitoneal mass is exceedingly rare. Serum tumor markers AFP and β-hCG are useful for diagnosis. Absence of a mass on physical examination of the testes should prompt the use of high-resolution scrotal ultrasound for diagnosis.

REFERENCES

Cheah WK, Clark OH, Horn JK et al: Laparoscopic adrenalectomy for pheochromocytoma. World J Surg 26: 1048–1051, 2002.

Comiter CV, Benson CJ, Capelouto CC et al: Nonpalpable intratesticular masses detected sonographically. J Urol 154:1367–1369, 1995.

Eilber FC, Eilber KS, Eilber FR: Retroperitoneal sarcomas. Curr Treat Options Oncol 1:274–278, 2000.

Kebebew E, Siperstein AE, Clark OH et al: Results of laparoscopic adrenalectomy for suspected and unsuspected malignant adrenal neoplasms. Arch Surg 137:948–951, 2002.

Kebebew E, Duh Q-Y: Operative strategies of adrenalectomy. In Doherty GM (ed): Surgical Endocrinology: A Clinical Syndromes Approach. Philadelphia: Lippincott Williams & Wilkins, 2000.

Lewis JJ, Leung D, Woodruff JM et al: Retroperitoneal soft-tissue sarcoma: Analysis of 500 patients treated and followed at a single institution. Ann Surg 228:355–365, 1998.

Quinn SF, Sheley RC, Nelson HA et al: The role of percutaneous needle biopsies in the original diagnosis of lymphoma: A prospective evaluation. J Vasc Interv Radiol 6:947–952, 1995.

Richie JP: Detection and treatment of testicular cancer. CA Cancer J Clin 43:151–175, 1993.

Schulick RD, Brennan MF: Adrenocortical carcinoma. World J Urol 17:26–34, 1999.

Storm FK, Mahvi DM, Hafez GR: Retroperitoneal masses, adenopathy and adrenal glands. Surg Oncol Clin 4:175–184, 1995.

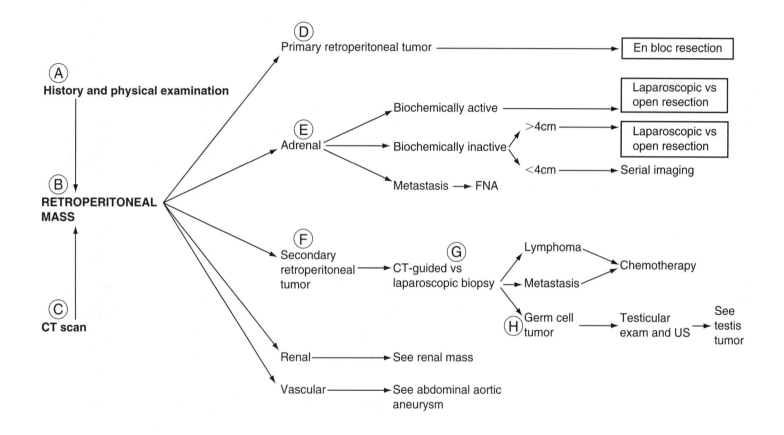

Chapter 85 *Melanoma*

MICHAEL BERGEN, MD • RENE GONZALEZ, MD

(A) The risk of developing melanoma increases with a family history of the disease, with sun exposure, and with a change in the size or appearance of a skin lesion. Pigmented skin changes are evaluated by the ABCDE system for *asymmetry*, irregular *border*, variegation of *color*, *diameter* greater than 6 mm, and *elevation*.

(B) Routine studies such as complete blood count (CBC), chest radiograph, and liver function tests (LFT) are performed routinely but are of unproven value. LDH is of some prognostic value. Detection of metastases before development of symptoms has no proven survival benefit, although some patients do quite well after complete resection of metastatic disease. Imaging studies are helpful only if disseminated disease is suspected.

(C) Early detection and treatment of primary melanoma improves prognosis. Lesions less than 2 cm in diameter should be excised for biopsy. Incisional biopsy is used only for large lesions. Shave biopsy is discouraged when melanoma is suspected because prognosis and survival are closely linked to the depth of the lesion and the width of margins on wide local excisions. Further, this information is used to make recommendations for sentinel lymph node biopsy and for consideration of adjuvant therapy.

(D) The Clark's system of microstaging is based on anatomic depth of lesions and has not correlated with survival as well as Breslow depth. The Breslow system quantifies depth of invasion or thickness of a lesion from the basal lamina, and subsequently is less subjective, easier to use, and correlates more accurately with prognosis than Clark's. The TNM classification and staging were recently revised and now place more emphasis on Breslow depth, ulceration, and the number (rather than dimensions) of lymph node metastases. A new convention was also defined that combines pathologic staging with information gained from intraoperative lymphatic mapping and sentinel lymph node biopsy (SLNB).

(E) Primary tumors that are 4 mm thick carry a high rate of local recurrence and mortality with local treatment alone.

(F) A palpable regional lymph node should be investigated with fine-needle aspiration (FNA) biopsy because open biopsy increases the risk of tumor spillage and subsequent local recurrence.

(G) Fewer than 5% of patients with metastatic melanoma survive 5 years.

(H) SLNB predicts involvement of regional nodes with melanoma and correlates strongly with survival. It must be performed before the wide local excision (WLE) of the primary lesion. SLNB can be used with radionuclide lymphatic mapping to facilitate discovery of the sentinel node. A blue dye and/or a radioisotope is injected around the tumor and followed to the regional node basin by the blue color and/or radioactivity counts. If the node shows no evidence of disease, there is a less than 10% chance that any regional nodes contain melanoma. If the node does have disease, a complete lymph node dissection is usually performed.

(I) Complete surgical excision (tumor-free margins) is the cornerstone of surgical treatment. Current recommendation for adequate margins by thickness of lesion: 0.5 cm for melanoma in situ; 1.0 cm for 0- to 1-mm melanoma; 1 to 2 cm for 1- to 4-mm thick melanomas; and 2 cm for lesions thicker than 4 mm. A margin greater than 1 cm offers no survival benefit but may decrease local recurrence.

(J) Occasionally, patients with a solitary metastasis may have a durable remission following local excision. Candidates for surgery may have skin, lymphatic, pulmonary, cerebral, or small bowel lesions. Stereotactic radiosurgery (also known as Gamma knife) is useful palliation for cerebral metastases. Radiation therapy to bony metastases and masses that are causing vascular or neurologic compression or pain can also be palliative.

(K) Dacarbazine (DTIC) is the standard chemotherapeutic agent, but it provides complete tumor response in fewer than 5% of patients and long-term survival in less than 2%. Multiagent chemotherapy gives higher response rates but does not improve survival. Interleukin-2 (IL-2) is also approved for stage IV melanoma and can produce durable complete responses in a small subset of patients. Biochemotherapy (IL-2, interferon plus chemotherapy) induces durable remissions in approximately 12% of patients but can be quite toxic and is not tolerated by elderly patients or those with significant comorbidities.

(L) Although immediate (prophylactic) regional lymph node dissection does not improve survival, therapeutic radical lymph node dissection appears to benefit patients with one or more positive regional nodes. Limited node dissection is not indicated because of the risk of recurrent, usually fatal, regional disease.

(M) There is little evidence that follow-up improves outcome. Examination includes palpation for local recurrence, in-transit metastases, and lymph nodes. The skin is inspected for new primaries and other skin cancers. A reasonable schedule for follow-up is every 3 to 4 months for 2 years, every 6 months for 3 years, and then yearly. Chest x-ray is obtained annually because the lungs are the most common site of visceral recurrence.

History and physical examination Ⓐ
Family history
Sun exposure
Increasing size
A B C D E system
Regional lymph nodes

SUSPICIOUS PIGMENTED LESION

Labs
CBC Ⓑ
Chest x-ray
LFT
LDH

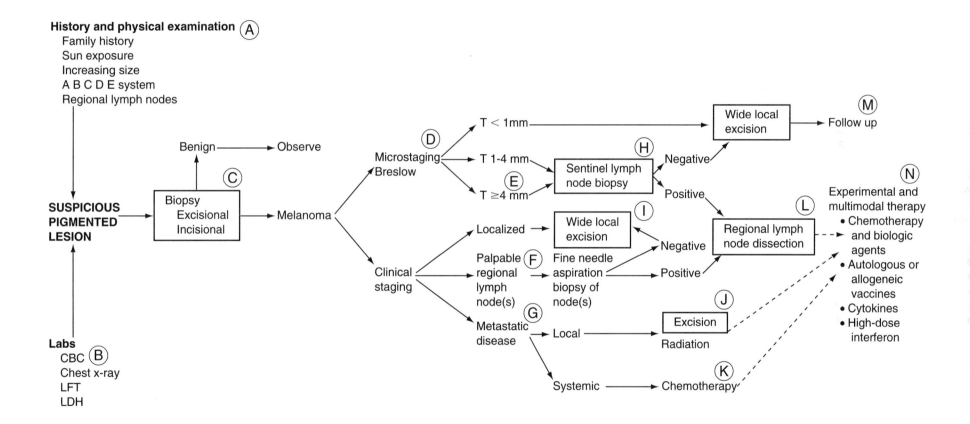

The common failure of therapy fuels the search for new treatments. Despite regional lymph node dissection, mortality in patients with only one involved node exceeds 50%. For patients with stage III melanoma, high-dose α-interferon probably improves disease-free survival but an overall survival advantage is less clear.

REFERENCES

Balch CM, Soong S, Bartolucci AA et al: Efficacy of an elective regional lymph node dissection of 1- to 4-mm thick melanomas for patients 60 years of age and younger. Ann Surg 224:255–263, 1996.

Balch CM, Soong S-J, Gershewald JE et al: Prognostic factor analysis of 17,600 melanoma patients: Validation of the American Joint Committee on Cancer melanoma staging system. J Clin Oncol 19:3622–3634, 2001.

Balch CM, Soong S-J, Ross MI et al: Long-term results of a multi-institutional randomized trial comparing prognostic factors and surgical results for intermediate thickness melanomas (1.0–4.0 mm). Ann Surg Oncol 7:87–97, 2000.

Caprio MG, Carbone G, Bracigliano A et al: Sentinel lymph node detection by lymphoscintigraphy in malignant melanoma. Tumori 88:S43–S45, 2002.

Carcoforo P, Soliani G, Bergossi L et al: Reliability and accuracy of sentinel node biopsy in cutaneous malignant melanoma. Tumori 88:S14–S16, 2002.

Cascinelli W, Belli F, Santinami M et al: Sentinel lymph node biopsy in cutaneous melanoma: The WHO Melanoma Program experience. Ann Surg Oncol 7:469–474, 2000.

Coit DC: Patient Survival and Follow-Up. In Balch CM, Hoaghton AN, Sober AJ et al (eds): Cutaneous Melanoma, 3rd ed. St Louis: Quality Medical Publishing, 1998.

DiBiase SJ, Chin LS, Ma L: Influence of gamma knife radiosurgery on the quality of life in patients with brain metastases. Am J Clin Oncol 25:131–134, 2002.

Lens MB, Dawes M, Goodacre T et al: Excision margins in the treatment of primary cutaneous melanoma: A systematic review of randomized controlled trials comparing narrow vs. wide excision. Arch Surg 137:1101–1105, 2002.

Lens MB, Dawes M: Interferon alpha therapy for malignant melanoma: A systematic review of randomized controlled trials. J Clin Oncol Apr 1:1818–1825, 2002.

Owens SA, Sanders LL, Edwards LJ et al: Identification of higher risk thin melanomas should be based on Breslow depth and not Clark level IV. Cancer 91:983–991, 2001.

Veronesi U, Cascinelli N, Adamus J et al: Thin stage primary cutaneous malignant melanoma: Comparison of excision with margins of 1 or 3 cm. N Engl J Med 318:1159, 1988.

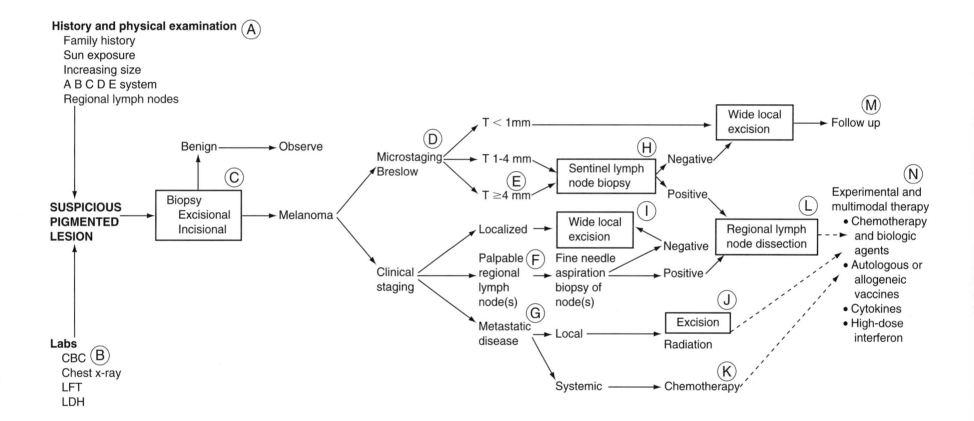

History and physical examination Ⓐ
Family history
Sun exposure
Increasing size
A B C D E system
Regional lymph nodes

SUSPICIOUS PIGMENTED LESION

Labs
CBC Ⓑ
Chest x-ray
LFT
LDH

Biopsy
Excisional
Incisional Ⓒ

Benign → Observe

Melanoma

Microstaging
Breslow Ⓓ

T < 1mm

T 1-4 mm

T ≥4 mm Ⓔ

Sentinel lymph node biopsy Ⓗ

Negative

Positive

Wide local excision

Follow up

Clinical staging

Localized

Palpable regional lymph node(s) Ⓕ

Metastatic disease Ⓖ

Fine needle aspiration biopsy of node(s)

Wide local excision Ⓘ

Negative

Positive

Regional lymph node dissection Ⓛ

Local

Excision Ⓙ
Radiation

Systemic → Chemotherapy Ⓚ

Experimental and multimodal therapy Ⓝ
• Chemotherapy and biologic agents
• Autologous or allogeneic vaccines
• Cytokines
• High-dose interferon

Chapter 86 *Soft Tissue Masses of the Extremities*

C. PARKER GIBBS, JR., MD ● MARK T. SCARBOROUGH, MD

(A) Most patients with an extremity soft tissue mass present with a painless, enlarging mass. A thorough history for syndromes that are associated with malignancies (e.g., Li Fraumeni, Mafucci's, Gardener's, and NF-1) should be taken. Patients often report a history of incidental trauma. This should be explored because significant trauma could indicate an underlying hematoma or myositis ossificans that might be managed with observation alone. Masses that both enlarge and shrink are more likely to be benign cysts originating from joints or tendon sheaths. Skin changes such as café au lait spots and axillary freckling can indicate neurofibromatosis and its associated tumors, both benign and malignant. The presence of an auscultatable bruit or palpable thrill should alert one to the possibility of an underlying aneurysm or arteriovenous malformation. A positive Tinel's sign may herald an underlying nerve sheath tumor or a major nerve juxtaposed to the mass in question. Patients with a longstanding, slowly growing mass are less likely to have a sarcoma than are those with a large, rapidly growing mass. However, it should be noted that some sarcomas (e.g., synovial sarcoma) can exist for years in a relatively indolent state.

The most important clues to the potential malignancy of a mass are its size and depth. Masses that are small (i.e., less than 5 cm) and superficial are likely to be benign. Those masses that are large or deep have significant malignant potential and should be evaluated as such. However, it should be noted that one-third of soft tissue sarcomas are small and superficial.

(B) The vast majority of soft tissue masses of the extremities are benign; however, appropriate evaluation is necessary to identify those that are malignant and thereby maximize the chances of successful limb-sparing surgery and cure (Table 86-1). Inappropriate biopsies and unplanned excisions of soft tissue masses can result in significant morbidity for the patient, including the need for flap coverage and amputation. The use of MRI has revolutionized

---

TABLE 86-1

Common Adult Soft Tissue Sarcomas
Malignant fibrous histiocytoma
Liposarcoma
Leiomyosarcoma
Synovial sarcoma
Malignant peripheral nerve sheath tumor

Common Benign Adult Soft Tissue Tumors
Lipoma
Ganglion cyst
Fibrous histiocytoma
Giant cell tumor of tendon sheath
Hemangioma
Schwannoma
Neurofibroma
Fibromatosis

---

the ability both to identify potentially dangerous neoplasms and to design appropriate surgical management. Biopsy is the final step in the local staging of these neoplasms following complete local evaluation including history, physical examination, and appropriate imaging.

(C) MRI is the standard of care in imaging soft tissue masses of the extremity. It can determine the local extent of disease and proximity to important neurovascular structures. It is essential in planning biopsy placement and subsequent surgical excision. It is often useful in evaluating the response to neoadjuvant radiation therapy or chemotherapy. Magnetic resonance imaging can differentiate between several tissue types, often obviating the need for biopsy. Lipomas have a characteristic bright signal on T1 weighted imaging and suppress with fat saturation sequences. If the diagnosis is made in this manner, the tumor can be either safely excised without biopsy or simply observed. Hemangiomas also have characteristic findings. They usually have serpiginous vascular channels and significant fat content. They occasionally contain flow voids. Aneurysms and pseudoaneurysms will often demonstrate flow artifact, suggesting

angiography as a better diagnostic tool than biopsy. Sarcomas have a nonspecific pattern on MRI. They are usually dark on T1 and bright on T2 sequences. Some have peritumoral edema. Because sarcomas grow in a centripetal fashion and compress the surrounding normal tissue into a pseudocapsule, they often appear encapsulated. This encapsulation in no way suggests indolent behavior. They most often push away major nerves and vascular structures as opposed to invading them.

(D) Subcutaneous masses that are less than 3 cm in greatest diameter and are not fixed to the underlying fascia can probably be excised without imaging, provided they are not immediately adjacent to important neurovascular structures such as in the antecubital or popliteal fossae. The surgeon should not violate the deep fascia because this can be used as the deep margin upon re-excision, should the mass prove to be malignant upon pathologic evaluation.

(E) Larger subcutaneous masses and all deep masses should be imaged with MRI before any surgical intervention. Should MRI not provide a diagnosis, a nonexcisional biopsy should be performed. Most soft tissue masses can be biopsied readily with a core needle under local anesthetic in the clinic, provided a pathologist with experience in mesenchymal tumors is available. Alternatively, fine-needle aspiration has been used successfully in a few large centers, and open incisional biopsy is still the gold standard for providing a diagnosis. An open incisional biopsy also provides an amount of fresh tissue that will allow the molecular diagnostic tests now performed on many soft tissue tumors. Any method of biopsy can leave malignant cells in the biopsy tract. This tract must then be excised at the time of the definitive procedure. Thus it is incumbent upon the surgeon performing the biopsy to have a complete understanding of the potential definitive limb-sparing resection options and the incisions that are required. Biopsy incisions in the extremities should be oriented longitudinally, and

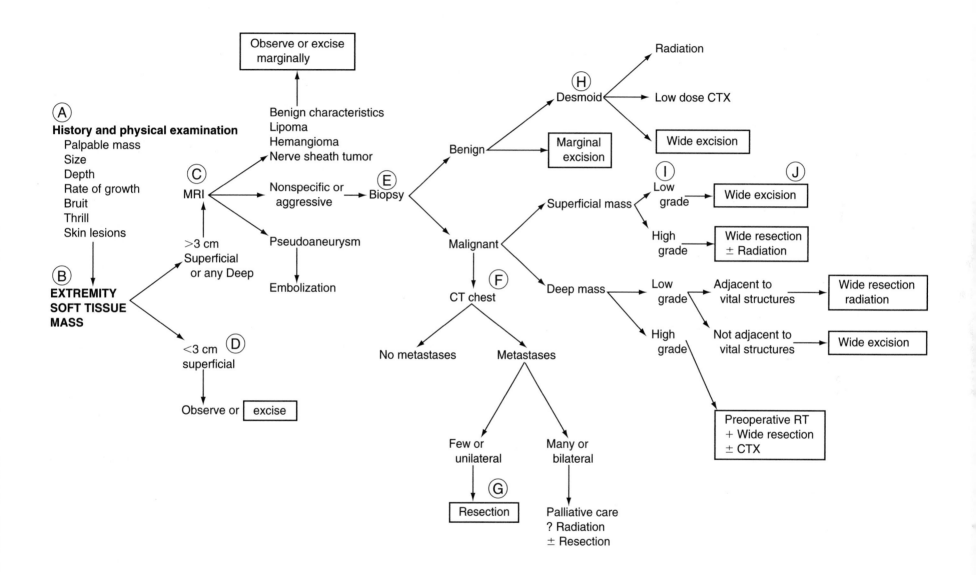

all drains should be brought out in line with and close to the incision to minimize contamination of surrounding tissue. The approach to the tumor should be direct and should not violate other compartments or expose neurovascular bundles. A frozen section should be obtained at the time of all open biopsies to determine that lesional tissue was obtained. Should the frozen section reveal a definitive benign diagnosis, the surgeon may proceed with definitive resection at that time. If, however, a malignant diagnosis is suggested, the surgeon should wait for complete staging before resection.

(F) Staging of soft tissue sarcomas includes the analysis of local imaging, size, depth, histologic grade, and presence of distant metastases. The majority (80%) of sarcoma metastases occur to the lung, and staging studies for most patients should include a CT of the chest. A few sarcomas (e.g., synovial, epithelioid, and rhabdomyosarcoma) can metastasize to lymph nodes and should therefore be staged with a CT of the chest, abdomen, and pelvis. PET scanning has not yet proven to be reliable in the staging of sarcomas.

(G) The treatment of those patients with pulmonary metastases is determined by the site and the number of the metastases. The 3-year survival of those patients with resectable disease is approximately 25%. Prognostic factors related to successful metastasectomy include complete resectability, fewer than five nodules, younger age, and prolonged disease-free interval.

(H) Most benign tumors can be managed with simple marginal excision through the pseudocapsule of the tumor (shelling out) or by observation, if asymptomatic. The exception is the extra-abdominal desmoid tumor (aggressive fibromatosis). This benign tumor behaves aggressively with a high rate of local recurrence even when wide surgical margins are obtained. Numerous authors have recommended radiotherapy alone or combined with surgery for optimal control. There are also reports of successful use of low-dose vinblastine-based chemotherapy in the management of these difficult tumors. The optimal management has not yet been elucidated.

(I) Histologic grade is the most important prognostic variable after presence of metastases. Sarcomas are practically defined as either high or low grade in most staging systems. Large tumors are usually defined as those greater than 5 cm and carry a worse prognosis than do small tumors.

(J) The management of soft tissue sarcomas is independent of the histologic subtype and depends on the grade, size, and depth of the mass as well as the presence or absence of metastases. In general, all sarcomas should be treated with wide local resection to include a zone of normal tissue between the mass and the plane of the resection. The addition of neoadjuvant or adjuvant radiation or chemotherapy depends on the grade, location, and margins obtained. One can divide tumors into superficial and deep types. Superficial low-grade tumors should be resected and do not need radiation or chemotherapy. Superficial high-grade tumors can also be resected without the use of radiation or chemotherapy unless margins are expected to be close, in which case preoperative radiation should be given. This is often the case near joints or major superficial nerves or vessels. Deep tumors are often large because their location allows them to be inconspicuous for a longer time as compared with their superficial counterparts. Low-grade deep tumors not adjacent to bone or neurovascular structures can be resected without the use of adjuvants. Patients with high-grade deep tumors and low-grade tumors near important structures should receive preoperative radiation therapy because this has been shown to greatly reduce the rate of local recurrence. Neoadjuvant or adjuvant chemotherapy can be considered in those patients with large, high-grade, deep tumors who are at especially high risk for distant metastases.

REFERENCES

Billingsley KG, Burt ME, Jara E et al: Pulmonary metastases from soft tissue sarcoma: Analysis of patterns of diseases and postmetastasis survival. Ann Surg 229:602–610, 610–612, 1999.

Janinis J, Patriki M, Vini L et al: The pharmacological treatment of aggressive fibromatosis: A systematic review. Ann Oncol 14:181–190, 2003.

Peabody TD, Monson D, Montag A et al: A comparison of the prognoses for deep and subcutaneous sarcomas of the extremities. J Bone Joint Surg 76-A:1167–1173, 1994.

Gibbs CP, Peabody TD, Mundt AJ et al: Oncological outcomes of operative treatment of subctaneous soft-tissue sarcomas of the extremities. J Bone Joint Surg 79-A:888–897, 1997.

Rydholm A, Berg NO: Size, site and clinical incidence of lipoma: Factors in the differential diagnosis of lipoma and sarcoma. Acta Orthop Scan 54:929–934, 1983.

Skapek SX, Hawk BJ, Hoffer FA et al: Combination chemotherapy using vinblastine and methotrexate for the treatment of progressive desmoid tumor in children. J Clin Oncol 16:3021–3027, 1998.

Tierney JF, Stewart LA, Parmar et al: Adjuvant chemotherapy for localized resectable soft-tissue sarcoma of adults: Meta-analysis of individual analysis. Lancet 350:1647–1654, 1997.

Van Geel AN, Pastorino U, Jauch KW et al: Surgical treatment of lung metastases: The European Organization for Research and Treatment of Cancer-Soft Tissue and Bone Sarcoma Group study of 255 patients. Cancer 77:675–682, 1996.

Virkus WW, Mollabashy A, Reith JD et al: Preoperative radiotherapy in the treatment of soft tissue sarcomas. Clinical Orthopaedic and Related Research 397:177–189, 2002.

Zlotecki RA, Scarborough MT, Morris CG et al: External beam radiotherapy for primary and adjuvant management of aggressive fibromatosis. Int J Radiat Oncol Biol Phys 54:177–181, 2002.

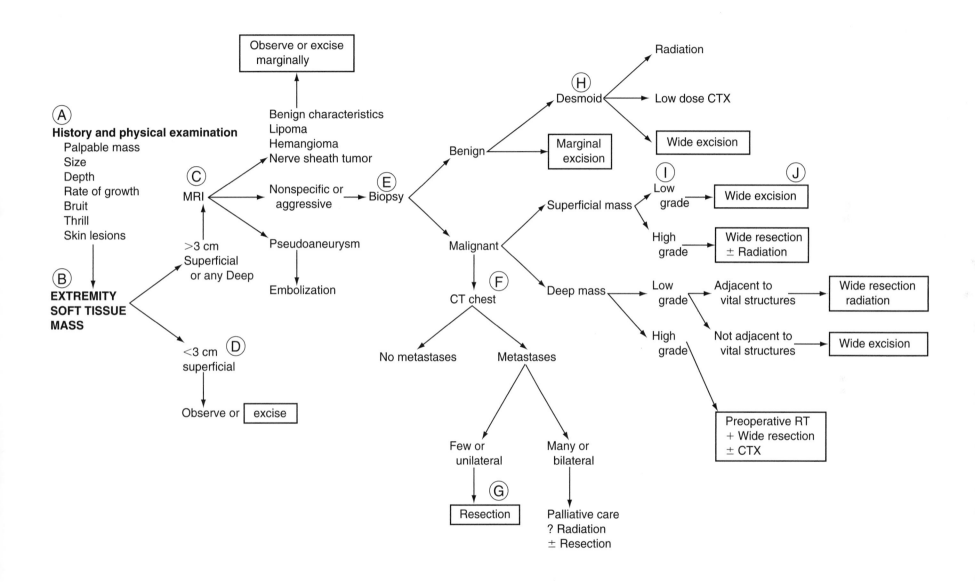

(A)
History and physical examination
Palpable mass
Size
Depth
Rate of growth
Bruit
Thrill
Skin lesions

(B)
EXTREMITY SOFT TISSUE MASS

(C) MRI

>3 cm
Superficial
or any Deep

<3 cm
superficial (D)

Observe or | excise |

Benign characteristics
Lipoma
Hemangioma
Nerve sheath tumor

Observe or excise
marginally

Nonspecific or
aggressive

Pseudoaneurysm

Embolization

(E) Biopsy

Benign

Malignant

Marginal
excision

Desmoid (H)

Radiation

Low dose CTX

Wide excision

CT chest (F)

No metastases

Metastases

Few or
unilateral

Many or
bilateral

Resection (G)

Palliative care
? Radiation
± Resection

Superficial mass

Low
grade (I) → Wide excision (J)

High
grade → Wide resection
± Radiation

Deep mass

Low
grade

High
grade

Adjacent to
vital structures → Wide resection
radiation

Not adjacent to
vital structures → Wide excision

Preoperative RT
+ Wide resection
± CTX

ENDOCRINE

Chapter 87 *Thyrotoxicosis*

BRYAN R. HAUGEN, MD • ROBERT C. MCINTYRE, JR., MD

(A) Thyroid-stimulating hormone (TSH) is the best initial test for suspected thyrotoxicosis. TSH suppression coupled with an elevated tetraiodothyronine (T_4) or triiodothyronine (T_3) value is diagnostic for thyrotoxicosis. Rarely, thyrotoxicosis is associated with normal or elevated TSH caused by a TSH-secreting pituitary tumor or by pituitary resistance to thyroid hormone.

(B) Free T_4 (FT_4) or free T_4 index (FT_4I) is the best measure of thyroid function in a patient with suppressed TSH. Many FT_4 tests are available, but equilibrium dialysis is the gold standard for free hormone. Remember that only 0.03% of T_4 is free and available to tissues, so total T_4 must always be measured with T_3 resin uptake (T_3RU), which reflects the amount of thyroxine-binding globulin. FT_4I, the product of T_4 and T_3RU, estimates the FT_4 level.

(C) After making a diagnosis of thyrotoxicosis (low TSH, high T_4), the radioactive iodine uptake test (RAIU) can differentiate among the many causes of the disorder. Thyroiditis, a destructive thyroid process, is marked by low RAIU because no new hormone is being produced and iodine is trapped. Factitious thyrotoxicosis, caused by excess exogenous T_4, also has a low RAIU that is caused by suppressed TSH and suppressed endogenous production of T_4. The Jod-Basedow phenomenon is hyperthyroidism caused by excess iodine (e.g., in contrast medium for computed tomography [CT] or angiography) presented to a nodular thyroid. The excess iodine blocks uptake of radioiodine and causes a low RAIU.

(D) Normal FT_4 or FT_4I with low TSH is not uncommon. The euthyroid "sick" syndrome, or nonthyroidal illness (NTI), commonly causes this biochemical picture during acute illness (e.g., trauma, burn, surgery, febrile illness, or myocardial infarction). These patients commonly have a normal FT_4, low total T_4, low T_3, and elevated reverse T_3 owing to altered deiodination of T_4. Subclinical hyperthyroidism, which is considered to be mild thyrotoxicosis with suppressed TSH and normal FT_4, can be caused by the same disorders as clinical thyrotoxicosis and should be considered if the patient is symptomatic or has a palpably abnormal thyroid. A total T_3 value should be obtained in a clinically thyrotoxic patient with a suppressed TSH and normal or low T_4 to evaluate for T_3 thyrotoxicosis.

(E) Hyperthyroidism, autonomous production of T_4 by the thyroid gland, is confirmed by suppressed TSH, elevated T_4, and elevated RAIU. A radioiodine scan can distinguish among types of hyperthyroidism caused by Graves' disease, toxic multinodular goiter (TMNG), or a solitary toxic nodule.

(F) Toxic thyroid nodules are best treated by surgery (lobectomy or subtotal thyroidectomy) or radioiodine (^{131}I). Antithyroid drug therapy (ATD) with propylthiouracil (PTU) or methimazole (MMI) is not recommended for long-term therapy for patients with toxic nodules. Ethanol injection under ultrasound guidance has become a popular and effective approach for the treatment of autonomous thyroid nodules in Europe, but it is rarely used in the United States. β-blockers can be used for symptomatic relief (e.g., of tachycardia or tremulousness) of thyrotoxicosis of all causes.

(G) ATD therapy is associated with a high rate of recurrence and is usually reserved for patients with mild hyperthyroidism and a small gland (40 g or less). Complications of ATD therapy include agranulocytosis (0.3%) and liver damage (less than 0.1%). PTU is the preferred therapy for pregnant women, although near-total thyroidectomy is useful in the second trimester.

(H) An adequate single dose of radioiodine produces remission in approximately 90% of Graves' patients. Hypothyroidism occurs in 50% to 80% of patients depending on the dose. Repeat doses can be given if hyperthyroidism recurs. The rates of thyroid cancer, secondary malignancies, and genetic damage are not increased by repeated radioiodine doses used to treat Graves' disease, even after 50 years of observation.

(I) Near-total thyroidectomy (leaving 1 to 2 g of tissue) is the best means of achieving euthyroidism in patients with large glands. Compared to subtotal thyroidectomy, near-total thyroidectomy avoids worsening of antithyroid autoimmunity and recurrence of hyperthyroidism. Surgery is indicated for the following: (1) patients who are unresponsive to or refuse radioiodine therapy; (2) women in the second trimester of pregnancy who are allergic to ATD or in whom ATD has failed; and (3) patients with severe hyperthyroidism and significant Graves' eye disease. Preparation for surgery includes treatment with ATD (if not allergic) for 2 weeks, β-blockers, and potassium iodide for 3 to 5 days. Complications of thyroidectomy for hyperthyroidism include mortality (0.3%), permanent hypoparathyroidism (1% to 3%), vocal cord paresis (less than 1%), and hemorrhage (2%).

REFERENCES

Fisher JN: Management of thyrotoxicosis. S Med J 95:493–505, 2002.

Franklyn JA: The management of hyperthyroidism. N Engl J Med 330:1731–1737, 1994.

Kang AS, Grant CS, Thompson GB et al: Current treatment of nodular goiter with hyperthyroidism (Plummer's disease): Surgery versus radioiodine. Surgery 132:916–923, 2002.

Miccoli P, Vitti P, Rago T et al: Surgical treatment of Graves' disease: Subtotal or total thyroidectomy? Surgery 120:1020–1024, 1996.

Monzani F, Caraccio N, Goletti O et al: Treatment of hyperfunctioning thyroid nodules with percutaneous ethanol injection: Eight years' experience. Exp Clin Endo Diab 106:S54–S58, 1998.

Singer PA, Cooper DS, Levy EG et al: Treatment guidelines for patients with hyperthyroidism and hypothyroidism.

Standards of Care Committee, American Thyroid Association. JAMA 273:808–812, 1995.

Soreide JA, van Heerden JA, Lo CY et al: Surgical treatment of Graves' disease in patients younger than 18 years. World J Surg 20:794–800, 1996.

Torring O, Tallstedt L, Wallin G et al: Graves' hyperthyroidism: Treatment with antithyroid drugs, surgery, or radioiodine: A prospective, randomized study. Thyroid Study Group. J Clin Endocrinol Metab 81:2986–2993, 1996.

Weetman AP: Graves' disease. N Engl J Med 343:1236–1248, 2000.

Witte J, Goretzki PE, Dotzenrath C et al: Surgery for Graves' disease: Total versus subtotal thyroidectomy—results of a prospective randomized trial. World J Surg 24:1303–1311, 2000.

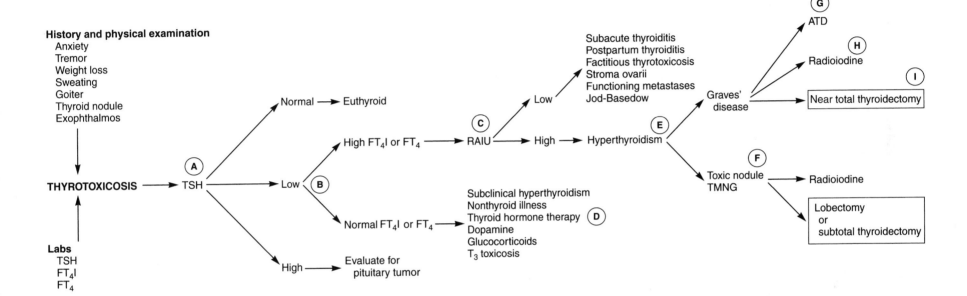

Chapter 88 *Thyroid Nodule*

ROBERT C. MCINTYRE, JR., MD • BRYAN R. HAUGEN, MD

(A) Important features of the history include age, sex, recent growth, local symptoms (e.g., stridor, dysphagia, and voice changes), other cervical masses, a history of radiation exposure, and a family history of thyroid disease. Clinical features suggesting carcinoma include a hard, fixed mass; hoarseness; and cervical lymphadenopathy. Symptoms of thyroid dysfunction should also be investigated.

(B) The examiner should determine the size and consistency of the nodule, fixation to surrounding tissues (by observing mobility on swallowing), and cervical lymphadenopathy.

(C) A screening serum thyroid-stimulating hormone (TSH) level should be obtained in all patients. A low TSH suggests thyrotoxicosis (see Chapter 87). A thyroxine (T_4) assay and thyroid scan should be performed. A high TSH suggests hypothyroidism or a rare pituitary tumor.

(D) Fine-needle aspiration (FNA) biopsy is the single most important diagnostic test for the evaluation of a thyroid nodule. This test predicts the need for surgery better than either ultrasound (US) or scintigraphy. Like US, FNA can determine if a nodule is solid or cystic. Solitary thyroid nodules and dominant nodules in a multinodular gland carry the same risk of cancer (5% to 10%) and should be biopsied. Unsatisfactory FNA biopsies should be repeated. Good technique and experience decrease the number of unsatisfactory FNA results. In most patients, the US and scan are unnecessary tests and only increase the cost of the evaluation. US determines the size of a nodule, can reveal nonpalpable nodules (50% in patients with solitary nodule on examination), and can be used to biopsy small nodules that are difficult to palpate. A thyroid scan can determine if a nodule is functioning.

(E) Benign thyroid nodules rarely respond to thyroid hormone therapy. If the serum TSH is elevated (greater than 2.5 to 3 mU/L), a trial of thyroid hormone therapy may be warranted (with a TSH goal 0.1 to 0.5 mU/L). A repeat biopsy is done at 6 to 12 months to confirm that a nodule is benign.

(F) Follicular neoplasms by FNA may be a follicular adenoma or a follicular carcinoma (20% to 30% risk of carcinoma). Like FNA, frozen section is unable to differentiate adenoma from carcinoma. Lobectomy and isthmusectomy or near total thyroidectomy are surgical options.

(G) Cytologic features suspicious for papillary carcinoma include a highly cellular aspirate with scant colloid; papillary structures; cellular pleomorphism and overlapping, nuclear inclusion bodies; and intranuclear grooves. Patients with minimal papillary cancer (younger than 45 years, less than 2 cm, no local invasion, no metastasis) may be treated with lobectomy and isthmusectomy. Others should have near-total thyroidectomy.

(H) Atypical, spindle-shaped cells on FNA should raise suspicion of medullary thyroid carcinoma (MTC). A calcitonin level should be obtained before thyroidectomy is undertaken. Patients with MTC require total thyroidectomy, and central neck and ipsilateral modified neck dissection. Contralateral modified neck dissection may also be necessary.

(I) If the fluid is cytologically benign and the cyst disappears with aspiration, the patient should be followed by clinical examination. Cysts that recur after two or three FNA should be treated by thyroidectomy. If the nodule fails to disappear, FNA of the remaining solid component should be performed. US may be useful to direct biopsy of solid components.

REFERENCES

Brooks AD, Shaha AR, DuMornay W et al: Role of fine-needle aspiration biopsy and frozen section analysis in the surgical management of thyroid tumors. Ann Surg Oncol 8:92–100, 2001.

Castro M, Caraballo P, Morris J: Effectiveness of thyroid hormone suppressive therapy in benign solitary thyroid nodules: A meta-analysis. J Clin Endocrinol Metab 87:4154–4159, 2002.

Chen H, Zeiger MA, Clark DP et al: Papillary carcinoma of the thyroid: Can operative management be based solely on fine-needle aspiration? J Am Coll Surg 184:605–610, 1997.

Fleming J, Lee J, Bouvet M et al: Surgical strategy for the treatment of medullary thyroid carcinoma. Ann Surg 230:697–707, 1999.

Gharib H, Goellner JR: Fine-needle aspiration biopsy of the thyroid: An appraisal. Ann Intern Med 118:282–289, 1993.

Hay ID, Grant CS, Bergstralh EJ et al: Unilateral total lobectomy: Is it sufficient surgical treatment for patients with AMES low-risk papillary thyroid carcinoma? Surgery 124:958–964, 964–966, 1998.

Mazzaferri EL: Management of a solitary thyroid nodule. N Engl J Med 328:553–559, 1993.

Mazzaferri EL, Kloos R: Current approaches to primary therapy for papillary and follicular thyroid cancer. J Clin Endocrinol Metab 86:1447–1463, 2001.

Moley JF, DeBenedetti MK: Patterns of nodal metastases in palpable medullary thyroid carcinoma: Recommendations for extent of node dissection. Ann Surg 229:880–887, 1999.

Singer PA, Cooper DS, Daniels GH et al: Treatment guidelines for patients with thyroid nodules and well-differentiated thyroid cancer: American Thyroid Association. Arch Intern Med 156:2165–2172, 1996.

Stojadinovic A, Hoos A, Ghossein RA et al: Hurthle cell carcinoma: A 60-year experience. Ann Surg Oncol 9:197–203, 2002.

Udelsman R, Westra WH, Donovan PI et al: Randomized prospective evaluation of frozen-section analysis for follicular neoplasms of the thyroid. Ann Surg 233:716–722, 2001.

History and physical examination
Age (A)
Sex
Growth
Toxicity
Stridor
Dysphagia
Hoarse
Radiation
Family history

THYROID NODULE

Exam
Size
Consistency (B)
Fixation
Lymphadenopathy

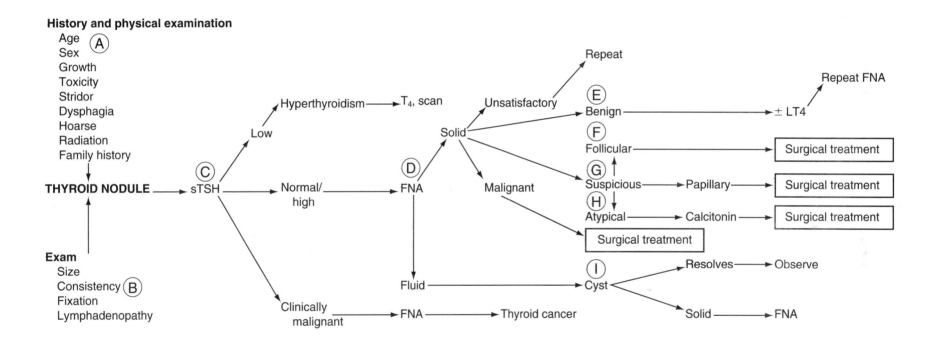

Chapter 89 *Thyroid Carcinoma*

CLIVE S. GRANT, MD

Ⓐ Four percent of the adult population of the United States has clinical thyroid nodules; fewer than 5% of these nodules are malignant. Approximately 17,000 new cases of thyroid cancer are diagnosed annually, making up 90% of all endocrine malignancies. Thyroid cancer is responsible for more deaths than all other endocrine cancers combined. Thyroid cancers derive primarily from follicular cells (i.e., papillary, follicular, Hürthle cell, and anaplastic) and parafollicular or C-cells.

Ⓑ About 25% of adult patients who had neck radiation in childhood have a palpable thyroid nodule. Of these, about a third (8.5% overall) have thyroid cancer, which may be occult and separate from the nodule. Although some clinicians advise total thyroidectomy for all irradiated patients with a nodule, conclusive data to support this advice are lacking.

Ⓒ A hot nodule on scintigraphy essentially excludes the chance of malignancy.

Ⓓ Fine-needle aspiration (FNA) is a safe, reliable, inexpensive, expedient, minimally invasive, and virtually risk-free technique for diagnosing thyroid nodules. Although this technique requires experience in thyroid FNA and an expert cytopathologist, it has become the standard of care in thyroid nodule diagnosis.

Ⓔ After a preoperative FNA finding of "positive" or "highly suspicious" for papillary or medullary thyroid carcinoma, cervical ultrasonography (US) is performed to image lateral jugular nodes. If they appear to be involved (e.g., are enlarged, rounded, containing microcalcifications, or cystic), node biopsy is performed. Positive histology prompts modified neck dissection.

Ⓕ Biochemical screening for medullary thyroid carcinoma (MTC) or C-cell hyperplasia provides early detection and reduces morbidity and mortality.

Ⓖ Mutation screening of RET proto-oncogene will discover 85% to 95% of inherited MTC (i.e., MEN2a, MEN 2b, and familial MTC).

Ⓗ With low-risk cancers, defined by classification systems such as the AMES (*age* of patient, presence of distant *m*etastatic lesions, and *extent* and *size* of the primary cancer), AGES (patient *age* and tumor *grade*, *extent*, and *size*), TNM (*tumor* characteristics, lymph *n*ode involvement, and distant *m*etastatic lesions), or MACIS (*m*etastatic lesions, patient *age*, *completeness* of resection, *invasion*, and *size* of tumor), 10- and 20-year survival rates approach 100%. For high-risk papillary thyroid cancer the 10-year survival may be only 40%.

Ⓘ Approximately 80% of follicular and Hürthle cell neoplasms by FNA prove to be benign by histology. Any papillary component of an otherwise follicular-appearing cancer behaves like and is classified as a papillary carcinoma. Follicular carcinomas are usually single, unilateral, and metastasize via the bloodstream rather than lymphatics. Prognosis correlates with patient age, degree of tumor invasion and presence of metastases, and tumor size. Hürthle cell cancers are best subclassified under follicular cancer, although lymph node metastases occur in about 25% of these patients. Ten-year and 20-year survival rates are both in the 90% to 95% range.

Ⓙ Family members of patients with medullary carcinoma should be screened for genetically caused MTC. Up to 20% may be index cases for this autosomal dominant disease. Because MTC is expressed in virtually 100% of hereditary MTC, the presence of a RET proto-oncogene mutation is sufficient to recommend thyroidectomy. For patients with MEN 2A, thyroidectomy should generally be undertaken by about age 5 to 6 years. For children with MEN 2B, thyroidectomy should be performed as soon as is considered safe. Approximately 75% are sporadic and 25% are hereditary. Characteristic cytologic features of MTC may be supplemented by immunostaining for calcitonin. Whereas total thyroidectomy and central neck lymphadenectomy is standard practice, the indications for lateral neck

dissection remain controversial. If disease is confined to the thyroid, 5- and 10-year survival rates are at least 97%. With higher stage disease, the 5-year survival rate is 65%. Postoperative elevation of calcitonin (and CEA) indicates residual disease whose biologic behavior ranges from indolent to aggressive.

Ⓚ There is no curative treatment for anaplastic thyroid cancer. Preoperative radiotherapy may permit palliative resection. Few patients survive 5 years.

Ⓛ With tumor in the thyroid only, the 5-year survival rate is 86%. When the tumor is extrathyroid, 5-year survival is 38%.

Ⓜ Nearly total thyroidectomy implies total lobectomy on the side of the cancer and contralateral subtotal or nearly total lobectomy, leaving only enough thyroid to protect the parathyroid vascular supply. Although controversial, this minimizes recurrent laryngeal nerve damage and hypoparathyroidism while excising multicentric lesions, facilitating radioiodine (^{131}I) ablation, and minimizing local recurrence in the thyroid.

Ⓝ Excision may be impossible. Debulking has questionable value. Tracheostomy may be required.

Ⓞ Dissection of the lateral internal jugular vein nodes from the base of the neck to the level of the hyoid bone or digastrics muscle may be necessary. The jugular vein, sternocleidomastoid muscle, and spinal accessory nerve are preserved, constituting a modified radical neck dissection.

Ⓟ Thyroid-stimulating hormone (TSH) levels are maximally stimulated after near-total or total thyroidectomy when T_4 has been withdrawn for 6 weeks, T_3 for 2 weeks, or after serial injections of recombinant human TSH (rhTSH). This new agent has been FDA approved for radioiodine scanning. It may be used in lieu of thyroid hormone withdrawal, often in conjunction with measurements of thyroglobulin (Tg) in follicular-cell thyroid cancer follow-up. ^{131}I thyroid remnant ablation has

History and physical examination
Thyroid nodule (A)
Neck node(s)
Paralyzed cord
Previous neck radiation (B)

**THYROID
CARCINOMA**

Labs

Chest x-ray

T_4

131I scan (C)

FNA cytology (D)

Ultrasound (E)

Calcitonin (F)

RET protooncogene (G)

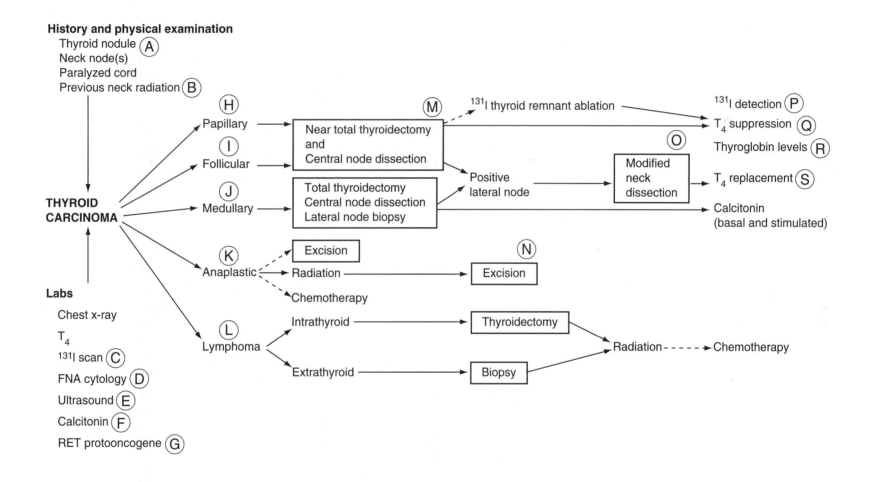

not proved to either diminish recurrence or prolong survival, but its use is reasonably supported in the literature and widely used in the United States and Europe. ^{131}I is useful for follow-up cancer detection.

^{131}I Doses for Scintigraphy and Therapy

Cervical scan	1 mCi
Whole-body scan	3 mCi
Thyroid remnant ablation	30 mCi
Metastasis therapy	100–200 mCi

Thyroid Hormone Doses

Short term	Cytomel (T$_3$), 25 µg PO twice a day
Long term	Synthroid (T$_4$) 0.125–0.3 mg/day PO

(Q) Experimental and clinical evidence support lifelong thyroid hormone suppression postoperatively for patients with papillary or follicular carcinoma.

(R) After elimination of thyroid tissue by total thyroidectomy or by a combination of surgical resection and radioactive ^{131}I ablation, increased Tg levels can be useful indicators of metastatic papillary or follicular cancer. Tg should be less than 2 ng/ml after successful thyroidectomy and postoperative radioiodine remnant ablation. Serum Tg concentrations are most reliable when serum TSH levels are high, either after levothyroxine withdrawal or utilizing rhTSH injections. When Tg antibodies are present, Tg measurements are unreliable.

(S) Thyroid hormone replacement therapy is necessary after total thyroidectomy for medullary carcinoma.

REFERENCES

Cobin R, Gharib H, Bergman D et al: AACE/AAES medical/surgical guidelines for clinical practice: Management of thyroid carcinoma. Endocrine Practice 7:203–220, 2001.

Grant CS, Hay ID, Gough IR et al: Local recurrence in papillary thyroid carcinoma: Is extent of surgical resection important? Surgery 104:954–962, 1988.

Grant CS, Hay ID, Gough IR et al: Long-term follow-up of patients with benign thyroid fine-needle aspiration cytologic diagnoses. Surgery 106:980–986, 1989.

Hay ID, Bergstralh EJ, Goellner JR et al: Predicting outcome in papillary thyroid carcinoma: Development of a reliable prognostic scoring system in a cohort of 1779 patients surgically treated at one institution during 1940 through 1989. Surgery 114:1050–1058, 1993.

Hay ID, Grant CS, Bergstralh EJ et al: Unilateral total lobectomy: Is it sufficient surgical treatment for patients with AMES low-risk papillary thyroid carcinoma? Surgery 124(6):958–966, 1998.

Herrera MF, Hay ID, Wu PS-C et al: Hürthle cell (oxyphilic) papillary thyroid carcinoma: A variant with more aggressive biologic behavior. World J Surg 16:669–675, 1992.

McIver B, Hay I, Giuffrida D et al: Anaplastic thyroid carcinoma: A 50-year experience at a single institution. Surgery 130:1028–1034, 2001.

Pyke CM, Hay ID, Goellner JR et al: Prognostic significance of calcitonin immunoreactivity, amyloid staining, and flow cytometric DNA measurements in medullary thyroid carcinoma. Surgery 110:964–971, 1991.

van Heerden JA, Grant CS, Gharib H et al: Long-term course of patients with persistent hypercalcitoninemia after apparent curative primary surgery for medullary thyroid carcinoma. Ann Surg 212:395–401, 1990.

van Heerden JA, Hay ID, Goellner JR et al: Follicular thyroid carcinoma with capsular invasion alone: A non-threatening malignancy. Surgery 112:1130–1136, 1992.

History and physical examination

Thyroid nodule (A)
Neck node(s)
Paralyzed cord
Previous neck radiation (B)

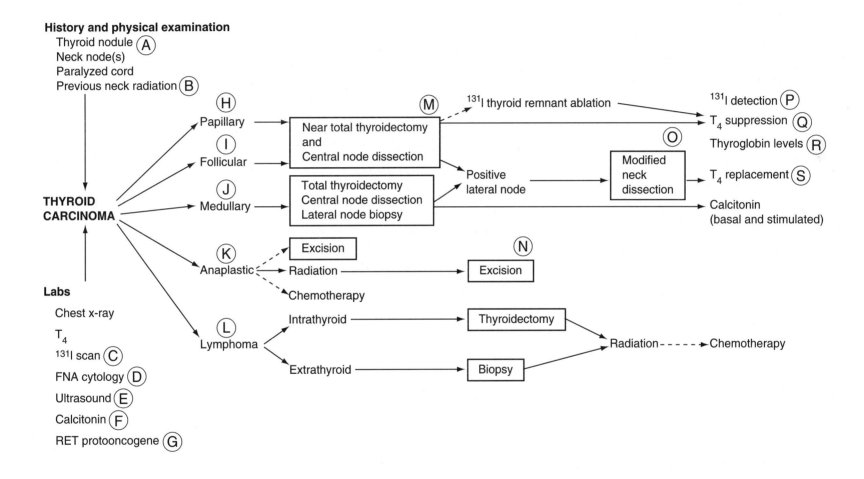

Labs

Chest x-ray

T₄

¹³¹I scan (C)

FNA cytology (D)

Ultrasound (E)

Calcitonin (F)

RET protooncogene (G)

Chapter 90 Hypercalcemia and Hyperparathyroidism

NORMAN W. THOMPSON, MD, PHD

(A) Primary hyperparathyroidism (PHPT) occurs in approximately 1 in 200 of the adult population, increasing with age, and is three times more common in women. The etiology of PHPT is a decreased expression of the calcium-sensing receptor protein (CaSR) located on the parathyroid cell membranes that control parathyroid hormone (PTH) release. The cause for this remains unknown in most cases, although previous neck irradiation and specific genetic mutations are factors in 10% to 15% of patients. Patients with familial PHPT usually have diffuse chief cell hyperplasia rather than a single gland adenoma, although one familial disorder (PHPT and jaw tumor) is associated with both adenoma and parathyroid carcinoma. When familial, the HPT may be associated with other endocrine gland involvement (MENI, MENIIa). Currently HPT is most commonly asymptomatic when first diagnosed. History and physical examination can exclude other causes of hypercalcemia such as malignant disease with or without bone involvement. Two diseases causing hypercalcemia can occur simultaneously.

(B) An elevated or high normal serum calcium level and an inappropriately elevated intact PTH level are the confirming diagnostic studies. Serum phosphorus levels are usually low and chloride levels are elevated in HPT when the renal function is normal. Urinary calcium and creatinine levels are measured to rule out benign familial (hypocalciuric) hypercalcemia (FHH), a rare entity that mimics HPT but requires no treatment. Urinary calcium levels less than 100 mg in a 24-hour collection and a reduced calcium-to-creatinine ratio strongly suggest the diagnosis of FHH. Unless the patient with HPT has specific symptoms, no radiographic studies are required, although dual energy x-ray absorptiometry (DEXA) bone densitometry is recommended to determine the degree of osteoporosis (cortical bone) present in three sites (i.e., forearm, spine, and hip). Parathyroid imaging (sestamibi scintiscan and/or cervical ultrasound) should be used for operative planning if a minimally invasive approach is to

be considered. A positive scan (70% to 90% of all cases) and the availability of rapid intact PTH assay are required for a high success rate. A positive localization study does not rule out multigland gland disease.

(C) A neck exploration is done after the diagnosis is established and localization studies are evaluated. A focused or minimally invasive procedure may be chosen and performed with local anesthesia and/or cervical block, or with general anesthesia, depending on the surgeon's preference. A classical four-gland exploration is still the procedure of choice for the 20% to 40% with negative localization studies, multiple gland visualization, familial HPT, or HPT caused by end-stage renal disease. Parathyroid adenomas arising in superior glands can always be excised through a cervical approach. Only 1% of inferior gland adenomas or hyperplastic glands require a subsequent deep mediastinal exploration.

(D) Most patients with HPT (80% to 85%) have a single enlarged gland (adenoma) that, when excised, "cures" the patient. When a focused or minimally invasive procedure is performed, this is confirmed by a rapid PTH fall of 50% or more from baseline after 10 minutes. Routine biopsy of normal-sized glands is avoided, and frozen section examination of a typical looking parathyroid adenoma is probably unnecessary in most cases.

(E) Double adenomas occur in about 2% to 4% of all HPT patients, but in those older than 65 years, the incidence is around 10%. The two remaining glands are histologically normal. Affected patients have neither a family history nor other endocrine syndrome. The possibility of double adenoma is the principal reason for exploring all four glands, particularly in older patients, when an intraoperative rapid PTH assay is unavailable.

(F) Normal superior glands are found most often just above the junction of the recurrent laryngeal nerve and the inferior thyroid artery. Adenomas are also found there, but in 40% or more patients

may migrate caudally to a paraesophageal site. They may also be encountered along or posterior to the superior thyroid pole beneath its sheath and obscured until the sheath has been incised. They are rarely, if ever, beneath the true thyroid capsule (intrathyroidal). Inferior parathyroid glands, if not found in approximation to the lower thyroid pole, can often be located in the upper thymus; or, less commonly, in the lower third of the thyroid gland (intrathyroidal); or undescended within the carotid sheath, usually at the level of the carotid bifurcation.

(G) Diffuse chief cell hyperplasia with approximate symmetry in size of all glands occurs sporadically or less often as an isolated familial endocrinopathy. Recurrence after a subtotal parathyroidectomy, leaving either a viable intact remnant (60 mg) or one gland intact, is unlikely. However, the MENI syndrome should be ruled out in all patients with hyperplasia, particularly younger ones (aged less than 50 years).

(H) Hyperplastic parathyroid glands in MENI patients are usually asymmetrically enlarged, a clue to the presence of the syndrome in patients who have no family history. Resection must be adequate, removing all glands with the exception of a viable 60 mg remnant, preferably an inferior gland tacked to the trachea with a metal clip. Because of the high frequency of a fifth supernumerary gland (15% to 20%), a cervical thymectomy should be done routinely in this group of patients. An optional procedure in MENI is a total parathyroidectomy, thymectomy, and forearm autotransplant. This procedure has lost favor because of a high incidence of permanent hypoparathyroidism.

(I) Patients with suspected MENI syndrome should have periodic follow-up for pituitary and pancreatic neuroendocrine tumors as well as possible recurrent HPT. Metachromous expression of disease is common. One the other hand, patients with single adenomas do not need routine studies for other endocrine gland disorders.

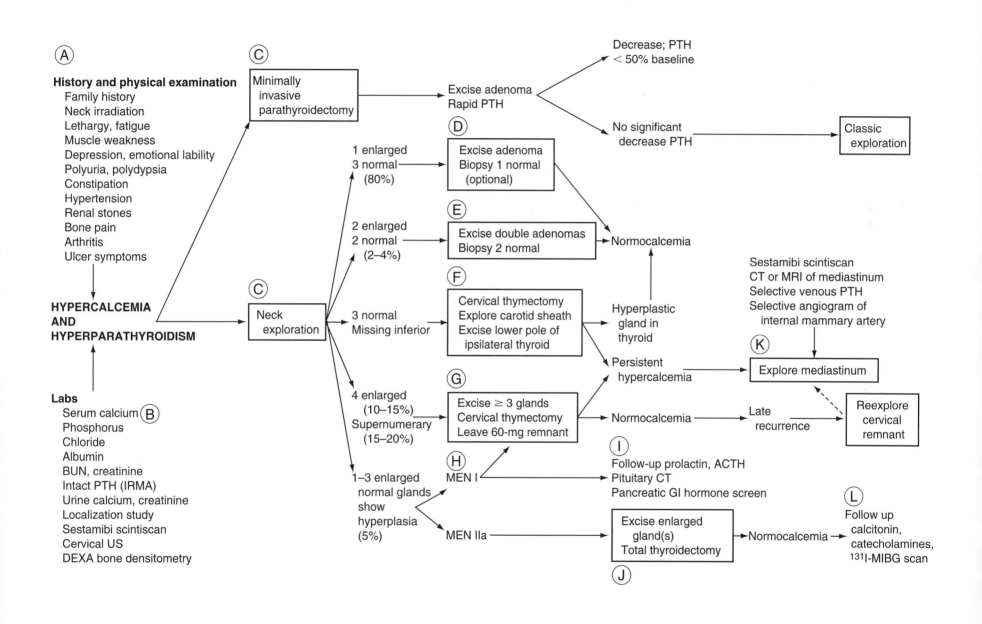

(A)

History and physical examination
Family history
Neck irradiation
Lethargy, fatigue
Muscle weakness
Depression, emotional lability
Polyuria, polydypsia
Constipation
Hypertension
Renal stones
Bone pain
Arthritis
Ulcer symptoms

**HYPERCALCEMIA
AND
HYPERPARATHYROIDISM**

Labs
Serum calcium (B)
Phosphorus
Chloride
Albumin
BUN, creatinine
Intact PTH (IRMA)
Urine calcium, creatinine
Localization study
Sestamibi scintiscan
Cervical US
DEXA bone densitometry

(C) Minimally invasive parathyroidectomy

Excise adenoma
Rapid PTH

Decrease; PTH
< 50% baseline

No significant
decrease PTH

Classic
exploration

(C) Neck exploration

1 enlarged
3 normal
(80%)

(D) Excise adenoma
Biopsy 1 normal
(optional)

2 enlarged
2 normal
(2–4%)

(E) Excise double adenomas
Biopsy 2 normal

Normocalcemia

3 normal
Missing inferior

(F) Cervical thymectomy
Explore carotid sheath
Excise lower pole of
ipsilateral thyroid

Hyperplastic
gland in
thyroid

Persistent
hypercalcemia

4 enlarged
(10–15%)
Supernumerary
(15–20%)

(G) Excise ≥ 3 glands
Cervical thymectomy
Leave 60-mg remnant

Normocalcemia

Late
recurrence

1–3 enlarged
normal glands
show
hyperplasia
(5%)

(H) MEN I

(I) Follow-up prolactin, ACTH
Pituitary CT
Pancreatic GI hormone screen

MEN IIa

(J) Excise enlarged
gland(s)
Total thyroidectomy

Normocalcemia

Sestamibi scintiscan
CT or MRI of mediastinum
Selective venous PTH
Selective angiogram of
internal mammary artery

(K) Explore mediastinum

Reexplore
cervical
remnant

(L) Follow up
calcitonin,
catecholamines,
^{131}I-MIBG scan

(J) HPT develops in only 20% to 30% of MENIIa patients and is usually mild and not prone to recurrence as in MENI. Subtotal or total parathyroidectomy and autotransplantation are not indicated for the HPT because usually only one or two glands are enlarged; it may be justified, however, if a total thyroidectomy and central neck dissection cannot be done without devascularizing the remaining glands. When only one or two enlarged glands have been removed, recurrences and hypoparathyroidism have been rare.

(K) Mediastinal exploration is required in only 1% to 2% of all patients with HPT, and only after the surgeon is convinced the diseased gland is not in the neck. Localization studies are clearly indicated in this group of patients, and reoperation should be deferred until one or more such studies are positive. Although most are in the anterior mediastinum (thymus), some are located in the middle mediastinum (aortopulmonary window or prebronchial); in these, an approach other than a sternal split may be more appropriate. A primary (initial operative) mediastinal exploration is done only in patients who have been in hypercalcemic crisis and in whom the adenoma was not found in the neck.

(L) MENIIa patients should have periodic evaluation for possible pheochromocytoma (40% to 50%). However, hypercalcemia in a patient with pheochromocytoma should be re-evaluated after its excision because some tumors secrete PTH-related peptide, and serum calciums subsequently may be normal.

REFERENCES

Boggs JE, Irvin GL III, Molinari AS et al: Intraoperative parathyroid hormone monitoring as an adjunct to parathyroidectomy. Surgery 120:954–958, 1996.

Carty SE, Worsey EJ, Virgi MA et al: Concise parathyroidectomy: The impact of preoperative SPECT 99mTc sestamibi scanning and intraoperative quick parathormone assay. Surgery 122:1107–1116, 1997.

Clark OH, Wilkes W, Siperstein AE et al: Diagnosis and management of asymptomatic hyperparathyroidism: Safety, efficacy, and deficiencies in our knowledge. J Bone Min Res 6:S135–S142, 1991.

Freeman JB, Sherman BN, Mason EF: Cervical thymectomy. Arch Surg 112:359–364, 1979.

Henry JF, Raffaelli M, Iacombone M et al: Video assisted parathyroidectomy via the lateral approach vs. conventional surgery in the treatment of sporadic primary hyperparathyroidism: Results of a case control study. Surg Endosc 15:1116–1119, 2001.

Irvin GL III, Carneior DM: Management changes in primary hyperparathyroidism. JAMA 284:934–936, 2000.

Monchik JM: Normocalcemic hyperparathyroidism. Surgery 118:917–923, 1995.

Monchik JM, Barellini L, Langer P et al: Minimally invasive parathyroid surgery in 103 patients with local/regional anesthesia, without exclusion criteria. Surgery 131:502–508, 2002.

Rao DS: Parathyroidectomy for asymptomatic primary hyperparathyroidism (PHPT): Is it worth the risk? J Endocrinol Invest 24:131–134, 2001.

Talpos GB, Bone HG III, Kleerekoper M et al: Randomized trial of parathyroidectomy in mild asymptomatic primary hyperparathyroidism: Patient description and defects on the SF-36 health survey. Surgery 128:1013–1021, 2000.

Thompson NW: The Techniques of Initial Parathyroid Exploration and Reoperative Parathyroidectomy. In Thompson NW, Vinik AK (eds): Endocrine Surgery Update. New York: Grune & Stratton, 1983.

Thompson NW, Eckhauser FE, Harness JK: The anatomy of primary hyperparathyroidism. Surgery 92:814–822, 1982.

Udelsman R: Six hundred fifty-six consecutive explorations for primary hyperparathyroidism. Ann Surg 235:665–672, 2002.

Vestergaard P, Mosekilde L: Fractures in patients with primary hyperparathyroidism: Nationwide follow-up study of 1201 patients. World J Surg 27:343–349, 2003.

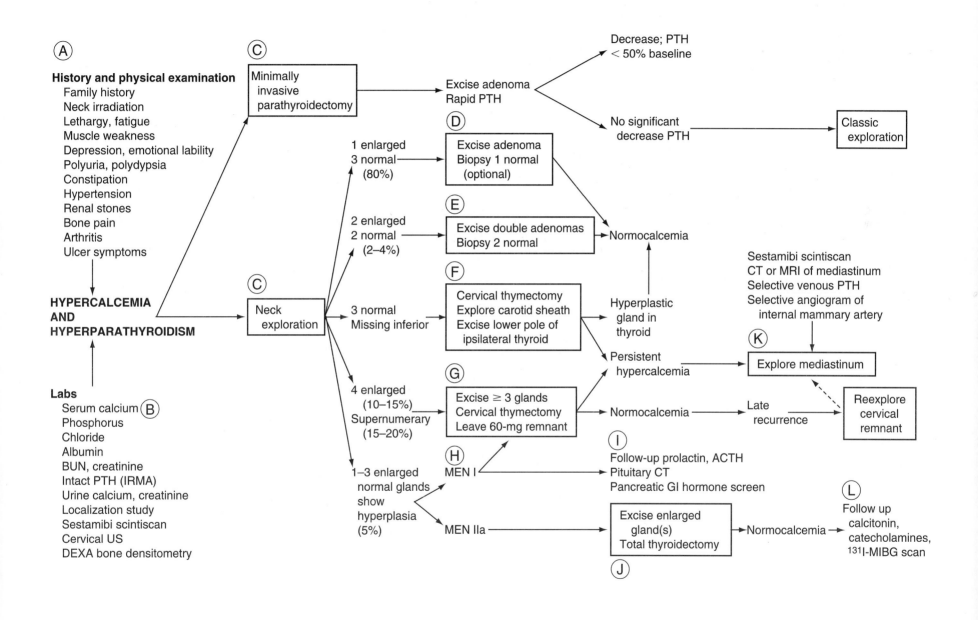

Ⓐ

History and physical examination
Family history
Neck irradiation
Lethargy, fatigue
Muscle weakness
Depression, emotional lability
Polyuria, polydypsia
Constipation
Hypertension
Renal stones
Bone pain
Arthritis
Ulcer symptoms

HYPERCALCEMIA AND HYPERPARATHYROIDISM

Labs
Serum calcium Ⓑ
Phosphorus
Chloride
Albumin
BUN, creatinine
Intact PTH (IRMA)
Urine calcium, creatinine
Localization study
Sestamibi scintiscan
Cervical US
DEXA bone densitometry

Ⓒ Minimally invasive parathyroidectomy

Excise adenoma
Rapid PTH

Decrease; PTH < 50% baseline

No significant decrease PTH → Classic exploration

Ⓒ Neck exploration

1 enlarged 3 normal (80%) → Ⓓ Excise adenoma Biopsy 1 normal (optional)

2 enlarged 2 normal (2–4%) → Ⓔ Excise double adenomas Biopsy 2 normal

3 normal Missing inferior → Ⓕ Cervical thymectomy Explore carotid sheath Excise lower pole of ipsilateral thyroid

4 enlarged (10–15%) Supernumerary (15–20%) → Ⓖ Excise ≥ 3 glands Cervical thymectomy Leave 60-mg remnant

1–3 enlarged normal glands show hyperplasia (5%)

Ⓗ MEN I

MEN IIa

Normocalcemia

Hyperplastic gland in thyroid

Persistent hypercalcemia

Normocalcemia → Late recurrence

Sestamibi scintiscan
CT or MRI of mediastinum
Selective venous PTH
Selective angiogram of internal mammary artery

Ⓚ Explore mediastinum

Reexplore cervical remnant

Ⓘ Follow-up prolactin, ACTH
Pituitary CT
Pancreatic GI hormone screen

Ⓙ Excise enlarged gland(s) Total thyroidectomy → Normocalcemia →

Ⓛ Follow up calcitonin, catecholamines, ¹³¹I-MIBG scan

Chapter 91 *Insulinoma*

GERARD M. DOHERTY, MD

(A) Symptoms of insulinoma include both neuroglycopenic and adrenergic complaints. Specifically, patients may present with diplopia, blurred vision, sweating, palpitations, weakness, confusion, abnormal behavior, unconsciousness, amnesia, or grand mal seizures. These symptoms and signs usually occur after either a prolonged fast or exercise.

(B) The diagnosis of insulinoma is made by documenting hypoglycemia (less than 40 mg/100 ml blood glucose) and simultaneous elevated plasma immunoreactive insulin levels (greater than 6 μU/ml) during supervised fasting (up to 48 hours). C-peptide levels (normal 0.5 to 3.0 μg/ml) and negative urine sulfonylurea levels are helpful in differentiating insulinoma from factitious hyperinsulinemia and hypoglycemia. Patients should also be evaluated for insulin antibodies, insulin receptor antibodies, and islet-stimulating antibodies that can elevate insulin levels.

(C) Radiologic evaluation should include abdominal computed tomography (CT) or abdominal ultrasound (US), which will localize the majority of insulinomas. In many centers, endoscopic US has now become an initial test of choice because of great sensitivity if someone with expertise in this technique is available.

(D) Surgical exploration consists of an extensive Kocher maneuver and examination of the head of the pancreas as well as the opening of the lesser sac and mobilization of the inferior and posterior aspects of the pancreatic body and tail. This allows bimanual palpation of the entire pancreas and thorough assessment by intraoperative ultrasound.

(E) Additional tests that may identify otherwise occult tumors include magnetic resonance imaging (MRI). If studies are negative, the patient may undergo pancreatic arteriography with calcium stimulation, although the author generally reserves this for the reoperative or MEN-1 settings. Because the combination of exploratory laparotomy and intraoperative US is very sensitive in localizing insulinomas, patients mainly need to have a very clear biochemical diagnosis.

(F) The choice of tumor enucleation or pancreatic resection is guided by the least morbid procedure that can completely remove the tumor. If a single tumor is localized to the head or body of the pancreas, simple enucleation can be performed. If, however, the tumor is in the very distal pancreas, then a spleen-sparing distal pancreatectomy may be a better choice. The patient with nesidioblastosis or multiple islet cell tumors of the pancreas should undergo subtotal pancreatectomy. Finally, should the patient have widely metastatic disease, tumor debulking, either by direct resection or by other ablative techniques such as cryoablation or radiofrequency ablation, may be helpful to reduce the symptoms of hypoglycemia.

(G) Widely metastatic disease from insulinoma can be treated with a combination of diazoxide and octreotide, and it may occasionally respond to systemic cytotoxic chemotherapy.

REFERENCES

Ardengh J, Rosenbaum P, Ganc A et al: Role of EUS in the preoperative localization of insulinomas compared with spiral CT. Gastrointestinal Endoscopy 51:552–555, 2000.

Bansal R, Tierney W, Carpenter S et al: Cost effectiveness of EUS for preoperative localization of pancreatic endocrine tumors. Gastrointestinal Endoscopy 49:19–25, 1999.

Cohen MS, Picus D, Lairmore TC et al: Prospective study of provocative angiograms to localize functional islet cell tumors of the pancreas. Surgery 122:1091–1100, 1997.

Doherty GM, Doppman JL, Shawker TH et al: Results of a prospective strategy to diagnose, localize, and resect insulinomas. Surgery 110: 989–996, 1991.

Hirshberg B, Livi A, Bartlett DL et al: 48-hour fast: The diagnostic test for insulinoma. J Clin Endocrinol Metabol 85:3222–3226, 2000.

Thompson GB, Service FJ, Andrews JC et al: Noninsulinoma pancreatogenous hypoglycemia syndrome: An update in 10 surgically treated patients. Surgery 128:937–944, 2000.

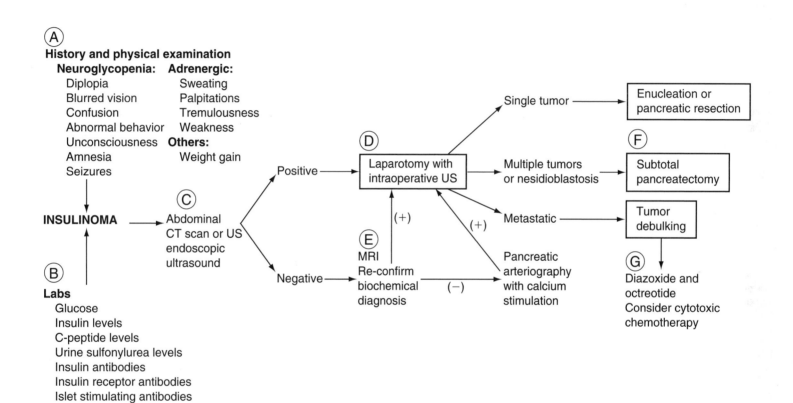

Ⓐ
History and physical examination
Neuroglycopenia: **Adrenergic:**
   Diplopia   Sweating
   Blurred vision   Palpitations
   Confusion   Tremulousness
   Abnormal behavior   Weakness
   Unconsciousness   **Others:**
   Amnesia   Weight gain
   Seizures

INSULINOMA

Ⓑ
Labs
   Glucose
   Insulin levels
   C-peptide levels
   Urine sulfonylurea levels
   Insulin antibodies
   Insulin receptor antibodies
   Islet stimulating antibodies

Ⓒ
Abdominal
CT scan or US
endoscopic
ultrasound

Positive

Negative

Ⓓ
Laparotomy with
intraoperative US

Ⓔ
MRI
Re-confirm
biochemical
diagnosis

(+)

(−)

Pancreatic
arteriography
with calcium
stimulation

(+)

Single tumor → Enucleation or
pancreatic resection

Multiple tumors
or nesidioblastosis

Ⓕ
Subtotal
pancreatectomy

Metastatic

Tumor
debulking

Ⓖ
Diazoxide and
octreotide
Consider cytotoxic
chemotherapy

Chapter 92 *Zollinger-Ellison Syndrome*

PETER MUSCARELLA, MD • E. CHRISTOPHER ELLISON, MD

(A) Hypergastrinemia results in peptic ulceration of the upper gastrointestinal tract in about 60% of the patients; it is commonly recurrent and occurs in atypical locations. The most common presenting symptom, occurring in 70% to 90% of patients, is abdominal pain related to ulcer disease. Diarrhea may be present in almost half of these patients, and 10% will present with diarrhea as the only manifestation of the syndrome. Although periods of quiescence may occur between exacerbations, most patients have a progressive and relentless course. Gastrinomas may arise sporadically or as part of the familial multiple endocrine neoplasia type 1 (MEN 1) syndrome in approximately 25% of cases. Conversely, 50% of MEN 1 patients will develop pancreatic endocrine tumors (PETs) and gastrinoma is the most common. Zollinger-Ellison syndrome (ZES) should be suspected in the following situations: (1) recurrent peptic ulcer disease despite adequate medical treatment or operation; (2) postbulbar ulcers; (3) prominent gastric rugal folds on upper endoscopy; (4) peptic ulcers with diarrhea; (5) patients with a strong family history of ulcer disease and/or endocrine disorders; (6) patients with ulcers at extreme ages (i.e., the very young and very old); and (7) patients with symptoms of both hyperparathyroidism and gastrointestinal ulceration.

(B) In 1955, Zollinger and Ellison were the first to describe the triad of peptic ulcerations in unusual locations, gastric hypersecretion despite therapy, and islet cell tumors of the pancreas. They hypothesized that an "ulcerogenic factor" secreted by the tumor caused the associated syndrome. Gastrin was subsequently isolated from tumor extracts, and pathophysiologic proof of its role as the proposed factor was provided. Although initially described as being associated with pancreatic islet cell tumors, primary gastrinomas are most commonly located in the duodenum (50%). Gastrinomas may also arise in the pancreas (25%), lymph nodes (10%), stomach, ovaries, or unknown locations. Cardiac tumors have even been described. Malignancy is determined by biological behavior rather than by histopathologic analysis. Lymph node and distant metastases are present in 55% and 10% of cases, respectively, with the liver being the most common location of distal dissemination.

(C) In suspected cases, the initial work-up should be targeted at making a biochemical diagnosis of ZES. Because the diagnosis of gastrinoma relies heavily on the identification of elevated serum gastrin levels, conditions that could result in hypergastrinemia should be included in the differential diagnosis. In the authors' series of 289 patients with hypergastrinemia, only 29% had gastrinomas; the majority of patients had either pernicious anemia or secondary hypergastrinemia related to omeprazole or renal failure. Other causes include G-cell hyperplasia, atrophic gastritis without pernicious anemia, retained gastric antrum, postvagotomy state, gastric outlet obstruction, and short gut syndrome. Acid-reducing medications should be withheld for 72 hours before testing. Fasting serum gastrin levels greater than 1000 pg/ml, with the presence of gastric hyperacidity, are usually diagnostic, and concentrations greater than 1500 pg/ml suggest metastatic disease. In patients with elevated serum gastrin concentrations, measurement of gastric acid secretion can assist in making the diagnosis. A fasting serum gastrin greater than 100 pg/ml and a basal acid output (BAO) greater than 15 mEq/hour are characteristic. BAO/MAO (maximal acid output with pentagastrin stimulation) ratios in excess of 0.6 also support the diagnosis. If a laboratory diagnosis of gastrinoma still cannot be made, provocative testing with secretin (2 U/kg IV) is indicated, and a paradoxical rise in serum gastrin concentration (200 pg/ml over baseline) is diagnostic of ZES. An alternative to secretin is a test meal; patients with gastrinoma will demonstrate at least a 50% increase in serum gastrin concentrations over baseline.

(D) All patients should be screened for other endocrinopathies associated with MEN 1 by analysis of serum calcium, parathyroid hormone (PTH), and prolactin concentrations. In patients who appear cushingoid, serum cortisol determinations are appropriate.

(E) Medical treatment with proton pump inhibitors (PPIs) is 100% effective in controlling acid secretion, and patients no longer die from acid-related causes. Standard doses of oral PPIs are begun, and these may be increased to control acid secretion. The average dosage of omeprazole is 65 mg/day. Vitamin B_{12} deficiency can occur in 6% of ZES patients treated with PPIs, and serum B_{12} levels should be evaluated periodically.

(F) Preoperative imaging studies are undertaken with the goal of identifying the location of the primary tumor. This information is extremely valuable for guiding surgical therapy, although surgical exploration is still warranted in patients with potentially resectable and biochemically proven ZES. In addition, special imaging studies are helpful for the evaluation of metastatic disease because the identification of unresectable metastatic disease before surgery may obviate the need for unnecessary exploration. Computed tomography (CT) scanning and somatostatin receptor scintigraphy (SRS) have been established as the initial localization studies. SRS clearly has superior accuracy, but CT allows for size measurement and assessment of tumor relation to surrounding structures. Endoscopic ultrasonography (EUS) is becoming increasingly utilized and should be considered as an initial tool for localization. Magnetic resonance imaging (MRI) may be most useful in patients with suspected bone metastases. Selective arteriography and transhepatic portal venous sampling are invasive and should be used only if all of the other tests are negative. The technique of selective intra-arterial provocation with secretin or calcium and measurement of hepatic vein gastrin concentrations is currently indicated for the evaluation of

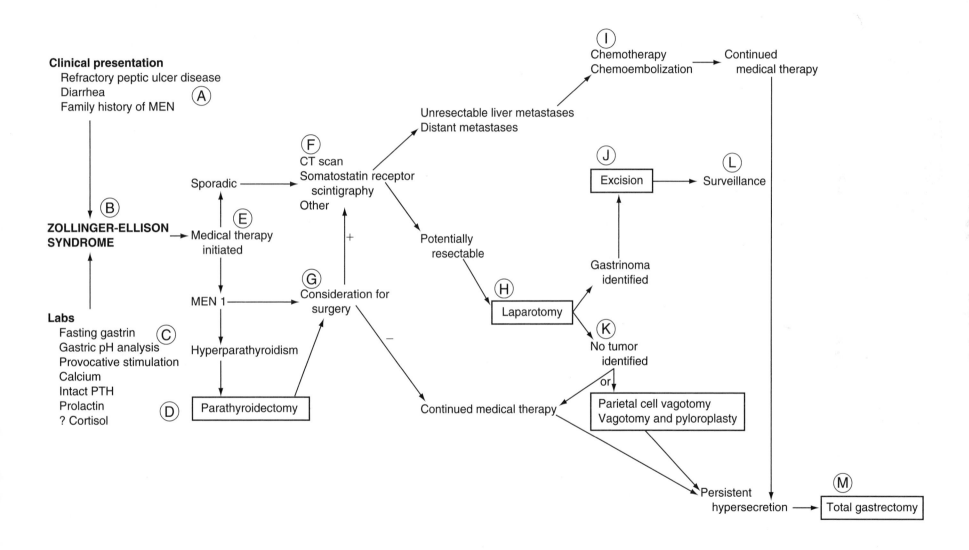

Clinical presentation
Refractory peptic ulcer disease
Diarrhea
Family history of MEN (A)

(B)
**ZOLLINGER-ELLISON
SYNDROME**

Labs
Fasting gastrin (C)
Gastric pH analysis
Provocative stimulation
Calcium
Intact PTH
Prolactin
? Cortisol (D)

(E) Medical therapy
initiated

MEN 1

Hyperparathyroidism

(D) Parathyroidectomy

Sporadic

(F)
CT scan
Somatostatin receptor
scintigraphy
Other

(G) Consideration for
surgery

+

−

Continued medical therapy

Unresectable liver metastases
Distant metastases

(I)
Chemotherapy
Chemoembolization

Continued
medical therapy

Potentially
resectable

(H)
Laparotomy

Gastrinoma
identified

(J)
Excision

(L)
Surveillance

(K)
No tumor
identified

or

Parietal cell vagotomy
Vagotomy and pyloroplasty

Persistent
hypersecretion

(M)
Total gastrectomy

gastrinomas that have not been localized by less invasive means.

(G) In cases of primary hyperparathyroidism, parathyroidectomy (subtotal leaving 60 mg viable tissue or 4 glands with autologous transplantation) is warranted to correct hypercalcemia, and has been demonstrated to result in decreased gastric acid secretion. Aggressive resection of gastrinomas in MEN 1 patients is currently controversial with Thompson and colleagues advocating duodenotomy and removal of mucosal tumors, pancreatic head tumor enucleation, peripancreatic lymph node dissection, and distal pancreatectomy. Eugastrinemia and failure to stimulate with secretin can be achieved in approximately 33% of patients using this approach, but the effects on survival are unclear. Long-term survival is actually quite good in patients with familial ZES, and many authors, including ourselves, favor a more conservative surgical approach or even observation for small lesions.

(H) Laparotomy is indicated for potentially resectable sporadic ZES and should be considered for patients in whom preoperative localization has been unsuccessful. Primary tumors are usually identified in the gastrinoma triangle. Adequate exploration includes complete pancreatic mobilization, bimanual palpation, and intraoperative ultrasonography. Evaluation of the duodenum may be facilitated by endoscopy with transillumination, but duodenotomy should be considered if no primary can be identified and in patients with MEN 1. Surgical resection can usually be accomplished by enucleation, but formal resection may be required for larger tumors. All suspicious lymph nodes should be removed, and resection of liver metastases is reserved for patients in whom extirpation of all disease can be safely performed. There are increasing data on the use of laparoscopic surgery for staging, intraoperative localization, and resection of ZES. Recently, a computer-assisted robotic resection of a pancreatic gastrinoma was performed successfully at the authors' institution.

(I) Hepatic arterial chemoembolization is indicated for the palliation of metastatic neuroendocrine tumors to the liver in the absence of other metastatic disease. Chemoembolization is performed with emulsified doxorubicin, followed by particulate embolization with absorbable gelatin powder or pledgets. Recent studies demonstrate symptomatic improvement of hormonal symptoms in up to 50% of patients, but the duration of the response may be limited. Chemotherapeutic recommendations are somewhat limited for metastatic ZES, and are usually reserved for patients who have failed all other modalities. Interferon-alpha (INF-α) has a direct antitumor effect and is an immunomodulator. Clinical and biologic responses are common (50%), but the median duration of the response is 20 months. Multidrug therapy with streptozotocin and doxorubicin is superior to streptozotocin plus fluorouracil, with objective response rates and remission times of 69% and 20 months versus 45% and 6.9 months, respectively. Chlorazotocin alone has a response rate of approximately 30%, and remission times are similar to those achieved using combination therapy with 5-FU and streptozotocin.

(J) Tumor resection delays the onset of metastatic disease and improves survival. Mortality rates are low (0% to 4%), whereas morbidity is considerable (11% to 27%). Tumor identification and resection is possible in 66% to 81% of patients. Surgical resection may result in eugastrinemia in 11% to 20% of patients, and medical management should be improved in the remainder. Gastrinoma excision is associated with a decrease in the incidence subsequent of liver metastases and an increase in long-term survival. Long-term survival following gastrinoma resection is excellent, and when deaths from other causes are excluded, 5- and 10-year survival rates are 100% are 95%, respectively.

(K) Some 10% to 15% of patients may have no tumor identified at surgical exploration. Blind pancreatic resection for gastrinomas that remain unlocalized is not currently recommended. These patients have an excellent long-term prognosis (90% 10-year survival). Acid-reducing operations such as parietal cell vagotomy or vagotomy and pyloroplasty may be considered.

(L) Long-term observation with yearly serum gastrin measurement is indicated for all patients. A rising gastrin concentration should prompt a search for metastases, and SRS imaging is the most useful study.

(M) Indications for total gastrectomy include failure of previous ulcer surgery or medical therapy, or complications of previous gastric surgery (e.g., gastrojejunal colic fistula). The presence of severe gastroesophageal reflux disease with stricture formation is challenging and may necessitate antireflux surgery or total gastrectomy.

REFERENCES

Ellison EC: Forty-year appraisal of gastrinoma: Back to the future. Ann Surg 222:511–521, 1995.

Gagner M, Pomp A, Herrera MF: Early experience with laparoscopic resections of islet cell tumors. Surgery 120: 1051–1054, 1996.

Jensen RT: Pancreatic endocrine tumors: Recent advances. Ann Oncol 10(Suppl 4):170–176, 1999.

Melvin WS, Johnson JA, Sparks J et al: Long-term prognosis of Zollinger-Ellison syndrome in multiple endocrine neoplasia. Surgery 114:1183–1188, 1993.

Norton JA, Fraker DL, Alexander HR et al: Surgery to cure the Zollinger-Ellison syndrome. N Engl J Med 341:635–644, 1999.

Norton JA, Alexander HR, Fraker DL et al: Comparison of surgical results in patients with advanced and limited disease with multiple endocrine neoplasia type 1 and Zollinger-Ellison syndrome. Ann Surg 234:495–505, 2001.

Schirmer WJ, Melvin WS, Rush RM et al: Indium-111-pentetreotide scanning versus conventional imaging techniques for the localization of gastrinoma. Surgery 118:1105–1113, 1995.

Thom AK, Norton JA, Doppman JL et al: Prospective study of the use of intra-arterial secretin injection and portal venous sampling to localize duodenal gastrinomas. Surgery 112:1002–1008, 1992.

Thompson NW: Current concepts in the surgical management of multiple endocrine neoplasia type 1 pancreatic-duodenal disease: Results in the treatment of 40 patients with Zollinger-Ellison syndrome, hypoglycaemia, or both. J Int Med 243:495–500, 1998.

Yu F, Venzon DJ, Serrano J et al: Prospective study of the clinical course, prognostic factors, causes of death, and survival in patients with long-standing Zollinger-Ellison syndrome. J Clin Oncol 17:615–630, 1999.

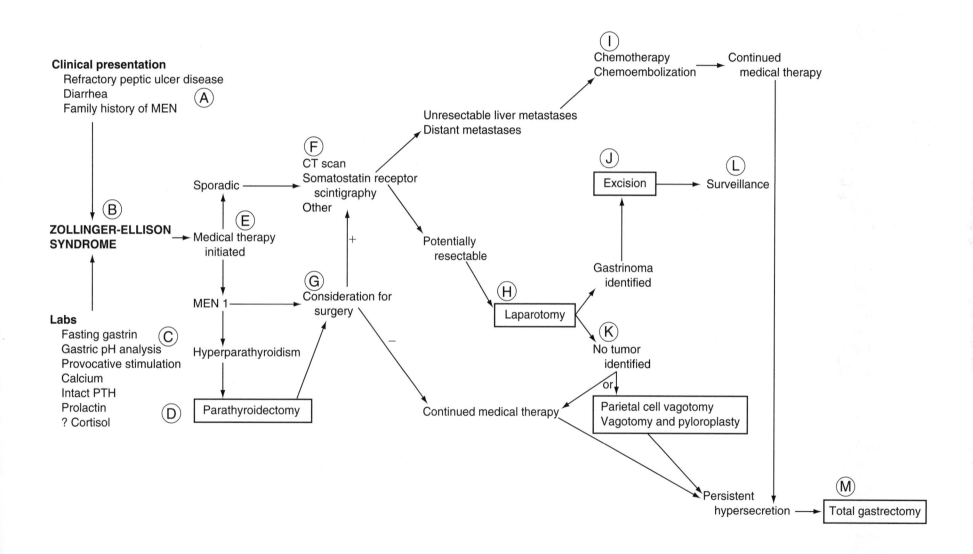

Clinical presentation
    Refractory peptic ulcer disease
    Diarrhea
    Family history of MEN   (A)

(B)

**ZOLLINGER-ELLISON
SYNDROME**

Labs
    Fasting gastrin   (C)
    Gastric pH analysis
    Provocative stimulation
    Calcium
    Intact PTH
    Prolactin
    ? Cortisol   (D)

Sporadic

(E)

Medical therapy
initiated

MEN 1

Hyperparathyroidism

Parathyroidectomy

(F)
CT scan
Somatostatin receptor
scintigraphy
Other

(G)
Consideration for
surgery

+

Unresectable liver metastases
Distant metastases

Potentially
resectable

(I)
Chemotherapy
Chemoembolization

Continued
medical therapy

(J)
Excision

(L)
Surveillance

Gastrinoma
identified

(H)
Laparotomy

(K)
No tumor
identified

or

Parietal cell vagotomy
Vagotomy and pyloroplasty

Continued medical therapy

−

Persistent
hypersecretion

(M)
Total gastrectomy

Chapter 93 Pheochromocytoma

DAVID R. FARLEY, MD • JON A. VAN HEERDEN, MD

(A) Pheochromocytoma, "the great mimic," may generate signs and symptoms compatible with many other diseases (e.g., hyperthyroidism, diabetes mellitus, mental illness, eclampsia of pregnancy, or gram-negative sepsis). Although hypertension remains the most prominent sign in patients with pheochromocytoma, owing to the sheer rarity of this disorder (incidence, 1:100,000 Americans, or 0.1% of all hypertensive patients), most patients with hypertension and associated complaints of headaches, palpitations, and flushing likely do not have a pheochromocytoma. The onus, however, remains on the physician to consider and rule out this rare disorder that has potentially lethal consequences.

(B) Modern radiologic studies (most often abdominal computerized tomography [CT] or magnetic resonance imaging [MRI]) performed for other reasons sometimes (around 3%) identify unsuspected adrenal neoplasms. It is imperative to investigate all such incidentalomas to rule out pheochromocytoma.

(C) Occasionally the suspicion of pheochromocytoma surfaces during medical intervention (e.g., hemodynamic instability during angiography, childbirth, or surgical intervention). Immediate blood pressure control during the untoward event is imperative, as is prompt completion or termination of the procedure. Thereafter, the diagnosis of pheochromocytoma must be ruled in or out. Unfortunately, as many as 800 Americans may die every year from unsuspected pheochromocytomas.

(D) Modern spiral CT (from diaphragm to pelvis) with thin sectioning (3 mm) accurately identifies most unilateral or bilateral pheochromocytomas and extra-adrenal paragangliomas. Ninety-eight percent of catecholamine-secreting tumors are intra-abdominal; 90% lie within the adrenal gland(s). Equivocal CT studies or familial syndromes (e.g., multiple endocrine neoplasia [MEN II] or von Hippel-Lindau) should prompt ^{123}I-meta-iodobenzylguanidine (MIBG) scintigraphy or MRI.

(E) Whether paroxysmal (about 45%) or sustained (about 50%), most hypertensive patients with pheochromocytomas secrete excessive catecholamines. Measurement of 24-hour urinary fractionated catecholamines (i.e., epinephrine, norepinephrine, and dopamine) and metanephrines identifies this disorder in more than 98% of patients, even including those without overt symptoms and signs of a pheochromocytoma. Measurement of fractionated plasma metanephrines is highly sensitive (around 99%) but lacks specificity (85% to 89%) when compared with the combination of 24-hour urinary total metanephrines and catecholamines. When biochemical testing is positive, potential causes of false-positive results such as medications (e.g., tricyclic antidepressants, levodopa, or drugs containing catecholamines) or clinical situations (e.g., physical stress or withdrawal from clonidine or other drugs) should be considered. Patients with a family history of adrenal or thyroid disorders should undergo genetic screening for MEN II syndrome (RET proto-oncogene).

(F) Patients with imaging evidence of an adrenal neoplasm, elevated 24-hour urinary metanephrines or catecholamines, and who are fit to tolerate general anesthesia warrant resection. Perioperative pharmacologic therapy lowers morbidity and mortality by minimizing intraoperative hemodynamic instability. A variety of regimens (e.g., prazosin, calcium channel blockers, and labetalol) have been used successfully. The authors' preference is for 7 to 10 days of outpatient nonselective α-adrenergic receptor blockade (phenoxybenzamine, 10 to 40 mg PO twice daily, titrated to normal blood pressure, resolution of spells, and onset of nasal congestion and mild orthostatic hypotension) with additional β-blockade over the last 3 preoperative days to minimize tachyarrhythmias (propranolol, 10 mg PO four times daily). Although α- and β-adrenergic blockade are useful, meticulous surgical technique and

an experienced anesthesiologist remain the cornerstones of successful intraoperative management.

(G) Laparoscopic unilateral or bilateral adrenalectomy is safe and efficacious. Deviations from this new gold standard of therapy seem logical if the adrenal lesion is larger than 8 cm or likely to be malignant (celiotomy indicated), or when previous upper abdominal or retroperitoneal operations might prove troublesome (i.e., posterior approach warranted). Identification of previously unsuspected metastatic disease is uncommon, but palliative resection, if safely accomplished, is beneficial. Although metastatic tumors respond poorly to radiation or chemotherapy, limited palliation with resection, radiation therapy (bony metastases), therapeutic ^{131}I MIBG, multi-dose chemotherapy, or radiofrequency ablation have been reported. The mainstay of treatment in such patients is control of hypertension with long-term α-adrenergic blockade.

(H) Hemodynamic stability is maximized by early adrenal vein ligation and judicious use of intravenous fluids and sodium nitroprusside (as indicated). Continuous arterial and central venous pressure monitoring allows the safest intraoperative management, with the ability to precisely measure changing hemodynamic parameters and react accordingly.

(I) With reasonable morbidity (less than 20%) and low mortality (less than 2%), most surgical interventions in patients with pheochromocytomas are successful. Histologic differentiation between malignant (around 10%) and benign neoplasms (around 90%) is nearly impossible. Diagnostic certainty requires long-term follow-up (5-year survival after pheochromocytoma resection is more than 90% for benign disease, less than 50% for a malignancy), which is best achieved by annual examination and rechecking urine catecholamines and metanephrines. Suspicion of MEN II and other familial syndromes associated with pheochromocytoma mandates all first-order relatives be screened for catecholamine hypersecretion.

REFERENCES

Baghai M, Thompson GB, Young WF Jr. et al: Pheochromocytomas and paragangliomas in von Hippel-Lindau disease: A role for laparoscopic and cortical-sparing surgery. Arch Surg 137:682–689, 2002.

Brunt LM, Lairmore TC, Doherty GM et al: Adrenalectomy for familial pheochromocytoma in the laparoscopic era. Ann Surg 235:713–721, 2002.

Eisenhofer G, Lenders JW, Pacak K: Choice of biochemical test for diagnosis of pheochromocytoma: Validation of plasma metanephrines. Curr Hypertens Rep 4:250–255, 2002.

Kercher KW, Park A, Matthews BD et al: Laparoscopic adrenalectomy for pheochromocytoma. Surg Endosc 16:100–102, 2002.

Kinney MAO, Warner ME, van Heerden JA et al: Perianesthetic risks and outcomes of pheochromocytoma and paraganglioma resection. Anesth Analg 91:1118–1123, 2000.

Neumann HP: Imaging vs. biochemical testing for pheochromocytoma. JAMA 288:314–315, 2002.

Orchard T, Grant CS, van Heerden JA et al: Pheochromocytoma: Continuing evolution of surgical therapy. Surgery 114:1153–1159, 1993.

van Heerden JA, Roland CF, Carney JA et al: Long-term evaluation following resection of apparently benign pheochromocytomas(s)/paraganglioma(s). World J Surg 14:325–329, 1990.

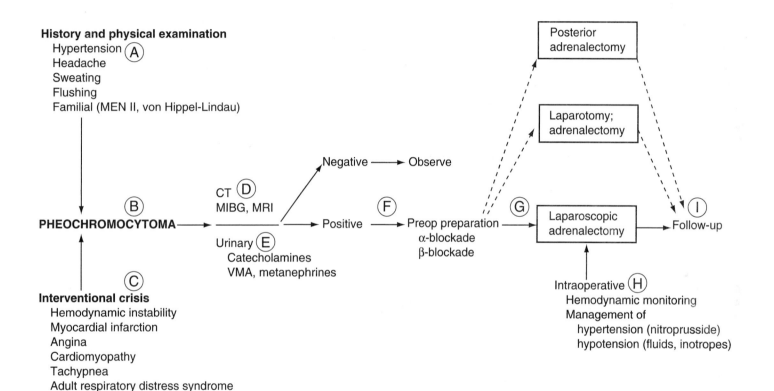

Chapter 94 *Cushing's Syndrome*

MICHEAL SEAN BOGER, MD, PHARM D • NANCY DUGAL PERRIER, MD

(A) Harvey Cushing (1869–1939), the Father of American Neurosurgery, is immortalized by his classic description of a reflex increase in blood pressure with increased intracranial pressure and his famous monograph on ACTH-secreting basophilic adenomas of the pituitary, known today as Cushing's disease. Cushing's syndrome is the more general state of hypercortisolism.

(B) The earliest consistent feature of Cushing's syndrome is the loss of negative feedback where adrenocorticotropic hormone (ACTH), and thus cortisol secretion is suppressed by elevation of cortisol or an analogous steroid. A positive 24-hour urine free cortisol, defined as greater than three times the upper limit of normal (reference range 20 to 100 µg/24 hr), should be further evaluated with the low-dose dexamethasone suppression test. Because cortisol hypersecretion is occasionally intermittent, a normal urinary cortisol should be repeated on several occasions if clinical suspicion is high.

(C) One mg of dexamethasone is given at 11 PM. Normally, plasma cortisol measured at 8 AM the next day should be less than 50% of that before the test and less than 10 µg/dl (reference range: 9 to 24 µg/dl at 8 AM, 3 to 12 µg/dl or approximately one-half of morning values at 4 PM, and less than 5 µg/dl at 11 PM). False-positive results may occur with agents accelerating dexamethasone metabolism (e.g., phenytoin, barbiturates, carbamazepine, and rifampin) and those elevating plasma cortisol-binding globulin (e.g., estrogens).

(D) To determine if Cushing's syndrome is ACTH-dependent, ACTH levels (reference range 8 to 25 pg/ml at 8 AM) are measured on two or three separate days (because of episodic secretion): more than 15 pg/ml is ACTH-dependent, whereas a level consistently less than 5 pg/ml is ACTH-independent. Levels greater than 100 pg/ml strongly suggest ectopic production.

(E) The high-dose dexamethasone suppression test (8 mg at 11 PM) differentiates an adrenal tumor from ACTH-related causes of Cushing's syndrome. ACTH is low and cortisol is not suppressed in the presence of an adrenal tumor. ACTH is normal or high, and cortisol is suppressed with ectopic ACTH syndrome or a pituitary tumor.

(F) With malignancy, computed tomography (CT) scanning demonstrates tumor irregularity or loss of margins between the adrenal gland and the vena cava, liver, kidney, or pancreas. Biochemical confirmation of Cushing's disease should be obtained before imaging studies to allow better interpretation of results. For example, up to 10% of such patients have benign macroscopic adrenal nodules that may otherwise be mistaken for a primary adrenal tumor.

(G) Scintigraphy with iodine-131 or NP-59 ([131]I-6β-iodomethyl-19-norcholesterol) provides functional information. Patients with bilateral adrenocortical hyperplasia have bilateral increased adrenal uptake, whereas those with cortisol-secreting adenomas, which suppress pituitary ACTH secretion, and therefore function of the contralateral gland, have unilateral tracer uptake. There is no tracer uptake in Cushing's syndrome resulting from an adrenocortical carcinoma.

(H) There are less commonly used procedures. Venous sampling (with aldosterone as a control for catheter placement) can lateralize a benign tumor. Venography can demonstrate invasion of the vena cava. Androgens may be elevated with malignancy (total testosterone greater than 8.67 nmol/L [reference range: male, total 280 to 800 ng/dl, free 47 to 244 pg/ml; female, total 12 to 82 ng/dl, free 0.6 to 6.8 pg/ml). Elevated dehydroepiandrosterone sulfate (DHEAS) greater than 16 µmol/L (reference range depends on age and sex) also has a high sensitivity and specificity.

(I) Laparoscopic adrenalectomy is the procedure of choice for small (less than 6 cm diameter), benign adrenal tumors. In a case-control study of 100 patients, there was statistically significant improvement in mean hospital stay, return to normal activity, narcotic use, patient satisfaction, late morbidity, and operating room time when compared with an open procedure. An open anterior or lateral approach should be used for tumors larger than 6 cm, local invasion, or lymphadenopathy.

(J) There is a high suspicion for malignant adrenal tumors when they are larger than 6 cm or if there is local invasion or distant disease. These malignant tumors are extremely aggressive, shortening life expectancy to only 50% at 2 years. Risks of laparoscopic surgery are seeding at the port site, tumor fracture, and incomplete resection leading to recurrence. Thus an open anterior or lateral approach is used for en bloc excision, node dissection, possible vascular reconstruction, and to identify metastases.

(K) Ectopic ACTH syndrome, accounting for 10% to 15% of cases of Cushing's syndrome, has multiple etiologies. Small cell lung cancer (SCLC) accounts for half of these cases, but only 1% to 5% of all SCLC have such potential. Other causes are tumors of foregut origin (35%), including carcinoid tumors (lungs, thymus, and gastrointestinal tract); pancreatic islet cell tumors; medullary thyroid carcinoma; pheochromocytomas (5%); ovarian tumors (2%); and ganglioneuromas.

(L) A pituitary tumor (usually a chromophobe microadenoma) results in ACTH overproduction and hypercortisolemia.

(M) The lateral transabdominal approach is most common and allows for a limited incision and flexibility with familiar anatomy. The lateral retroperitoneal approach allows a large working space and avoids abdominal adhesions, whereas the posterior retroperitoneal approach is useful in patients with prior laparotomy, intraabdominal adhesions, history of peritonitis, or bilateral adrenal tumors. Overall patient outcomes are similar in all three methods, and choice depends on the surgeon's experience. Exogenous corticosteroid replacement for several months may be necessary for hypothalamic pituitary adrenal (HPA) axis recovery.

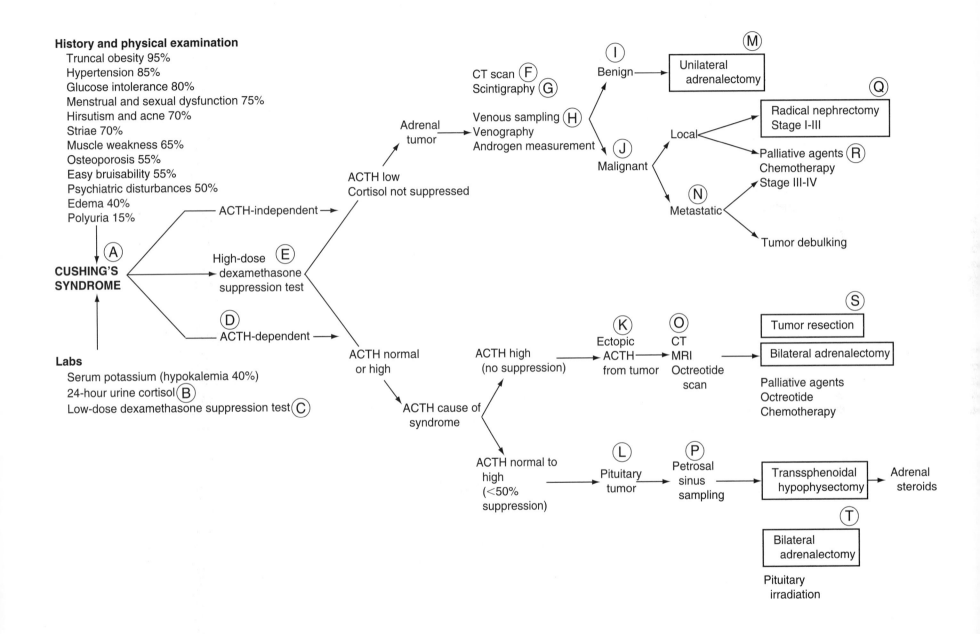

History and physical examination
Truncal obesity 95%
Hypertension 85%
Glucose intolerance 80%
Menstrual and sexual dysfunction 75%
Hirsutism and acne 70%
Striae 70%
Muscle weakness 65%
Osteoporosis 55%
Easy bruisability 55%
Psychiatric disturbances 50%
Edema 40%
Polyuria 15%

Ⓐ

CUSHING'S SYNDROME

Labs
Serum potassium (hypokalemia 40%)
24-hour urine cortisol Ⓑ
Low-dose dexamethasone suppression test Ⓒ

ACTH-independent →

High-dose dexamethasone suppression test Ⓔ

Ⓓ ACTH-dependent →

Adrenal tumor →

ACTH low
Cortisol not suppressed

ACTH normal or high

ACTH cause of syndrome

CT scan Ⓕ
Scintigraphy Ⓖ

Venous sampling Ⓗ
Venography
Androgen measurement

Benign Ⓘ →

Malignant Ⓙ

ACTH high (no suppression) →

Ectopic Ⓚ ACTH from tumor →

ACTH normal to high (<50% suppression) →

Pituitary tumor Ⓛ →

Ⓜ
Unilateral adrenalectomy

Local

Metastatic Ⓝ

Ⓠ
Radical nephrectomy
Stage I-III

Palliative agents Ⓡ
Chemotherapy
Stage III-IV

Tumor debulking

CT Ⓞ
MRI
Octreotide scan

Ⓢ
Tumor resection

Bilateral adrenalectomy

Palliative agents
Octreotide
Chemotherapy

Petrosal Ⓟ sinus sampling →

Transsphenoidal hypophysectomy → Adrenal steroids

Ⓣ
Bilateral adrenalectomy

Pituitary irradiation

Ⓝ Metastatic disease is almost always accompanied by persistence or recurrence of Cushing's syndrome. Palliative agents (discussed in R) and tumor debulking are options.

Ⓞ High-resolution chest CT localizes most tumors, but magnetic resonance imaging (MRI) may be preferable because it can better denote small bronchial carcinoids. Octreotide scanning may identify responsible neuroendocrine tumors but has a substantial false-positive rate and should only be performed after CT or MRI.

Ⓟ The diagnosis of a pituitary adenoma must be based on endocrine rather than radiographic studies because MRI does not have adequate sensitivity or specificity. Petrosal sinus catheterization shows a petrosal sinus-to-peripheral vein ACTH concentration gradient greater than 2:1 before or greater than 3:1 after corticotropin-releasing hormone (CRH) administration. This may allow tumor lateralization, permitting partial anterior hypophysectomy.

Ⓠ Radical nephrectomy has supplanted simple adrenalectomy, appearing to yield somewhat better results. With evidence of distant disease, tumor debulking may be valuable. Surgical resection is the principal therapy for stage I to III disease.

Ⓡ Limited information is available on palliative therapy. Mitotane, an adrenocorticolytic agent, is directly cytotoxic to the adrenal gland and has long-lasting effects. However, large randomized prospective trials are lacking, and its use results in adrenal insufficiency, requiring replacement of cortisol and aldosterone. Aminoglutethimide, ketoconazole, and metyrapone inhibit cytochrome P450 enzymes involved in adrenocorticosteroid synthesis but have no proven long-term efficacy.

Ⓢ A minority of ectopic ACTH-secreting tumors can be resected. Bilateral laparoscopic adrenalectomy is a more effective and definitive therapy. Tumor response to chemotherapy may be monitored by changes in ACTH. When the source of ACTH cannot be determined or removed, other options have been used with limited experience. Inhibitors of cortisol production are used for palliation but are less successful in the setting of ectopic ACTH because of more potent adrenal stimulation from higher ACTH levels. Octreotide inhibits ACTH secretion and has been used with moderate success to decrease cortisol levels from disseminated tumors. Mitotane may stabilize the condition of some patients preoperatively.

Ⓣ The treatment of choice is transsphenoidal hypophysectomy. If pituitary surgery fails, bilateral laparoscopic adrenalectomy is a reasonable alternative to prevent the high risk of panhypopituitarism with additional cranial surgery. In either case, replacement of adrenal steroids, often a prolonged course of supraphysiologic dosing, is mandatory to prevent postoperative Addisonian crisis. Primary therapy with pituitary irradiation is not optimal in patients with significant hypercortisolism because the mean onset of action is 18 months. Furthermore, pituitary insufficiency commonly results.

REFERENCES

Aniszeweski JP, Young WF, Thompson GB et al: Cushing syndrome due to ectopic adrenocorticotrophic hormone secretion. World J Surg 25:934–940, 2001.

Bonjer HJ, Kazemier G, De Herder WW: Retroperitoneal Endoscopic Adrenalectomy. In Gagner M, Inabnet WB (eds): Minimally Invasive Endocrine Surgery. Philadelphia: Lippincott, 2002.

Clutter WE: Cushing's syndrome: Hypercortisolism. In Doherty GM, Skogseid B (eds): Surgical Endocrinology. Philadelphia: Lippincott, 2001.

Jay V: The legacy of Harvey Cushing. Arch Pathol Lab Med 125:1539–1541, 2001.

Kebebew E, Duh QY: Operative Strategies for Adrenalectomy. In Doherty GM, Skogseid B (eds): Surgical Endocrinology. Philadelphia: Lippincott, 2001.

Kebebew E, Siperstein AE, Clark OH et al: Results of laparoscopic adrenalectomy for suspected and unsuspected malignant adrenal neoplasms. Arch Surg 137:948–951, 2002.

Kebebew E, Siperstein AE, Duh QY: Laparoscopic adrenalectomy: The optimal surgical approach? J Laparoendosc Adv Surg Tech 11:409–413, 2001.

Kendrick ML, Lloyd R, Erickson L et al: Adrenocortical carcinoma: Surgical progress or status quo? Arch Surg 136:543–549, 2001.

Siperstein AE, Berber E, Engle KL et al: Laparoscopic posterior adrenalectomy: Technical considerations. Arch Surg 135:967–971, 2000.

Starr FL, Prinz RA: Transabdominal Laparoscopic Adrenalectomy. In Gagner M, Inabnet WB (eds): Minimally Invasive Endocrine Surgery. Philadelphia: Lippincott, 2002.

Thompson GB, Grant CS, van Heerden JA et al: Laparoscopic versus open posterior adrenalectomy: A case-control study of 100 patients. Surgery 122:1132–1136, 1997.

Tsigos C, Kamilaris TC, Chrousos GP: Adrenal Diseases. In Moore WT, Eastman RC (eds): Diagnostic Endocrinology. St. Louis: Mosby, 1996.

Vella A, Thompson GB, Grant CS et al: Laparoscopic adrenalectomy for adrenocorticotropin-dependent Cushing's syndrome. J Clin Endoc Metab 86:1596–1599, 2001.

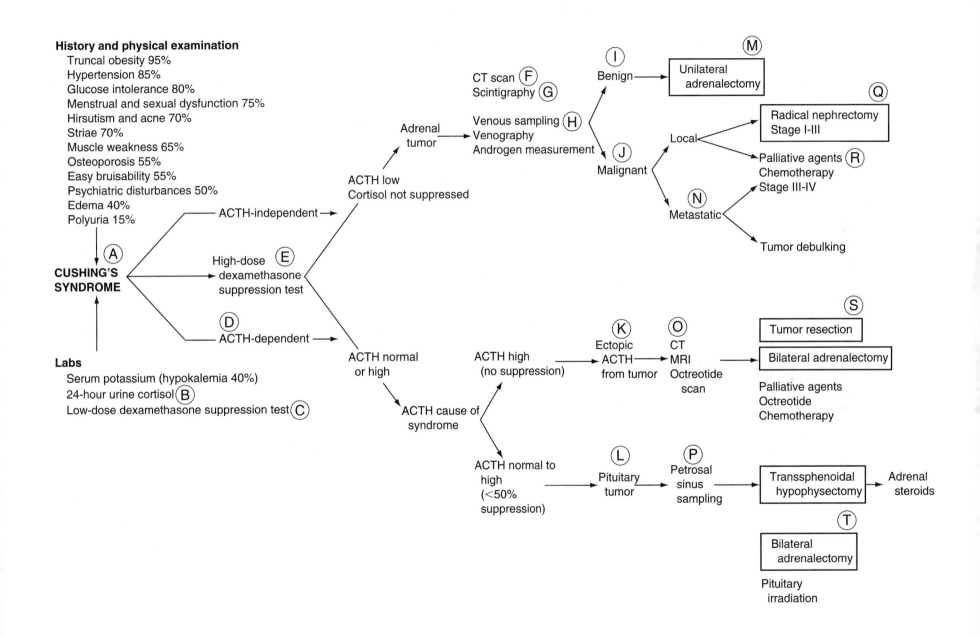

History and physical examination
Truncal obesity 95%
Hypertension 85%
Glucose intolerance 80%
Menstrual and sexual dysfunction 75%
Hirsutism and acne 70%
Striae 70%
Muscle weakness 65%
Osteoporosis 55%
Easy bruisability 55%
Psychiatric disturbances 50%
Edema 40%
Polyuria 15%

Ⓐ

CUSHING'S SYNDROME

Labs
Serum potassium (hypokalemia 40%)
24-hour urine cortisol Ⓑ
Low-dose dexamethasone suppression test Ⓒ

ACTH-independent →

High-dose Ⓔ
dexamethasone
suppression test

Ⓓ
ACTH-dependent →

Adrenal
tumor →

ACTH low
Cortisol not suppressed

ACTH normal
or high

ACTH cause of
syndrome

CT scan Ⓕ
Scintigraphy Ⓖ

Venous sampling Ⓗ
Venography
Androgen measurement

Ⓘ
Benign →

Ⓙ
Malignant

Ⓜ
Unilateral
adrenalectomy

Local

Ⓝ
Metastatic

Ⓠ
Radical nephrectomy
Stage I-III

Palliative agents Ⓡ
Chemotherapy
Stage III-IV

Tumor debulking

ACTH high
(no suppression) →

Ⓚ
Ectopic
ACTH →
from tumor

Ⓞ
CT
MRI
Octreotide
scan

Ⓢ
Tumor resection

Bilateral adrenalectomy

Palliative agents
Octreotide
Chemotherapy

ACTH normal to
high
(<50%
suppression) →

Ⓛ
Pituitary
tumor →

Ⓟ
Petrosal
sinus
sampling →

Transsphenoidal
hypophysectomy →

Adrenal
steroids

Ⓣ
Bilateral
adrenalectomy

Pituitary
irradiation

Chapter 95 *Primary Hyperaldosteronism*

JULIE K. HEIMBACH, MD • C. CLAY COTHREN, MD • ROBERT C. MCINTYRE, JR., MD

(A) The incidence of primary hyperaldosteronism (PHA) accounts for only 1% to 2% of patients with hypertension, so screening has not been recommended unless a patient was either hypokalemic (3.5 mEq or less) associated with kaliuresis, or had resistant hypertension. However, at least 20% of patients with PHA have a normal serum potassium. Thus recent reports suggest the incidence may be as high as 8% to 15% in hypertensive patients. Symptoms other than hypertension are rare.

(B) The most common cause of elevated aldosterone is secondary hyperaldosteronism caused by an elevated plasma rennin. PHA associated with a suppressed rennin activity is most commonly caused by an aldosterone-producing adenoma (APA), which is typically a small (less than 2 cm), unilateral, benign nodule more commonly found in women. The second most common cause of hyperaldosteronism is bilateral adrenal hyperplasia or idiopathic hyperaldosteronism (IHA), occurring in 20% to 30% of patients with hyperaldosteronism; it is more common in older males. Rare causes of hyperaldosteronism are primary adrenal hyperplasia, adrenal carcinoma, and glucocorticoid-remediable aldosteronism (GRA). GRA is caused by an autosomal dominant chimeric gene that allows ACTH to stimulate aldosterone synthesis. This is most common in hypertensive children or young patients with a family history of hyperaldosteronism.

(C) The most widely utilized screening test is the ratio of plasma aldosterone (PA) to plasma renin activity (PRA), with elevated results considered to be above 30 ng/dl:ng/ml/hour. This test should be done after holding diuretics for 2 weeks and spironolactone for 6 weeks. Labs are drawn in the morning with the patient in the upright position. The sensitivity and specificity of this test have been challenged, though no clear alternative screening tool is available.

(D) Confirmatory testing involves sodium loading (2 to 3 g with each meal for 3 days) followed by urinary aldosterone excretion. A 24-hour urine is collected for aldosterone, sodium, potassium, and cortisol levels. Sodium excretion over 200 mEq/24 hours confirms sodium loading. Aldosterone less than 12 µg/24 hours rules out hyperaldosteronism. Urinary potassium excretion is generally greater than 40 mEq/24 hours. Alternative confirmatory tests include saline infusion (2 L in 4 hours) followed by plasma aldosterone level (less than 8.5 ng/dl rules out hyperaldosteronism), or fludrocortisone suppression testing.

(E) Postural testing differentiates aldosteronoma from IHA. A plasma aldosterone level is drawn after 4 hours in the upright position following an overnight in the supine position. Patients with APA will have a small reduction or slight increase in aldosterone in the upright position. Patients will have a greater than 33% increase in aldosterone levels owing to angiotensin II stimulation of IHA. However, about 20% of patients with an aldosteronoma are responsive to angiotensin II and thus have a rise in aldosterone with postural testing. Plasma 18-hydroxycortisol is elevated in patients with APA compared with IHA (a cutoff of 100 ng/dl). Adrenal venous sampling, though invasive, is the most sensitive and specific test to differentiate aldosteronoma from IHA.

(F) A plasma aldosterone level that remains stable or decreases with postural testing is indicative of an APA.

(G) An increased plasma aldosterone level is diagnostic of IHA.

(H) Patients with suspected aldosteronoma should proceed to CT scanning. If there is evidence of a solitary nodule, and postural testing suggests APA, the patient may proceed to adrenalectomy.

Patients with a negative or equivocal CT scan should undergo selective venous sampling (SVS) for both aldosterone levels and cortisol levels. If levels of aldosterone are unilaterally elevated, the patient should proceed to adrenalectomy. If aldosterone levels are low bilaterally, with elevated cortisol levels (confirming sampling within the adrenal vein), patients should undergo medical management of hyperaldosteronism.

(I) Laparoscopic adrenalectomy decreases hospital stay and recovery time when compared with the open technique, and has been shown to be safe. Spironolactone therapy for 3 weeks before surgery may replace potassium stores and reduce postoperative hypoaldosteronism.

(J) Medical management of IHA consists of spironolactone (50 mg/day) in combination with other antihypertensive agents (e.g., ACE inhibitors or calcium-channel blockers) if needed.

REFERENCES

Bornstein SR, Stratakis CA, Chrousos GP: Adrenocortical tumors: Recent advances in basic concepts and clinical management. Ann Intern Med 130:759–771, 1999.

Ganguly A: Primary aldosteronism. N Engl J Med 339:1828–1834, 1998.

Schwartz DL, Chapman AB, Boerwinkle E et al: Screening for primary aldosteronism: Implication of an increased plasma aldosterone/renin ratio. Clin Chem 48:1919–1923, 2002.

Gordon RD, Stowasser M, Rutherford JC: Primary aldosteronism: Are we diagnosing and operating on too few patients? World J Surg 25:941–947, 2001.

Lo CY, Tam PC, Kung AW et al: Primary aldosteronism: Results of surgical treatment. Ann Surg 224:125–130, 1996.

Sawka AM, Young WF, Thompson GB et al: Primary aldosteronism: Factors associated with normalization of blood pressure after surgery. Ann Intern Med 135:258–261, 2001.

Thakkar RB, Oparil S: Primary aldosteronism: A practical approach to diagnosis and treatment. J Clin Hypertens 3:189–195, 2001.

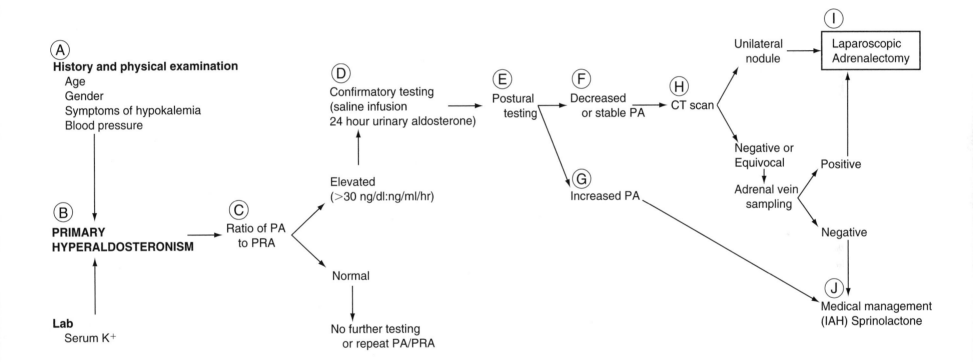

(A) **History and physical examination**
　　Age
　　Gender
　　Symptoms of hypokalemia
　　Blood pressure

(B) **PRIMARY HYPERALDOSTERONISM**

Lab
　　Serum K+

(C) Ratio of PA to PRA

Elevated
(>30 ng/dl:ng/ml/hr)

Normal

No further testing
or repeat PA/PRA

(D) Confirmatory testing
(saline infusion
24 hour urinary aldosterone)

(E) Postural testing

(F) Decreased or stable PA

(G) Increased PA

(H) CT scan

Unilateral nodule

Negative or Equivocal

Adrenal vein sampling

Positive

Negative

(I) Laparoscopic Adrenalectomy

(J) Medical management
(IAH) Sprinolactone

Chapter 96 *Adrenal Incidentaloma*

CHRISTOPHER J. SONNENDAY, MD • MARTHA A. ZEIGER, MD

(A) The initial evaluation of a previously clinically inapparent adrenal tumor should include a history and physical examination for signs and symptoms suggestive of glucocorticoid, mineralocorticoid, catecholamine, or adrenal sex hormone excess. A history of malignancy may suggest an adrenal metastasis.

(B) An adrenal incidentaloma is defined as an adrenal mass measuring more than 1 cm in diameter that is discovered at the time of an imaging procedure performed for an otherwise unrelated clinical indication. The majority of incidentalomas are benign; however, it is incumbent upon the clinician to assess whether the mass is hormonally active and/or malignant. Autopsy series reveal an incidence of 1.4% to 9% in patients without evidence of adrenal disease before death. Imaging studies identify clinically inapparent adrenal tumors in 0.4% to 4.4%.

(C) All patients with an adrenal incidentaloma must be tested for evidence of hypercortisolism, hyperaldosteronism, and pheochromocytoma. Subclinical Cushing's syndrome is the most common abnormality associated with these lesions and is found in 5% to 10% of cases.

(D) Hypercortisolism is associated with increased risk of cardiovascular, metabolic, and psychiatric diseases, and with adrenal insufficiency after adrenalectomy. The best screening test for the diagnosis of occult hypercortisolism is the 1 mg overnight dexamethasone suppression test. In normal patients, a serum cortisol level drawn the following morning should be less than 3 to 5 µg/dl. Confirmation of autonomous cortisol hypersecretion should be obtained with a 2-day low-dose or high-dose dexamethasone suppression test as well as measurement of plasma ACTH level. Lack of dexamethasone suppression and a low ACTH level support the diagnosis of a cortisol-producing adrenal adenoma.

(E) The second-most common functioning incidentalomas are pheochromocytomas, which represent about 5% of cases. Measurement of 24-hour urinary metanephrines and total catecholamines will detect the majority of pheochromocytomas; however, sensitivity of plasma-free metanephrines has been recently reported to be as high as 99% and is now recommended as the test of choice. These tumors also exhibit a characteristic radiologic phenotype, appearing heterogeneous on noncontrast CT and bright on T2-weighted MRI scans. All patients with pheochromocytoma should undergo adrenalectomy after α-adrenergic blockade.

(F) Classically, screening for this rare diagnosis has included measurement of patient blood pressure and serum potassium only; however, at least 20% of patients with hyperaldosteronism have normal serum potassium. The best screening test in patients with an adrenal incidentaloma and hypertension is measurement of ambulatory morning plasma aldosterone concentration (ng/dl) to plasma renin activity (ng/ml per hour) ratio (PAC/PRA ratio). A PAC/PRA ratio greater than 20 and a plasma aldosterone level greater than 15 ng/dl are highly suggestive of hyperaldosteronism. Patients need to discontinue spironolactone for 6 weeks before testing. A confirmatory test should include measurement of 24-hour urinary aldosterone secretion with oral salt loading or saline infusion. Persistently elevated urinary aldosterone and renin levels characterize hyperaldosteronism. Patients with confirmation of hyperaldosteronism and a unilateral adrenal mass should be considered for adrenalectomy; they generally are good candidates for the laparoscopic approach.

(G) As imaging techniques have improved, phenotypic descriptions of benign and malignant adrenal masses have emerged. CT is the primary adrenal imaging modality, and evaluation of adrenal lesions depends on morphology and density, measured in Hounsfield units (HU). Adrenal adenomas tend to have low attenuation (less than 10 HU) on a noncontrast CT scan and are well-circumscribed, homogeneous lesions. Adrenal adenomas typically exhibit low signal intensity on T2-weighted images.

Chemical-shift MRI may also confirm the diagnosis of adrenal adenomas, which have higher lipid content and typically show a reduction in signal intensity during the opposed phase.

(H) Adrenal carcinomas typically have higher attenuation (greater than 18 HU) and have characteristic irregular borders with a nonhomogeneous appearance. MRI has been advocated as an alternative to CT in the diagnosis of adrenal lesions. Adrenal metastases exhibit a bright intensity and pheochromocytomas, a hyperintense signal.

(I) In the absence of abnormal hormone production or worrisome radiologic features, recommendations for adrenalectomy for incidentalomas are based on the size of the lesion or its growth over time. The majority of adrenal incidentalomas less than 4 cm in diameter are benign adenomas, and adrenal carcinomas smaller than 4 cm have been rarely reported. The risk of adrenal carcinoma is significantly associated with increasing mass size, with approximately 25% of clinically silent masses greater than 6 cm found to be primary carcinomas. Therefore, all patients with unilateral adrenal lesions greater than 4 cm in diameter or a documented increase in size should undergo surgical resection. The presence of a radiographic phenotype worrisome for malignancy is an additional indication for adrenalectomy.

(J) Fine-needle aspiration biopsy (FNA) is most commonly used in the evaluation of a patient for metastatic cancer, and only in those cases in which the diagnosis would alter clinical management. A hormonal evaluation is essential, even in patients with a previous history of cancer, because percutaneous biopsy of an undiagnosed pheochromocytoma may be associated with hypertensive crisis or hemorrhage. Routine FNA is not recommended in the evaluation of patients with an incidentaloma because FNA of adrenal masses carries a significant risk of complications, and cytologic analysis will not distinguish among primary adrenal tumors.

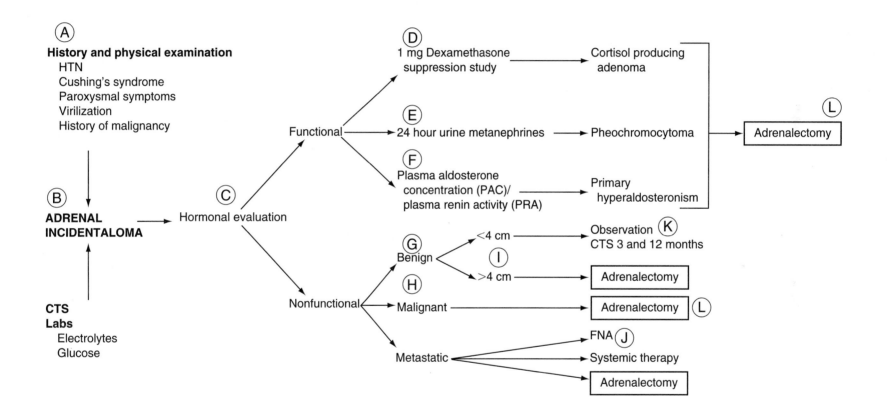

(A)

History and physical examination
    HTN
    Cushing's syndrome
    Paroxysmal symptoms
    Virilization
    History of malignancy

(B)

ADRENAL INCIDENTALOMA

(C) Hormonal evaluation

CTS
Labs
    Electrolytes
    Glucose

Functional

(D) 1 mg Dexamethasone suppression study → Cortisol producing adenoma

(E) 24 hour urine metanephrines → Pheochromocytoma

(F) Plasma aldosterone concentration (PAC)/ plasma renin activity (PRA) → Primary hyperaldosteronism

(L) Adrenalectomy

Nonfunctional

(G) Benign
    <4 cm → Observation (K) CTS 3 and 12 months
    (I)
    >4 cm → Adrenalectomy

(H) Malignant → Adrenalectomy (L)

Metastatic
    FNA (J)
    Systemic therapy
    Adrenalectomy

(K) In patients with nonfunctional unilateral masses less than 4 cm without malignant radiologic features, observation is the best management option. Most centers recommend follow-up imaging with CT or MRI at least once in the first 3 to 6 months, followed by repeat imaging at 12 and 24 months. Any interval increase in tumor size or change in radiologic appearance suggestive of malignancy should be treated with adrenalectomy. There is some evidence that incidentalomas require long-term follow-up because a significant percentage will grow in size or become functional.

(L) All patients with functional unilateral adrenal masses, unilateral masses greater than 4 cm, and unilateral masses with concerning radiologic features (particularly when greater than 4 cm) should be considered for adrenalectomy by either an open or laparoscopic approach. Laparoscopic adrenalectomy has the advantages of shortened recovery time and decreased postoperative pain. Preoperative suspicion of adrenal carcinoma is considered a relative contraindication for laparoscopic adrenalectomy. Adrenalectomy for isolated metastases from a nonadrenal primary has been reported in individual cases, but there is no evidence that resection of adrenal metastases improves patient survival.

REFERENCES

Barzon L, Scaroni C, Sorino N, et al: Risk factors and long-term follow-up of adrenal incidentalomas. J Clin Endocrinol Metab 84:520–526, 1999.

Brunt LM, Moley JF: Adrenal incidentaloma. World J Surg 25:905–913, 2001.

Caoili EM, Korobkin M, Francis IR, et al: Adrenal masses: Characterization with combined unenhanced and delayed enhanced CT. Radiology 222:629–633, 2002.

Grumbach MM, Biller BM, Braunstein GD et al: Management of the clinically inapparent adrenal mass (incidentaloma). Ann Intern Med 138:424–429, 2003.

Lenders JW, Pacak K, Walther MM, et al: Biochemical diagnosis of pheochromocytoma: Which test is best? JAMA 287: 1427–1434, 2002.

Libe R, Dall' Asta C, Barbetta L, et al: Long-term follow-up study of patients with adrenal incidentalomas. Eur J Endocrinol 147:489–494, 2002.

Young WF Jr.: Management approaches to adrenal incidentalomas: A view from Rochester, Minnesota. Endocrinol Metab Clin North Am 29:159–185, 2000.

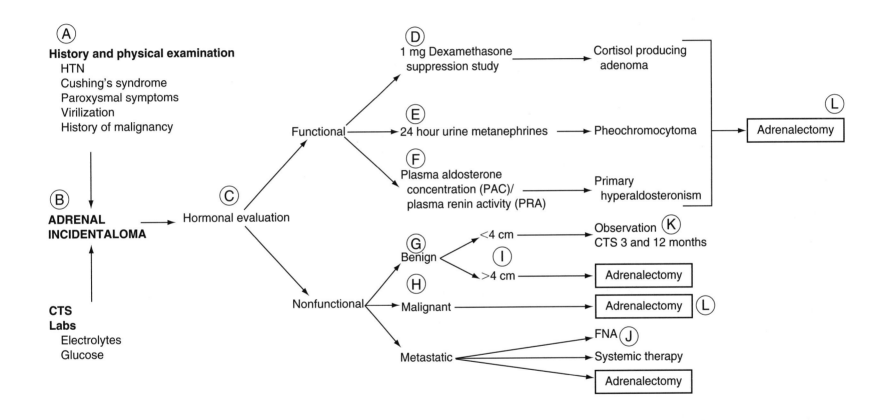

A **History and physical examination**
HTN
Cushing's syndrome
Paroxysmal symptoms
Virilization
History of malignancy

B **ADRENAL INCIDENTALOMA**

CTS
Labs
Electrolytes
Glucose

C Hormonal evaluation

Functional

D 1 mg Dexamethasone suppression study → Cortisol producing adenoma

E 24 hour urine metanephrines → Pheochromocytoma

F Plasma aldosterone concentration (PAC)/plasma renin activity (PRA) → Primary hyperaldosteronism

L Adrenalectomy

Nonfunctional

G Benign
<4 cm → K Observation CTS 3 and 12 months
I >4 cm → Adrenalectomy

H Malignant → Adrenalectomy L

Metastatic
J FNA
Systemic therapy
Adrenalectomy

VASCULAR

Chapter 97 *Thoracic Outlet Syndrome*

DAVID RIGBERG, MD • JULIE FREISCHLAG, MD

(A) Neurogenic thoracic outlet syndrome (TOS) is the most common, and controversial, variant. Although patients of any age can be affected, the usual case involves a young to middle-aged adult in otherwise good health. Paresthesia of the upper extremity is the most common presentation (90%). Pain of the upper extremity occurs in 80% of patients, the most common site being the area over the back of the shoulder. Arm pain may be focal or generalized. Ulnar symptoms dominate the former (ring and small fingers), representing C8-T1 impingement. Pain is usually exacerbated by stress positioning, particularly in patients whose disease is work-related. Headache may occur in up to 65% of patients. Occasionally, ipsilateral hyperhidrosis may be a component of TOS. For all of these patients, the history needs to include details of previous injuries, occupation information, and activities that exacerbate symptoms. In addition to providing evidence to support the presence of TOS, the physical examination is critical for ruling out other diagnoses. Although muscle atrophy may be present, most patients have nearly normal gross baseline sensory and motor examinations. The region overlying the anterior scalene muscle is commonly tender. The elevated arm stress test (EAST) is a controversial diagnostic maneuver designed to constrict the costoclavicular space and bring on TOS symptoms. Patients are asked to clench and unclench their fists while holding them in the "hold up" position. Pulses should also be assessed in all of these patients, although blood pressure measurements are much more sensitive and specific than Adson's test. Most cases of neurogenic TOS can be diagnosed through the combination of history and physical examination. Objective testing is helpful in confirming the diagnosis and in ruling out other causes of symptoms.

(B) Paget-Schroetter syndrome (axillo-subclavian venous or "effort" thrombosis) usually presents suddenly in previously healthy patients with no symptoms of neurogenic TOS. The typical patient is a young athlete or worker in an activity requiring prolonged or repetitive stressful positioning of the arms. Patients usually seek medical attention immediately. Physical examination discloses discoloration of the extremity, ranging from rubor to cyanosis. Dilated collateral veins may be found around the shoulder and upper arm.

(C) Arterial symptoms in TOS are the most varied because subclavian artery compression can lead to a number of different injuries. Cold sensitivity, Raynaud's syndrome, or other conditions may lead to an errant diagnosis of a collagen vascular disease. Others present with upper extremity "claudication." Acute occlusion of the subclavian artery can lead to rest pain, although limb threat is exceedingly rare in this setting. Emboli to the hand and fingers are commonly found.

(D) Objective testing for neurogenic TOS should start with a chest x-ray and cervical spine films. These tests can identify cervical ribs, elongated transverse processes of C7, and other conditions.

(E) MRI and CT scanning have some utility in the setting of neurogenic TOS, both in ruling out other conditions and in securing the diagnosis. Studies of MRI and CT for TOS are ongoing. For neurogenic TOS, a variety of neurodiagnostic tests can be used. These include nerve conduction velocity (NCV) studies, electromyelography (EMG), F-wave studies, and somatosensory-evoked potentials (SSEP). The tests are used selectively by most practitioners and are generally more useful for ruling out other causes of patient symptoms. EMG-guided scalene block is the most useful ancillary study. If the test is positive, there is a 94% positive predictive value for good outcomes if surgery is undertaken.

(F) For Paget-Schroetter syndrome, routine chest x-ray and cervical spine films are obtained. Noninvasive duplex ultrasound and dynamic venography (with provocative positioning) are used to secure the diagnosis. The role of magnetic resonance venography (MRV) is still being defined.

(G) The work-up of arterial TOS is highly dependent on the presentation and may involve digital plethysmography; upper extremity duplex examination; or angiography of the aortic arch, and the subclavian and axillary arteries. This study may require provocative positioning to be diagnostic. If distal embolization is suggested, the target sites should be included in the angiography.

(H) Therapy for neurogenic TOS is nonoperative in 60% of patients. Treatment starts with a minimum of 6 weeks of physical therapy designed to strengthen muscle groups that open the thoracic outlet (i.e., trapezius, levator scapulae, and sternocleidomastoid) and relax those that close it (i.e., middle scalene, subclavius, and pectoralis). If this is not successful, therapeutic blockade of the scalene muscle with botulinum toxin is advocated by some groups. This is usually only a temporizing measure but may allow for extended periods of physical therapy or other adjustments such as in the patient's ergonomics at work.

(I) Paget-Schroetter patients should receive prompt treatment. Arm elevation and heparinization are the initial maneuvers, followed by expeditious catheter-directed lysis of the clot. tPA and urokinase have similar profiles in this setting. Coumadin anticoagulation is subsequently started and a 1- to 3-month period has traditionally been allowed for venous intimal healing to occur before undertaking first rib resection. Others now advocate first rib resection at the time of the initial hospitalization, reporting equally good results and a decreased disability period for most patients. In either protocol, venography following surgery can identify any remaining problems, and catheter-based venoplasty can be performed if indicated. Prompt treatment of Paget-Schroetter syndrome can prevent the repeated venous problems seen in 75% of patients when immobilization and anticoagulation constituted full therapy.

(J) Treatment of arterial TOS varies with the underlying problem. For most situations,

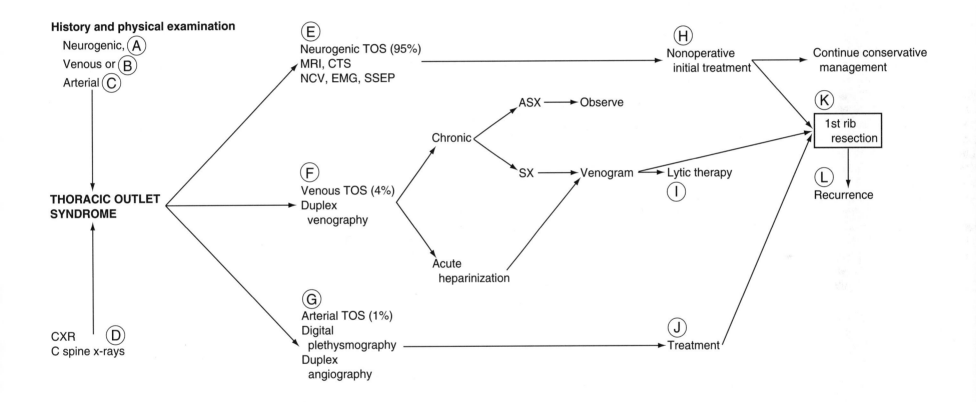

History and physical examination

Neurogenic, (A)
Venous or (B)
Arterial (C)

**THORACIC OUTLET
SYNDROME**

CXR (D)
C spine x-rays

(E)
Neurogenic TOS (95%)
MRI, CTS
NCV, EMG, SSEP

(F)
Venous TOS (4%)
Duplex
venography

(G)
Arterial TOS (1%)
Digital
plethysmography
Duplex
angiography

ASX → Observe

Chronic

SX → Venogram → Lytic therapy (I)

Acute
heparinization

(H)
Nonoperative
initial treatment

Continue conservative
management

(K)
1st rib
resection

(L)
Recurrence

(J)
Treatment

transaxillary first rib resection followed by arterial repair remains the treatment of choice. The retroscalene subclavian to prepectoral region of the axillary artery is the most commonly involved segment. If treating a patient with embolic disease, catheter-based thrombolysis is usually necessary before addressing their source. Complex regional pain syndrome (causalgia) may occasionally be present in TOS patients, and cervicodorsal or cervicothoracic sympathectomy can be performed. Aneurysms in the setting of arterial TOS are treated with resection and graft reconstruction.

(K) Operative management of TOS involves first rib resection, usually by either the transaxillary or supraclavicular approach. Some surgeons omit the rib resection when using the supraclavicular route, opting to perform only scalenectomy. There are also advocates of thoracoscopic first rib resection. Division of the anterior scalene, subclavius tendon, and first intercostal muscle attachments is required to remove the first rib. Cervical ribs, if present, are resected. Studies report a 59% to 94% improvement in symptoms following surgery.

(L) Recurrent TOS symptoms may be secondary to a faulty initial diagnosis, so special emphasis is placed on ruling out other causes. Iatrogenic injury to the brachial plexus, carpal tunnel syndrome, tendinitis, arthritis, and spine injury must be sought before treatment is initiated. A conservative plan is initially undertaken, although improvement is much less likely than what would be expected in initial treatment. Further surgery can follow if this treatment fails. If the original operation was by the transthoracic route, a supraclavicular operation is undertaken now. If any remaining first rib is found, it is resected back to the transverse processes. If the initial operation was supraclavicular scalenectomy without first rib resection, the rib is now removed via the transaxillary approach. Most surgeons add some form of neurolysis to the reoperation, whereby the scar around the nerves is carefully removed. Some surgeons remove the middle scalene during the course of re-exploration. In one series, 86% of patients with status of post-reoperation still reported subjective benefit at the 5- to 10-year interval.

REFERENCES

Aligne C, Barral X: Rehabilitation of patients with thoracic outlet syndrome. Ann Vasc Surg 6:381–389, 1992.

Angle N, Gelabert HA, Farooq MM et al: Safety and efficacy of early surgical decompression of the thoracic outlet for Paget-Schroetter syndrome. Ann Vasc Surg 15:37–42, 2001.

Feugier P, Aleksic I, Salari R et al: Long-term results of venous revascularization for Paget-Schroetter syndrome in athletes. Ann Vasc Surg 15:212–218, 2001.

Franklin GM, Fulton-Kehoe D, Bradley C et al: Outcome of surgery for thoracic outlet syndrome in Washington State Workers' Compensation. Neurology 54:1252–1257, 2000.

Jordan SE, Ahn SS, Freischlag JA: Selective botulinum chemo-denervation of the scalene muscles for treatment of neurogenic thoracic outlet syndrome. Ann Vasc Surg 14:365–369, 2000.

Machleder HI: Thoracic outlet syndromes: New concepts from a century of discovery. Cardiovasc Surg 2:137–145, 1994.

Machleder HI, Mill F, Nuwer M et al: Somatosensory-evoked potentials in the assessment of thoracic outlet compression syndrome. J Vasc Surg 6:177–184, 1987.

Perler BA, Mitchell SE: Percutaneous transluminal angioplasty and transaxillary first rib resection: A multidisciplinary approach to the thoracic outlet syndrome. Am Surg 52:485–488, 1986.

Roos DB: Recurrent thoracic outlet syndrome after first rib resection. Acta Chir Belg 79:363–372, 1980.

Roos DB, Owens JC: Thoracic outlet syndrome. Arch Surg 93:71–74, 1966.

Sanders RJ, Jackson CGR, Baushero N et al: Scalene muscle abnormalities in traumatic thoracic outlet syndrome. Am J Surg 159:231–236, 1990.

Sharp WJ, Nowak LR, Zamani T et al: Long-term follow-up and patient satisfaction after surgery for thoracic outlet syndrome. Ann Vasc Surg 15:32–36, 2001.

Siivola J, Myllyla VV, Sulg I et al: Brachial plexus and radicular neurography in relation to cortical evoked responses. J Neurol Neurosurg Psychiatry 42:1151–1158, 1979.

Tilney ML, Griffiths HJ, Edwards EA: Natural history of major venous thrombosis of the upper extremity. Arch Surg 101:792–796, 1970.

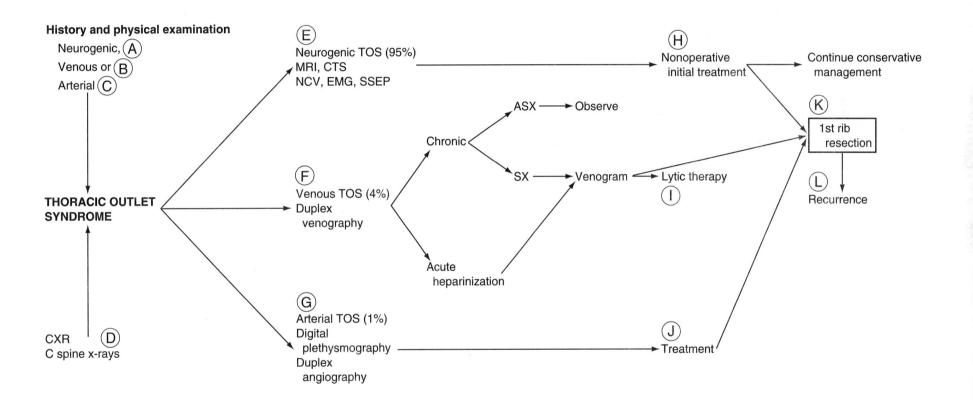

History and physical examination

Neurogenic, (A)

Venous or (B)

Arterial (C)

THORACIC OUTLET SYNDROME

CXR
C spine x-rays (D)

(E)
Neurogenic TOS (95%)
MRI, CTS
NCV, EMG, SSEP

(F)
Venous TOS (4%)
Duplex
venography

(G)
Arterial TOS (1%)
Digital
plethysmography
Duplex
angiography

Chronic

ASX → Observe

SX → Venogram → Lytic therapy
(I)

Acute
heparinization

(H)
Nonoperative
initial treatment

Continue conservative
management

(K)
1st rib
resection

(L)
Recurrence

(J)
Treatment

Chapter 98 *Intermittent Claudication*

THOMAS A. WHITEHILL, MD

A Claudication is classically characterized by the commencement of reproducible pain, tension, and weakness in the calf musculature after walking is begun; intensification of the condition until walking becomes impossible; and the disappearance of the symptoms after a short period of rest. Patients can typically walk only 1 to 3 blocks before they must stop and rest. The most common cause of claudication in most Western populations is atherosclerosis. Risk factors for peripheral arterial disease include cigarette smoking, diabetes mellitus, hypertension, dyslipidemia, abnormalities of hemostatic function, and abnormalities of homocysteine metabolism. Complications of atherosclerosis (e.g., myocardial infarction and stroke) cause most of the deaths in claudicants, who die at a rate of roughly 7% per year. The prevalence of claudication sharply increases in late middle age and is somewhat higher among men than women.

B Physical examination reveals absent or diminished peripheral pulses, and sometimes reveals aortic or femoral arterial bruits. Pallor with elevation and rubor with dependency of the affected extremity, along with decreased skin temperature and atrophy of skin appendages (e.g., hairless with dry skin) suggests a significant dysvascular state. Occasionally with noncritical aortoiliac arterial stenosis, femoral and distal pulses are normal at rest. The ankle-brachial index (ABI) corroborates the pulse examination findings. Patients with evidence of peripheral arterial disease (PAD) should undergo a careful examination of the entire cardiovascular system. Abdominal examination should be carried out because 9% of claudicants will have an abdominal aortic aneurysm. Neurologic examination includes motor, sensory, and reflex testing of both lower extremities. The lumbar spine and paraspinous muscles are examined for point tenderness, spasm, and pain on hyperextension or straight leg raising.

C Noninvasive vascular laboratory (NIVL) tests aid in the determination of the level of arterial occlusive disease and can monitor response to treatment. Tests include Doppler ultrasonography, segmental limb blood pressure measurement, pulse volume recording, exercise treadmill testing, postocclusive reactive hyperemia testing, and color-assisted duplex ultrasound imaging. Tests can be used individually or in combination to obtain information about the hemodynamic and functional severity of peripheral atherosclerosis.

D Medical therapies can effectively modify the natural history of atherosclerotic lower extremity arterial occlusive disease. Aggressive risk factor modification and antiplatelet therapy (e.g., aspirin or clopidogrel) are primary goals because they may decrease not only the progression of disease in the lower extremities but also the risk of death from systemic atherosclerotic complications. Diabetes, smoking, and hypertension are recognized to be associated with an increased risk of death and of disease progression in the lower extremities. These factors, as well as hypercholesterolemia, should be controlled if possible. Smoking cessation is most likely to succeed in the context of a supervised program. Pain-free walking distance may not improve on cessation of smoking alone; it is therefore unwise to predict such a benefit with smoking cessation.

Patients with a moderate walking disability or a moderate need to walk farther are the ideal candidates for a trial of an exercise program. Exercise rehabilitation can improve functional capacity in persons with claudication. Meta-analysis showed that pain-free walking time increased 180% and maximal walking time increased 120% in claudicants who participated in an exercise program. Substantial improvements have been found in walking speeds and distances (65% and 44%, respectively), caloric expenditure (31%), and physical functioning (67%). Success has been greater with supervised exercise than with home-based programs. Weight reduction decreases the demand on the circulation and improves functional walking ability. These strategies can decrease claudication, forestall the onset of limb-threatening events, decrease rates of invasive interventional therapies, and improve long-term survival.

E Intermittent claudication is considered to be only a relative indication for vascular reconstruction, and then only after an adequate trial of nonsurgical therapy.

F Surgeons disagree about the advisability of operation for claudicative symptoms alone. Decisions must be individualized. Age, associated medical disease, employment requirements, and lifestyle preferences are taken into consideration. Claudication that jeopardizes the livelihood of a patient or that significantly impairs the desired lifestyle of an otherwise low-risk patient may be considered to be a reasonable indication for surgical correction. The surgeon should have followed the patient conservatively for a time, and the patient should have demonstrated a commitment to controlling risk factors (notably, quitting smoking and losing weight). In general, operations for isolated proximal inflow disease are more commonly performed than are operations for distal disease in the femoropopliteal arterial segments.

G Claudication progresses to limb-threatening ischemia in only a small percentage of patients. Surgical or radiologic interventions are justified only if they are safe, effective, and durable; and if they are performed after the long-term prognosis for both life and limb is considered. Because the complication rate of operative therapy is slightly higher than that of nonoperative treatment, surgery should not be performed without an adequate trial of nonoperative therapy.

H If the symptoms and clinical findings indicate sufficient disability or threat to limb survival, arteriography is in order. Arteriography is employed for the anatomic information it provides the surgeon in selecting and planning an operation. It can determine when occlusive disease is amenable to

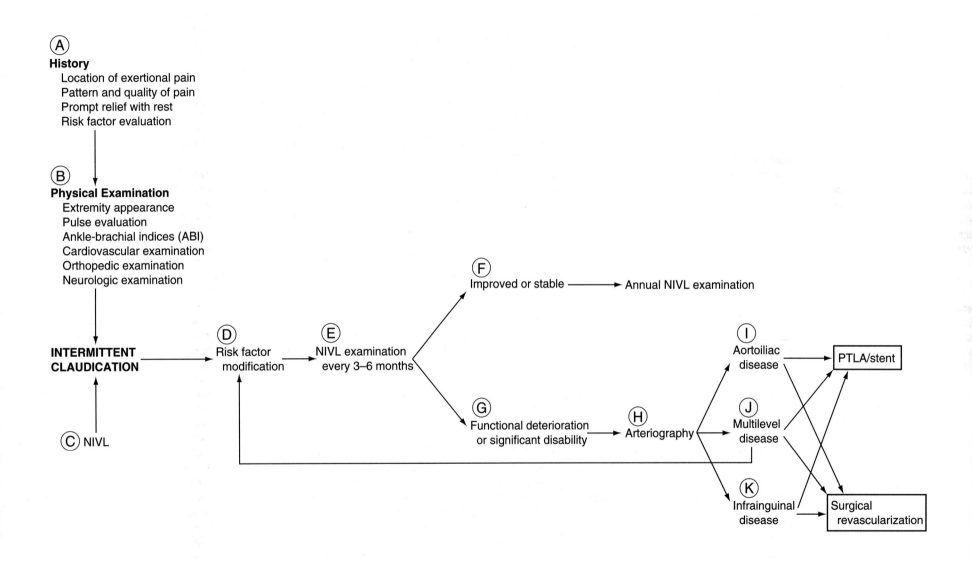

Ⓐ
History
   Location of exertional pain
   Pattern and quality of pain
   Prompt relief with rest
   Risk factor evaluation

Ⓑ
Physical Examination
   Extremity appearance
   Pulse evaluation
   Ankle-brachial indices (ABI)
   Cardiovascular examination
   Orthopedic examination
   Neurologic examination

**INTERMITTENT
CLAUDICATION**

Ⓒ NIVL

Ⓓ Risk factor
   modification

Ⓔ NIVL examination
   every 3–6 months

Ⓕ
Improved or stable ⟶ Annual NIVL examination

Ⓖ
Functional deterioration
or significant disability

Ⓗ Arteriography

Ⓘ
Aortoiliac
disease

Ⓙ
Multilevel
disease

Ⓚ
Infrainguinal
disease

PTLA/stent

Surgical
revascularization

percutaneous transluminal balloon angioplasty (PTLA).

(I) Focal stenosis of the common iliac artery less than 10 cm long (prevalence 10% to 15% of patients) is the most favorable situation for PTLA and has excellent early and late patency rates. PTLA is not recommended for diffuse diseased or totally occluded iliac disease unless the patient is a poor surgical candidate. This is because of the high incidences of complications and recurrent occlusions. Endovascular stents might provide more durable vascular dilation than PTLA, particularly when the patient is at high risk for restenosis. Stents are useful for PTLA-induced dissection, especially of the external iliac artery. PTLA in the femoropopliteal region is associated with a higher risk of failure and with poor durability because lesions are usually long and totally occlusive.

(J) Aortofemoral reconstruction is often used to treat claudication because of the perception that claudication in patients with aortoiliac disease may progress to critical ischemia. Five-year patency is 85% to 90%; operative mortality is less than 5%. Femoropopliteal bypass grafting has a low operative risk but also carries a lower long-term patency.

Infrainguinal bypass for disabling claudication carries an overall 5-year patency rate of 57% to 72%. Patients with claudication and good distal runoff generally have better results than do those who have more advanced occlusive disease (5-year patency rates as high as 82% and operative mortality rates of less than 3%). Complications after all types of lower extremity bypass include hemorrhage (less than 3%), graft thrombosis (2% to 20%), and graft infection (2% to 6%).

(K) In the presence of hemodynamically-significant multilevel PAD, decision-making is more complex. One must consider the relative contributions of each level of occlusive disease to the overall reduction in flow and the likelihood of clinical success after each interventional or surgical procedure. Careful risk-benefit analysis must be discussed with the patient's full understanding. If complex or multilevel open intervention is required to achieve the patient's goals, many patients and physicians opt for medical and/or exercise therapy.

REFERENCES

Girolami B, Bernardi E, Prins M et al: Treatment of intermittent claudication with physical training, smoking cessation, pentoxyphylline, or nafronyl: A meta-analysis. Arch Intern Med 159:337–345, 1999.

Hunnick MGM, Wong JB, Donaldson MC et al: Revascularization for femoropopliteal disease: A decision and cost-effectiveness analysis. JAMA 274:165–171, 1995.

Kent KC, Donaldson MC, Attinger CE et al: Femoropopliteal reconstruction for claudication. Arch Surg 123:1196–1198, 1998.

Money S, Herd J, Isaacson J et al: Effect of cilostazol on walking distances in patients with intermittent claudication caused by peripheral vascular disease. J Vasc Surg 27:267–275, 1998.

Nawaz S, Cleveland T, Gaines P et al: Aortoiliac stenting: Determinants of clinical outcome. Eur J Vasc Endovasc Surg 17:351–359, 1999.

Patterson R, Pinto B, Marcus B et al: Value of a supervised exercise program for the therapy of intermittent claudication. J Vasc Surg 25:312–319, 1997.

Powell R, Fillinger M, Walsh D et al: The durability of endovascular treatment of diffuse iliac occlusive disease. J Vasc Surg 31:1178–1184, 2000.

Rutherford R, Baker J, Ernst C et al: Recommended standards for reports dealing with lower extremity ischemia: Revised version. J Vasc Surg 26:517–538, 1997.

Weitz JI, Byrne J, Clagett GP et al: Diagnosis and treatment of chronic arterial insufficiency of the lower extremities: A critical review. Circulation 94:3026–3049, 1996.

Zannetti S, L'Italien GJ, Cambria RP: Functional outcome after surgical treatment for intermittent claudication. J Vasc Surg 24:65–73, 1996.

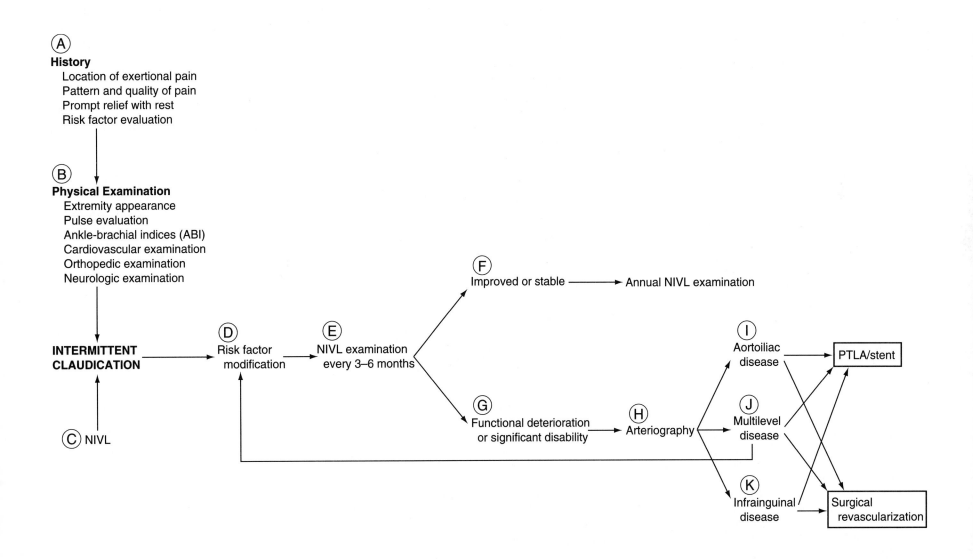

Ⓐ
History
    Location of exertional pain
    Pattern and quality of pain
    Prompt relief with rest
    Risk factor evaluation

Ⓑ
Physical Examination
    Extremity appearance
    Pulse evaluation
    Ankle-brachial indices (ABI)
    Cardiovascular examination
    Orthopedic examination
    Neurologic examination

INTERMITTENT CLAUDICATION

Ⓒ NIVL

Ⓓ Risk factor modification

Ⓔ NIVL examination every 3–6 months

Ⓕ Improved or stable ⟶ Annual NIVL examination

Ⓖ Functional deterioration or significant disability

Ⓗ Arteriography

Ⓘ Aortoiliac disease

Ⓙ Multilevel disease

Ⓚ Infrainguinal disease

PTLA/stent

Surgical revascularization

Chapter 99 *Peripheral Arterial Embolism*

MATTHEW J. EAGLETON, MD • KENNETH OURIEL, MD

(A) It is estimated that 10% of peripheral arterial emboli affect the visceral circulation, 20% involve the cerebral circulation, and 70% involve the extremities. The lower extremities are affected five times more often than are the upper extremities and will be the focus of this chapter.

Patients with peripheral arterial emboli present with acute limb ischemia with any or all of the following signs and symptoms: pain, pulselessness, paralysis, poikilothermia, pallor, and paresthesia. There are multiple etiologies of acute limb ischemia that may mimic peripheral arterial embolism including acute thrombosis of native artery or bypass graft, acute arterial dissection, severe vasospastic disease, and severe heart failure superimposed on chronic peripheral arterial occlusive disease.

A careful history and physical examination can help to determine the etiology of acute limb ischemia. In particular, the chronology of the onset of symptoms should be elicited as well as any associated complaints. A past history of coronary artery disease, hypercoagulable state, cardiac dysrhythmias, claudication or rest pain, and previous vascular procedures (both open and percutaneous) should be investigated. A thorough physical examination should be performed with particular emphasis on the pulse deficit, skin color, limb temperature, and motor and sensory function. Doppler interrogation of ankle and pedal vessels is imperative. Comparison with the contralateral limb is important because in many patients with peripheral emboli the contralateral vascular examination is normal.

(B) Viability of the extremity is determined utilizing the Society for Vascular Surgery/International Society for Cardiovascular Surgery revised reporting standards. Limbs are classified into one of the following four categories, each of which has prognostic and therapeutic implications:

Class I: Viable (not immediately threatened: no sensory or motor loss and audible arterial signals)

Class IIa: Marginally threatened (salvageable if promptly treated; minimal [toes] or no sensory loss, no motor loss, and inaudible arterial signals)

Class IIb: Immediately threatened (salvageable with immediate revascularization; sensory loss [more than toes] associated with rest pain, mild/moderate muscle weakness, inaudible arterial signals)

Class III: Irreversible (major tissue loss or permanent nerve damage inevitable; profound sensory loss with anesthetic limb, profound motor loss/paralysis [rigor], inaudible arterial and venous signals)

(C) Appropriate laboratory tests include hematocrit, platelet count, electrolytes, and creatine phosphokinase levels. Coagulation studies are also helpful. If a hypercoagulable state is considered, blood is drawn for the appropriate laboratory studies before anticoagulation is administered.

(D) Patients presenting with peripheral arterial embolization should be anticoagulated with heparin at a dose of 100 IU/kg IV. This prevents thrombus propagation and possibly controls embolic sources. If subsequent therapy is to be delayed, continuous heparin infusion is begun.

(E) Viable limbs (Class I) allow the surgeon to fully evaluate the patient under close observation. This includes stabilization of comorbidities and formal angiographic evaluation.

(F) Marginally threatened limbs (Class IIa) can tolerate additional ischemic time without developing irreversible damage. These patients can generally be taken to the angiography suite. The operating room is a suitable alternative provided the equipment for fluoroscopically directed thromboembolectomy or intraoperative thrombolysis is available.

(G) Immediately threatened limbs (Class IIb or early Class III) should prompt the surgeon to take the patient immediately to the operating room for revascularization.

(H) Irreversibly ischemic limbs (late Class III) may require amputation. Irreversible damage can begin in 4 to 6 hours, but limb salvage is possible even with a 12-hour delay. Clinical judgment must be applied to determine the likely success of attempted limb salvage balanced with the patient's comorbidities and ability to tolerate the systemic insult sustained with reperfusion of a severely ischemic leg.

(I) The absence of bilateral femoral pulses suggests the presence of a saddle embolus. Both femoral arteries should be explored and the surgeon must be prepared to obtain inflow from the abdominal aorta or an extra-anatomic bypass utilizing the axillary artery.

(J) When the femoral pulse is absent on only one side, an iliofemoral thromboembolus should be suspected. Again, if thromboembolectomy is not successful, the surgeon should be prepared to obtain an alternate source of inflow whether that is the aorta, the contralateral femoral artery (femoral-femoral bypass), or the ipsilateral axillary artery.

(K) A palpable femoral pulse with an absent popliteal pulse suggests an embolus or thrombus at the level of the femoral bifurcation (or a thrombosed femoral stenosis at the level of Hunter's canal). Again, the femoral artery is explored through a groin incision.

(L) When the clot is lodged at the popliteal trifurcation, there will be femoral and popliteal artery pulses present bilaterally with absent pedal pulses. The below-the-knee popliteal artery is explored with control of all three outflow vessels. The surgeon should be prepared to explore the pedal vessels for both antegrade and retrograde thromboembolectomy.

(M) For isolated common femoral embolism with minimal propagation, femoral embolectomy may be performed under local anesthesia.

(N) When propagation of embolism involves the distal branches, thrombolytic therapy provides more complete dissolution of the thrombus. Catheter-directed thrombolysis allows for the resolution of

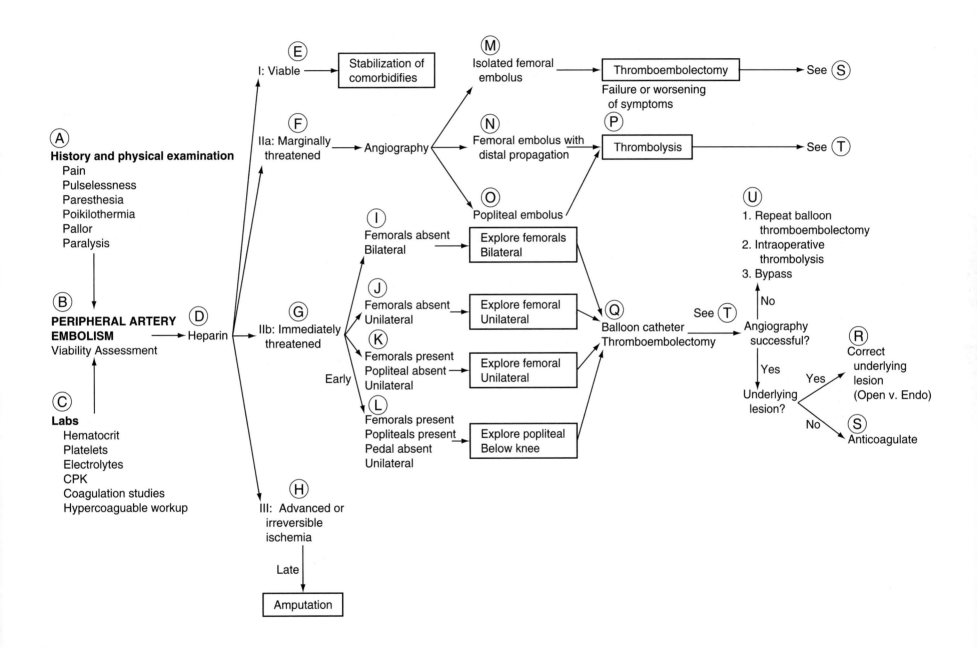

thrombus from distal run-off vessels and angiographic control of the process. The luxury of time, however, is a necessity with this process because it can often take 6 to 12 hours before reperfusion is achieved.

(O) Thrombolysis can be continued as far distally as required, and with subsequent proximal clot resolution the thrombolytic catheters are advanced distally into unlysed thrombus.

(P) Catheter directed thrombolysis currently is performed with t-PA, reteplase, or urokinase. In the STILE trial, thrombolytic therapy was successful at restoring patency in 81% of the bypass grafts and 69% of native arteries. In 56% of the cases there was a subsequent reduction in the planned surgical intervention. The Rochester trial noted a decrease in cardiopulmonary complications in patients undergoing thrombolytic therapy compared with surgical revascularization. Percutaneous thrombectomy is another option that can be used alone or in combination with thrombolysis. The simplest method is suction thrombectomy, but more advanced systems are under evaluation. These systems include devices such as the Angiojet Rheolytic Thrombectomy System (Possis Medical, Minneapolis, MN) and the Hydrolyser Percutaneous Thrombectomy Catheter (Cordis, Miami, FL).

(Q) Balloon catheter thromboembolectomy combined with heparin therapy has been shown to improve limb salvage rates to nearly 95%. Recent data suggest that fluoroscopically guided balloon catheter thromboembolectomy may improve outcomes. Most blind passes with a thromboembolectomy catheter pass distally through the peroneal artery. Fluoroscopic guidance can aid in directing the catheter into the posterior tibial artery and anterior tibial artery as well. Over-the-wire thromboembolectomy catheters can aid in this process. Thromboembolectomy catheters need to be passed until no residual thrombus is returned.

(R) If, on completion of arteriography, underlying lesions are identified, these should be treated. Short-segment, localized lesions may be amenable to balloon angioplasty with or without stent placement. More diffuse disease may require bypass surgery.

(S) The patient needs to be evaluated for an embolic source. Cardiac sources are best evaluated with transesophageal echocardiography whereas aortic sources can be evaluated with ultrasound, computed tomography scan, and magnetic resonance angiography. Embolic sources such as abdominal aortic aneurysms and "shaggy" aortas can be operatively or endovascularly managed. Until such time, patients should remain on heparin anticoagulation. Patients with cardiac sources or hypercoagulable states will require long-term anticoagulation with oral Coumadin.

(T) Completion arteriography is the only way to adequately determine full thrombus removal, whether the patient has undergone thrombolysis or thromboembolectomy.

(U) If thrombus remains in the outflow vessels after balloon catheter thromboembolectomy, intraoperative thrombolysis should be used. High doses of thrombolytic agent are injected into the arterial system through the exposed artery over a period of 5 to 30 minutes. The inflow vessel may or may not be occluded with a clamp or proximal tourniquet.

If residual thrombus is found during thrombolytic therapy, the duration of the therapy may need to be continued, keeping in mind that the risk of a bleeding complication increases with the duration of therapy. Catheters and wires may need to be advanced more distally into the thrombus. Continued failure at removal of thrombus may necessitate bypass surgery.

REFERENCES

Ouriel K, Shorell CK, DeWeese JA et al: A comparison of thrombolytic therapy with operative revascularization in the initial treatment of acute peripheral arterial ischemia. J Vasc Surg 19:1021–1030, 1994.

Parsons RE, Marin ML, Veith FJ et al: Fluoroscopically assisted thromboembolectomy: An improved method for treating acute arterial lesions. Ann Vasc Surg 10:201–210, 1996.

Rutherford RB, Baker JD, Ernst C et al: Recommended standards for reports dealing with lower extremity ischemia: Revised version. J Vasc Surg 26:517–538, 1997.

Rutherford RB: Acute Limb Ischemia. In Cronenwett JL, Rutherford RB (eds): Decision Making in Vascular Surgery. Philadelphia: WB Saunders, 2001.

STILE Investigators: Results of a prospective randomized trial evaluating surgery versus thrombolysis for ischemia of the lower extremity. Ann Surg 220:251–268, 1994.

Tawes RL, Beaver JP, Schribnre RG: Value of postoperative heparin therapy in peripheral arterial thromboembolism. Am J Surg 146:213–215, 1983.

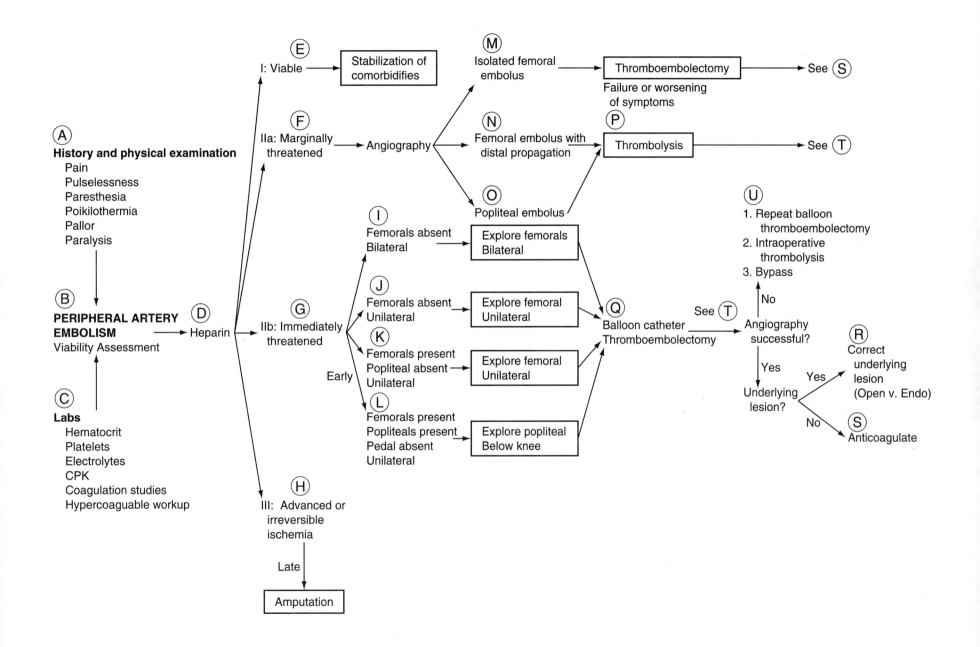

Chapter 100 *Abdominal Aortic Aneurysm*

MARK R. NEHLER, MD • JENNIFER ST. CROIX, MD

(A) An abdominal aortic aneurysm (AAA) is defined by the Society for Vascular Surgery as a 50% or greater increase in normal aortic diameter. Normal infrarenal aortic diameter in the Abdominal Aortic Aneurysm and Management (ADAM) study screening program was 2.0 cm for men, with minimal variability caused by factors such as sex, weight, and race. Therefore, a definition of AAA as 3.0 cm in diameter or larger seems appropriate. The incidence of AAA varies according to the population selected, ranging from 1.5% in autopsy series to 3.2% in unselected adult patients screened with ultrasound.

(B) The incidence of AAA increases when examining more selected patient populations with vascular disease. Coexistent AAA ranges from 5% in patients with known coronary artery disease to almost 10% in patients with known peripheral vascular disease. However, this data suffers from a lack of conformity regarding the definition of an aneurysm.

(C) Multiple reports describe a familial subgroup of AAA. These aneurysms seem to behave differently than "sporadic" types, with a higher risk of rupture even at smaller diameters. Screening of the AAA patient's first-degree male relatives older than 50 years seems prudent. Two prospective studies demonstrated AAA incidence in these relatives of about 30%. The proposed genetic defect has been linked to abnormal type III collagen.

(D) Multiple aneurysms are seen most commonly in patients with peripheral aneurysms. Some 40% to 50% of patients with a popliteal artery aneurysm will harbor an AAA. Also, 50% to 90% of patients with a femoral artery aneurysm will have an AAA. Patients with thoracic aneurysms have a 20% to 25% chance of having a simultaneous AAA. In addition, approximately 3% to 8% of patients will develop aortic aneurysms proximal to their graft during follow-up after infrarenal AAA repair.

(E) The aortic bifurcation is at the level of the umbilicus. The pulsatile mass of an AAA is located in the epigastrium. On physical examinations, only relatively large AAAs can be detected in obese patients; tortuous or hyperdynamic nonaneurysmal aortas can be mistaken for AAAs in thin patients. Physical examination only allows for a very approximate estimation of aneurysm diameter.

(F) In about 20% of cases, plain abdominal or lumbar spine radiographs will detect occult AAA. A thin rim of calcification identifies the aneurysmal aortic wall. Most aneurysms do not have sufficient calcium to be visualized by this method. Plain films are not accurate for aneurysm diameter determination because of variable magnification.

(G) Abdominal ultrasound (US) is the best screening method for detecting AAA. Measurement accuracy is within 0.3 cm, and US provides information in both cross-sectional and longitudinal dimensions. It does not provide significant anatomic detail (particularly the relationship of the proximal aneurysmal neck and the renal arteries) to plan operative management without other imaging modalities.

(H) The contrast-enhanced computed tomography (CT) scan is currently the best overall study for the preoperative evaluation of AAA architecture. Diameter measurements are accurate within 0.2 cm. Venous anomalies that dramatically alter operative approach (e.g., retroaortic or circumaortic left renal vein, inferior vena cava duplication, and left-sided inferior vena cava) are well visualized on CT. CT is excellent at detecting aneurysmal rupture or leak (92% accuracy and 100% specificity). CT is less useful for predicting suprarenal aneurysm involvement (83% sensitive, 90% specific, positive predictive value 48%).

(I) Ruptured aneurysms are antecedently diagnosed less than one-third of the time. The sudden onset of abdominal pain is the most common presenting symptom (82%). The classic diagnostic triad (present in only half) is abdominal/back pain, hypotension, and pulsatile abdominal mass. The diagnosis is much more difficult when the patient presents with abdominal pain alone. Less than 5% of patients presenting with abdominal pain to an emergency room have ruptured AAAs. Rapidly establishing the correct diagnosis is critical and can reduce the mortality rate from 75% to 35%. At a minimum, patients should have an electrocardiogram to rule out myocardial infarction. Less common symptomatic presentations include embolization to the legs, caval fistula with lower extremity edema and acute heart failure, compression of adjacent cava with deep venous thrombosis, and acute AAA thrombosis with leg and pelvic ischemia.

(J) Patients who suffer profound shock and cardiac arrest at the time of presentation have little chance of survival. Many authorities maintain that extreme age, dementia, metastatic cancer, and other severe end-stage medical problems should also preclude operation.

(K) Approximately 50% of patients with a ruptured AAA die before reaching the hospital. Another 25% who make it to the hospital die before they can be brought to the operating room. Unstable patients suspected of the diagnosis should be resuscitated en route to the operating room in preparation for immediate laparotomy. The patient should not be anaesthetized until completely prepped and draped and ready for immediate incision because the blood pressure may fall dramatically upon induction.

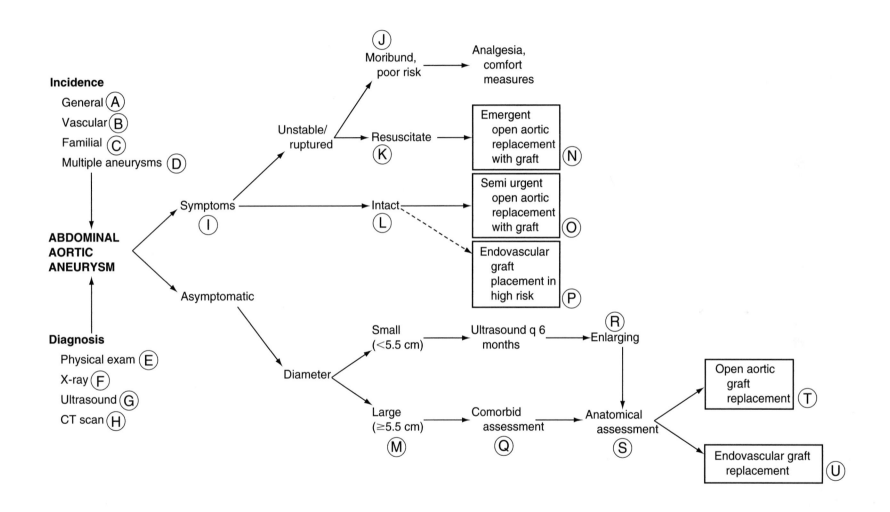

Incidence

General (A)

Vascular (B)

Familial (C)

Multiple aneurysms (D)

(L) A hemodynamically stable patient should have the diagnosis confirmed by CT scan with intravenous contrast. The ability of CT scan to rule out rupture has been well documented (see preceding). Other intra-abdominal organs that may produce similar symptoms (particularly the pancreas) can be visualized. Symptomatic nonleaking AAAs are either inflammatory or rapidly expanding with increased risk for rupture.

(M) The recent multicenter Veterans Administration Aneurysm Diagnosis and Management Trial demonstrated an annual risk of rupture of 0.6% in patients with aneurysms smaller than 5.5 cm. There was no mortality benefit from early operative repair for AAAs smaller than 5.5 cm despite an impressively low perioperative mortality rate of 2%. A similar annual risk of rupture in 5-cm AAAs was demonstrated in the United Kingdom Small Aneurysm Trial. The perioperative mortality for AAA repair in that study was 5.8%, again demonstrating no mortality benefit for early repair. In addition, the large aneurysm trial demonstrated an annual incidence of AAA rupture of 10% for AAAs 5.5 to 7.0 cm, and increased to 32% for AAAs larger than 7.0 cm.

(N) Rapid proximal aortic control is the key to successful outcome of operations for ruptured AAA. This can be at the diaphragm (in an unstable patient with either free intraperitoneal bleeding or a retroperitoneal hematoma that extends proximal to the left renal vein) or at the infrarenal aortic segment (in a stable patient with a lower retroperitoneal hematoma). With free intraperitoneal rupture, intraluminal balloon occlusion of the aorta can be useful. Once control is obtained, the patient is resuscitated and clamps are moved to the standard infrarenal location. Distal control can be performed with balloons or packs to prevent iliac venous injury. Heparin use, if any, is limited. Standard grafting techniques are performed. Major causes of operative death are venous injuries and coagulopathy. Operative mortality rates range from 40% to 75%.

(O) Although management is slightly controversial, most agree that symptomatic but intact AAAs should be repaired expediently. Emergent operation on presentation often combines unprepared patients, tired surgeons, and random on-call anesthesiologists. Of note, the operative mortality rate for urgent nonruptured AAA repair is about 20%, far higher than the standard elective repair.

(P) Endovascular prosthetic grafts have been successfully placed in high-risk patients with symptomatic AAAs or contained ruptures in either the aortic and aortoiliac position, but a variety of prefabricated endoluminal grafts are unavailable in most medical centers.

(Q) The extent of cardiac assessment appropriate for these patients is extremely controversial. Clearly the incidence of coronary disease in these patients is high, and the primary cause of postoperative and long-term mortality in these patients is cardiac disease. Equally high, however, is the mortality from coronary interventions in this elderly subgroup. Current strategies range from cardiac evaluation (using dipyridamole thallium scanning, most commonly followed by coronary angiography in those patients with reversible defects) in all patients to only in selected patients with defined clinical risk factors or only patients who have significant concomitant coronary symptoms.

(R) The average expansion rate of all AAAs is 0.4 cm/year. However, 15% to 20% of all AAAs show no change in size over time. Conversely, 15% to 20% expand at a rate greater than 0.5 cm/year. The rate of expansion is variable among individuals, with quiescent periods of months to years followed by rapid expansion. Rapid expansion (0.5 cm or more in 6 months) is considered to be an indication for repair. Patient subgroups (e.g., those with uncontrolled hypertension, postcardiac transplant, chronic obstructive pulmonary disease, or familial AAA) have higher rates of expansion (see preceding). In addition, the extent of intraluminal thrombus on CT has

been proposed as a predictor of rapid aneurysm expansion.

(S) As stated previously, CT scanning can be inaccurate for determination of proximal extent of juxtarenal and suprarenal aneurysms because of the difficulty of obtaining cross sectional images in a commonly tortuous region of the aorta. Traditionally, angiography has been used in patients when there is concern regarding the proximal neck, concomitant visceral occlusive disease, renal anomalies, a prior colectomy with need to visualize the visceral circulation, or lower extremity occlusive or aneurysmal disease. Most recently, spiral CT with 3-dimensional reconstruction has provided dramatic anatomical images of aneurysmal geometry and visceral arterial anatomy. The major disadvantage is the up-front investment cost to the hospital for purchase of the technology, the time required to create the images, and the requirement for substantial amounts of intravenous contrast. The major advantage is the potential benefit in planning and performing endovascular aortic grafting procedures. Magnetic resonance angiography has also been used to visualize the visceral vessels and aortoiliac system, but the need for patient breath-holding to eliminate respiratory artifacts is a potential problem.

(T) Elective aortic graft placement can be carried out equally well via a transperitoneal or extraperitoneal approach. The former has the advantage of better pelvic exposure and avoids the occasional lateral muscle bulge seen postoperatively with the extraperitoneal incision. The extraperitoneal approach provides superior exposure of the suprarenal aorta and may provide improved postoperative pulmonary management. Operative mortality rates range from 0% in individual series to up to 10% in state and community-wide surveys. There does appear to be significant near-term functional impairment for older patients with open AAA repair.

(U) Results of endovascular AAA repair have been mixed. Currently three FDA-approved grafts are being used. Perigraft leaks (endoleaks)

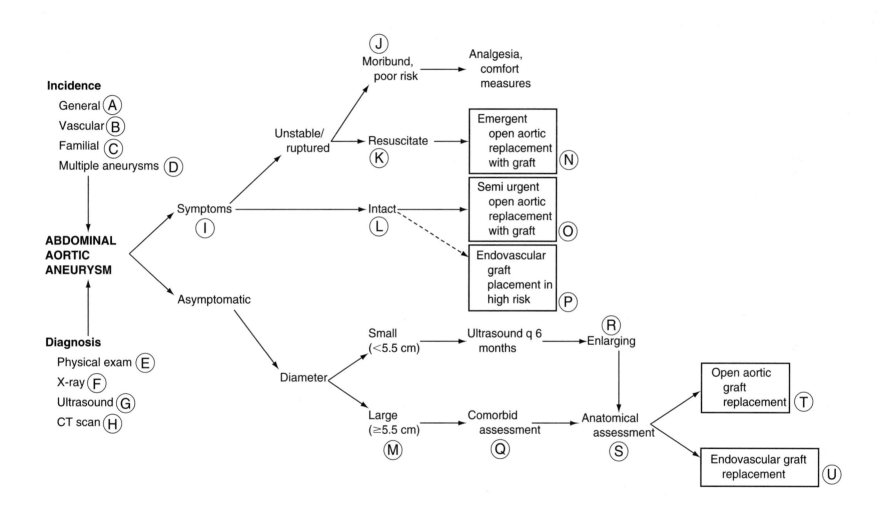

can occur following implantation in up to 20% of patients, making postoperative surveillance CT scanning a requirement. Ruptures caused by unrecognized leaks have been reported with grafts in place; however, these reports remain rare. A major issue currently is the greater cost of endografts, particularly when the surveillance CT scans are factored in. The majority of patients too ill to undergo open AAA repair will die from other causes, and repairing their AAAs, unless markedly large, does not change their poor natural history.

REFERENCES

Hallett JWJ, Marshall DM, Petterson TM et al: Graft-related complications after abdominal aortic aneurysm repair: Reassurance from a 36-year population-based experience. J Vasc Surg 25:277–284, 1997.

Lederle FA, Johnson GR, Wilson SE et al: Veterans Affairs Cooperative Study #417 investigators: Rupture rate of large abdominal aortic aneurysms in patients refusing or unfit for elective repair. JAMA 287:2968–2972, 2002.

Lederle FA, Wilson SE, Johnson GR et al: Aneurysm Detection and Management Veterans Affairs Cooperative Study Group: Immediate repair compared with surveillance of small abdominal aortic aneurysms. N Engl J Med 346:1437–1444, 2002.

The UK Small Aneurysm Trial participants: Mortality results for randomised controlled trial of early elective surgery or ultrasonographic surveillance for small abdominal aortic aneurysms. Lancet 352:1649–1655, 1998.

Williamson WK, Nicoloff AD, Taylor LM Jr. et al: Functional outcome after open repair of abdominal aortic aneurysm. J Vasc Surg 33:913–920, 2001.

Zarins CK, White RA, Hodgson KJ et al: Endoleak as a predictor of outcome after endovascular aneurysm repair: AneuRx multicenter clinical trial. J Vasc Surg 32:90–107, 2000.

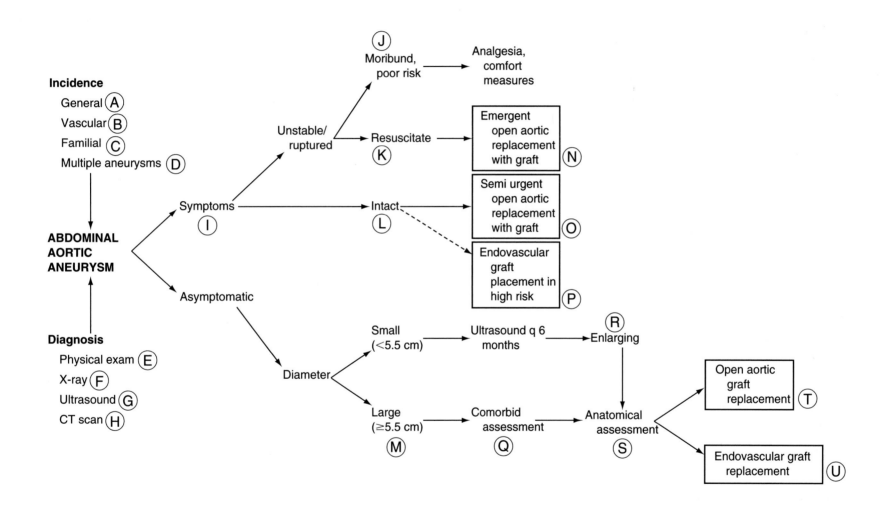

Chapter 101 *Extracranial Cerebrovascular Disease*

WESLEY S. MOORE, MD

(A) Risk factors for cerebrovascular disease include smoking, hypertension, diabetes mellitus, hyperlipidemia, family history, the presence of arteriosclerotic lesions in other distributions (including coronary and peripheral arterial systems), and age greater than 70 years. The presence of two or more risk factors, even in the absence of symptoms, suggests the likelihood of significant lesions in the bifurcation. A history of carotid territory transient ischemic attacks (TIA) with ocular or hemispheric symptoms is important to elicit. Posterior circulation symptoms are more difficult to differentiate. A history of stroke in the carotid distribution may indicate significant carotid bifurcation disease. An acute presentation of stroke or stroke in evolution speaks for itself. In the absence of specific symptoms, the physical findings of a carotid bruit, a difference (gradient) in blood pressure (BP) between the two arms, or subtle persistence of a neurologic deficit suggest the possibility of cerebrovascular insufficiency.

(B) The term "extracranial cerebrovascular disease" describes lesions in the circulation from the level or the aortic arch to the base of the skull. The lesions are primarily atherosclerosis but may also include such disease processes as fibromuscular dysplasia and arteritis. The most common site of disease is the area of the carotid bifurcation, but lesions of the aortic arch trunks and vertebral arteries are also important.

(C) Routine laboratory studies may elicit abnormalities such as elevated red blood cell count or erythrocyte sedimentation rate (ESR) suggestive of hematopoietic factors that can predispose to cerebrovascular manifestations. Arrhythmia, particularly atrial fibrillation, is important and can be identified on a routine electrocardiogram (ECG). Symptoms of cardiac origin should be evaluated by echocardiography looking for mural thrombus.

(D) Noninvasive testing is particularly important. Carotid duplex scanning using a color format is most helpful in identifying plaque in the carotid bifurcation and in determining flow compromise by velocity criteria. Plaque characteristics, including areas of increased echolucency and irregularity suggestive of ulceration, can be identified. Symptomatic patients should undergo brain imaging with either computed tomography (CT) or magnetic resonance imaging (MRI). If MRI is chosen, imaging of the extracranial and intracranial circulation with the MR angiography (MRA) format provides important additional information.

(E) When duplex scan information is inconclusive, either because of difficulty in imaging or interpretation, further imaging studies are required. CT angiography has been the most accurate alternative to direct catheter-based angiography. MRA with gadolinium enhancement yields clear images but often overestimates the percentage of stenosis at the carotid bifurcation.

(F) Lesions involving the origin of the vertebral arteries can often be diagnosed with carotid duplex scanning. Failure to visualize a vertebral artery or reversal of flow direction is indicative of a lesion in the vertebral or proximal subclavian artery. Increased flow velocities in the proximal common carotid arteries suggest lesions in the innominate or proximal left common carotid artery at the level of the aortic arch.

(G) When duplex scanning, perhaps supplemented with MRA, indicates occlusive stenotic or ulcerative disease in the carotid bifurcation, it is seldom necessary to obtain more imaging information. The data obtained from a qualified laboratory are often all that is necessary to make a decision for carotid bifurcation operation.

(H) Contrast angiography used to be considered the hallmark of diagnosis and a prerequisite to carotid bifurcation endarterectomy. Contrast angiography carries significant risk, including approximately 1% risk of stroke in patients with significant carotid bifurcation disease. In addition, carotid angiography is expensive and anxiety producing for the patient. Fortunately, it is possible to manage the majority of patients with noninvasive imaging. Contrast angiography can be applied selectively in the uncommon case in which noninvasive testing is not diagnostic.

(I) The designation of a critical lesion of the carotid bifurcation depends on the presence or absence of symptoms. In asymptomatic patients, to be considered critical, carotid bifurcation disease must produce a lesion that is more than 60% diameter-reducing by contrast angiography or more than 80% diameter-reducing by duplex scan. Lesions in patients with territorial TIA in either the ocular or hemisphere distribution are considered critical at the level of 50% diameter-reducing stenosis, and they may be critical with lesser degrees of stenosis when medical therapy has failed.

(J) Asymptomatic patients with lesions smaller than 60% or symptomatic patients with lesions smaller than 50% are usually considered for medical management and careful follow-up, including a visit combined with noninvasive testing every 6 months or every year.

(K) Antiplatelet therapy with aspirin or Plavix is the most common form of treatment for the medical management of symptomatic patients or for pre- and postsurgical management. Occasionally, it is necessary to add anticoagulation with warfarin, particularly for patients with cardiac arrhythmias.

(L) The most common operation on the extracranial system is carotid bifurcation endarterectomy carried out for stenosis or ulceration of an atherosclerotic plaque. Carotid endarterectomy has been proven to be the treatment of choice for both symptomatic and asymptomatic lesions of the carotid bifurcation. This is based upon level-one evidence from multiple prospective randomized clinical trials.

Recently, the use of balloon angioplasty with stenting has been proposed as an alternative to carotid endarterectomy. Anecdotal evidence suggests that angioplasty performed with an appropriate

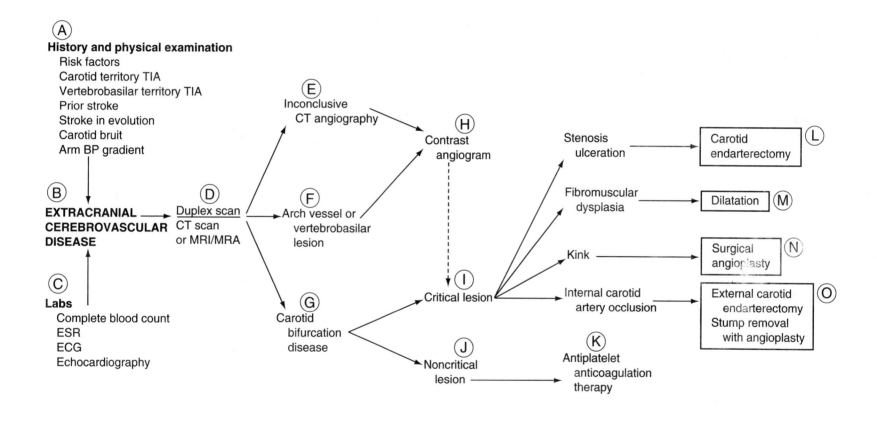

(A)
History and physical examination
Risk factors
Carotid territory TIA
Vertebrobasilar territory TIA
Prior stroke
Stroke in evolution
Carotid bruit
Arm BP gradient

(B)
EXTRACRANIAL CEREBROVASCULAR DISEASE

(C)
Labs
Complete blood count
ESR
ECG
Echocardiography

(D)
Duplex scan
CT scan
or MRI/MRA

(E)
Inconclusive
CT angiography

(F)
Arch vessel or
vertebrobasilar
lesion

(G)
Carotid
bifurcation
disease

(H)
Contrast
angiogram

(I)
Critical lesion

(J)
Noncritical
lesion

(K)
Antiplatelet
anticoagulation
therapy

Stenosis
ulceration

Fibromuscular
dysplasia

Kink

Internal carotid
artery occlusion

Carotid
endarterectomy (L)

Dilatation (M)

Surgical
angioplasty (N)

External carotid
endarterectomy
Stump removal
with angioplasty (O)

antiembolism adjunctive device can be done with safety comparable to that of endarterectomy. In order to test the utility of carotid angioplasty, a prospective randomized trial entitled Carotid Endarterectomy versus Angioplasty for Symptomatic Carotid Stenosis (CREST) has been initiated. In 5 years we should have the comparative data regarding safety, efficacy, and durability of the two techniques.

(M) Symptomatic fibromuscular dysplasia that does not respond to medical management can be treated with surgical angioplasty using progressive arterial dilation or balloon angioplasty with an antiembolism protective device.

(N) Anatomic abnormalities, including kinking with recurrent symptoms, can be treated with surgical angioplasty technique.

(O) Finally, patients with totally occluded internal carotid arteries whose symptoms persist, and who have either associated stenosis of the external carotid artery or a stump off the internal carotid artery that could serve as a nidus for embolization, can be managed with external carotid endarterectomy and removal of the occluded stump with appropriate angioplasty. If there is evidence that the symptoms are flow related, an extracranial to intracranial bypass can be considered.

REFERENCES

Barnett HJM, Taylor DW, Eliasziw M et al: The benefit of carotid endarterectomy in patients with symptomatic moderate or severe stenosis. New Engl J Med 339:1415–1425, 1998.

Caracci BF, Zukowski AF, Hurley JJ et al: Asymptomatic severe carotid stenosis. J Vasc Surg 9:361–366, 1989.

European Carotid Surgery Trialists' Collaborative Group: Medical Research Council European Carotid Surgery Trial: Randomized trial of endarterectomy for recently symptomatic carotid stenosis: Final results of the MRC European Carotid Surgery Trial (ECST). Lancet 351:1379–1387, 1998.

Executive Committee for the Asymptomatic Carotid Atherosclerosis (ACAS) Study: Endarterectomy for asymptomatic carotid artery stenosis. JAMA 273:1421–1428, 1995.

Geuder JW, Lamparello PJ, Riles TS et al: Is duplex scanning sufficient evaluation before carotid endarterectomy? J Vasc Surg 9:193–201, 1989.

Hobson RW II, Weiss DG, Fields WS et al, for the Veterans Affairs Asymptomatic Cooperative Study Group: Efficacy of carotid endarterectomy for asymptomatic carotid stenosis. N Engl J Med 328:221–227, 1993.

Langsfeld M, Gray-Weale AC, Lusby RJ: The role of plaque morphology and diameter reduction in the development of new symptoms in asymptomatic carotid arteries. J Vasc Surg 9:548–557, 1989.

Mackey WC, O'Donnell TF, Callow AD: Cardiac risk in patients undergoing carotid endarterectomy: Impact on peri-operative and long-term mortality. J Vasc Surg 11:226–234, 1990.

North American Symptomatic Carotid Endarterectomy Trial collaborators: Beneficial effect of carotid endarterectomy in symptomatic patients with high-grade carotid stenosis. N Engl J Med 325:445–453, 1991.

Piotrowski JJ, Bernard VM, Rubin JR et al: Timing of carotid endarterectomy after acute stroke. J Vasc Surg 11:45–52, 1990.

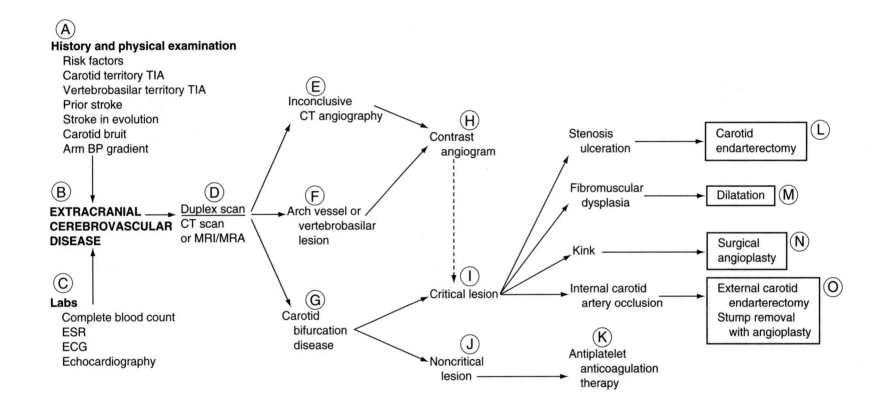

Ⓐ
History and physical examination
    Risk factors
    Carotid territory TIA
    Vertebrobasilar territory TIA
    Prior stroke
    Stroke in evolution
    Carotid bruit
    Arm BP gradient

Ⓑ
EXTRACRANIAL CEREBROVASCULAR DISEASE

Ⓒ
Labs
    Complete blood count
    ESR
    ECG
    Echocardiography

Ⓓ
Duplex scan
CT scan
or MRI/MRA

Ⓔ
Inconclusive
CT angiography

Ⓕ
Arch vessel or
vertebrobasilar
lesion

Ⓖ
Carotid
bifurcation
disease

Ⓗ
Contrast
angiogram

Ⓘ
Critical lesion

Ⓙ
Noncritical
lesion

Ⓚ
Antiplatelet
anticoagulation
therapy

Stenosis
ulceration

Fibromuscular
dysplasia

Kink

Internal carotid
artery occlusion

Ⓛ
Carotid
endarterectomy

Ⓜ
Dilatation

Ⓝ
Surgical
angioplasty

Ⓞ
External carotid
endarterectomy
Stump removal
with angioplasty

Chapter 102 Renovascular Disease

KIMBERLEY J. HANSEN, MD • MATTHEW S. EDWARDS, MD

(A) No symptom or sign is both sensitive and specific for renovascular disease contributing to hypertension (i.e., renovascular hypertension [RVH]) or excretory renal insufficiency (i.e., ischemic nephropathy [IN]). Considering all cases of hypertension, RVH is rare, but it is most prevalent among those with severe hypertension, especially at the extremes of age. IN is associated with severe hypertension and rapid decline in kidney function. An elevation in serum creatinine may occur after initiation of converting enzyme inhibitors or angiotensin receptor antagonists.

(B) Screening studies for renovascular disease may be either anatomic or functional. The authors prefer anatomic screening studies, particularly renal duplex sonography (RDS). When performed by a skilled sonographer, RDS is both sensitive (93%) and specific (98%) for main renal artery stenosis or occlusion. These results are not affected by concomitant aortic disease or IN.

RDS requires only an overnight fast and is usually an outpatient study. The primary limitation of RDS is the inability to detect branch or polar renal artery disease. The clinical importance of this limitation varies with the indication for study. A negative RDS or a normal CTA/MRA effectively excludes IN, whereas a negative RDS does not exclude polar or branch vessel disease contributing to RVH. In the latter instance, especially in children or young adults, the authors proceed with angiography when hypertension is severe. CTA/MRA alone is associated with an unacceptable incidence of false positive studies.

(C) When screening studies are positive, or when clinical suspicion remains high despite negative screening studies, RA anatomy is most commonly defined by angiography. Selective RA angiography is used to define branch artery disease. Digital subtraction angiography may decrease contrast load. For patients with IN, carbon dioxide

(CO_2) and gadolinium (GAD) angiography may be useful alternatives.

(D) Hypertension is a prerequisite for RA intervention; however, the presence of unilateral RA disease does not ensure a causal relationship with hypertension. In most cases of unilateral RA disease, the authors perform renal vein renin assays to define the lesion's physiologic significance. Simultaneous sampling from both renal veins is positive when a renin ratio greater than or equal to 1.5 exists after sodium depletion and cessation of confounding antihypertensive medication. Empiric intervention when functional studies are negative or have not been performed is reserved for young patients and for adults with severe (i.e., 80% or greater diameter reduction) stenosis associated with severe hypertension.

(E) Virtually all hypertension can be controlled medically with the currently available antihypertensive agents. In the case of RA disease, however, decreased glomerular filtration may lead to a decline in excretory function. There are no functional studies that relate correctable RA lesions with renal function response in IN. Clinical correlates of improved renal function after operative intervention include severe hypertension, severe (i.e., greater than 80% diameter reduction and occlusion) bilateral RA lesions, rapid decline in renal function, and bilateral renal artery repair.

(F) Bilateral atherosclerotic lesions to multiple renal arteries are often treated by transaortic thromboendarterectomy (35%).

(G) When the RA is redundant, reimplantation is the simplest method of repair (10%).

(H) Extra-anatomic (i.e., splanchnorenal) bypass avoids aortic control but is limited by coexisting stenosis of the celiac axis in 40% of patients.

(I) Direct aortorenal bypass with autologous saphenous vein is the most versatile method of surgical repair. Polytetrafluoroethylene (PTFE;

6-mm, thin-walled) is a satisfactory alternative when the RA exceeds 4 mm in diameter.

(J) Ex vivo techniques are employed for branch RA repair when warm renal ischemia exceeds 40 minutes.

(K) Nephrectomy is reserved for a nonfunctioning kidney with an unreconstructible distal RA contributing to severe hypertension.

(L) Although widely applied, renal artery percutaneous transluminal angioplasty (RA-PTA), with or without endoluminal stents, has not been compared prospectively with surgical therapy in randomized trials. In three recent prospective randomized trials comparing medical management and RA-PTA with or without endoluminal stents, each concluded that catheter-based intervention provided no benefit over medical management.

The authors advise PTA for fibromuscular dysplasia of a medial fibroplasia type in a main renal artery and non-ostial RA atherosclerosis. The authors will advise RA-PTA with or without endoluminal stenting in older adults with severe hypertension and unilateral renal artery disease.

Collective review of reports describing RA-PTA with endoluminal stents for IN demonstrate results inferior to selected surgical series. Collectively RA-PTA with stents appears to improve renal function in 15% to 20% of patients, whereas 15% to 20% of patients are worsened. Although the 60% to 70% of patients remaining unchanged are often considered "preserved," surgical series indicate that only patients with an immediate increase in renal function demonstrate improved dialysis-free survival.

(M) Regardless of the method of intervention, RDS is used to follow the result of repair. After surgical repair, intraoperative RDS is used to exclude technical defects. Major B-scan defects are associated with hemodynamic stenosis in 10%, and these are revised immediately. Direct aortorenal reconstruction provides 96% primary patency at 5 and 10 years. Recurrent stenosis after RA-PTA and stenting for ostial stenosis is observed in 20% to 25% at 12 months. The mortality/morbidity of surgical management varies directly with the complexity of repair and is increased by increased patient age, presence of clinical congestive heart failure, and azotemia. Overall, beneficial blood pressure response is observed in 90% of patients and improved renal function is observed in 60% to 70% of patients after bilateral renal artery repair. After percutaneous techniques, beneficial blood pressure and renal function response are observed in 65% and 15% to 20%, respectively.

REFERENCES

Benjamin ME, Dean RH: Techniques in renal artery reconstruction: Part I. Ann Vasc Surg 10:306–314, 1996.

Benjamin ME, Dean RH: Techniques in renal artery reconstruction: Part II. Ann Vasc Surg 10:409–414, 1996.

Cherr GS, Hansen KJ, Craven TE et al: Surgical management of atherosclerotic renovascular disease. J Vasc Surg 35:236–245, 2002.

Hansen KJ, Cherr GS, Craven TE et al: Management of ischemic nephropathy: Dialysis-free survival after surgical repair. J Vasc Surg 32:472–482, 2000.

Motew SJ, Cherr GS, Craven TE et al: Renal duplex sonography: Main renal artery versus hilar analysis. J Vasc Surg 32:462–471, 2000.

Plouin PF, Chatellier G, Darne B et al: Blood pressure outcome of angioplasty in atherosclerotic renal artery stenosis: A randomized trial. Essai Multicentrique Medicaments vs Angioplastie (EMMA) Study Group. Hypertension 31:823–829, 1998.

van Jaarsveld BC, Krijnen P, Pieterman H et al: The effect of balloon angioplasty on hypertension in atherosclerotic renal artery stenosis. Dutch Renal Artery Stenosis Intervention Cooperative Group. N Engl J Med 342:1007–1014, 2000.

Webster J, Marshall F, Abdalla M et al: Randomised comparison of percutaneous angioplasty vs. continued medical therapy for hypertensive patients with atheromatous renal artery stenosis. Scottish and Newcastle Renal Artery Stenosis Collaborative Group. J Hum Hypertens 12:329–335, 1998.

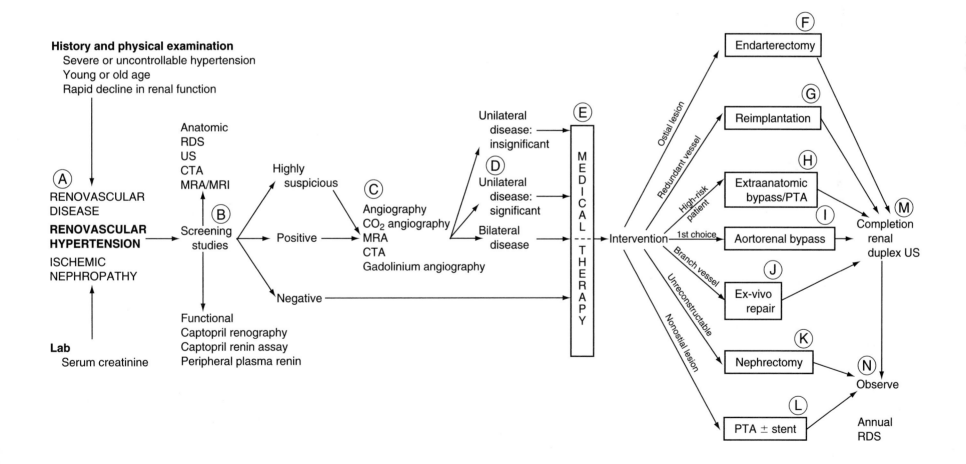

Chapter 103 *Varicose Veins*

MARK R. NEHLER, MD • JENNIFER ST. CROIX, MD

(A) The potential heredity mechanisms include a collagen defect in the venous wall or an absence of a "sentinel" valve in the common femoral vein just proximal to the saphenofemoral junction (supported by the significantly higher percentage of duplex confirmed saphenofemoral reflux in children of patients with primary varicose veins compared with control children). Regardless of the inherited defect, added stress is usually needed to produce significant varicosities. The most common of these stresses is pregnancy.

(B) Varicose veins often present during pregnancy (70% to 80% in the first trimester), perhaps related to high levels of progesterone and resultant alterations in distensibility. Other factors include proximal iliac vein obstruction secondary to compression by the gravid uterus, an increase in intra-abdominal pressure, and an increase in total blood volume and extremity flow. In this setting, incompetence at the saphenofemoral junction causes distention of distal segments and progressive serial retrograde valve incompetence. The saphenous vein thus becomes incompetent through much of its length, but rarely becomes varicose itself. It is the thin-walled tributaries that undergo this aneurysmal change.

(C) On examination, varicose veins can be classified into three types based on appearance and location: (1) trunk varicosities, in the distribution of long and short saphenous veins; (2) reticular, which are dilated, tortuous subcutaneous veins not belonging to major branches of the long or short saphenous distribution; and (3) telangectasias, intradermal venules in any location that are less than 1 mm.

(D) Superficial thrombophlebitis often is associated with varicose veins. Particularly susceptible are varicosities surrounding a venous ulcer, and long-standing varicosities in older patients. Patients with superficial thrombophlebitis have a 15% to 20% incidence of associated deep venous thrombosis and should undergo duplex examination of the deep veins.

(E) Patients often complain of a dull ache or heaviness in the legs that is worse at the end of the day. Symptoms may be exacerbated by menstruation or pregnancy. The CEAP classification system for venous disease involves clinical signs, etiology information, anatomic information, and pathophysiology information. This system has been in place in the last decade to improve standardization of disease severity for comparative trial and outcome research.

(F) Venous telangectasias are primarily a cosmetic rather than a functional problem. Cosmesis is not an unreasonable indication for local, small-dose sclerotherapy. The patient must understand potential complications however, including long-standing pigmentation in areas of extravasation or thrombosis, and occasional ulceration at the injection site.

(G) Up to 15% of patients with a venous ulcer will be found on duplex examination to have valvular reflux isolated to the superficial venous system only and may benefit from vein stripping or perforator ligation. This is commonly caused by secondary perforator incompetence from retrograde saphenous flow when standing.

(H) Patients with prior deep venous thrombosis and deep venous incompetence will usually not benefit from surgical vein stripping because of the high recurrence rate and the failure to affect post-thrombotic changes in the deep system.

(I) The two most common venous malformation syndromes are Klippel-Trenaunay and Sturge-Weber. Both have hypoplasia or aplasia of the deep venous system, varicosities of the superficial venous system, and capillary dermal malformations of port wine stain. Superficial vein ablation therapy in these patients can lead to disaster because these may be the only significant veins draining the limb.

(J) Venous duplex examination (using the distal cuff deflation method) to determine sites of valvular reflux is generally only indicated if the patient has lipodermatosclerosis, ulceration, or other manifestations of severe chronic venous insufficiency; or as dictated by the PPG test carried out with tourniquet application (see K), where perforator mapping may be relevant. Venous duplex is not necessary for most cases treated with sclerotherapy alone, particularly telangectasias.

(K) Secondary varicosities are most commonly caused by valvular reflux in the deep venous system and/or the perforators, and these limbs commonly have skin changes, edema, and/or venous ulcers. These may be congenital, but are usually post-thrombotic. These patients are best managed with compression therapy, although improved ulcer healing following periulcer sclerotherapy and compression has been reported. Other rare causes of secondary varicosities are arteriovenous fistulas (e.g., Parkes-Weber syndrome) or venous malformations (e.g., Klippel-Trenaunay syndrome).

(L) Venous recovery time (VRT) using photoplethysmography (PPG) is a useful and relatively inexpensive test to evaluate patients with varicose veins. Abbreviated VRTs (i.e., less than 13 seconds, or significantly faster than a contralateral normal leg) that correct with upper cuff alone indicate isolated saphenofemoral incompetence. Correction with a lower thigh tourniquet may indicate an incompetent low thigh perforator in addition to saphenofemoral incompetence. Correction with an upper calf tourniquet may be explained by lesser saphenous incompetence. Limb VRTs that do not correct with a tourniquet at any level indicate perforator or deep venous valvular incompetence and are an indication for adjunctive Duplex scanning (see J).

(M) Sclerotherapy is effective for veins less than 0.5 cm diameter. Larger veins are treated first, followed by smaller ones, working proximal to distal. Inject small volumes (0.25 to 0.5 ml) to reduce extravasation. A solution of 1% sodium tetradecyl (0.1 to 0.2 ml of 0.3% for telangectasias)

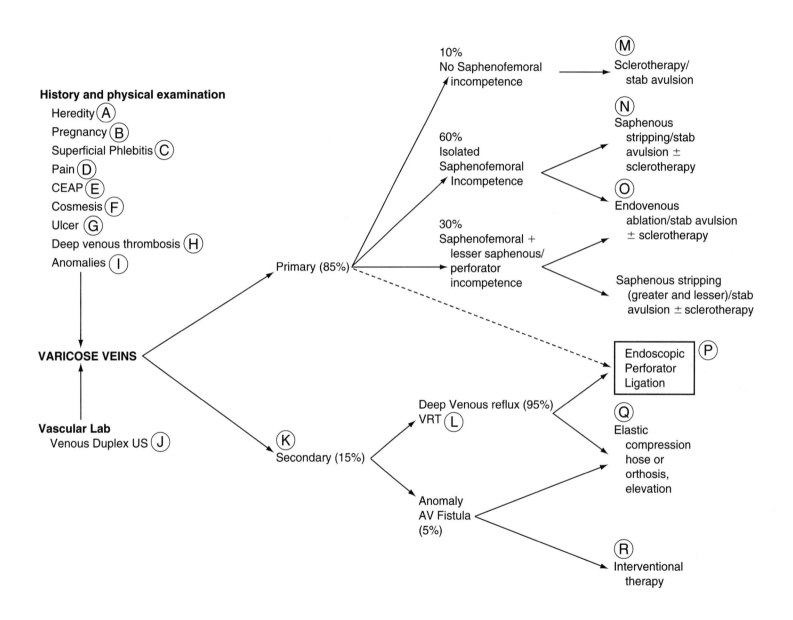

History and physical examination

Heredity (A)
Pregnancy (B)
Superficial Phlebitis (C)
Pain (D)
CEAP (E)
Cosmesis (F)
Ulcer (G)
Deep venous thrombosis (H)
Anomalies (I)

VARICOSE VEINS

Vascular Lab
Venous Duplex US (J)

Primary (85%)

10%
No Saphenofemoral
incompetence

(M)
Sclerotherapy/
stab avulsion

60%
Isolated
Saphenofemoral
Incompetence

(N)
Saphenous
stripping/stab
avulsion ±
sclerotherapy

(O)
Endovenous
ablation/stab avulsion
± sclerotherapy

30%
Saphenofemoral +
lesser saphenous/
perforator
incompetence

Saphenous stripping
(greater and lesser)/stab
avulsion ± sclerotherapy

Endoscopic
Perforator
Ligation (P)

Secondary (15%) (K)

Deep Venous reflux (95%)
VRT (L)

Elastic
compression
hose or
orthosis,
elevation (Q)

Anomaly
AV Fistula
(5%)

(R)
Interventional
therapy

hypertonic (10%) saline, or polidocanol (in Europe) can be used as agents. Injection is performed in the recumbent position. Compression hosiery or Ace bandages should be worn from 3 days to 1 week following injection to promote more effective fibrosis, to decrease the fullness of thrombus formed in the injected vessel, and to prevent extension of thrombus into the deep venous system.

(N) Both high ligation of the saphenous vein with division of the two to seven branches in the groin (either with or without saphenous vein stripping) have been advocated to deal with saphenofemoral reflux. However, several reports indicate increased recurrence rates for ligation alone compared with ligation and stripping. The saphenous vein normally does not need to be stripped much below the knee (this avoids potential saphenous neuralgia, and the important perforators below the knee are connected to the posterior arch circulation). Vein stripping to below the knee where the anterior and posterior arch tributaries join the greater saphenous often exposes the origins of the major varicosities and even allows access for subfascial perforator interruption. Up to one-third of patients develop further varicose veins within 5 to 10 years, possibly caused by neovascularization at the saphenofemoral junction.

(O) Radiofrequency ablation uses an intravenous probe to obliterate the vein by controlled thermal injury. Early results demonstrate efficacy in obliteration of the saphenous vein and branches. A small, randomized trial demonstrated improved return to function despite increased cost of endovenous ablation compared with open vein stripping surgery.

(P) Endoscopic perforator ligation, or simple open modifications of this procedure using a horizontal incision and long endoscopic instruments, have emerged as promising new approaches to manage incompetent perforators. The Linton concept is used without having the wound complications associated with that procedure. Multiple ongoing registries demonstrate effective ulcer healing rates of 80% or greater at 1 year, but recurrence of ulcers over time is a significant issue.

(Q) Compression is the cornerstone of treatment for lipodermatosclerosis and venous ulceration. The key issue is patient compliance. Elastic compression hosiery is commonly difficult for patients to put on. Zippered stockings; assist devices; and, most recently, the legging orthosis consisting of easy to adjust and remove velcro straps, are helping to improve compliance. In addition, periodic elevation of the legs during the day is important (ideally, every 2 hours for 10 minutes).

(R) Patients with congenital AV fistula are best managed by interventional methods utilizing embolotherapy. These techniques are usually palliative only. Surgery in these patients often eliminates important vascular routes necessary for interventional access and complicates future therapy.

REFERENCES

Ad Hoc Committee, American Venous Forum: Classification and grading of chronic venous disease in the lower limbs: A consensus statement. J Cardiovasc Surg (Torino) 38:437–441, 1997.

Bergan JJ: Causes of venous varicosities and telangectasias: Implications for treatment. J Vasc Biol Med 1995.

Chandler JG, Pichot O, Sessa C et al: Defining the role of extended saphenofemoral junction ligation: A prospective comparative study. J Vasc Surg 32:941–953, 2000.

Edgar SA: Etiology of varicose veins. Postgrad Med 6:234, 1949.

Gloviczki P, Bergan JJ, Rhodes JM et al: Mid-term results of endoscopic perforator vein interruption for chronic venous insufficiency: Lessons learned from the North American subfascial endoscopic perforator surgery registry. The North American Study Group. J Vasc Surg 29:489–502, 1999.

Gloviczki P, Stanson AW, Stickler GB et al: Klippel-Trenaunay syndrome: The risks and benefits of vascular interventions. Surgery 110:469–479, 1991.

Hanrahan LM, Araki CT, Rodriguez AA et al: Distribution of valvular incompetence in patients with venous stasis ulceration. J Vasc Surg 13:805–811, 1991.

Iafrati MD, Pare GJ, O'Donnell TF et al: Is the nihilistic approach to surgical reduction of superficial and perforator vein incompetence for venous ulcer justified? J Vasc Surg 36:1167–1174, 2002.

Merchant RF, DePalma RG, Kabnick LS: Endovascular obliteration of saphenous reflux: A multicenter study. J Vasc Surg 35:1190–1196, 2002.

Munn SR, Morton JB, Macbeth WA et al: To strip or not to strip the long saphenous vein? A varicose veins trial. Br J Surg 68:426–428, 1981.

Queral LA, Criado FJ, Lilly MP et al: The role of sclerotherapy as an adjunct to Unna's boot for treating venous ulcers: A prospective study. J Vasc Surg 11:572–575, 1990.

Rautio T, Ohinmaa A, Perala J et al: Endovenous obliteration versus conventional stripping operation in the treatment of primary varicose veins: A randomized controlled trial with comparison of the costs. J Vasc Surg 35:958–965, 2002.

Reagan B, Folse R: Lower limb venous dynamics in normal persons and children of patients with varicose veins. Surg Gynecol Obstet 132:15–18, 1971.

Rose, SS, Ahmed A: Some thoughts on the aetiology of varicose veins. J Cardiovasc Surg (Torino) 27:534–543, 1986.

Sarin S, Scurr JH, Coleridge Smith PD: Assessment of stripping the long saphenous vein in the treatment of primary varicose veins. Br J Surg 79:889–893, 1992.

Skillman JJ, Kent KC, Porter DH et al: Simultaneous occurrence of superficial and deep thrombophlebitis in the lower extremity. J Vasc Surg 11:818–823, 1990.

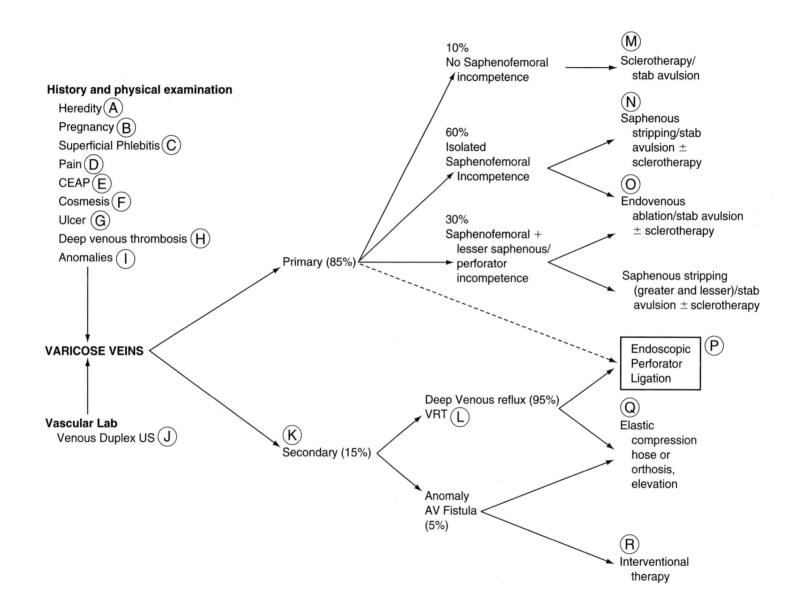

History and physical examination
Heredity (A)
Pregnancy (B)
Superficial Phlebitis (C)
Pain (D)
CEAP (E)
Cosmesis (F)
Ulcer (G)
Deep venous thrombosis (H)
Anomalies (I)

VARICOSE VEINS

Vascular Lab
Venous Duplex US (J)

Primary (85%)

Secondary (15%) (K)

10%
No Saphenofemoral
incompetence

60%
Isolated
Saphenofemoral
Incompetence

30%
Saphenofemoral +
lesser saphenous/
perforator
incompetence

Deep Venous reflux (95%)
VRT (L)

Anomaly
AV Fistula
(5%)

(M)
Sclerotherapy/
stab avulsion

(N)
Saphenous
stripping/stab
avulsion ±
sclerotherapy

(O)
Endovenous
ablation/stab avulsion
± sclerotherapy

Saphenous stripping
(greater and lesser)/stab
avulsion ± sclerotherapy

Endoscopic
Perforator
Ligation (P)

(Q)
Elastic
compression
hose or
orthosis,
elevation

(R)
Interventional
therapy

Chapter 104 *Deep Vein Thrombosis*

THOMAS A. WHITEHILL, MD

(A) Thorough clinical assessment delineates the need for serial duplex ultrasound studies and the duration of anticoagulant therapy. Using signs and symptoms, associated thrombotic risk factors, and the plausibility of alternative diagnoses, it is possible to stratify patients to a high, moderate, or low pre-ultrasound probability group. Major outpatient risk factors for deep venous thrombosis (DVT) include active malignancy, trauma, paralysis or limb immobilization, prolonged bedrest or recent surgery, and a strong family history.

(B) DVT of the lower extremity involves either the proximal veins (e.g., popliteal vein to the inferior vena cava) or the deep calf veins (e.g., anterior/posterior tibial or peroneal). The diagnosis of acute DVT is important because delayed anticoagulant therapy is associated with pulmonary embolism (PE). Inappropriate anticoagulant treatment carries the inconvenience, expense, and risk of hemorrhage. Unfortunately, the bedside diagnosis of DVT is often inaccurate because the clinical findings of pain, swelling, and tenderness are unreliable. The diagnosis of DVT requires duplex ultrasound scanning. Unless contraindicated, initial empiric anticoagulation with intravenous heparin is advised.

(C) Duplex ultrasonography has largely replaced venography in the diagnosis of DVT. More than 80% of symptomatic lower extremity venous thromboses involve the easily interrogated proximal veins. Consistently high sensitivities of 93% to 97% and specificities of 94% to 99% can be achieved in a dedicated noninvasive vascular laboratory.

(D) Strategies for withholding anticoagulation based upon duplex ultrasound examination alone require serial testing because 3% to 7% of documented thromboses show initial findings that are negative for proximal thrombosis. Initial diagnostic failure rates may be higher among inpatients and those with persistent symptoms. However, the incidence of thromboembolism within 6 months of serially negative ultrasound scans is less than 2%, and withholding anticoagulation in the symptomatic patient with two negative scans 5 to 7 days apart has proven safe. Strategies combining clinical assessment with duplex ultrasonography have been the most extensively evaluated. Using distinct inpatient and outpatient criteria, groups with low, moderate, and high pretest probabilities can be defined as having respective DVT prevalences of 10%, 20%, and 76% for inpatients and 5%, 33%, and 85% for outpatients. Anticoagulation may be safely withheld in moderate probability patients with two negative scans, whereas contrast venography should be considered either before or after a second negative scan in patients with a high clinical suspicion of venous thrombosis.

(E) Most patients with an acute DVT associated with identifiable risk factors require no further evaluation; however, patients with idiopathic DVT need to be evaluated for an underlying hypercoagulability state or an occult malignancy. The search for a congenital or an acquired thrombophilic state is appropriate when the patient has an idiopathic DVT and is younger than 50 years, a family history of DVT, an unusual site of thrombosis, or recurrent fetal loss. DVT may herald a previously undetected malignancy in up to 20% of patients with idiopathic thrombosis, with the incidence of occult malignancy diagnosed within 6 to 12 months being 2.2 to 5.3 times higher than that expected in the general population. Although the positive cost-benefit of an intensive search for occult malignancy has not been demonstrated, directed screening is certainly warranted.

(F) Without timely treatment, pulmonary embolism may complicate up to 50% of proximal DVT, whereas as many as two thirds of patients may experience the long-term manifestations of the postphlebitic syndrome –(i.e., pain, edema, hyperpigmentation, or chronic ulceration). Although the incidence of these complications is lower with isolated calf vein thrombosis, it is not trivial, and these thromboses should not be ignored. Approximately 20% of calf vein thromboses will propagate proximally, carrying a theoretical 2% risk of fatal PE and 5% to 10% risk of symptomatic PE. Approximately 25% of patients with isolated calf vein thrombosis will have persistent postphlebitic symptoms during follow-up.

(G) Options for the management of symptomatic, isolated calf vein thrombosis include anticoagulation versus serial noninvasive follow-up with anticoagulation only in the event of proximal extension. Based upon the risk of proximal propagation and the associated risk of PE and the postthrombotic syndrome, the benefits of anticoagulation exceed the risk and inconvenience for most patients. Anticoagulation may be particularly warranted in patients with a previous history of DVT, in whom recurrence rates of 50% have been documented; and also in those patients with malignancy or multiple thrombotic risk factors, in whom the risk of proximal thrombosis is high. Serial duplex scans may be a reasonable alternative in patients with contraindications to anticoagulation, if they can be reliably monitored. Follow-up testing at 2- to 3-day intervals for 10 to 14 days after initial presentation is recommended.

(H) Anticoagulation therapy is the standard of care for patients with proximal DVT. Placement of an inferior vena cava (IVC) filter is appropriate for patients with contraindications or complications of anticoagulation. Recurrent thrombosis despite adequate anticoagulation is the other indication for IVC filter placement.

(I) Anticoagulation with unfractionated heparin, followed by warfarin, remains the standard therapy for acute DVT. An initial IV bolus of 80 IU/kg of heparin should be followed by a maintenance infusion of 18 IU/kg per hour, with subsequent dosage adjustments to maintain the aPTT within the therapeutic range. Failure to achieve an aPTT above 1.5 times the control value within 24 hours is associated with a significantly higher risk of recurrent thrombotic events. Intermittent adjusted-dose subcutaneous heparin therapy is an option for the

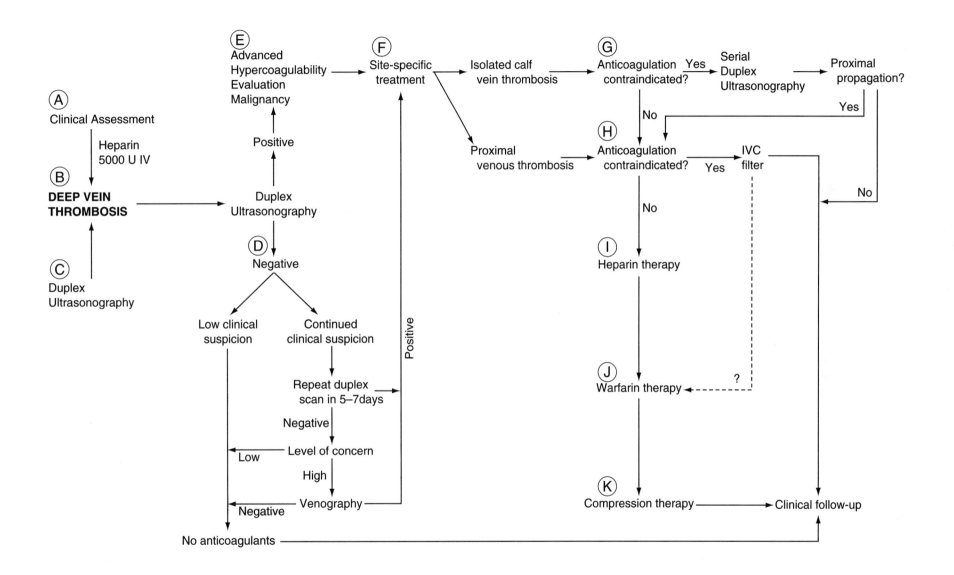

ambulatory patient, but only for the short term (1 to 2 weeks). Platelet counts should be monitored daily to watch for the possibility of heparin-induced thrombocytopenia (HIT). The availability of low-molecular weight heparins (LMWH) and other antico-agulants has expanded treatment options in selected patient populations. Because of its predictable dose-response relationship, LMWH therapy does not require monitoring of its anticoagulant effect. The advantages of LMWH over standard heparin preparations include a lower risk of bleeding compli-cations and thrombocytopenia, and a lower risk of osteopenia.

Ⓙ Warfarin is used following an initial course of unfractionated or LMW heparin. Warfarin is dosed to achieve and maintain an International Normalized Ratio (INR) of 2.0 to 3.0. Combined therapy with heparin and warfarin should be con-tinued for 5 to 7 days until the INR is therapeutic for 2 consecutive days. The appropriate duration of anticoagulation after an episode of acute DVT is based upon balancing the risks of hemorrhage with those of recurrent thrombo-embolism. The optimal duration of anticoagulation therapy remains unre-solved in many patients. In patients with isolated calf

vein thrombosis, 3 months of warfarin is recom-mended. In those patients with a first episode of DVT and either heterozygous factor V Leiden mutation or reversible risk factors, a 3- to 6-month course is recommended. Patients with an idiopathic DVT should receive 6 months of therapy. Patients with recurrent DVT or a first DVT in association with malignancy, congenital anticoagulant deficien-cies, persistent antiphospholipid antibodies, or homozygous factor V Leiden mutation should receive at least 12 months if not lifelong warfarin anticoagulation.

Ⓚ Prevention of the post-thrombotic syndrome is the second objective in the treatment of acute DVT. Although anticoagulation is important, randomized trials have also shown that the use of graded elastic compression stockings (40 mm Hg at the ankle) reduces the incidence of objectively doc-umented post-thrombotic syndrome by approxi-mately 50%.

REFERENCES

Birdwell B, Raskob G, Whitsett T et al: The clinical validity of normal compression ultrasonography in outpatients sus-pected of having deep venous thrombosis. Ann Intern Med 128:1–7, 1998.

Brandjes D, Buller H, Heijboer H et al: Randomized trial of effect of compression stockings in patients with symptomatic proximal-vein thrombosis. Lancet 349:759–762, 1997.

Decousus H, Leizorovicz A, Parent F et al: A clinical trial of vena cava filters in the prevention of pulmonary embolism in patients with proximal deep-vein thrombosis. N Engl J Med 338:409–415, 1998.

Glover JL, Bendick PJ: Appropriate indications for venous duplex ultrasonic examinations. Surgery 120:725–730, 1996.

Hirsh J: The optimal duration of anticoagulant therapy for venous thrombosis. N Engl J Med 332:1710–1711, 1995.

Hyers TM: Management of venous thromboembolism: Past, present, and future. Ann Int Med 14:759–768, 2003.

Meissner M, Caps M, Bergelin R et al: Early outcome after isolated calf vein thrombosis. J Vasc Surg 26:749–756, 1997.

Perrier A, Desmarais S, Miron MJ et al: Non-invasive diagnosis of venous thromboembolism in outpatients. Lancet 353: 190–195, 1999.

Siragusa S, Cosmi B, Piovella F et al: Low-molecular weight heparins and unfractionated heparin in the treatment of patients with acute venous thromboembolism: Results of a meta-analysis. Am J Med 100:269–277, 1996.

Sorensen HT, Mellemkjaer L, Steffensen FH et al: The risk of a diagnosis of cancer after primary deep venous thrombosis or pulmonary embolism. N Engl J Med 338:1169–1173, 1998.

Yusen RD, Haraden BM, Gage BF et al: Criteria for outpatient management of proximal lower extremity deep venous thrombosis. Chest 115:972–979, 1999.

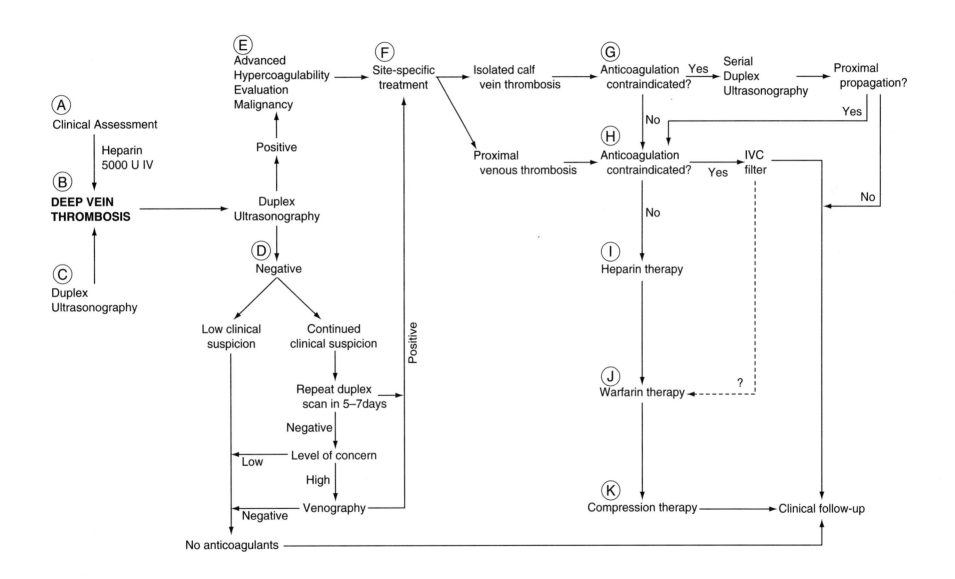

Chapter 105 *Venous Stasis Ulcer*

MANJU KALRA, MBBS • PETER GLOVICZKI, MD

(A) Chronic venous disease is a spectrum classified into six major classes (C) as follows: telangiectasia (C_1), varicose veins (C_2), edema (C_3), skin changes (C_4), healed ulcer (C_5), and active venous ulcers (C_6). The incidence of venous ulcers is estimated to be 18 per 100,000 person years, with women more commonly affected than men (20.4 vs. 14.6). The incidence of ulcers has not changed in the past two decades in females, and it recently increased in males. In the United States each year over 20,000 new ulcer patients are treated, 12% require hospitalization, and the associated costs are high ($150 million to $1 billion). Two pathologic processes, valvular incompetence and venous obstruction, result in ambulatory venous hypertension, the final common pathway to chronic venous insufficiency (CVI). Reflux caused by valvular incompetence is responsible for 90% of cases, whereas deep venous obstruction secondary to deep venous thrombosis (DVT) is less common, accounting for 10%. Primary valvular incompetence is a more common cause (70%) than is secondary incompetence following DVT (30%) because of valvular destruction.

(B) The clinical examination is supplemented by a hand-held, continuous-wave Doppler examination. The extent of edema, varicosities, lipodermatosclerosis with brawny induration and discoloration, dermatitis, and ulceration are documented. Most venous ulcers occur medially in the "gaiter area," from 2.5 cm distal to the medial malleolus to the point where the calf muscles become visible. Arterial ischemic ulcers are usually located at or distal to the ankle in high-pressure areas or in the toes; they are deeper, usually have a necrotic base, and are more painful. Pulses should be documented and the ankle-brachial index (ABI) determined. Decreased ABI (less than 0.9) suggests mixed (arterial and venous) ulcer. Continuous wave Doppler evaluation will identify great saphenous vein incompetence. Patients with history of recurrent thrombophlebitis or DVT merit a detailed coagulation profile including antithrombin level, protein C and S, anticardiolipin antibodies, lupus anticoagulant, homocysteine levels, and factor V Leiden assay to identify and treat hypercoagulability syndromes.

(C) All patients with venous ulcer should undergo duplex scanning to determine the sites of obstruction and incompetence (reflux) of superficial, deep, and perforating veins. Duplex examination provides qualitative information about the anatomic presence of obstruction or reflux; however, it cannot quantitate it or assess its hemodynamic significance. Plethysmography (air or strain-gauge) can be performed to evaluate calf pump function, global reflux, or outflow obstruction. Contrast venography is performed only in patients with deep venous obstruction, if endovenous or open treatment is planned, or in those patients with incompetence who may undergo treatment for deep vein valvular incompetence.

(D) The traditional treatment of venous ulceration remains nonoperative, is time-intensive, and requires strict patient compliance. Recommendations include bedrest, frequent leg elevation or decrease of daily ambulation, local care of the ulcer, and enforcement of elastic compression of the leg with graduated elastic stockings (30 to 40 mm Hg gradient). Edema and cellulitis are treated with leg elevation and antibiotic therapy. Alternative treatment is weekly application of Unna paste boots. Adjuvant topical agents (e.g., platelet-derived growth factor and human recombinant epidermal growth factor); oral agents (e.g., defibrotide, aspirin, or pentoxifylline); and systemic agents (e.g., prostaglandin E_1) have all shown some effectiveness for ulcer healing. The role of topical antiseptics, antibiotics, pharmacologic agents, enzymes, or growth factors is not conclusively established. Several clinical trials of medical management report success in healing most ulcers over time (92% to 100%). Ulcer recurrence rates following medical treatment range from 29% to 41% in compliant patients, to 71% to 100% in noncompliant patients.

(E) If compression therapy fails or if the ulcer recurs, treatment depends on the cause (i.e., incompetence or obstruction). Surgical, endovenous, or endoscopic treatment needs to be individualized for each patient based on the results of noninvasive and invasive investigation of the venous system (i.e., superficial, perforator, and deep).

(F) For superficial incompetence alone, ablation is performed by high ligation and stripping of the incompetent portion of the saphenous vein from the groin to the knee using the inversion technique. Avulsion of branch varicosities is performed simultaneously. Endovenous saphenous vein obliteration by radiofrequency (closure) or laser ablation techniques (endovenous laser therapy or EVLT) offers a shorter postoperative recovery and faster return to work; however, long-term results are awaited. Duplex-guided foam sclerotherapy has been reported for saphenous reflux ablation. At a mean follow-up of 3 to 5 years, 71% to 90% of patients after stripping and high ligation have functional and hemodynamic improvement. Recurrent varicose veins develop in up to 25% of patients on long-term follow-up, the incidence increasing with the length of follow-up. The most common complication of stripping is saphenous neuralgia that may occur in 4% to 8% of patients. Hematoma, cellulitis, edema, or thrombophlebitis can also occur. Deep venous thrombosis or pulmonary embolism is very rare.

(G) SEPS (subfascial endoscopic perforator vein surgery) is now the preferred method of interrupting incompetent perforator veins. It utilizes endoscopic instruments to interrupt incompetent perforators through one or two endoscopic ports placed remotely from the active ulcer area. It is associated with a quicker recovery and much lower wound complication rate compared with the open technique, which uses one long or several small incisions along the medial aspect of the leg. Ulcer healing rates of 90% and recurrence rates of 27% at 5 years have been reported following SEPS and superficial reflux ablation. Patients with advanced

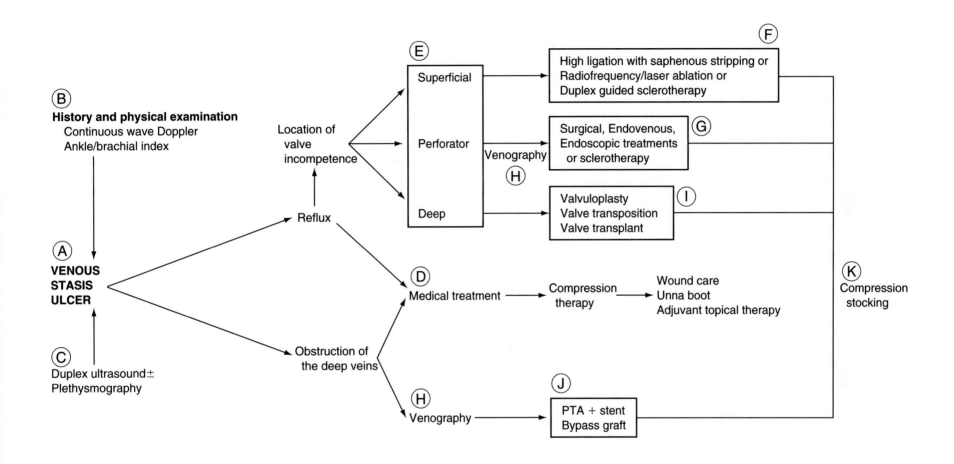

Ⓑ **History and physical examination**
   Continuous wave Doppler
   Ankle/brachial index

Ⓐ **VENOUS STASIS ULCER**

Ⓒ Duplex ultrasound±
   Plethysmography

Reflux

Location of valve incompetence

Obstruction of the deep veins

Ⓔ Superficial

Perforator

Deep

Ⓕ High ligation with saphenous stripping or
   Radiofrequency/laser ablation or
   Duplex guided sclerotherapy

Venography Ⓗ

Ⓖ Surgical, Endovenous,
   Endoscopic treatments
   or sclerotherapy

Ⓘ Valvuloplasty
   Valve transposition
   Valve transplant

Ⓓ Medical treatment

Compression therapy

Wound care
Unna boot
Adjuvant topical therapy

Ⓗ Venography

Ⓙ PTA + stent
   Bypass graft

Ⓚ Compression stocking

CVI and perforator incompetence because of primary valvular incompetence benefit most from SEPS; results in patients with postthrombotic syndrome are poorer. Duplex-guided foam sclerotherapy of perforator veins has recently emerged as treatment option, but long-term results are not available.

(H) Ascending venography is performed to exclude venous obstruction. Descending venography confirms the presence, location, and magnitude of valvular reflux. Patients with Kistner's grade 3 or 4 reflux down through popliteal veins into the tibial veins are considered suitable candidates for ablation of deep venous reflux. Venous pressures are measured to assess the severity of the occlusion; a pressure difference of 5 mm Hg between the two femoral veins in unilateral iliac disease, or between the femoral and the central pressures, or a 5 mm Hg increase in femoral vein pressure after exercise indicates a hemodynamically significant lesion.

(I) Patients with primary valvular incompetence are usually candidates for either internal or external valvuloplasty. Valvuloplasty is achieved by either an open procedure or closed technique, with or without angioscopic assistance. The redundant, floppy valve cusps are plicated with fine monofilament sutures to restore competence. In spite of demonstrable reflux in multiple valves in the deep system, only one valve is usually repaired, most commonly the first valve of the femoral vein. If the profunda femoris vein valve is also incompetent it also has to be repaired. An alternative is repair of an incompetent valve at the popliteal vein level to prevent reflux into the popliteal and tibial veins. Postthrombotic limbs often demonstrate destruction of the valves, and direct valve repair is usually not feasible. Options include valve transposition by transposing the incompetent vein to the adjacent competent great saphenous vein or profunda femoris vein. Other procedures include transplantation of an axillary or brachial vein that contains a valve; and attempts at de-novo valve reconstruction. Deep vein valve reconstructions continue to be challenging and rarely performed; however, good clinical outcome is reported in as many as 80% of patients undergoing direct valve reconstructions. Results of vein transplantations and

transpositions are less obvious; benefit has been reported in 50% of patients.

(J) Endovascular treatment with venous stents is used more and more commonly for iliac vein obstruction and is now the first option for treating deep venous obstruction if technically feasible. The low pressure venous system is more amenable to balloon dilatation, and a previously occluded vein can be dilated to 14 to 16 mm with careful attention to wall resistance. The flexibility and self-expansion of Wallstents makes them particularly suitable for venous stenting. Early rethrombosis occurs in 10% of patients and pulmonary embolism in less than 1%. Patients with May-Thurner syndrome (compression of left common iliac vein by right common iliac artery) with no evidence of prior DVT demonstrate better results than those with complicating thrombosis. Initial technical success is more than 90% patency at 1 year, ranging from 79% to 94% in series reporting treatment of acute and chronic lesions.

For patients with unilateral iliac vein obstruction who are not suitable for or who fail endovascular treatment, the cross-pubic venous bypass (Palma-Dale procedure) remains the best open surgical technique for autologous reconstruction. Clinical improvement has been observed in 75% to 86% of patients. Only patients with significant disability should be considered for femoral-iliac or femoral-caval bypass grafts. Expanded polytetrafluoroethylene (PTFE) continues to be the best prosthetic material for reconstruction of the vena cava, and short, large-diameter grafts have the best long-term patency. A femoral arteriovenous fistula is recommended for prosthetic grafts anastomosed to the femoral vein and for iliocaval grafts longer than 10 cm. fistula is closed by open or endovascular means 3 to 6 months after the operation. Functional improvement and patency rates are 50% to 60%. For femoropopliteal venous obstruction, saphenopopliteal bypass (May-Husni procedure) can occasionally be considered. The ipsilateral/contralateral great saphenous vein, if available, is the conduit of choice, followed by arm veins.

(K) Split thickness skin grafts, and more recently Apligrafs (a biosynthetic human skin equivalent) have been reported to hasten ulcer healing,

especially of large ulcers. Once ulcers heal, patients are fitted for $Class_3$ (30 to 40 mm Hg) below-knee, graduated compression stockings, which should be worn during the day.

REFERENCES

Goren G, Yellin AE: Invaginated axial saphenectomy by a semi-rigid stripper: Perforate-invaginate stripping. J Vasc Surg 20:970–977, 1994.

Heit JA, Rooke TW, Silverstein MD et al: Trends in the incidence of venous stasis syndrome and venous ulcer: A 25-year population-based study. J Vasc Surg 33:1022–1027, 2001.

Jost CJ, Gloviczki P, Cherry KJ Jr. et al: Surgical reconstruction of iliofemoral veins and the inferior vena cava for nonmalignant occlusive disease. J Vasc Surg 33:320–332, 2001.

Gloviczki P, Bergan JJ, Rhodes JM et al: Mid-term results of endoscopic perforator vein interruption for chronic venous insufficiency: Lessons learned from the North American subfascial endoscopic perforator surgery registry. The North American Study Group. J Vasc Surg 29:489–502, 1999.

Kalra M, Gloviczki P, Noel AA et al: Subfascial endoscopic perforator vein surgery in patients with postthrombotic venous insufficiency: Is it justified? Vasc Endovasc Surg 36:41–50, 2002.

Kistner RL: Definitive diagnosis and definitive treatment in chronic venous disease: A concept whose time has come. J Vasc Surg 24:703–710, 1996.

Korn P, Patel ST, Heller JA et al: Why insurers should reimburse for compression stockings in patients with chronic venous stasis. J Vasc Surg 35:950–957, 2002.

Lurie F, Creton D, Eklof B et al: Prospective randomized study of endovenous radiofrequency obliteration (closure procedure) versus ligation and stripping in a selected patient population (EVOLVeS Study). J Vasc Surg 38:207–217, 2003.

Lurie F, Kistner RL, Eklof B: Surgical management of deep venous reflux. Semin Vasc Surg 15:50–56, 2002.

Mayberry JC, Moneta GL, Taylor LM Jr. et al: Fifteen-year results of ambulatory compression therapy for chronic venous ulcers. Surgery 109:575–581, 1991.

Merchant RF, DePalma RG, Kabnick LS: Endovascular obliteration of saphenous reflux: A multicenter study. J Vasc Surg 35:1190–1196, 2002.

Neglen P, Einarsson E, Eklof B: The functional long-term value of different types of treatment for saphenous vein incompetence. J Cardiovasc Surg 34:295–301, 1993.

Neglen P, Raju S: Balloon dilation and stenting of chronic iliac vein obstruction: Technical aspects and early clinical outcome. J Endovasc Ther: Off J Inter Soc Endovasc Special 7:79–91, 2000.

Nelzen O: Prospective study of safety, patient satisfaction, and leg ulcer healing following saphenous and subfascial endoscopic perforator surgery. Br J Surg 87:86–91, 2000.

Perrin M: Reconstructive surgery for deep venous reflux: A report on 144 cases. Cardiovasc Surg 8:246–255, 2000.

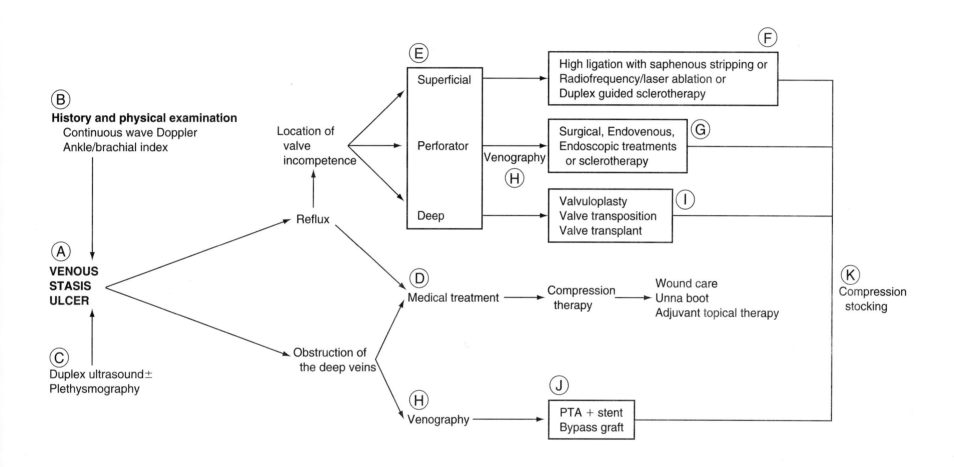

Ⓔ Superficial

Ⓕ High ligation with saphenous stripping or
Radiofrequency/laser ablation or
Duplex guided sclerotherapy

Ⓑ **History and physical examination**
Continuous wave Doppler
Ankle/brachial index

Ⓐ **VENOUS STASIS ULCER**

Ⓒ Duplex ultrasound±
Plethysmography

Location of
valve
incompetence

Perforator

Ⓖ Surgical, Endovenous,
Endoscopic treatments
or sclerotherapy

Venography

Ⓗ

Deep

Ⓘ Valvuloplasty
Valve transposition
Valve transplant

Reflux

Ⓓ Medical treatment

Compression
therapy

Wound care
Unna boot
Adjuvant topical therapy

Obstruction of
the deep veins

Ⓗ Venography

Ⓙ PTA + stent
Bypass graft

Ⓚ Compression
stocking

Pierik EG, van Urk H, Hop WC et al: Endoscopic versus open subfascial division of incompetent perforating veins in the treatment of venous leg ulceration: A randomized trial. J Vasc Surg 26:1049–1054, 1997.

Porter JM, Moneta GL, International Consensus Committee on Chronic Venous Disease: Reporting standards in venous disease: An update. J Vasc Surg 21:635–645, 1995.

Proebstle TM, Lehr HA, Kargl A et al: Endovenous treatment of the greater saphenous vein with a 940-nm diode laser: Thrombotic occlusion after endoluminal thermal damage by laser-generated steam bubbles. J Vasc Surg 35:729–736, 2002.

Raju S: New approaches to the diagnosis and treatment of venous obstruction. J Vasc Surg 4:42–54, 1986.

Raju S, Fredericks RK, Neglen PN et al: Durability of venous valve reconstruction techniques for "primary" and post-thrombotic reflux. J Vasc Surg 23:357–366, 1996.

Raju S, Owen S Jr., Neglen P: The clinical impact of iliac venous stents in the management of chronic venous insufficiency. J Vasc Surg 35:8–14, 2002.

Rooke TW, Felty C: The Medical Management of Venous Ulcers. In Gloviczki P, Bergan JJ (eds): Atlas of Endoscopic Perforator Vein Surgery. London: Springer-Verlag, 1998.

Rutgers PH, Kitslaar PJ: Randomized trial of stripping versus high ligation combined with sclerotherapy in the treatment of the incompetent greater saphenous vein. Am J Surg 168:311–315, 1994.

Sottiurai VS: Results of deep vein reconstruction. Vasc Surg 31:276–278, 1997.

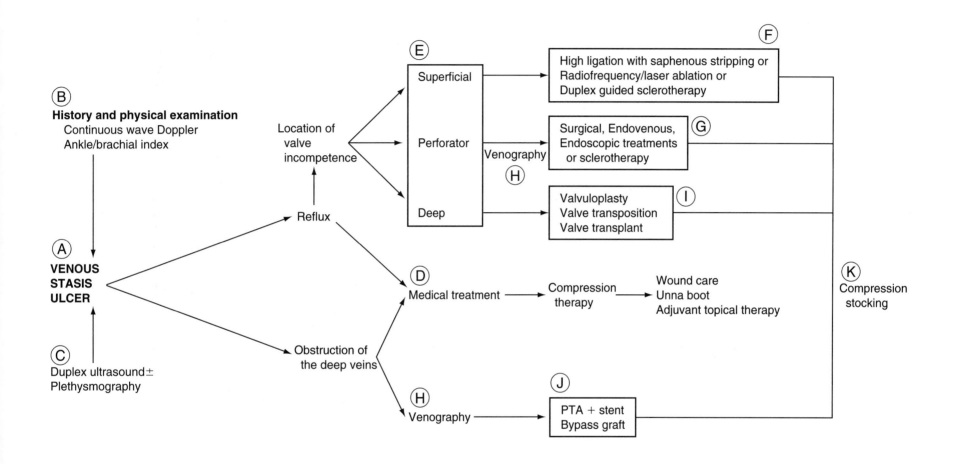

B **History and physical examination**
Continuous wave Doppler
Ankle/brachial index

A **VENOUS STASIS ULCER**

C Duplex ultrasound±
Plethysmography

Reflux

Obstruction of the deep veins

Location of valve incompetence

E Superficial
Perforator
Deep

F High ligation with saphenous stripping or
Radiofrequency/laser ablation or
Duplex guided sclerotherapy

Venography H

G Surgical, Endovenous,
Endoscopic treatments
or sclerotherapy

I Valvuloplasty
Valve transposition
Valve transplant

D Medical treatment

Compression therapy

Wound care
Unna boot
Adjuvant topical therapy

H Venography

J PTA + stent
Bypass graft

K Compression stocking

Chapter 106 *Chronic Limb-Threatening Ischemia*

GREGORY J. LANDRY, MD

(A) Symptomatic patients with chronic arterial insufficiency have a spectrum of discomfort ranging from intermittent claudication to critical limb ischemia, defined as the presence of rest pain or ischemic ulcerations or gangrene. Patient history should focus on the presence of atherosclerotic risk factors (e.g., smoking, diabetes, and hyperlipidemia); other signs of systemic atherosclerosis (e.g., a history of coronary artery or cerebrovascular disease); and the degree of life impairment. Physical examination is essential in the patient evaluation process, with specific attention paid to extremity pulse status, discoloration, swelling, erythema, ulceration, and localized tenderness. The ankle-brachial index (ABI) provides an objective measurement of lower extremity bloodflow. The ABI is calculated by dividing the highest systolic pressure in either the dorsalis pedis or posterior tibial arteries by the highest arm systolic blood pressure. An ABI from 0.5 to 0.9 is consistent with intermittent claudication. An ABI less than 0.5 is generally required for critical limb ischemia.

(B) Segmental four-cuff pressure measurement throughout the limb provides an objective assessment of circulation. This test provides approximate localization of occlusive lesions, accurate assessment of degree of ischemia, and valuable predictive information regarding interventions. An important adjunct is exercise treadmill testing with ABI determination. The vascular lab diagnosis of claudication requires a 20% drop in ABI with exercise to the point of pain.

(C) Other causes of claudication and rest pain include neurogenic, venous, and arthritic pain, each of which manifests a symptomatic pattern distinctly different from arterial ischemia.

(D) Smoking cessation is by far the most important treatment for intermittent claudication. Patient symptoms will likely not progress and may even improve once smoking is stopped. Regular walking exercise results in a measurable improvement in walking distance in the majority of patients with claudication. Currently two drugs, pentoxifylline (Trental) and cilostazol (Pletal), have been approved by the FDA for the treatment of patients with intermittent claudication. A modest improvement in claudication symptoms can be anticipated in patients treated with pentoxifylline. The usual dose of pentoxifylline is 400 mg PO tid. To date, three randomized, multicenter, placebo-controlled trials have demonstrated superiority of treatment with cilostazol over placebo in improving initial and absolute claudication distances in patients with intermittent claudication. The usual dose of cilostazol is 100 mg PO bid. One randomized, prospective trial comparing pentoxifylline to cilostazol has recently been published; it reports significantly greater walking distance in patients receiving cilostazol as compared with pentoxifylline or placebo.

(E) Patients who are nonambulatory should not be considered for lower extremity revascularization. Additionally, patients may have significant comorbidities (e.g., malignancy, severe coronary artery disease, or chronic obstructive pulmonary disease) that would put them at high risk for surgical revascularization. The results of arteriography may show inadequate distal targets for a revascularization procedure, or the patient may have inadequate conduit for performing a bypass. The judgment of the surgeon is essential in determining the candidacy of each individual patient for surgical revascularization.

(F) The natural history of critical limb ischemia is not necessarily one of inevitable progression to gangrene and limb loss. This was clearly shown in two large, prospective, placebo-controlled clinical trials of treatment with prostaglandins in patients with limb-threatening ischemia, in which approximately 50% of patients with rest pain or ulcer improved on placebo. In situations in which patients refuse surgery or are not surgical candidates, small ulcers or rest pain improve on occasion without operative therapy. No currently available pharmacologic therapy has been shown to augment wound healing in this patient population.

The determination of amputation level should be done with consideration for the patient's anticipated degree of activity. If patients are expected to subsequently ambulate, an attempt should be made to preserve the knee joint. Nonambulatory patients, in general, should undergo above-knee amputations to optimize wound healing and to avoid subsequent flexion contractures at the knee that may necessitate a higher level amputation.

(G) Contrast arteriography remains the gold standard for preoperative assessment of critical limb ischemia. Arteriography should consist of an aortogram with runoff of the affected extremity to identify inflow lesions as well as the optimal sites for proximal and distal graft anastomoses. Magnetic resonance and computerized tomography angiography are emerging techniques that may ultimately supplant contrast arteriography as the methods of choice for lower extremity arterial imaging.

(H) Endovascular techniques (e.g., thrombolytic therapy, angioplasty, and arterial stenting) presently have only a limited role in the treatment of critical limb ischemia. Angioplasty and stenting of focal iliac lesions is often recommended to improve arterial inflow to the affected leg. Because patients with critical limb ischemia almost always have multilevel disease, treatment of iliac lesions alone is rarely sufficient in improving patient symptoms. Angioplasty, with or without stenting, of infrainguinal vessels for the treatment of arterial occlusive disease cannot be recommended currently because of reported high recurrence rates. Thus endovascular techniques for critical limb ischemia may be used adjunctively with surgical revascularization but are rarely definitive therapy.

(I) Extensive cardiac evaluation in a patient scheduled to undergo major vascular surgery should not be performed routinely but rather should be undertaken on the merit of symptoms or ECG findings. Prophylactic coronary revascularization prior to vascular surgery is not associated with improved cardiac outcome and may, in fact, be

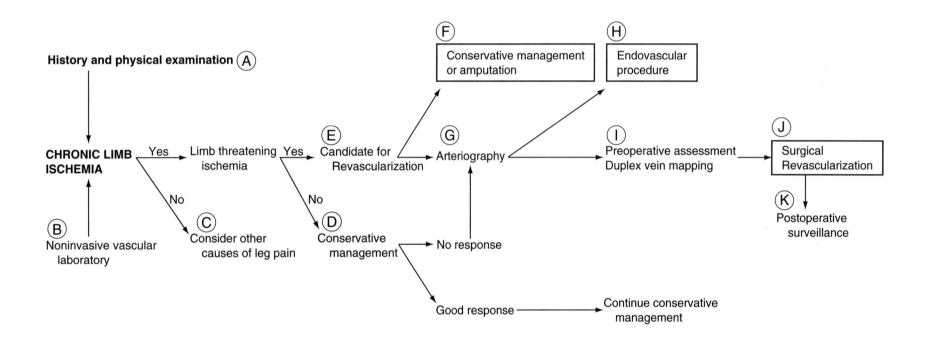

History and physical examination (A)

CHRONIC LIMB ISCHEMIA — Yes → Limb threatening ischemia — Yes → (E) Candidate for Revascularization → (G) Arteriography

No → (C) Consider other causes of leg pain

No → (D) Conservative management

(B) Noninvasive vascular laboratory

Conservative management → No response

Good response → Continue conservative management

(F) Conservative management or amputation

(H) Endovascular procedure

(I) Preoperative assessment Duplex vein mapping → (J) Surgical Revascularization → (K) Postoperative surveillance

associated with increased overall morbidity following the subsequent major vascular surgery. Because coronary artery disease is ubiquitous in the patient population with APVD, recent research has focused on optimizing medical management in the perioperative period. It is clear that the perioperative use of ß-blockers in patients undergoing surgery for APVD should become the standard of practice. Perioperative aspirin therapy is also recommended to reduce coronary morbidity and also to possibly improve graft patency.

Duplex vein mapping is a useful adjunct to identify available autogenous conduit. This is particularly true in patients who may require the use of alternate conduit such as lesser saphenous or arm vein.

(J) Over the past three decades, data obtained about patency, limb salvage, and patient survival has repeatedly supported aggressive revascularization in patients with chronic lower extremity ischemia. Data have also supported revascularization in difficult subsets of patients including those requiring alternate conduit, patients who have had multiple previous failed attempts at limb revascularization, the elderly, diabetics, and patients with end-stage renal disease. When possible, autogenous vein is the preferred conduit. In experienced hands, reversed autogenous vein and in situ vein bypass are equally effective (as, perhaps, is nonreversed translocated vein conduit) in terms of patency and limb salvage.

(K) Approximately 20% of lower extremity vein grafts will develop stenoses requiring revision, the majority within the first year following bypass. Most stenoses are asymptomatic but can be detected with an aggressive program of postoperative duplex graft surveillance. Surveillance every 3 months the first year following bypass and every 6 months thereafter is recommended.

REFERENCES

Beebe HG, Dawson DL, Cutler BS et al: A new pharmacologic treatment for intermittent claudication: Results of a randomized, multicenter trial. Arch Int Med 159:2041–2050, 1999.

Brothers TE, Rios GA, Robison JG et al: Justification of intervention for limb-threatening ischemia: A surgical decision analysis. Cardiovasc Surg 7:62–69, 1999.

Gray BH, Sullivan TM, Childs MB et al: High incidence of restenosis/reocclusion of stents in the percutaneous treatment of long-segment superficial femoral artery disease after suboptimal angioplasty. J Vasc Surg 25:74–83, 1997.

Hiatt WR, Regensteiner JG, Wolfel EE et al: Effect of exercise training on skeletal muscle histology and metabolism in peripheral arterial disease. J Appl Physiol 81:780–788, 1996.

Landry GJ, Moneta GL, Taylor LM Jr. et al: Long-term outcome of revised lower extremity bypass grafts. J Vasc Surg 35:56–63, 2002.

McDermott MM, Greenland P, Liu K et al: Leg symptoms in peripheral arterial disease: Associated clinical characteristics and functional impairment. JAMA 286:1599–1606, 2001.

Nicoloff AD, Taylor LM Jr., McLafferty RB et al: Patient recovery after infrainguinal bypass grafting for limb salvage. J Vasc Surg 27:256–266, 1998.

Taylor LM Jr., Edwards JM, Porter JM: Present status of reversed vein bypass grafting: Five-year results of a modern series. J Vasc Surg 11:193–205, 1990.

Visser K, Idu MM, Buth J et al: Duplex scan surveillance during the first year after infrainguinal autologous vein bypass grafting surgery: Costs and clinical outcomes compared with other surveillance programs. J Vasc Surg 33:123–130, 2001.

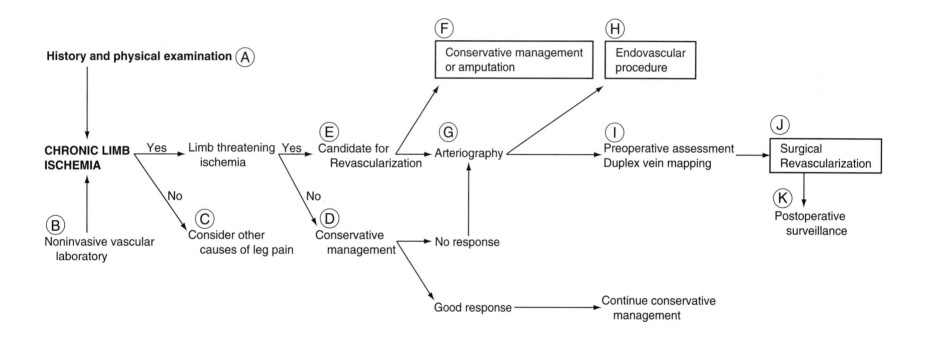

History and physical examination (A)

CHRONIC LIMB ISCHEMIA

(B)
Noninvasive vascular laboratory

Yes → Limb threatening ischemia

No → (C) Consider other causes of leg pain

Yes → (E) Candidate for Revascularization

No → (D) Conservative management

(F) Conservative management or amputation

(G) Arteriography

→ No response

→ Good response ──────── Continue conservative management

(H) Endovascular procedure

(I) Preoperative assessment Duplex vein mapping

(J) Surgical Revascularization

(K) Postoperative surveillance

PEDIATRICS

Chapter 107 *Tracheoesophageal Fistula/ Esophageal Atresia*

RICHARD J. HENDRICKSON, MD • FREDERICK M. KARRER, MD

(A) Tracheoesophageal malformations occur in 1 in 4000 births. Some 25% to 40% of these neonates are premature or of low birth weight.

(B) Fifty percent of infants have associated congenital defects, the most common ones being cardiac malformations (35%), GU malformations (20%), and GI malformations (24%). The acronym VACTERL (*v*ertebral defects, *a*norectal malformations, *c*ardiovascular anomalies, *t*racheoesophageal fistula, *e*sophageal atresia, *r*enal anomalies, *l*imb defects) summarizes possible defects. Prenatal diagnosis by maternal ultrasound is possible in the presence of polyhydramnios and a small stomach bubble.

(C) Respiratory distress (e.g., choking, coughing, and regurgitation with the first feeding) is the most characteristic sign of esophageal atresia. There is often gastric distention secondary to air inspired through the tracheoesophageal fistula (TEF). More subtle signs include desaturation with nippling associated with noisy breathing.

(D) The current classification describes the anatomic defect rather than being a complex categorization by number and letter. The most common types of tracheoesophageal malformation are proximal esophageal atresia with distal fistula (85%), isolated esophageal atresia (10%), and H-type TEF without esophageal atresia (5%).

(E) Radiographs of the chest and abdomen may demonstrate pneumonitis; air in the GI tract (which rules out isolated esophageal atresia); and associated anomalies such as duodenal atresia ("double bubble"), vertebral and sacral malformations, and other skeletal anomalies. Preoperative echocardiography allows assessment of cardiac structural anomalies (e.g., atrial or ventricular septal defect, valvular anomalies, and patent ductus arteriosus) that could have an impact on anesthesia management. The position of the aortic arch (5% right-sided) can also be determined. Renal ultrasound can be delayed until after esophageal repair but should be performed to identify possible renal anomalies (obstructive uropathy) that may require further intervention and/or follow-up.

(F) A soft, radiopaque catheter, No. 6 to 10 Fr, passed through the mouth or nose into the esophagus as far as it will go, with lateral x-ray confirmation, determines the level of the proximal esophageal remnant. If repair is going to be delayed, a small amount of barium sulfate (1 to 2 ml) should be instilled into the esophagus to rule out a proximal TEF.

(G) Air in the stomach on an abdominal radiograph distinguishes isolated esophageal atresia from proximal esophageal atresia with distal TEF. A stomach bubble suggests a distal TEF with proximal esophageal atresia. Absence of intestinal air suggests isolated esophageal atresia.

(H) Preoperatively, elevating the head of the bed to 45 degrees and Replogle tube sump suction help to prevent aspiration. H_2-blockers minimize gastric acid reflux into the bronchial tree. Primary extrapleural anastomosis of esophageal segments can be performed in the first 24 hours of life in the absence of associated life-threatening malformations or pneumonitis. Traditionally, a right thoracotomy with an extrapleural approach is used. Recently, thoracoscopic repair has been reported to be safe and effective. The goals of operative repair include a tension-free anastomosis with good blood supply. A chest tube or drain is left in the chest until a leak has been ruled out, either clinically or radiographically.

(I) Gastrostomy, sump aspiration of the proximal esophageal segment, and total parenteral nutrition (TPN) feeding until clinical status improves is the optimal approach for low–birth weight infants (less than 1500 gm), infants with associated life-threatening anomalies, and those with significant respiratory compromise. Occasionally, in infants with severely compromised pulmonary status whose TEF prevents adequate oxygenation, the fistula is ligated as a temporizing measure until delayed repair becomes feasible. Fistula ligation can be performed either via right thoracotomy or thoracoscopy. In addition, a gastrostomy tube may be inserted to allow enteral nutrition. Another approach is Fogarty or Foley catheter occlusion of the fistula via bronchoscopy or gastrostomy. This method stabilizes the patient without thoracotomy, avoiding violation of the chest until definitive repair.

(J) In isolated esophageal atresia, there is commonly a long gap between the two segments of the esophagus. The gap should be evaluated with a contrast study after a gastrostomy tube has been placed. A short distal esophagus makes primary repair impossible. Gastrostomy feedings are then instituted, along with sump aspiration of the proximal pouch. After several weeks of gastrostomy feedings, elongation of the proximal and distal esophageal pouches may permit end-to-end anastomosis.

(K) An H-type fistula commonly occurs in the cervical esophagus. The lesion often escapes detection in infancy and is usually discovered later in infancy or childhood because of repeated episodes of pneumonia. Bronchoscopy can be diagnostic. Passing a No. 4 or 5 Fr catheter across the fistula during bronchoscopy allows easier identification during right transcervical exploration. Thoracotomy is rarely necessary but is indicated for unusual fistulas in the thorax.

(L) When the esophageal gap is still too long for anastomosis, cervical esophagostomy is occasionally necessary. Gastrostomy feedings are continued and the esophagus is replaced with stomach, colon, or jejunum.

(M) Morbidity and mortality rates for immediate primary repair and for staged repair are not substantially different. Waterston's risk classification helped to predict outcome based on birth weight, pneumonia, and associated congenital anomalies. The modern Spitz classification for prediction of

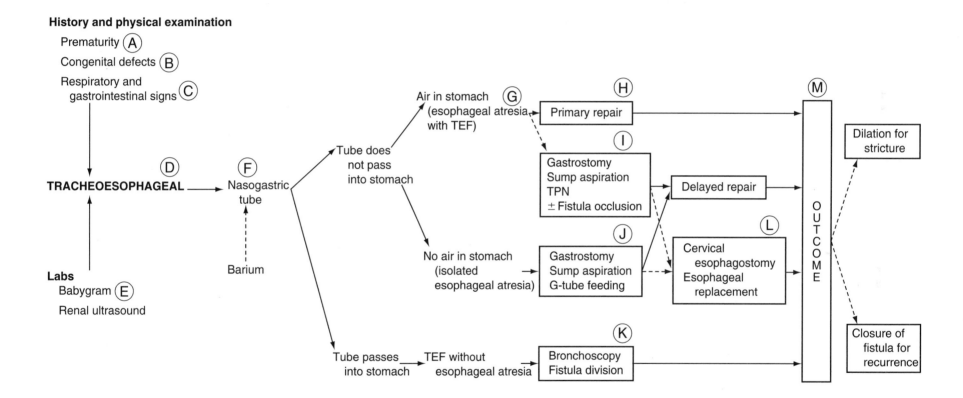

History and physical examination

Prematurity (A)

Congenital defects (B)

Respiratory and
   gastrointestinal signs (C)

Air in stomach (G)
(esophageal atresia
with TEF)

(H) Primary repair

(M)

TRACHEOESOPHAGEAL (D) → Nasogastric (F)
tube

Tube does
not pass
into stomach

(I) Gastrostomy
Sump aspiration
TPN
± Fistula occlusion

Delayed repair

Dilation for
stricture

Barium

No air in stomach
(isolated
esophageal atresia)

(J) Gastrostomy
Sump aspiration
G-tube feeding

(L) Cervical
esophagostomy
Esophageal
replacement

OUTCOME

Labs

Babygram (E)

Renal ultrasound

Tube passes → TEF without → (K) Bronchoscopy
into stomach   esophageal atresia   Fistula division

Closure of
fistula for
recurrence

survival is based upon birth weight and major cardiac disease. Postoperatively, a contrast swallow is performed to identify a leak or stricture. If no leak is identified, then enteral feeds are initiated with chest tube or drain removal. Complications after repair include abnormal motility (100%), esophageal stricture (10% to 25%), gastroesophageal reflux (40% to 70%), anastomotic leak (8% to 12%), and recurrent fistula and significant tracheomalacia (both 3% to 5%). Anastomotic leaks usually seal spontaneously, but they contribute to stricture. In most cases, strictures are managed successfully by dilation during the first postoperative year. Recurrent fistula requires reoperation. Clinical tracheomalacia may require aortopexy in infants with TEF. Gastroesophageal reflux is initially treated with acid reduction and/or prokinetic agents but may require fundoplication in up to 25%. Replacement of the esophagus with stomach, jejunum, or colon is associated with mortality rates of 2% to 9% and with increased morbidity, including leak (10% to 30%), stricture (12% to 15%), and revision after failure (10% to 18%). Late complications include intestinal obstruction (5% to 10%) and dysphagia (20% to 40%). Mortality after repair of H-type fistula is very rare, and morbidity from the neck incision or leak is minor.

REFERENCES

Brown AK, Tam PKH: Measurement of gap length in esophageal atresia. A simple predictor of outcome. J Am Coll Surg 182:41–45, 1996.

Hirschl RB, Yardeni D, Olkham K et al: Gastric transposition for esophageal replacement in children: Experience with 41 consecutive cases with special emphasis on esophageal atresia. Ann Surg 236:531–539, 2002.

Kallen K, Mastroiacovo P, Castilla EE et al: VATER non-random association of congenital malformations: Study based on data from four malformation registers. Am J Med Genet 101:26–32, 2001.

Rothenberg SS: Thoracoscopic repair of tracheoesophageal fistula in newborns. J Pediatr Surg 37:869–872, 2002.

Spitz L, Kiely EM, Morecroft JA et al: Oesophageal atresia: At-risk groups for the 1990s. J Pediatr Surg 29:723–725, 1994.

Spitz L: Esophageal atresia: Past, present, and future. J Pediatr Surg 31:19–25, 1996.

Stringer MD, McKenna KM, Goldstein RB et al: Prenatal diagnosis of esophageal atresia. J Pediatr Surg 30:1258–1263, 1995.

Waterston DJ, Carter RT, Aberdeen E: Tracheoesophageal fistula: A study of survival in 218 infants. Lancet 1:819–826, 1962.

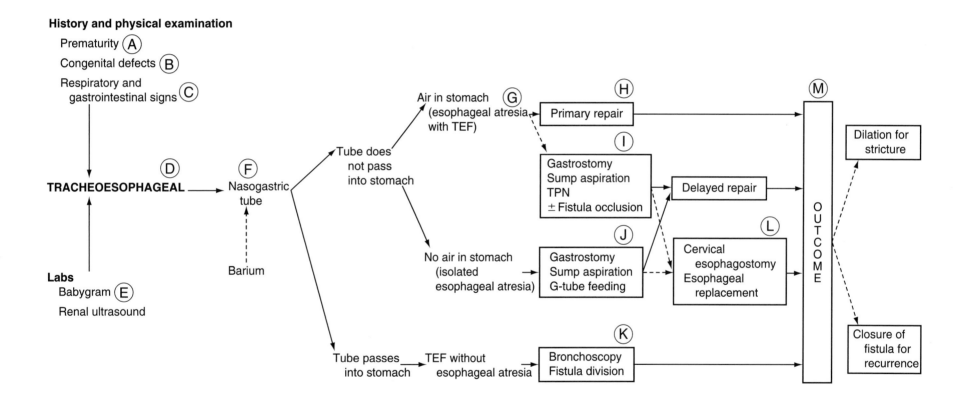

History and physical examination

Prematurity (A)

Congenital defects (B)

Respiratory and
gastrointestinal signs (C)

TRACHEOESOPHAGEAL (D) → Nasogastric (F) tube

Barium

Labs
Babygram (E)

Renal ultrasound

Tube does
not pass
into stomach

Air in stomach (G)
(esophageal atresia
with TEF)

Primary repair (H)

Gastrostomy (I)
Sump aspiration
TPN
± Fistula occlusion

No air in stomach
(isolated
esophageal atresia)

Gastrostomy (J)
Sump aspiration
G-tube feeding

Delayed repair

Cervical (L)
esophagostomy
Esophageal
replacement

Tube passes
into stomach

TEF without
esophageal atresia

Bronchoscopy (K)
Fistula division

OUTCOME (M)

Dilation for
stricture

Closure of
fistula for
recurrence

Chapter 108 *Infantile Hypertrophic Pyloric Stenosis*

RICHARD J. HENDRICKSON, MD • DENIS D. BENSARD, MD

(A) The diagnosis of hypertrophic pyloric stenosis (HPS) is suggested by a history of a healthy infant who initially feeds normally, but at 4 to 6 weeks of age suffers the onset of intermittent nonbilious emesis that progresses to projectile emesis with each feeding. The infant appears hungry and often refeeds immediately despite the repeated vomiting. Signs of dehydration (e.g., sunken fontanelle, dry mucous membranes, or poor skin turgor) are late findings.

(B) Physical examination is focused on palpation of a thickened and enlarged pylorus, referred to as an "olive" for its size and shape. Palpation of an olive requires skill and patience. Unequivocal palpation of the pyloric olive, possible in 75% to 90% of infants with pyloric stenosis, eliminates the need for additional diagnostic tests; allows prompt preparation for operative treatment; and, therefore, minimizes cost. Associated findings are rare, but mild jaundice occurs in 5% of infants because of reduced glucuronyl transferase activity.

(C) Hypertrophic pyloric stenosis is the most common surgical cause of emesis in infants, affecting 1:300 to 1:900 newborns. Thickening of the circular muscle layer of the pylorus produces an elongation and obstruction of the pyloric channel. The cause of HPS remains unknown. The incidence is greatest in boys (4:1) and in offspring of an affected parent. Offspring of an affected parent have an increased incidence of HPS (10%); the highest rate occurs in males born to an affected mother (20%).

(D) Electrolytes are often normal, but long-standing vomiting will eventually result in hypokalemic, hypochloremic metabolic alkalosis because of the loss of gastric acid (HCl). Earlier consideration of the diagnosis has led to a significant reduction in this classic triad of electrolyte abnormalities at presentation. Dehydration is corrected with either 5% Dextrose (DS) 0.9% NaCl or, in less severe cases, DS 0.45% NaCl with 20 meq/liter KCl. Once dehydration and electrolytes are corrected, pyloromyotomy is performed.

(E) If diagnosis is uncertain, B-mode ultrasound examination is done. Pyloric diameter greater than 1.4 cm, wall thickness greater than 4 mm, and pyloric channel length greater than 1.6 cm are diagnostic of HPS (sensitivity, specificity, positive predictive value greater than 90%).

(F) Barium upper GI contrast study is reserved for infants who remain symptomatic despite a nondiagnostic ultrasound or in whom another diagnosis is suspected. Pyloric channel narrowing, bulging of the hypertrophic pylorus into the gastric antrum, and gastric outlet obstruction characterize the contrast findings of HPS. Current analyses suggest that UGI is the most cost-effective initial radiologic diagnostic test because, unlike ultrasound, alternative causes of nonbilious vomiting (e.g., gastroesophageal reflux, malrotation, and duodenal stenosis) can be identified.

(G) Surgical correction of pyloric stenosis is not an emergency procedure, but in general, only significant dehydration or serum bicarbonate greater than 30 meq/dl precludes immediate operative correction. Infants who present early without significant dehydration or electrolyte abnormalities can be operated upon early. In more severely affected infants, correction of fluid and electrolyte abnormalities requires 12 to 24 hours. Current data fail to demonstrate benefit of prophylactic antibiotics.

(H) When pyloric stenosis has been excluded, other causes of nonbilious vomiting should be investigated. Gastroesophageal reflux is common in infants and is often confused with HPS. Less common causes of nonbilious vomiting in an infant include malrotation, duodenal stenosis, and intestinal duplication. All of these abnormalities are identifiable by barium upper GI contrast studies.

(I) Pyloromyotomy is performed by dividing the hypertrophic pylorus muscle from the pyloric vein to the antrum. Complete pyloromyotomy is suggested by bulging mucosa and mobile pyloric muscle with independent movement of the two halves when they are pulled in opposite directions.

Laparoscopic pyloromyotomy is performed through three small incisions (3 mm) in the epigastrium. Comparative studies suggest that laparoscopic pyloromyotomy is equal to open pyloromyotomy with comparable outcomes. Initial reports of higher complication rates are likely related to the learning curve associated with minimally invasive surgery. The increased operative costs of laparoscopic pyloromyotomy will diminish with operative experience and a reduction in operative time. This, in conjunction with shortened hospitalization, is likely to eliminate cost differences in the future.

(J) Open pyloromyotomy (Fredet-Ramstedt pyloromyotomy) is the conventional approach to surgical correction of HPS. The procedure is performed via a transverse, right upper quadrant incision (preferred); or by a circumferential, supraumbilical incision. Infiltration with local anesthetic at the time of closure can enhance recovery and promote earlier feeding, offsetting the advantage of the laparoscopic approach. Postoperative wound infection occurs in 1% to 5% of patients.

(K) In performing pyloromyotomy, inadvertent mucosal perforation can occur (1% to 3%). Care must be taken to avoid perforation of the underlying mucosa. Failure to recognize a mucosal perforation can be catastrophic, and perforation must be ruled out before closure. Injection of 60 ml of air into the stomach via a nasogastric tube following pyloromyotomy facilitates diagnosis of mucosal perforation. If mucosal perforation is identified, the opening is repaired and covered with an omental patch; or the myotomy is closed and repeated after rotating the pylorus 180 degrees (preferred).

(L) Feedings are started 3 hours postoperatively. Ad lib feeding or gradual advancement of feeds may be employed. Full feeding is achieved within 18 to 24 hours. Small episodes of emesis are common in the early postoperative period and should not delay the progression of feeding. A disadvantage of ad lib feeding is the greater frequency

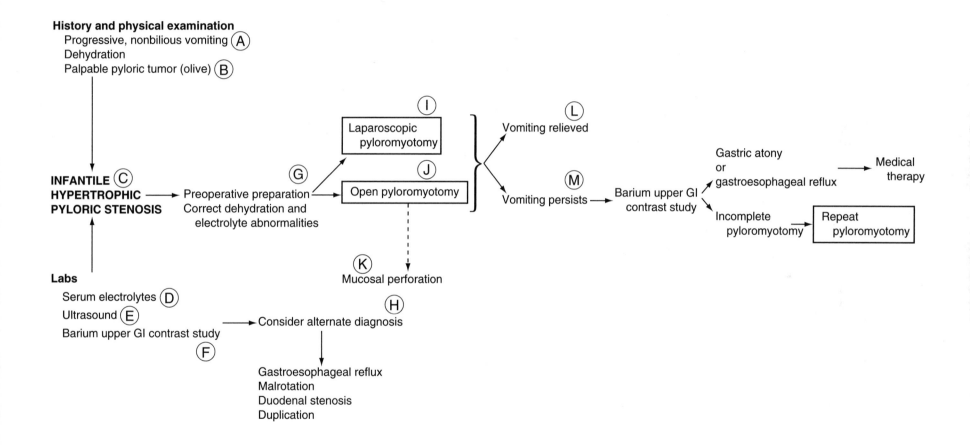

History and physical examination
   Progressive, nonbilious vomiting (A)
   Dehydration
   Palpable pyloric tumor (olive) (B)

INFANTILE (C)
HYPERTROPHIC
PYLORIC STENOSIS

Preoperative preparation
Correct dehydration and
   electrolyte abnormalities

(G)

(I)
Laparoscopic
pyloromyotomy

(J)
Open pyloromyotomy

(K)
Mucosal perforation

(L)
Vomiting relieved

(M)
Vomiting persists

Barium upper GI
contrast study

Gastric atony
or
gastroesophageal reflux

Medical
therapy

Incomplete
pyloromyotomy

Repeat
pyloromyotomy

Labs
   Serum electrolytes (D)
   Ultrasound (E)
   Barium upper GI contrast study
   (F)

(H)
Consider alternate diagnosis

Gastroesophageal reflux
Malrotation
Duodenal stenosis
Duplication

of postoperative emesis, which should be discussed with the parent in advance.

Ⓜ Persistent postoperative vomiting (longer than 48 hours), although uncommon (3%), warrants further evaluation. A trial of antireflux therapy should be implemented. If symptoms continue, a barium upper GI study is obtained to assess gastric emptying and to exclude gastroesophageal reflux. Unfortunately, incomplete pyloromyotomy cannot be identified radiographically because the images of the hypertrophic pylorus before and after myotomy are similar. Because incomplete myotomy is rare, the infant is supported with peripheral hyperalimentation for 10 to 14 days or until symptoms resolve. A repeat barium study demonstrating gastric outlet obstruction or persistent symptoms despite an adequate period of observation warrants re-exploration for presumptive incomplete pyloromyotomy.

REFERENCES

Campbell BT, McLean K, Barnhart DC et al: A comparison of laparoscopic and open pyloromyotomy at a teaching hospital. J Pediatr Surg 37:1068–1071, 2002.

Chen EA, Luks FI, Gilchrist BF et al: Pyloric stenosis in the age of ultrasonography: Fading skills, better patients? J Pediatr Surg 31:829–830, 1996.

Garza JJ, Morash D, Dzakovic A et al: Ad libitum feeding decreases hospital stay for neonates after pyloromyotomy. J Pediatr Surg 37:493–495, 2002.

Hernanz SM, Sells LL, Ambrosino MM et al: Hypertrophic pyloric stenosis in the infant without a palpable olive: Accuracy of sonographic diagnosis. Radiology 193:771–776, 1994.

Hulka F, Harrison MW, Campbell TJ et al: Complications of pyloromyotomy for infantile hypertrophic pyloric stenosis. Am J Surg 173:450–452, 1997.

Miozzari HH, Tonz M, von Vigier RO et al: Fluid resuscitation in infantile hypertrophic pyloric stenosis. Acta Paediatr 90:511–514, 2001.

Royal RE, Linz DN, Gruppo DL et al: Repair of mucosal perforation during pyloromyotomy: Surgeon's choice. J Pediatr Surg 30:1430–1432, 1995.

Yoshizawa J, Eto T, Higashimoto Y et al: Ultrasonographic features of normalization of the pylorus after pyloromyotomy for hypertrophic pyloric stenosis. J Pediatr Surg 36:582–586, 2001.

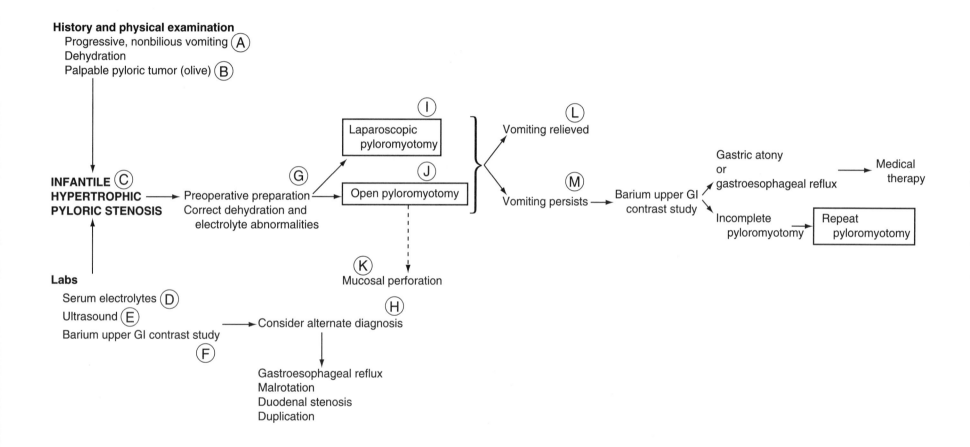

History and physical examination
Progressive, nonbilious vomiting (A)
Dehydration
Palpable pyloric tumor (olive) (B)

INFANTILE (C)
HYPERTROPHIC
PYLORIC STENOSIS → Preoperative preparation
Correct dehydration and
electrolyte abnormalities

(G)

(I) Laparoscopic
pyloromyotomy

(J) Open pyloromyotomy

(K)
Mucosal perforation

(L) Vomiting relieved

(M) Vomiting persists → Barium upper GI
contrast study

Gastric atony
or → Medical
gastroesophageal reflux therapy

Incomplete → Repeat
pyloromyotomy pyloromyotomy

Labs
Serum electrolytes (D)
Ultrasound (E) → Consider alternate diagnosis (H)
Barium upper GI contrast study
(F)

Gastroesophageal reflux
Malrotation
Duodenal stenosis
Duplication

Chapter 109 *Neonatal Bowel Obstruction*

RICHARD J. HENDRICKSON, MD • DENIS D. BENSARD, MD

(A) A prenatal diagnosis of fetal bowel obstruction is suggested by polyhydramnios. Several forms of intestinal obstruction are variably observed with genetic conditions such as trisomy 21 (e.g., duodenal atresia, malrotation, and Hirschsprung's disease) and cystic fibrosis (e.g., meconium ileus). Associated anomalies of the heart, vertebrae, kidneys, or limbs may also be identified. Bilious emesis in a newborn suggests mechanical bowel obstruction and will be confirmed in approximately 40% to 50% of neonates. Nonsurgical causes of bilious emesis include metabolic disorders (e.g., hypokalemia, hypothyroidism, hypermagnesemia, and hypoglycemia); dysmotility (e.g., mitochondrial pathology); and infections.

(B) The need for adequate volume replacement and correction of electrolyte derangements may be inferred from clinical laboratory studies. Evaluation begins with an abdominal radiograph. Air visualized in a dilated stomach and proximal duodenum ("double bubble") without distal air suggests duodenal obstruction (e.g., duodenal atresia or malrotation with volvulus). Abdominal radiographs demonstrating several dilated loops suggest proximal intestinal obstruction (e.g., jejunoileal atresia), whereas multiple dilated loops suggest distal intestinal obstruction. Contrast studies are indicated in stable infants without indications for emergent laparotomy (e.g., perforation or shock). If malrotation obstruction is suspected, an upper GI contrast series should be obtained to exclude midgut volvulus. More distal intestinal obstruction is best evaluated with contrast enema.

(C) Suspected neonatal bowel obstruction requires cessation of enteral feeding and gastric decompression. The latter is more effective with relatively proximal obstructions. IV fluid resuscitation and correction of electrolyte abnormalities constitute initial resuscitation. Empiric antibiotic therapy, especially when bowel perforation or necrosis is suspected, should be initiated.

(D) Proximal obstruction often presents early (less than 24 hours) in the newborn period and is characterized by emesis or feeding intolerance. Distal obstruction often presents later (more than 24 hours) with the development of abdominal distention and delayed or failed passage of meconium.

(E) Obstruction of the stomach results from neonatal gastroparesis or acquired outlet obstruction. Anatomic obstruction is rare. Pyloric webs are three times more common than antral membranes. Ectopic pancreatic rests can also cause pyloric obstruction. Feeding intolerance and nonbilious, projectile emesis suggest gastric outlet obstruction. Respiratory compromise may result from extreme gastric dilatation but improves rapidly with gastric decompression. Radiographic features include a large gastric air bubble. Contrast studies facilitate the distinction of gastroparesis from structural lesions.

(F) Congenital duodenal obstruction can be partial or complete and intrinsic or extrinsic. Extrinsic obstruction may be caused by malrotation, preduodenal portal vein, intestinal duplication, pancreatic cyst, or annular pancreas. The latter is invariably associated with intrinsic duodenal obstruction (atresia or stenosis). Intrinsic obstruction evolves from failed recanalization of the duodenum during first-trimester organogenesis (incidence is 1:7000) and accounts for half of all small bowel atresias. Postampullary obstruction accounts for 80% of obstructing lesions. Because an insult occurs early in gestation, associated congenital anomalies are common (50% to 80%). The VACTERL complex (*v*ertebral, *a*nal, *c*ardiac, *t*racheoesophageal, *r*enal, and *l*imb anomalies) or trisomy 21 is evident in 30% of affected infants. Postampullary obstruction is manifested as bilious emesis in the absence of abdominal distention within the first 24 hours of life. Radiographs reveal the classic double bubble sign of dilated stomach and proximal duodenal bulb. Differentiation of duodenal obstruction from malrotation is essential. Contrast studies permit differentiation of duodenal atresia from malrotation with midgut volvulus, the latter a surgical emergency.

(G) Duodenal webs may escape diagnosis in the newborn period. Identifying the site of deformity is difficult. With either an orogastric or nasogastric tube in place, the tube can be advanced by the anesthesiologist until it causes an indentation in the duodenum, which is distal to the site of the membrane origin. This technique permits correct placement of the duodenotomy. Membrane deformities may be associated with anomalies of the common bile duct, such as termination of ductules within the web.

(H) Sites of jejunoileal atresia and stenosis are equally distributed from the ligament of Treitz to the ileocecal valve. Up to 20% of children have more than one affected area. Associated extraintestinal anomalies are uncommon. Abdominal distention and bilious emesis, in conjunction with a history of failure to pass meconium, suggests the diagnosis. In selected cases passage of meconium may occur despite obstruction if the lesion occurred as a result of a late vascular accident in utero. Radiographs demonstrate distended, air-filled loops of bowel with a paucity of distal gas. Contrast enema reveals a microcolon without reflux of contrast into the dilated, proximal bowel.

(I) Congenital colonic atresias account for less than 5% of all intestinal atresias. Contrast enema demonstrates the level of colonic obstruction. Surgical treatment is limited segmental resection with primary or staged reconstruction. A colostomy and delayed reconstruction is preferred if there is significant disparity between the dilated proximal segment and nondilated distal segment.

(J) Anomalies of rotation and fixation of the midgut can lead to volvulus and extensive bowel loss. Midgut volvulus accounts for nearly 20% of short bowel syndrome cases. Diagnosis is

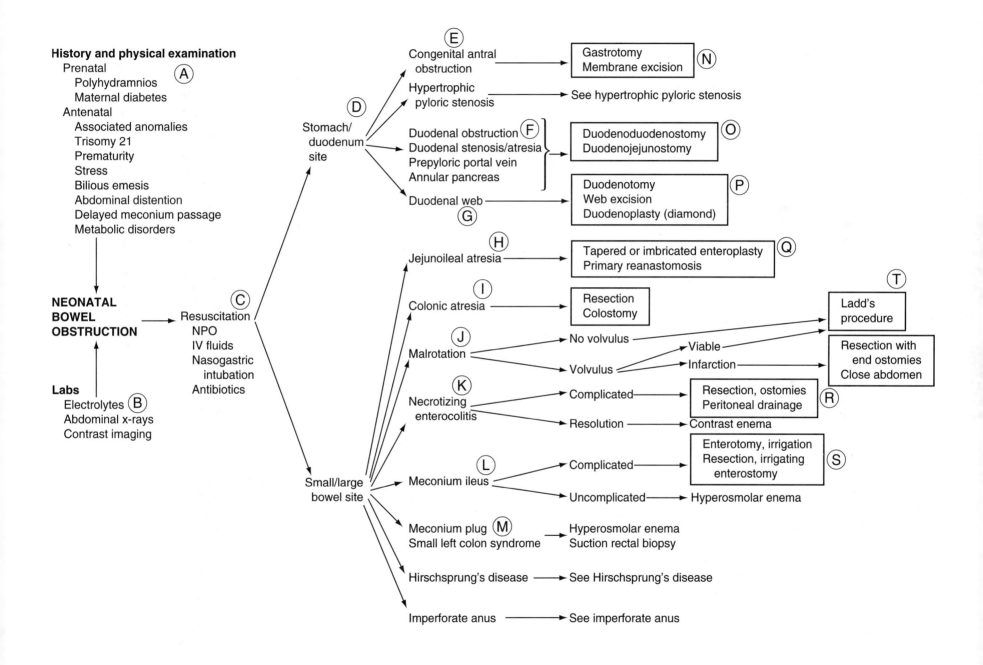

History and physical examination
Prenatal (A)
    Polyhydramnios
    Maternal diabetes
Antenatal
    Associated anomalies
    Trisomy 21
    Prematurity
    Stress
    Bilious emesis
    Abdominal distention
    Delayed meconium passage
    Metabolic disorders

NEONATAL BOWEL OBSTRUCTION

Labs
Electrolytes (B)
Abdominal x-rays
Contrast imaging

Resuscitation (C)
NPO
IV fluids
Nasogastric intubation
Antibiotics

Stomach/duodenum site (D)
    Congenital antral obstruction (E) → Gastrotomy / Membrane excision (N)
    Hypertrophic pyloric stenosis → See hypertrophic pyloric stenosis
    Duodenal obstruction (F)
    Duodenal stenosis/atresia
    Prepyloric portal vein
    Annular pancreas → Duodenoduodenostomy / Duodenojejunostomy (O)
    Duodenal web (G) → Duodenotomy / Web excision / Duodenoplasty (diamond) (P)

Small/large bowel site
    Jejunoileal atresia (H) → Tapered or imbricated enteroplasty / Primary reanastomosis (Q)
    Colonic atresia (I) → Resection / Colostomy
    Malrotation (J)
        No volvulus → Ladd's procedure (T)
        Volvulus → Viable → Ladd's procedure
        Volvulus → Infarction → Resection with end ostomies / Close abdomen
    Necrotizing enterocolitis (K)
        Complicated → Resection, ostomies / Peritoneal drainage (R)
        Resolution → Contrast enema
    Meconium ileus (L)
        Complicated → Enterotomy, irrigation / Resection, irrigating enterostomy (S)
        Uncomplicated → Hyperosmolar enema
    Meconium plug (M) / Small left colon syndrome → Hyperosmolar enema / Suction rectal biopsy
    Hirschsprung's disease → See Hirschsprung's disease
    Imperforate anus → See imperforate anus

made by emergent upper gastrointestinal contrast study. Malrotation or nonrotation is always associated with congenital diaphragmatic hernia or abdominal wall defect and is observed in as many as 30% of infants with duodenal or jejunoileal atresia.

(K) Necrotizing enterocolitis (NEC) is a condition of premature or low–birth weight infants that affects any segment of the GI tract. The cause is unknown, but the triad of immature gut, bacteria, and substrate (feeds) appears central to the development of NEC. Approximately 30% of infants require operation for complications of NEC, including necrosis or perforation. NEC is suggested by abdominal distention, lethargy, feeding intolerance, bilious emesis, and rectal bleeding. Radiographs often demonstrate the pathognomonic finding of *Pneumatosis intestinalis*. Portal vein gas suggests extensive intestinal gangrene and a poor prognosis. Indications for operation include perforation (pneumoperitoneum); a fixed abdominal mass; a radiographically fixed, dilated loop of intestine; abdominal wall erythema or edema; and clinical deterioration as manifested by progressive thrombocytopenia, leukocytosis or leucopenia, and septic shock.

(L) Meconium ileus (MI) produces intestinal obstruction from inspissated meconium secondary to pancreatic exocrine insufficiency. It is the earliest clinical manifestation of cystic fibrosis. Uncomplicated meconium ileus causes distal ileal obstruction with proximal bowel dilatation. Complicated meconium ileus results in volvulus, perforation with meconium peritonitis, or intestinal atresia. Failure to pass meconium within 24 hours with associated abdominal distention and bilious emesis are the clinical features of MI. Radiographs reveal intestinal obstruction, often with a coarse, granular (ground-glass), or soapy appearance of air trapped in meconium. Complicated meconium ileus may present with findings of pneumoperitoneum, extraluminal intraperitoneal calcifications or cysts, and ascites. Contrast enema with hyperosmolar

agents is both diagnostic and therapeutic in up to 60%. If gastrograffin enema is unsuccessful or associated with complications, laparotomy and evacuation of the obstructing meconium becomes necessary.

(M) Meconium plug may result from either functional inertia of prematurity; small left colon syndrome; or, rarely, from cystic fibrosis and Hirschsprung's disease. Maternal eclampsia requiring magnesium administration or hyperglycemia as a consequence of maternal diabetes induces fetal intestinal hypomotility and resultant obturation of the colon by normal meconium. Delayed passage of meconium is noted with a patent anus. Water-soluble contrast enema is diagnostic and often therapeutic. A suction rectal biopsy should be performed to identify the 5% to 10% of infants who have underlying Hirschsprung's disease. The evaluation is completed by obtaining DNA analysis or sweat chloride test to exclude cystic fibrosis.

(N) Antral webs are corrected by gastrotomy with membrane excision and transverse closure. Alternatively, antral excision with primary gastro-duodenostomy may be performed and is generally curative. Gastrojejunostomy is poorly tolerated by neonates and should be avoided.

(O) The preferred surgical treatment is diamond end-to-end duodenoduodenostomy.

(P) Longitudinal incision of the duodenum at the membrane origin followed by partial membrane excision is the preferred treatment. Anomalous biliary radicles should be identified and preserved. Resection is limited to the antimesenteric portion of the membrane. Primary closure is performed using a standard Heineke-Mikulicz repair.

(Q) At laparotomy, distal intestinal patency is confirmed. Reestablishment of intestinal continuity with preservation of bowel length is the mainstay of operative therapy. An anastomosis is created between dilated, proximal bowel and decompressed distal bowel with a technique such as tapered or imbricated proximal enteroplasty and end-to-back anastomosis.

(R) Gangrenous bowel is excised, stomas are exteriorized, and attempts to conserve bowel length are indicated. Resection with primary anastomosis is rarely indicated because of the absence of clear benefit or improved outcome. Up to 25% of very premature infants (less than 1000 g) can be managed with primary peritoneal drainage at the bedside. Advantages include comparable survival, improved intestinal preservation, and elimination of emergent laparotomy in critically ill premature infants. Postoperative management is focused upon control of sepsis, nutritional support, correction of electrolyte imbalances, and identification of intestinal stricture. Some 15% to 25% of surviving infants treated medically or surgically will develop late intestinal stricture. Therefore contrast enema is indicated in infants suffering severe NEC treated medically, or before stoma closure in those treated by surgery.

(S) Operative management is by enterotomy, evacuation of inspissated meconium, saline irrigation, and primary closure. Selected patients may require intestinal resection and creation of an irrigating enterostomy (Bishop-Koop procedure).

(T) During initial abdominal exploration, volvulus is first identified. Counterclockwise detorsion of the twisted intestine is performed. Viability of intestine is assessed with the goal of preserving bowel length. Equivocal segments are preserved and reevaluated at second-look laparotomy. The treatment for uncomplicated malrotation is Ladd's procedure: (1) division of abnormal peritoneal bands (Ladd's bands) crossing the duodenum; (2) widening of the mesentery; (3) positioning of the duodenum and small bowel to the right and the colon to the left; and (4) incidental appendectomy. Laparoscopic Ladd's procedure can be performed in the absence of midgut volvulus, and preliminary results suggest comparable efficacy to laparotomy. Cecopexy or duodenopexy do not reduce the risk of recurrent volvulus (5%) and are discouraged.

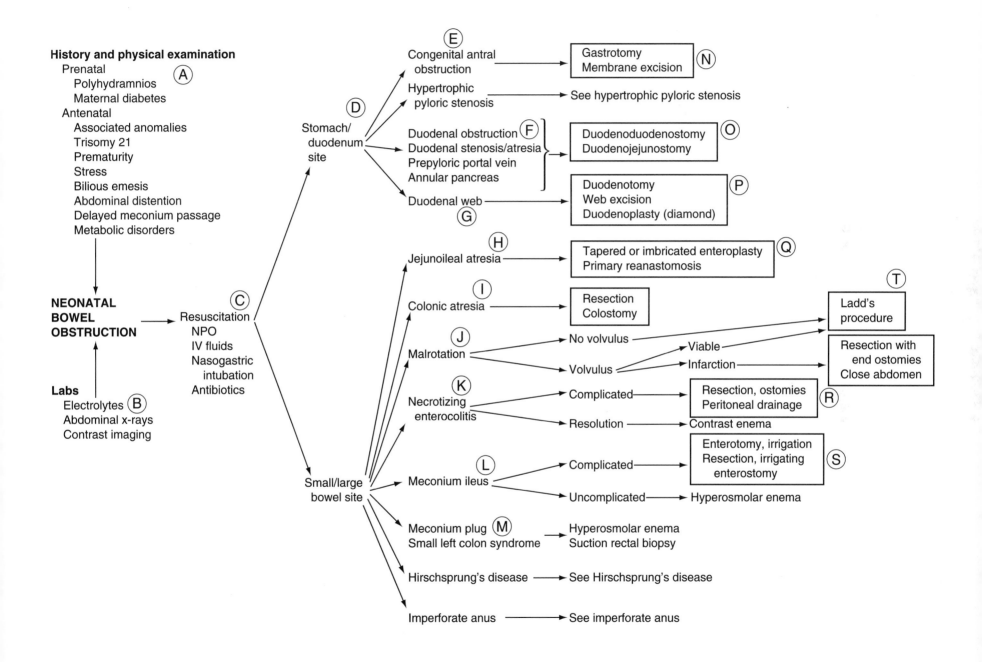

History and physical examination

Prenatal (A)
- Polyhydramnios
- Maternal diabetes

Antenatal
- Associated anomalies
- Trisomy 21
- Prematurity
- Stress
- Bilious emesis
- Abdominal distention
- Delayed meconium passage
- Metabolic disorders

NEONATAL BOWEL OBSTRUCTION

Labs (B)
- Electrolytes
- Abdominal x-rays
- Contrast imaging

(C) Resuscitation
- NPO
- IV fluids
- Nasogastric intubation
- Antibiotics

(D) Stomach/duodenum site

(E) Congenital antral obstruction → Gastrotomy / Membrane excision (N)

Hypertrophic pyloric stenosis → See hypertrophic pyloric stenosis

(F) Duodenal obstruction / Duodenal stenosis/atresia / Prepyloric portal vein / Annular pancreas → Duodenoduodenostomy / Duodenojejunostomy (O)

(G) Duodenal web → Duodenotomy / Web excision / Duodenoplasty (diamond) (P)

Small/large bowel site

(H) Jejunoileal atresia → Tapered or imbricated enteroplasty / Primary reanastomosis (Q)

(I) Colonic atresia → Resection / Colostomy

(J) Malrotation
- No volvulus → Ladd's procedure (T)
- Volvulus → Viable → Ladd's procedure / Infarction → Resection with end ostomies / Close abdomen

(K) Necrotizing enterocolitis
- Complicated → Resection, ostomies / Peritoneal drainage (R)
- Resolution → Contrast enema

(L) Meconium ileus
- Complicated → Enterotomy, irrigation / Resection, irrigating enterostomy (S)
- Uncomplicated → Hyperosmolar enema

(M) Meconium plug / Small left colon syndrome → Hyperosmolar enema / Suction rectal biopsy

Hirschsprung's disease → See Hirschsprung's disease

Imperforate anus → See imperforate anus

REFERENCES

Bass KD, Rothenberg SS, Chang JH: Laparoscopic Ladd's procedure in infants with malrotation. J Pediatr Surg 33:279–281, 1998.

Cheu HW, Sukarochana K, Lloyd DA: Peritoneal drainage for necrotizing enterocolitis. J Pediatr Surg 23:557–561, 1988.

Clatworthy HW, Howard WHR, Lloyd J: The meconium plug syndrome. Surgery 39:131–142, 1956.

Cragen JD, Martin ML, Moore CA et al: Descriptive epidemiology of small intestinal atresia in Atlanta, GA. Teratology 48: 441–450, 1993.

Del Pin CA, Czyrko C, Ziegler MM et al: Management and survival of meconium ileus: A 30-year review. Ann Surg 215:179–185, 1992.

Godbole P, Stringer MD: Bilious vomiting in the newborn: How often is it pathologic? J Pediatr Surg 37:909–911, 2002.

Grosfeld JL, Rescorla FJ: Duodenal atresia and stenosis. World J Surg 17:301–309, 1993.

Kosloske AM, Musemeche CA, Ball WS et al: Necrotizing enterocolitis: The value of radiographic findings. Am J Roentgenol 151:771–774, 1988.

Messineo A, MacMillan JH, Palder SB et al: Clinical factors affecting mortality in children with malrotation of the intestine. J Pediatr Surg 27:1343–1345, 1992.

Rescorla FJ, Shedd FJ, Grosfeld JL et al: Anomalies of intestinal rotation in childhood: Analysis of 447 cases. Surgery 108:710–715, 1990.

Stringer MD, Spitz L: Surgical management of necrotizing enterocolitis. Arch Dis Child 69:269–271, 1993.

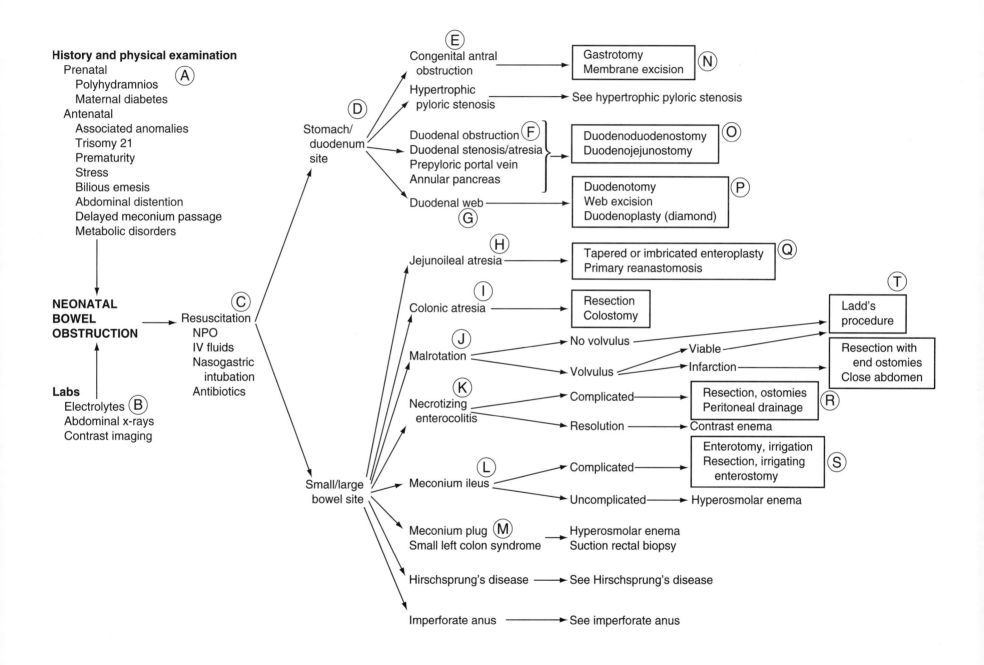

History and physical examination
Prenatal ⒶA
  Polyhydramnios
  Maternal diabetes
Antenatal
  Associated anomalies
  Trisomy 21
  Prematurity
  Stress
  Bilious emesis
  Abdominal distention
  Delayed meconium passage
  Metabolic disorders

NEONATAL BOWEL OBSTRUCTION

Labs
Electrolytes ⒷB
Abdominal x-rays
Contrast imaging

Resuscitation ⒸC
NPO
IV fluids
Nasogastric
  intubation
Antibiotics

Stomach/duodenum site ⒹD

Small/large bowel site

Congenital antral obstruction ⒺE → Gastrotomy / Membrane excision ⓃN

Hypertrophic pyloric stenosis → See hypertrophic pyloric stenosis

Duodenal obstruction ⒻF
Duodenal stenosis/atresia
Prepyloric portal vein
Annular pancreas → Duodenoduodenostomy / Duodenojejunostomy ⓄO

Duodenal web ⒼG → Duodenotomy / Web excision / Duodenoplasty (diamond) ⓅP

Jejunoileal atresia ⒽH → Tapered or imbricated enteroplasty / Primary reanastomosis ⓆQ

Colonic atresia ⒾI → Resection / Colostomy

Malrotation ⒿJ
  No volvulus → Ladd's procedure ⓉT
  Volvulus
    Viable → Ladd's procedure ⓉT
    Infarction → Resection with end ostomies / Close abdomen

Necrotizing enterocolitis ⓀK
  Complicated → Resection, ostomies / Peritoneal drainage ⓇR
  Resolution → Contrast enema

Meconium ileus ⓁL
  Complicated → Enterotomy, irrigation / Resection, irrigating enterostomy ⓈS
  Uncomplicated → Hyperosmolar enema

Meconium plug ⓂM
Small left colon syndrome → Hyperosmolar enema / Suction rectal biopsy

Hirschsprung's disease → See Hirschsprung's disease

Imperforate anus → See imperforate anus

Chapter 110 *Hirschsprung's Disease*

RICHARD A. FALCONE, JR., MD • BRAD W. WARNER, MD

⏤⏤⏤

(A) Hirschsprung's disease is diagnosed in the newborn period in more than 90% of patients with the disease. Passage of meconium delayed beyond the first 24 to 48 hours of life should raise the suspicion of Hirschsprung's disease. Other presenting signs include constipation, abdominal distention, poor feeding, and emesis. In older children, chronic constipation, abdominal distention, or enterocolitis may be present.

(B) Hirschsprung's disease occurs with an incidence of approximately 1 in 5000 live births, ranking third behind intestinal atresia and meconium ileus as a cause of neonatal intestinal obstruction. The male-to-female ratio is generally considered to be 4:1 in favor of males; however, in long segment disease (extending proximally from the rectum to involve the entire colon and varying degrees of small bowel), the ratio approaches 1:1. A positive family history of Hirschsprung's disease may be present and is more common with long segment involvement. It is important that the pediatric surgeon caring for these patients be aware of associated abnormalities including Down syndrome (5% to 15%), intestinal atresias, and trisomy 18.

(C) Plain radiographs of the abdomen commonly show distended loops of bowel and may demonstrate a paucity of air within the rectum. This study should be followed by a contrast enema. In the newborn, this diagnostic intervention is best performed before a rectal examination or rectal irrigation because these interventions might distort the important features. In a normal contrast enema study, the rectum is larger in caliber than the sigmoid colon. In patients with Hirschsprung's disease, spasm of the distal colon usually results in a smaller caliber rectum when compared with the more proximal sigmoid colon. Identification of a transition zone (evolution between the dilated normal bowel to the smaller caliber, aganglionic bowel) may be quite helpful. However, the radiographic determination of the location of this zone is relatively inaccurate and should not be relied upon as the sole determinant of the site of transition. Failure to completely evacuate the instilled contrast material after 24 hours would also be consistent with Hirschsprung's disease and may provide additional diagnostic yield. In older infants and children the contrast enema has a higher likelihood of revealing a transition zone.

(D) The contrast enema is very useful to exclude other important causes for abdominal distention and obstipation in the newborn period such as meconium ileus, distal ileal or colonic atresia, or small left colon syndrome (as seen with infants of diabetic mothers). Alternate diagnoses should be treated accordingly.

If the contrast enema study is normal, and the infant begins to stool normally, no further work-up may be needed. If a large meconium plug is passed, the patient should undergo genetic and/or sweat chloride testing to exclude cystic fibrosis.

(E) Even with a normal contrast enema, either the failure to improve or the recurrence of symptoms is an indication for a rectal biopsy.

(F) If the contrast enema is suspicious and/or the history is concerning for Hirschsprung's disease, then a rectal biopsy is necessary to definitively establish the diagnosis. For neonates and infants less than 6 months of age, a suction rectal biopsy can be easily performed at the bedside. This technique is quick, painless, and is associated with low morbidity. A full thickness mucosal biopsy under general anesthesia is indicated in situations in which a prior suction rectal biopsy is equivocal or in a patient older than 6 months. Using either method, the biopsy should be taken approximately 2 cm proximal to the dentate line. At least two specimens should be obtained using suction rectal biopsy, whereas one specimen is usually adequate with a full thickness biopsy.

(G) The pathologic criteria for Hirschsprung's disease include the absence of ganglion cells in both the submucosal (Meissner's plexus) as well as the intermuscular (Auerbach's) plexus. Further, there is a marked hypertrophy of nerve fibers. Finally, robust immunohistochemical staining for acetylcholinesterase within the hypertrophied nerve trunks is usually present. If the biopsy reveals Hirschsprung's disease, several options exist for definitive treatment and should be presented to the family.

(H) If the biopsy is equivocal and/or the clinical suspicion for Hirchsprung's disease is high, a repeat rectal biopsy should be performed. The most common reasons for a false negative biopsy include an inadequate specimen or a biopsy taken too far proximal to the transition zone (within normally ganglionated bowel). In some specialized pediatric centers, anorectal manometry may help provide the diagnosis in selected situations. The classic manometric finding is failure of the internal sphincter to relax when the rectum is distended with a balloon.

(I) If the biopsy is negative, continued investigation into an alternative diagnosis should be made. The accuracy of a properly performed biopsy has been reported to be as high as 99.7%.

(J) In a newborn or in an infant younger than 6 months, the leveling procedure may be the most conservative approach, followed by a definitive procedure at a later date.

(K) In older patients (greater than 6 to 12 months of age) a leveling colostomy should be the initial intervention. This may also be the procedure of choice as a more conservative approach for newborns.

(L) In a newborn or in a young infant (younger than 6 months) with no evidence for enterocolitis, rectal irrigations with 5 to 10 cc/kg of normal saline utilizing a soft-tipped catheter may afford successful decompression of the distended proximal colon. These can be performed every 6 hours with serial abdominal examinations. Failure to decompress the infant with rectal irrigations or the development of enterocolitis would direct a more conservative approach by initial leveling colostomy, followed by a definitive pull-through.

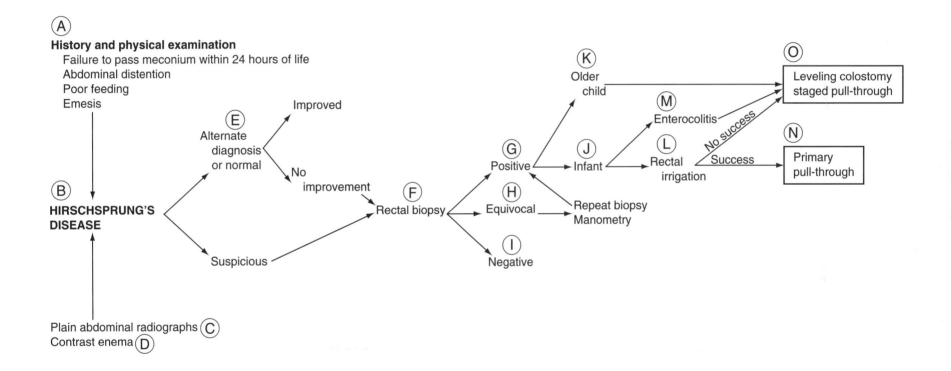

(A) **History and physical examination**
Failure to pass meconium within 24 hours of life
Abdominal distention
Poor feeding
Emesis

(B) **HIRSCHSPRUNG'S DISEASE**

(C) Plain abdominal radiographs
(D) Contrast enema

(E) Alternate diagnosis or normal → Improved

No improvement

Suspicious

(F) Rectal biopsy

(G) Positive

(H) Equivocal → Repeat biopsy Manometry

(I) Negative

(K) Older child

(J) Infant

(M) Enterocolitis

(L) Rectal irrigation

No success

Success

(O) Leveling colostomy staged pull-through

(N) Primary pull-through

(M) Enterocolitis associated with Hirschsprung's disease remains a major cause of morbidity and mortality. Enterocolitis generally presents with explosive diarrhea, abdominal distention, and fever; it is felt to occur secondary to intestinal stasis and bacterial overgrowth. Medical management includes rectal irrigations and decompression, as well as intravenous broad-spectrum antibiotics. The lack of rapid clinical improvement or presence of any sign of deterioration is an indication for an initial decompressive ostomy and leveling procedure, followed by definitive pull-through at a later date.

(N) If the rectal irrigations are successful, a primary pull-through procedure without a protective colostomy may be performed using one of several techniques. The timing for this intervention is dictated by such factors as the ability of the parents to perform the irrigations at home and the overall health of the child. One approach is via a conventional open laparotomy with resection of the aganglionic distal colon to the peritoneal reflection. At this point, an endorectal mucosectomy is performed to the anal verge and the normal ganglionated colon is pulled through the muscular rectal cuff and a coloanal anastomosis performed (Soave procedure). In another technique, the colon is mobilized laparoscopically from the abdomen. A rectal mucosectomy is then performed for a distance, and the full thickness of the bowel is transected. At this point, the aganglionic bowel is delivered through the anus and transected proximal to the transition zone and a coloanal anastomosis performed. Recently, this technique has been performed entirely through a transanal approach without the need for laparoscopic colon mobilization. Along these lines, the choice of procedure should also be directed by the suspected site of the transition zone. The perineal approach, with or without laparoscopic assistance, can be very difficult if not impossible if the transition zone is identified to be proximal to the splenic flexure. The vast majority of

infants, by whatever procedure, enjoy normal continence and lifestyle. The mortality rate for each operation is in the range of 3% to 6% and is higher for infants younger than 4 months. Normal continence is achieved in 80% to 90% of infants. Some children require 10 years or more to become totally continent and may also require a postoperative bowel regimen such as stool softeners and/or enemas. Anastomotic leaks occur in 5% to 9%. When a leak is immediately treated with a diverting colostomy, it generally seals spontaneously, and the colostomy can be closed after 6 to 8 weeks. Anastomotic strictures occur in 6% to 12% of cases. Few of these require operative treatment because most will respond to dilation regimens. Postoperative enterocolitis occurs episodically in about 25% and may require intravenous resuscitation, rectal irrigations, and systemic antibiotics. Daily rectal irrigations or anal dilations for 4 to 6 months after the definitive procedure may decrease the incidence of enterocolitis. The reoperation rate is about 2% to 3%. Urinary and sexual dysfunction rarely occurs.

(O) A leveling procedure consists of a limited laparotomy to obtain serial seromuscular biopsies extending proximally from the rectum to the transition zone into normally ganglionated colon. Using frozen section interpretation, the site of normally ganglionated bowel just proximal to the transition zone is identified; this dictates the appropriate location on the colon to exteriorize as a loop colostomy. Permanent sections after the leveling procedure, coupled with a normally functioning colostomy, definitively establish the exact location of the transition zone. Several months after the creation of the ostomy, a definitive corrective procedure is performed. There are three basic procedures that require a combined abdominal and perineal approach. The Swenson procedure consists of removal of the aganglionic bowel down to the level of the internal sphincters followed by

a coloanal anastomosis to normally ganglionated proximal colon on the perineum. In the Duhamel procedure, the aganglionic rectal stump is left in place and the ganglionated, normal colon is pulled behind this stump. A stapling device is then inserted through the anus with one arm within the normal, ganglionated bowel posteriorly and the other in the aganglionic rectum anteriorly. Finally, the Soave technique involves an endorectal mucosal dissection within the aganglionic distal rectum. The normally ganglionated colon is then pulled through the remnant muscular cuff and a coloanal anastomosis is performed.

REFERENCES

Albanese CT, Jennings RW, Smith B et al: Perineal one-stage pull-through for Hirschsprung's disease. J Pediatr Surg 34:377–380, 1999.

Coran AG, Teitelbaum DH: Recent advances in the management of Hirschsprung's disease. Am J Surg 180:382–387, 2000.

Georgeson KE, Cohen RD, Hebra A et al: Primary laparoscopic-assisted endorectal colon pull-through for Hirschsprung's disease: A new gold standard. Ann Surg 229:678–682, 1999.

Jasonni V, Martucciello G: Total colonic aganglionosis. Semin Pediatr Surg 7:174–180, 1998.

Kusafuka T, Puri P: Genetic aspects of Hirschsprung's disease. Semin Pediatr Surg 7:148–155, 1998.

Stockmann PT, Philippart AI: The Duhamel procedure for Hirschsprung's disease. Semin Pediatr Surg 7:89–95, 1998.

Swenson O: Hirschsprung's disease: A review. Pediatrics 109:914–918, 2002.

Teitelbaum DH, Cilley RE, Sherman NJ et al: A decade of experience with the primary pull-through for Hirschsprung's disease in the newborn period: A multicenter analysis of outcomes. Ann Surg 232:372–380, 2000.

Teitelbaum DH, Coran AG: Enterocolitis. Semin Pediatr Surg 7:162–169, 1998.

Van Leeuwen K, Geiger JD, Barnett JL et al: Stooling and manometric findings after primary pull-throughs in Hirschsprung's disease: Perineal versus abdominal approaches. J Pediatr Surg 37:1321–1325, 2002.

Weinberg G, Boley SJ: Endorectal pull-through with primary anastomosis for Hirschsprung's disease. Semin Pediatr Surg 7:96–102, 1998.

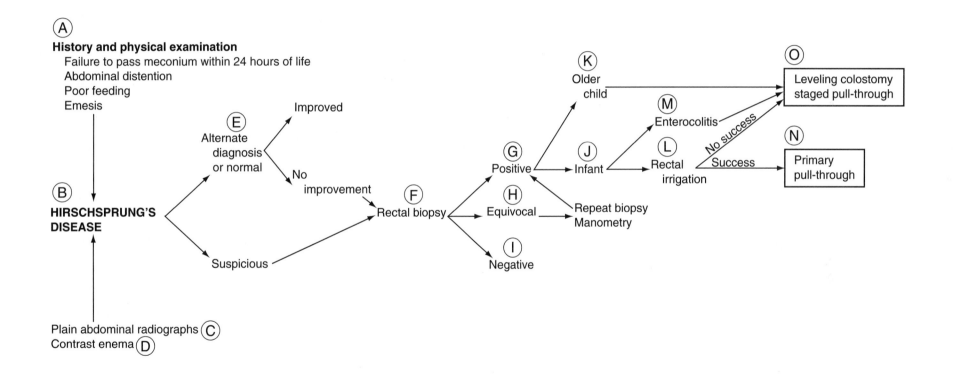

(A)

History and physical examination
Failure to pass meconium within 24 hours of life
Abdominal distention
Poor feeding
Emesis

(B)

**HIRSCHSPRUNG'S
DISEASE**

Plain abdominal radiographs (C)
Contrast enema (D)

(E) Alternate
diagnosis
or normal

Improved

No
improvement

Suspicious

(F) Rectal biopsy

(G) Positive

(H) Equivocal

(I) Negative

Repeat biopsy
Manometry

(K) Older
child

(J) Infant

(M) Enterocolitis

(L) Rectal
irrigation

No success

Success

(O) Leveling colostomy
staged pull-through

(N) Primary
pull-through

Chapter 111 *Imperforate Anus*

J. LAURANCE HILL, MD • ERIC D. STRAUCH, MD

(A) Imperforate anus is life-threatening because of sepsis, bowel obstruction, or associated congenital anomalies. The latter two conditions are readily recognized. Sepsis is less obvious and is the result of either contamination of the urinary tract through a rectourinary fistula, or translocation of organisms secondary to stasis in a rectal pouch with no outlet or with a tiny fistula that affords inadequate decompression. Sepsis is diagnosed by thermal instability, lethargy, falling platelet counts, abdominal distention, and positive blood cultures. Treatment is systemic antibiotics followed by relief of obstruction.

(B) The mortality rate for imperforate anus is low. Genitourinary anomalies are responsible for 30% of deaths. Cardiac, central nervous system, and GI defects (e.g., esophageal atresia) each cause 10% of deaths.

(C) In the absence of a perineal fistula and meconium staining, ultrasonography (US) is the procedure of choice to differentiate high and low lesions.

(D) The Rice-Wangensteen inversion "babygram" can be performed in infants older than 18 hours to determine the level of obstruction. A lateral x-ray is made with the baby inverted, its knees flexed, and an opaque marker at the anal "wink" or dimple.

(E) The pubococcygeal line indicates the level of the levator ani. Gas in the rectal pouch 2 cm or more above the pubococcygeal line (supralevator) excludes the possibility of primary anoplasty. Meconium in the rectal pouch can cause error on the "high pouch" side.

(F) For an intermediate (vestibular) fistula, the condition of the neonate and the degree of anterior angulation of the fistula indicate whether primary anoplasty or a colostomy should be performed.

(G) For "low" perineal and fourchette fistulas, anoplasty can be performed without a colostomy.

(H) A urinary fistula is assumed for all high pouches until it can be ruled out. It is diagnosed by the finding of meconium in urine (culture or microscopic); by the escape into the urine of carmine red instilled into the gut; or by cystoscopy, voiding cystourethrography, colostography, or vaginography. Urinary fistula demands total fecal diversion by colostomy with separated stomas.

(I) Supralevator obstruction requires a separated stoma (double-barreled) sigmoid colostomy. In the absence of pediatric anesthesia expertise, a transverse colostomy can be done using local anesthesia. This carries higher risks of distal limb stasis with translocation or urinary sepsis, hyperchloremic acidosis, stomal prolapse with partial obstruction, and failure to thrive.

(J) Septicemia can be avoided by irrigating the rectal pouch with 0.1% neomycin in Ringer's lactate solution through the distal limb of the colostomy and by administering systemic antibiotics.

(K) Contraindications to anoplasty are prematurity and poor condition of the infant secondary to delayed diagnosis, sepsis, or associated anomalies.

(L) Programmed neorectal dilations for 6 to 12 months are an essential part of care after all repairs of imperforate anus.

(M) After the infant is 3 to 6 months old, the second-stage repair can be done with relative safety. Laparoscopic assist has been introduced as part of the second stage repair when an abdominal dissection is required for a high fistula, or to provide length preliminary to the pull-through. The anterior perineal approach of Mollard and the posterior (sagittal anorectoplasty) procedures of Stephens and Smith or of deVries and Pena have anatomic and functional advantages if length is not an issue.

(N) Colostomy closure occurs 6 to 12 weeks after the neoanus is constructed.

(O) Functional assessments at least 5 years after treatment (with more objective data from manometry, electromyography, and magnetic resonance imaging) demonstrate that continence depends on anatomic level and sacral integrity rather than on the technical differences among the perineal operations. Higher defects are associated with high rates of incontinence and constipation; lower defects have a better prognosis.

(P) Cost is proportional to the severity of the anomaly. The least expensive scenario is discharge to trustworthy parents 3 days after a simple anoplasty with the expectation of complete continence by age 3 years. The greatest cost is associated with at least three major operations, laparoscopic assist, 3 to 5 weeks of initial hospitalization, numerous complications from infection or associated anomalies, and constant incontinent soiling with the attendant psychosocial difficulties for the child and the parents.

(Q) For patients with fecal incontinence or severe constipation, the antegrade continence enema (ACE) enables return to normal social function. Access into the right colon is established by appendicostomy or bowel tube (Malone method). Self-controlled intermittent catheterization once or twice daily evacuates the colon and alleviates constipation or, worse, embarrassing incontinence.

REFERENCES

DeVries PA, Pena A: Posterior sagittal anorectoplasty. J Pediatr Surg 17:638–643, 1982.

Kiesewetter WB, Chang JHT: Imperforate anus: A 5- to 30-year follow-up perspective. Prog Pediatr Surg 10:111–120,1977.

Malone PS, Rangley PG, Kiely EM: Preliminary report: The antegrade continence enema. Lancet 336:1217–1218, 1990.

Mollard P, Marechal JM, deBeaujeu MJ et al: Anterior perineal approach. J Pediatr Surg 13:499–504, 1978.

Pena A: Posterior sagittal anorectoplasty: A unified concept; results in the management of 332 cases of anorectal malformation. Pediatr Surg Int 3:82–104, 1988.

Rehbein F: Imperforate anus: Experience with abdomino-perineal and abdomino-sacroperineal pull-through procedures. J Pediatr Surg 2:99–105, 1967.

Santulli TB, Schullinger JN, Kiesewetter WB et al: Imperforate anus: A survey from the members of the Surgical Section of the American Academy of Pediatrics. J Pediatr Surg 6:484–487, 1971.

Stephen FD, Smith ED: Anorectal Malformations in Children: Update 1988. New York: Alan R. Liss, 1988.

Sydorak RM, Albanese CT: Laparoscopic repair of high imperforate anus. Semin Pediatr Surg 11:217–225, 2002.

Wangensteen OH, Rice CO: Imperforate anus. Ann Surg 92: 77–81, 1930.

History and physical examination

Sepsis (A)
Bowel obstruction
Other anomalies (B)

**IMPERFORATE
ANUS**

Labs
US (C)
Rice-Wangensteen (D)
Inverted x-ray

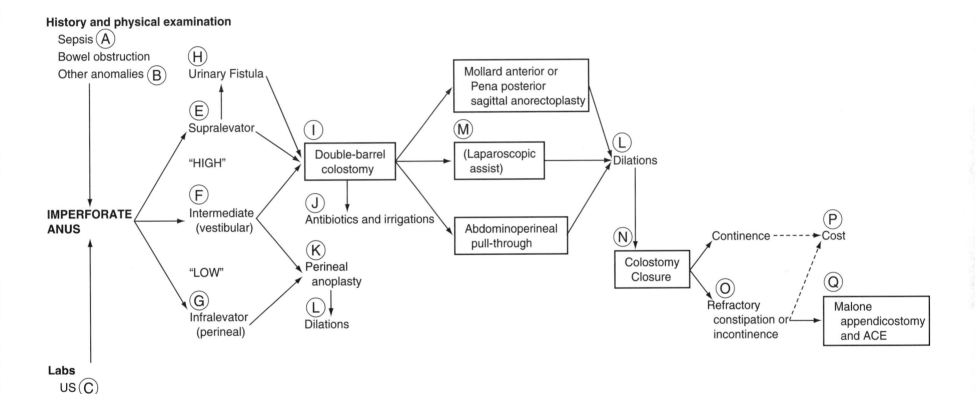

(H)
Urinary Fistula

(E)
Supralevator

"HIGH"

(F)
Intermediate
(vestibular)

"LOW"

(G)
Infralevator
(perineal)

(K)
Perineal
anoplasty

(L)
Dilations

(I)
Double-barrel
colostomy

(J)
Antibiotics and irrigations

Mollard anterior or
Pena posterior
sagittal anorectoplasty

(M)
(Laparoscopic
assist)

Abdominoperineal
pull-through

(L)
Dilations

(N)
Colostomy
Closure

Continence

(O)
Refractory
constipation or
incontinence

(P)
Cost

(Q)
Malone
appendicostomy
and ACE

Chapter 112 Surgical Jaundice in Infancy

RICHARD J. HENDRICKSON, MD • FREDERICK M. KARRER, MD

(A) Acholic stools are typical of biliary atresia (BA). Stool color can be misleading. Infants with BA may pass normal meconium or yellow-green stools at birth. An infant's stools are never completely acholic, even in the absence of bile excretion.

(B) About 10% of infants with BA have a peculiar constellation of associated anomalies: polysplenia, bilobed liver, situs inversus, absence of the inferior vena cava, preduodenal portal vein, and intestinal malrotation. "Butterfly" vertebrae and peripheral pulmonary stenosis suggest the diagnosis of Alagille syndrome, a familial disease marked by a paucity of intrahepatic bile ducts.

(C) Splenomegaly occurs with hematologic disorders, neonatal hepatitis, and sepsis. In early infancy, splenic enlargement from biliary atresia is unusual.

(D) Ascites can be caused by spontaneous perforation of the bile duct resulting in loculated fluid collections around the porta hepatis or free bilious ascites.

(E) Jaundice in the newborn that persists longer than 2 weeks is no longer considered to be physiologic. Among the myriad of diagnostic possibilities, the most important distinction is between mechanical/obstructive causes and hepatocellular dysfunction (e.g., infectious, hematologic, metabolic, or genetic).

(F) Neonatal jaundice with elevated levels of conjugated bilirubin is never physiologic and signifies disease of the liver or biliary tract. Unconjugated hyperbilirubinemia suggests hemolysis (caused by Rh incompatibility or red cell defects), Crigler-Najjar syndrome, or Gilbert's syndrome.

(G) Elevated alkaline phosphatase and γ-glutamyl transferase levels suggest mechanical biliary obstruction, whereas elevated transaminase values suggest parenchymal damage (e.g., neonatal hepatitis). Unfortunately, the prevalence of crossover makes it impossible to rely solely on these generalizations.

(H) Leukocytosis suggests an infectious cause of jaundice. Anemia and abnormal red cell forms on peripheral smear suggest a hemolytic disorder.

(I) About 7% to 10% of infants with cholestasis have α_1-antitrypsin deficiency. This autosomal-recessive trait causes liver disease in 20% of homozygous persons with this deficiency. The manifestations have a bimodal pattern: neonatal cholestasis and, later in childhood, cirrhosis. No specific therapy can prevent the consequences of liver disease, but liver transplantation can be curative.

(J) Coagulation studies, TORCH (toxoplasmosis, other infections, rubella, cytomegalovirus, herpesvirus) titers, sweat chloride, thyroid function tests, and a metabolic screen (urine-reducing substances and urine and serum amino acids) rule out a host of other diagnoses.

(K) Hepatobiliary scintigraphy using iminodiacetic acid (IDA) correctly discriminates obstructive from hepatocellular jaundice in 70% of patients. With biliary atresia, hepatocyte function is intact early; therefore uptake of the isotope is unimpaired, but it is not excreted. In parenchymal disease, hepatocellular function is poor. Uptake, therefore, is sluggish, and excretion may or may not be appreciated. Oral phenobarbital (5 mg/kg for 5 days) can enhance excretion of the nucleotide and increase the sensitivity of the procedure.

(L) Ultrasound evaluates gallbladder size (with biliary atresia usually very small or absent), bile duct size (dilated with choledochal cyst), and fluid collections (as in spontaneous perforation of the common bile duct).

(M) Percutaneous liver biopsy is a safe diagnostic procedure. It accurately detects liver disease in as many as 90% of cases. There is considerable overlap between the most common diagnoses (i.e., biliary atresia, neonatal hepatitis, and TPN cholestasis).

(N) When extrahepatic obstruction is suspected, surgical exploration, either laparoscopically or with a limited right upper quadrant incision, should be performed with operative cholangiography and liver biopsy (needle and wedge).

(O) If cholangiography shows a patent but hypoplastic biliary tree, the incision is closed. In many cases of hepatocellular jaundice (e.g., neonatal hepatitis, Alagille syndrome, cystic fibrosis, and α_1-antitrypsin deficiency) the absence of bile production results in a diminutive biliary duct system from disease atrophy.

(P) Biliary atresia is the most common and life-threatening cause of cholestasis-related jaundice in infancy. Diagnosis before age 2 months is optimal. The treatment success rate drops dramatically after age 90 days. In the most common form, the entire extrahepatic tree is a fibrous cord and the gallbladder either has no lumen or is tiny and filled with "white bile." Occasionally a bile cyst is encountered at the liver hilum. The cyst, which has no epithelial lining, is resected, and a standard portoenterostomy is performed.

(Q) A choledochal cyst is treated by excision and Roux-en-Y hepaticojejunostomy. Cyst drainage alone is associated with increased risk of malignancy and a propensity for stricture formation with cholangitis.

(R) Spontaneous perforation usually occurs at the junction of the cystic duct with the common bile duct. Treatment by drainage alone often results in sealing of the perforation. A cholecystostomy catheter can be left in place for postoperative cholangiography to confirm closure of the perforation. Distal obstruction may require biliary reconstruction with a Roux-en-Y.

(S) Kasai's operation (portoenterostomy) attempts to produce drainage from minute bile duct remnants in the fibrous cord of the biliary remnant near the liver hilum. A Roux-en-Y limb of jejunum

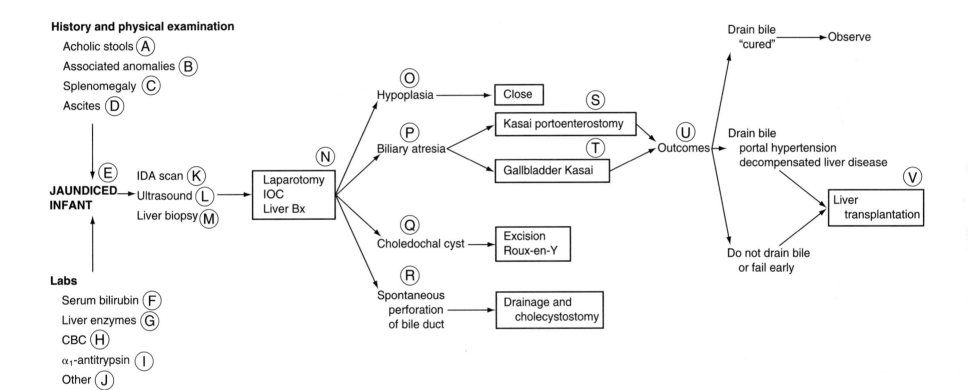

is constructed and sutured to the transected porta hepatis. Postoperatively, evaluation of the stool is crucial. If the stool is green (success), the patients are observed. If no green stools are observed, then a course of steroids is administered. All patients are placed on ursodiol and fat-soluble vitamins.

Ⓣ In 10% to 20% of patients there is a small patent lumen of the gallbladder, cystic duct, and common bile duct. The proximal extrahepatic ducts are still fibrotic from the liver hilum to the cystic duct. In these cases, the gallbladder can be carefully mobilized and used for anastomosis to the transected porta. These children have fewer episodes of cholangitis and a better chance for survival.

Ⓤ Outcomes: Short-term bile flow dependent on age at Kasai: younger than 60 days, 80%; aged 60 to 90 days, 50%; older than 90 days, 10% to 20%. Overall long-term survival is 30% to 40% without transplantation, 30% to 40% never drain bile or fail early, and 30% to 40% drain and become anicteric but develop portal hypertensive complications or decompensated liver disease in later childhood.

Ⓥ Liver transplantation is reserved for those children whose disease is diagnosed late, who fail to drain bile after portoenterostomy, or whose disease progresses to decompensated liver disease and portal hypertension. Approximately 80% will require liver transplantation.

REFERENCES

Bezerra JA, Balistreri WF: Cholestatic syndromes of infancy and childhood. Semin Gastrointest Dis 12:54–65, 2001.

Chardot C, Iskandarani F, DeDrenzy O et al: Spontaneous perforation of the biliary tract in infancy: A series of 11 cases. Eur J Pediatr Surg 6:341–346, 1996.

Howard ER: Surgery for Biliary Atresia. In Spitz L, Coran A (eds): Rob and Smith's Operative Surgery, 5th ed. London: Chapman and Hall Medical, 1995.

Karrer FM, Lilly JR: Biliary Atresia. In Oldham K, Columbani P, Foglia R (eds): Surgery of Infants and Children: Scientific Principles and Practices. Philadelphia: Lippincott-Raven, 1997.

Lilly JR: Total excision of choledochal cyst. Surg Gynecol Obstet 146:254–256, 1978.

Ohi R, Nio M, Chiba T et al: Long-term follow-up after surgery for patients with biliary atresia. J Pediatr Surg 25:442–445, 1990.

Ryckman F, Fisher F, Pedersen R et al: Improved survival in biliary atresia in the present era of liver transplantation. J Pediatr Surg 28:382–385, 1993.

Senyuz OF, Yesildag E, Emir H et al: Diagnostic laparoscopy in prolonged jaundice. J Pediatr Surg 36:463–465, 2001.

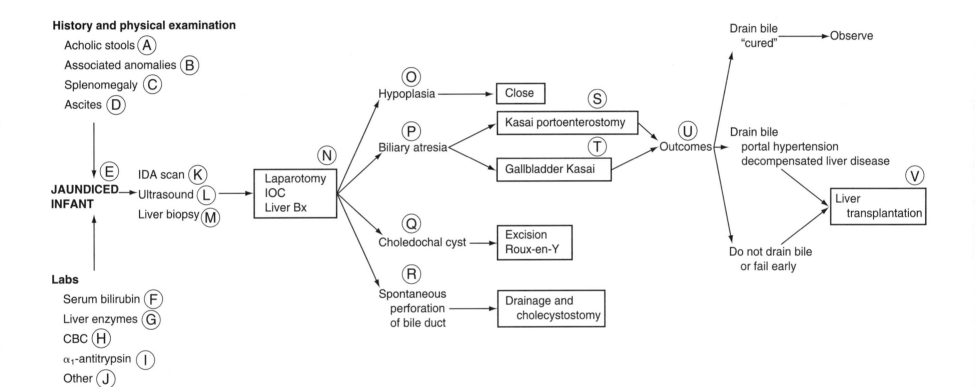

History and physical examination

Acholic stools (A)

Associated anomalies (B)

Splenomegaly (C)

Ascites (D)

JAUNDICED INFANT

IDA scan (K)

Ultrasound (L)

Liver biopsy (M)

(E)

Labs

Serum bilirubin (F)

Liver enzymes (G)

CBC (H)

α_1-antitrypsin (I)

Other (J)

Laparotomy
IOC
Liver Bx (N)

Hypoplasia → Close (O)

Biliary atresia (P)

Kasai portoenterostomy (S)

Gallbladder Kasai (T)

Choledochal cyst (Q) → Excision
Roux-en-Y

Spontaneous perforation of bile duct (R) → Drainage and cholecystostomy

Outcomes (U)

Drain bile "cured" → Observe

Drain bile portal hypertension decompensated liver disease

Do not drain bile or fail early

Liver transplantation (V)

Chapter 113 *Abdominal Mass in Childhood*

DANIEL J. OSTLIE, MD ● GEORGE K. GITTES, MD

(A) Abdominal masses in children more than 2 years old raise concerns for family members and surgeons alike. In the absence of trauma, the presentation is usually that of a painless mass found incidentally by the family or by their pediatrician during a routine visit. Commonly the mass will be quite large, and occasionally a rapid increase in size will have occurred secondary to bleeding into the mass. Systemic symptoms are rare, and usually physical examination will not provide a diagnosis or identify the origin of the mass.

(B) The mass can arise from intra-abdominal or retroperitoneal structures. The initial evaluation should include a US or CT of the abdomen, pelvis, and retroperitoneum. US can provide mass characteristics (e.g., cystic or solid) and its relationship with surrounding organs. US is considered by some to be superior for adnexal and pelvic masses, but there are operator-dependent limitations when used for diagnostic purposes. Color flow Doppler should be included to evaluate for thrombus in the inferior vena cava and/or renal veins, especially if a renal origin is identified. CT scan is the gold standard for evaluating abdominal masses and should be performed in all patients. Helical scanners with advanced computer software are highly sensitive and provide fine details of the mass, including its extent and 3-D reconstruction in relation to surrounding viscera and vascular involvement. MRI is not routinely obtained; however, it is useful in the evaluation of retroperitoneal masses suspected to be of neurogenic origin. After determining the location of the mass (i.e., retroperitoneal or intra-abdominal), the differential diagnosis narrows quickly.

(C) Intra-abdominal (nonretroperitoneal) masses can be divided into hepatic and extrahepatic masses.

(D) Retroperitoneal masses can be divided into renal and extrarenal origins. Further subdivision according to their radiographic characteristics (i.e., cystic, solid, or mixed) allows for simplification of the differential diagnosis.

(E) Most hepatic masses in children (about 70%) are malignant, and about half of these are hepatoblastomas. The mean age at presentation is 18 months, and failure to thrive is commonly encountered. Two laboratory values are of significant use in patients with hepatoblastoma. First, alpha-fetoprotein is a well established marker useful for the diagnosis as well as for monitoring of disease after treatment. Second, thrombocytosis with platelet counts in the millions is commonly associated with untreated hepatoblastoma. Survival is contingent on complete removal of the primary tumor. In all but stage I hepatoblastoma with fetal histology, adjuvant chemotherapy (e.g., doxorubicin, vincristine, 5-FU, cisplatin, and ifosfamide) in various combinations is utilized. Survival is 60% to 70% for patients with stage I to III disease (excluding anaplastic histology) and drops precipitously for stage IV. Hepatocellular carcinoma accounts for approximately one quarter of malignant hepatic tumors. AFP levels are elevated but not to the degree seen with hepatoblastoma. Survival is only possible with complete resection. Overall survival for children with hepatocellular carcinoma is dismal.

(F) Benign hepatic tumors include vascular lesions, hamartomas, focal nodular hyperplasia (FNH), adenomas, and benign cysts. Vascular lesions usually spontaneously regress by 1 year of age; however, hepatic artery embolization or ligation occasionally will be needed when spontaneous regression does not occur. Overall prognosis is excellent. FNH and adenoma occur rarely and are more common in females. The classic highlighted capsule on imaging studies facilitates diagnosis. All should be resected because of the possibility of malignant degeneration, and resection with negative margins is virtually always curative. Hamartomas are more common in males and usually require anatomic resection for optimal outcome. Cysts are very rare in the pediatric population and are usually found incidentally by US or CT performed for other reasons. Observation can safely be undertaken.

(G) Extrahepatic intra-abdominal masses can be subdivided into cystic and solid/mixed. Completely cystic lesions are virtually always intestinal duplications. Rarely, these entities present as obstruction, intussusception, peptic ulcer, or perforation. When symptoms do occur, they are related to the location and type of duplication. Regardless of the location/type, surgical intervention is required and involves resection of the duplication with reconstruction of the involved portion of the alimentary tract.

(H) Three diagnoses encompass intra-abdominal masses of predominantly solid or mixed cystic/solid characteristics. In females these cystic/solid masses are of adnexal etiology and can be malignant or benign. It is important to remember that the ovaries do not become pelvic until after puberty, and thus ovarian torsion will often present as an abdominal mass preceded by, and associated with, abdominal pain. Classification of ovarian neoplasms is based on their cell of origin and, when malignant, the stage is determined by operative findings including nodal status, capsular rupture, peritoneal seeding, and metastasis. Surgical management of ovarian masses is determined by the diagnosis and pathology. Ovarian torsion commonly results in gonadal ischemia necessitating oophorectomy. Occasionally, however, detorsion of the affected ovary allows for revascularization and obviates gonad removal. For benign tumors, enucleation with preservation of unaffected ovarian tissue should be the goal. However, if any concern regarding malignant potential exists, salpingo-oophorectomy is indicated. In males (and females without an adnexal etiology) with mixed/solid intra-abdominal tumors, lymphoma of the non-Hodgkin's lymphoma (NHL) type should be suspected. CT scans in NHL commonly show a mass with a necrotic center. Diagnosis is made by incisional biopsy, and treatment is based on the subtype and stage with directed chemotherapy. Fortunately, these tumors are highly chemosensitive, and more

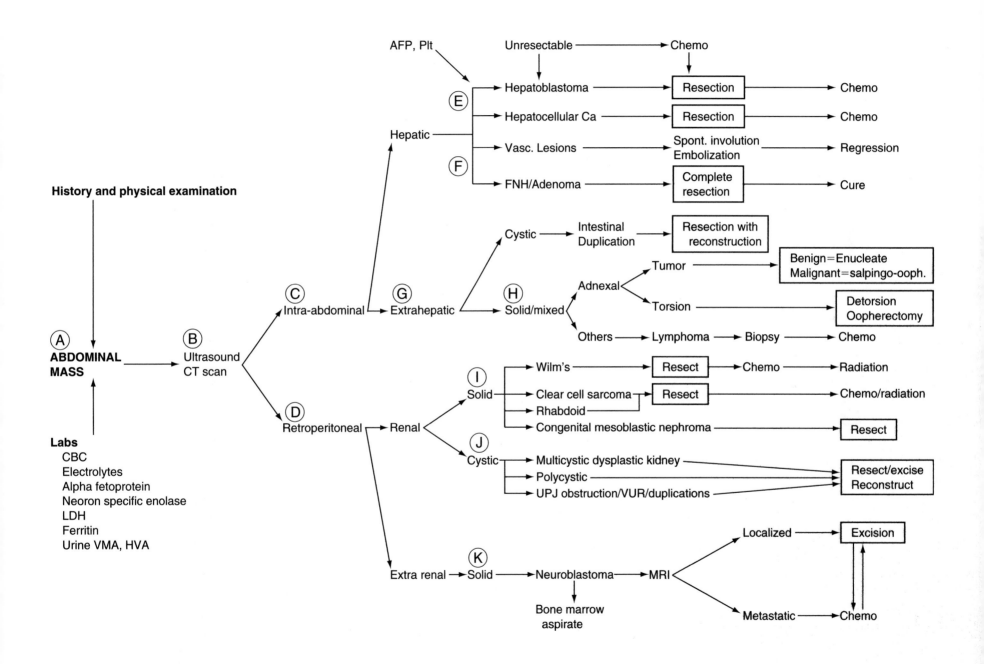

than 90% of pediatric patients with NHL can be expected to achieve complete remission.

(I) As with intra-abdominal masses, solid retroperitoneal tumors are more often malignant. Wilms' tumor is the most common solid mass of renal origin, with clear-cell sarcoma, rhabdoid tumors, and congenital mesoblastic nephroma rarely occurring. CT scans of the abdomen, pelvis, and chest are mandatory. If there is any concern of venous extension into the renal vein or IVC, doppler US should be performed; occasionally echocardiogram should be performed to evaluate for right atrial extension. Surgical intervention has two specific goals: to accomplish a complete resection of all viable tumor; and to provide accurate staging information. Radical nephroureterectomy is the surgery of choice in most cases. Exceptions include local invasion not amenable to complete resection, and bilateral renal involvement. The contralateral kidney must be visually inspected and palpated to determine the presence of bilateral disease (7% to 10%). Radiologic imaging alone is not reliable, with US missing about 45% and CT missing about 15% of contralateral tumors. Almost all patients receive chemotherapy, and radiation therapy is used in advanced disease. With regard to survival, the most powerful predictor remains the histologic subtype. Patients with favorable histology have the best prognosis (more than 90% 3-year survival), whereas those with anaplastic, sarcomatous, and rhabdoid tumors have greatly diminished survival.

(J) Cystic lesions of the kidney are rarely malignant. The most common diagnosis is multicystic dysplastic kidney in the newborn period; this is followed by polycystic kidney disease, ureteropelvic junction obstruction, vesicoureteral reflux, and renal collecting system duplications in older children. Diagnostic modalities include US and CT scan in combination with voiding cystourethrogram and nuclear medicine studies to determine anatomy and function. Surgical intervention should focus on resection with anatomic reconstruction when indicated.

(K) The presence of a solid extrarenal mass in a child should immediately lead a surgeon to suspect neuroblastoma, the most common solid tumor in children. These tumors arise from neuroblasts of the sympathetic nervous system and accordingly can occur anywhere sympathetic nerves are found. The most common site (more than 50%) is the adrenal medulla. Elevated serum levels of neuron specific enolase, lactate dehydrogenase, and ferritin are all associated with advanced disease and poorer outcome. Also, vanillylmandelic acid and homovanillic acid are usually present in the urine. The presence of dystrophic calcifications on plain abdominal x-rays is seen in more than 50% of cases. Accurate anatomic detail and extent is determined via CT or MRI. MRI is valuable in this instance to evaluate for intraspinal extension when the tumor arises from the paraspinal sympathetic nerves. Unique to neuroblastoma, bone scan and bone marrow aspirate is usually obtained because of the high likelihood of metastatic disease at the time of presentation. Only about 25% of patients presenting with neuroblastoma

will have localized stage I or II disease. Surgical management of neuroblastoma depends on extent of disease and presence of metastasis. The most important predictor of survival is age, and patients older than 1 year have an overall survival of more than 85% regardless of stage; but this falls to less than 25% for children with distant disease.

REFERENCES

Alvarado CS, London WB, Look AT et al: Natural history and biology of stage A neuroblastoma: A Pediatric Oncology Group study. J Pediatr Hematol Oncol 22:197–205, 2000.

Chow SN, Yang JH, Lin YH et al: Malignant ovarian germ cell tumors. Int J Gynecol Obstet 53:151–158, 1996.

Grundy P, Coppes M: An overview of the clinical and molecular genetics of Wilms' tumor. Med Pediatr Oncol 27:394–397, 1996.

Holcomb GW III, Gheissari A, O'Neill JA Jr. et al: Surgical management of alimentary tract duplications. Arch Surg 209:167–174, 1989.

Huffman JW, Dewhurst DJ, Capraro VJ: Ovarian Tumors in Children and Adolescents, 2nd ed. Philadelphia: WB Saunders, 1981.

Lack EE, Neave C, Vawter GF: Hepatoblastoma: A clinical and pathologic study of 54 cases. Am J Surg Pathol 6:693–705, 1982.

Lampkin BC, Wong KY, Kalinyak KA et al: Solid malignancies in children and adolescents. Surg Clin North Am 65:1351–1386, 1985.

Ni YH, Chang MH, Hsu HY et al: Hepatocellular carcinoma in childhood: Clinical manifestations and prognosis. Cancer 68:1737–1741, 1997.

Ritchey ML, Shamberger RC, Haase G et al: Surgical complications after primary nephrectomy for Wilms' tumor: report from the National Wilms' Tumor Study Group. J Am Coll Surg 192:63–68, 2001.

Sandlund JT, Downing JR, Crist WM: Non-Hodgkin's lymphoma in childhood. N Engl J Med 334:1238–1248, 1996.

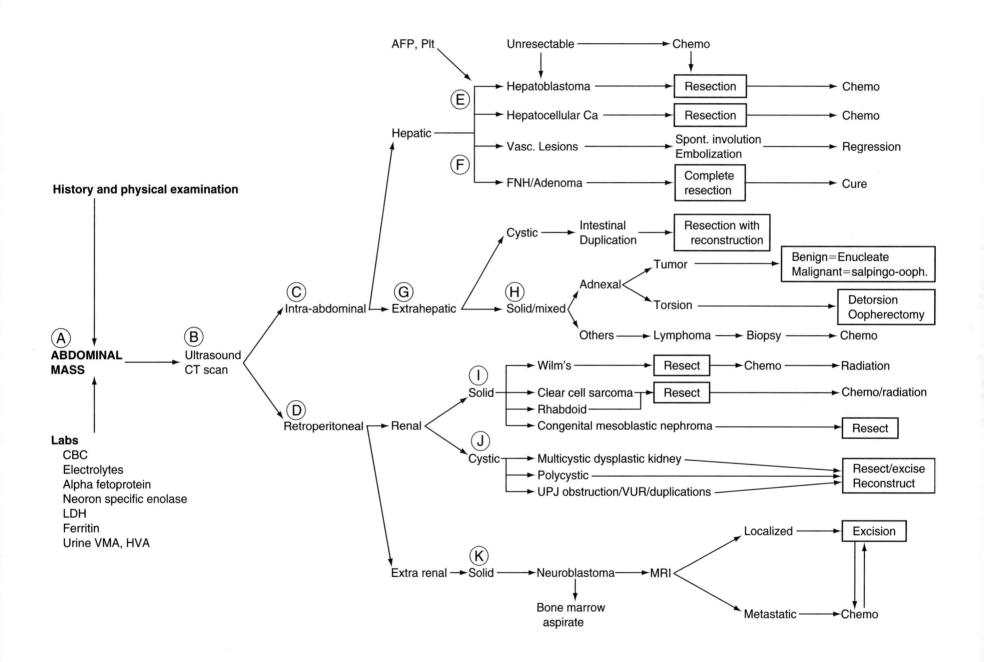

History and physical examination

Ⓐ

**ABDOMINAL
MASS**

Labs
  CBC
  Electrolytes
  Alpha fetoprotein
  Neoron specific enolase
  LDH
  Ferritin
  Urine VMA, HVA

Ⓑ
Ultrasound
CT scan

Ⓒ
Intra-abdominal

Ⓓ
Retroperitoneal

Ⓖ
Extrahepatic

Hepatic

AFP, Plt

Ⓔ

Ⓕ

Unresectable ⟶ Chemo

Hepatoblastoma ⟶ | Resection | ⟶ Chemo

Hepatocellular Ca ⟶ | Resection | ⟶ Chemo

Vasc. Lesions ⟶ Spont. involution
Embolization ⟶ Regression

FNH/Adenoma ⟶ | Complete resection | ⟶ Cure

Ⓗ

Cystic ⟶ Intestinal Duplication ⟶ | Resection with reconstruction |

Solid/mixed

Adnexal ⟶ Tumor ⟶ | Benign=Enucleate Malignant=salpingo-ooph. |

Torsion ⟶ | Detorsion Oopherectomy |

Others ⟶ Lymphoma ⟶ Biopsy ⟶ Chemo

Renal

Ⓘ
Solid

Wilm's ⟶ | Resect | ⟶ Chemo ⟶ Radiation

Clear cell sarcoma ⟶ | Resect | ⟶ Chemo/radiation

Rhabdoid

Congenital mesoblastic nephroma ⟶ | Resect |

Ⓙ
Cystic

Multicystic dysplastic kidney

Polycystic

UPJ obstruction/VUR/duplications ⟶ | Resect/excise Reconstruct |

Extra renal ⟶ Ⓚ Solid ⟶ Neuroblastoma ⟶ MRI

Localized ⟶ | Excision |

Metastatic ⟶ Chemo

Bone marrow aspirate

Chapter 114 *Inguinal and Scrotal Conditions in Children*

DAVID A. PARTRICK, MD

(A) Physicians often need to rely on historical information from parents concerning appearance of a groin mass and changes in size when crying or straining. The physician should question any history of trauma to the perineum. Examine patients in a standing position; ask them to blow up a balloon as a Valsalva maneuver. Feel for a sliding sensation in the spermatic cord (silk glove sign) or a thickened cord. The most crucial characteristic is if the mass is reducible. A hydrocele will not extend upwards to the inguinal canal and is typically spherical and mobile. The upward margin of a hernia is not clearly defined. Verify both testes are in the scrotum.

(B) Additional studies are rarely necessary. X-rays may reveal bowel gas below the inguinal ligament. Ultrasound may help differentiate a hernia from a hydrocele and can document blood flow to the testicle.

(C) A child with an incarcerated inguinal hernia will present with a painful groin mass that may extend into the scrotum. This may be associated with vomiting, and the child will be irritable.

(D) Reduction under sedation can be attempted. If successful, repair should proceed within 48 hours after edema has resolved to prevent recurrent incarceration. If unsuccessful or if there is evidence of strangulation, urgent groin exploration and repair is necessary.

(E) If a testicle is not palpable in the base of the scrotum, it may be located in the inguinal canal and can be palpated with careful manipulation. Scrotal asymmetry with a hypoplastic hemiscrotum is suggestive of cryptorchidism. Imaging studies are rarely useful for testicular localization.

(F) Spontaneous testicular descent is rare after 6 months of age, and histologic deterioration of the undescended testis appears to begin within the first year of life.

(G) Nonpalpable testes can be located laparoscopically. This technique also facilitates a staged Fowler-Stephens approach in which the testicular vessels are ligated laparoscopically as the first stage. Subsequent testicular mobilization is performed relying on enlarged collateral circulation from the artery to the vas deferens and cremasteric vessels. A single-stage laparoscopic-assisted orchiopexy can also be performed.

(H) Hernia repair is performed using high ligation and excision of the indirect inguinal hernia sac. Laparoscopy through the opened hernia sac allows examination of the contralateral internal inguinal ring and diagnosis of a patent processus vaginalis, if present. Laparoscopy is recommended for children less than 5 years old or in any child with clinical concerns of bilateral inguinal hernias. Approximately 50% of infants less than 1 year old will have a contralateral patent processus vaginalis; this decreases after infancy to 40%, and to 15% or less after 5 years.

(I) A tender scrotal mass of acute onset is testicular torsion until proven otherwise. Early diagnosis is key to successful treatment. Doppler ultrasound, if readily available, can demonstrate bloodflow to the testicle. Management involves urgent surgical exploration through a scrotal approach. A blue spot seen through the skin at the upper pole of the testis (blue dot sign) may indicate torsion of a testicular appendage, which requires no surgical intervention.

(J) Epididymitis is extremely rare in childhood and occurs in association with a urinary tract infection. The diagnosis of epididymitis is doubtful in the presence of a sterile urine analysis or culture; therefore further radiographic and cystoscopic evaluation is indicated.

(K) In contrast to inguinal hernias, the cranial border of a hydrocele can be defined and does not extend into the inguinal canal. Hydroceles will transilluminate, but so will dilated air-filled intestine. An isolated cord hydrocele may also be present separate from the testis.

(L) Most congenital hydroceles will resolve spontaneously within the first year of life. Operative repair is therefore avoided during the first year unless hernia cannot be excluded. Repair should proceed if there are no signs of resolution or if there is continued evidence of communication by 18 to 24 months of age.

(M) A nontender scrotal mass that does not transilluminate and is inseparable from the testis may represent a testicular tumor.

(N) Examining patients supine and erect will delineate a varicocele. Because 95% are left-sided, a right-sided varicocele should prompt evaluation for an abdominal tumor. Surgical repair is indicated for chronic pain or if a greater than 30% difference in testicular size develops with the left testis being smaller.

REFERENCES

Burd RS, Heffington SH, Teague JL: The optimal approach for management of metachronous hernias in children: A decision analysis. J Pediatr Surg 36:1190–1195, 2001.

Geisler DP, Jegathesan S, Parmley MC et al: Laparoscopic exploration for the clinically undetected hernia in infancy and childhood. Am J Surg 182:693–696, 2001.

Greenfield SP, Seville P, Wan J: Experience with varicoceles in children and young adults. J Urol 168:1684–1688, 2002.

Jordan GH: Laparoscopic management of the undescended testicle. Urol Clin North Am 28:23–29, 2001.

Levitt MA, Ferraraccio D, Arbesman MD et al: Variability of inguinal hernia surgical technique: A survey of North American pediatric surgeons. J Pediatr Surg 37:745–751, 2002.

McAndrew HF, Pemberton R, Kikiros CS et al: The incidence and investigation of acute scrotal problems in children. Pediatr Surg Int 18:435–437, 2002.

Munden MM, Trautwein LM: Scrotal pathology in pediatrics with sonographic imaging. Curr Prob Diag Radiol 29:185–205, 2000.

Skoog SJ: Benign and malignant pediatric scrotal masses. Pediatr Clin N Am 44:1229–1250, 1997.

Varlet F, Becmeur F: Groupe d'etudes en cardiochirugie infantile: laparoscopic treatment of varicoceles in children. Multicentric prospective study of 90 cases. Eur J Pediatr Surg 11:399–403, 2001.

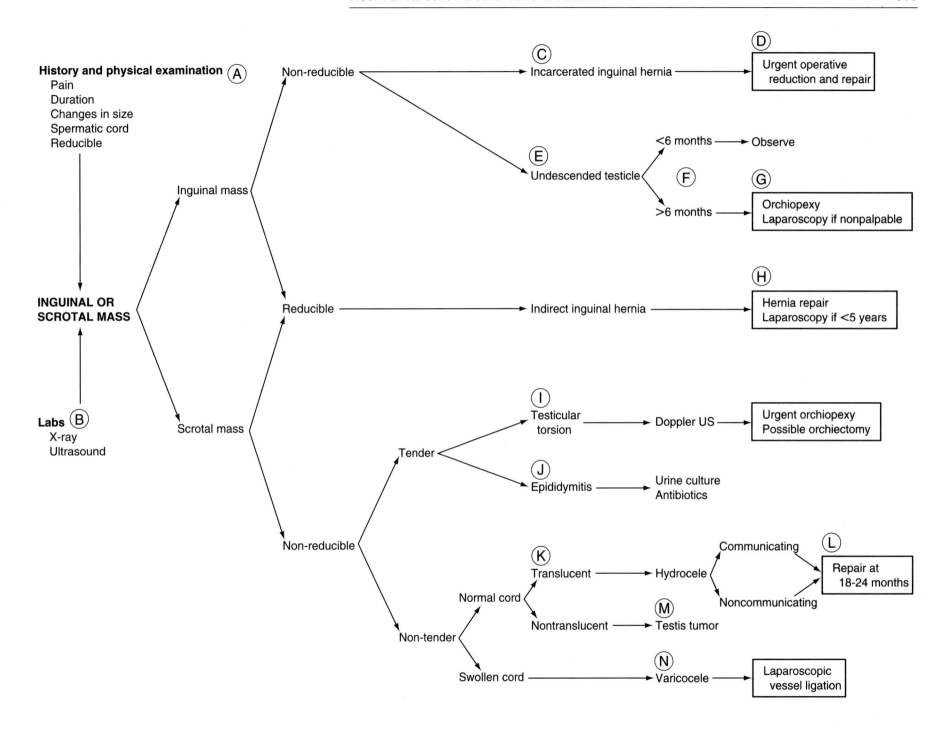

Chapter 115 *Congenital Diaphragmatic Hernia*

GARRETT ZALLEN, MD • PHILIP L. GLICK, MD

(A) Most congenital diaphragmatic hernias (CDHs) can be diagnosed with prenatal ultrasound. The most common finding is absence of the stomach bubble below the diaphragm. Other findings include loops of bowel in the chest; polyhydramnios; mediastinal shift; and, in severe cases, fetal hydrops. At present there is no evidence to support changing the mode of delivery (i.e., vaginal vs. C-section) based on the CDH alone; however, delivery should be performed at a tertiary care facility with neonatal specialists and pediatric surgeons. In prenatally diagnosed CDH, amniocentesis should be preformed before elective delivery. If the amniocentesis shows immature lungs, administration of steroids to the pregnant mother may be helpful in aiding the maturation of the fetal lungs.

Clinical presentation varies significantly with the severity of the CDH. The classical presentation is respiratory distress and a scaphoid abdomen, but this may not present for up to 24 hours (the so-called "honeymoon period"). Signs of persistent fetal circulation caused by high pulmonary artery pressures may also be present.

(B) CDH occurs in approximately 1 in 3000 to 1 in 5000 live births. The actual incidence of CDH is higher because almost 10% of all fetuses with CDH will spontaneously abort or die shortly after delivery, usually because of other life-threatening associated anomalies (most commonly cardiac). Females are affected more often than males. The most common side for CDH is the left and almost 90% are posteriolateral (Bochdalek's hernia). The next most common location is retrosternal (Morgagni's hernia), midline posterior to the sternum. The third most common area is through the esophageal hiatus. The major pathophysiological consequence of CDH is lung hypoplasia characterized by a decrease in lung size, a reduction in the number bronchial divisions, a decrease in the number of alveoli, pulmonary hypertension, decreased surfactant synthesis and release, and decreased antioxidant production.

(C) A chest x-ray is usually diagnostic, with loops of bowel seen in the chest and mediastinal shift if the CDH is large. Placement of a nasogastric tube may aid in the identification of the stomach in the chest. Other congenital anomalies can mimic the radiographic appearance of CDH (e.g., congenital cystic adenomatoid malformation, teratomas, and bronchogenic cysts.

(D) Treatment of CDH has changed dramatically over the years. Initially it was felt that the mass effect of the bowel was responsible for the newborn's symptoms, and therefore the bowel should be reduced and the hernia fixed immediately. It has now become apparent that symptoms are caused by the lung hypoplasia, surfactant deficiency, hypoxia, and the resultant pulmonary hypertension. Focus has now shifted to correcting these abnormalities and then performing surgery when the infant is stable. Surgery is commonly delayed for days or even weeks.

(E) Fetal surgery for CDH has been performed at limited centers; it consists of tracheal occlusion to stimulate lung development. Selection of patients for fetal surgery (i.e., those who would not survive to delivery) has been a challenging issue for fetal surgery. At this time it remains an experimental procedure and has a high mortality rate.

(F) The prophylactic administration of surfactant (preferably before the infant takes his or her first breath) may be beneficial. Most infants will require endotracheal intubation. A nasogastric tube should be placed to aid in decompressing the stomach and small bowel. Bag mask ventilation should be avoided to prevent distension of the bowel. An echocardiogram should be obtained to look for concurrent heart deformities. If conventional ventilation fails to prevent acidosis or hypoxia, then jet ventilation or high frequency ventilation may be necessary.

(G) Surgery for CDH usually entails primary closure of the defect through a trans-abdominal approach. If the defect is too large, a PTFE patch can be used to cover the defect. The bowel can usually be replaced into the abdominal cavity, but occasionally a silo must be constructed to avoid abdominal compartment syndrome.

(H) Although historically a ventilation strategy of hyperventilation and hyperoxia has been used, conventional wisdom now is a strategy of gentle ventilation and permissive hypercapnia. Avoiding severe hypoxia is paramount because it produces more pulmonary hypertension, which can lead to persistent fetal circulation and worsen hypoxia. Occasionally the use of inotropes, which raise systemic pressure to reverse shunting, is necessary.

(I) Barotrauma is not uncommon in these infants because of high airway pressures, but the recent use of permissive hypercapnia has decreased the incidence of barotrauma. Partial liquid ventilation (not FDA approved) and the use of nitric oxide have also been tried and have had been found to be beneficial but inconsistent.

(J) If the infant cannot be ventilated, extracorporeal membrane oxygenation (ECMO) should be considered. The selection criteria for ECMO is somewhat institution dependant, but any infant with a predicted mortality of 80% or greater (oxygen index of 50 to 60) on maximal ventilation should be placed on ECMO if no other significant contraindications exist (e.g., intracranial hemorrhage, gestational age less than 32 weeks, or non-survivable associated anomalies).

(K) Timing of repair of CDH is performed after the infant has stabilized from the pulmonary hypertension. If the infant has to be placed on ECMO, the timing of repair is controversial. Some centers will repair the infant while on ECMO; some will repair it when the ECMO run is nearly complete; and others will wait until the infant is back on conventional ventilation. Bleeding is the main complication of fixing a CDH on ECMO because of the systemic heparinization necessary to run the ECMO circuit. The use of Amicar decreases operative bleeding complications.

REFERENCES

Bohn DJ, Pearl R, Irish MS et al: Postnatal management of congenital diaphragmatic hernia. Clin Perinatol 23:843–872, 1996.

Bollman R, Kalache K, Mau H et al: Associated malformations and chromosomal defects in congenital diaphragmatic hernia. Fetal Diag Ther 10:52–59, 1995.

Boloker J, Bateman DA, Wung JT et al: Congenital diaphragmatic hernia in 120 infants treated consecutively with permissive hypercapnia/spontaneous respiration/elective repair. J Pediatr Surg 37:357–366, 2002.

Breaux CWJ, Rouse TM, Cain WS et al: Congenital diaphragmatic hernia in an era of delayed repair after medical and or extracorporeal membrane oxygenation stabilization: A prognostic and management classification. J Pediatr Surg 27:1192–1196, 1992.

Geggel RL, Murphy JD, Langleben D et al: Congenital diaphragmatic hernia: Arterial structural changes and persistent pulmonary hypertension after surgical repair. J Pediatr 107:457–464, 1985.

Harrison MR, Adzick NS, Flake AW et al: Correction of congenital diaphragmatic hernia in utero VI: Hard-learned lessons. J Pediatr Surg 28:1411–1417, 1993.

Irish MS, Holm BA, Glick PL: Congenital diaphragmatic hernia: A historical review. Clin Perinatol 23:625–653, 1996.

Langham MR, Kays DW, Ledbetter DJ et al: Congenital diaphragmatic hernia: Epidemiology and outcome. Clin Perinatol 23:671–688, 1996.

Wilcox DT, Glick PL, Karamanoukian HL et al: Contributions by individual lungs to the surfactant status in congenital diaphragmatic hernia. Pediatr Res 41:686–691, 1997.

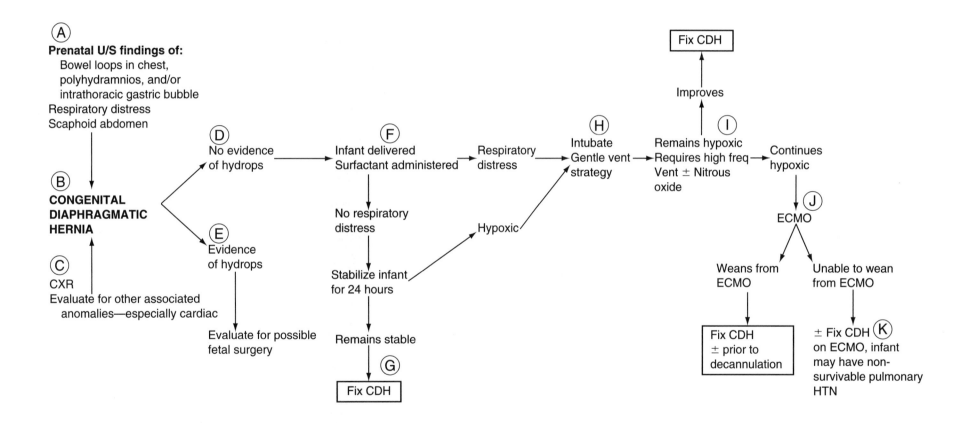

Ⓐ **Prenatal U/S findings of:**
Bowel loops in chest, polyhydramnios, and/or intrathoracic gastric bubble
Respiratory distress
Scaphoid abdomen

Ⓑ **CONGENITAL DIAPHRAGMATIC HERNIA**

Ⓒ CXR
Evaluate for other associated anomalies—especially cardiac

Ⓓ No evidence of hydrops

Ⓔ Evidence of hydrops
Evaluate for possible fetal surgery

Ⓕ Infant delivered
Surfactant administered
No respiratory distress
Stabilize infant for 24 hours
Remains stable

Ⓖ Fix CDH

Respiratory distress
Hypoxic

Ⓗ Intubate
Gentle vent strategy

Remains hypoxic
Requires high freq
Vent ± Nitrous oxide

Ⓘ Continues hypoxic

Improves

Fix CDH

Ⓙ ECMO

Weans from ECMO
Fix CDH ± prior to decannulation

Unable to wean from ECMO

Ⓚ ± Fix CDH on ECMO, infant may have non-survivable pulmonary HTN

TRANSPLANTATION

Chapter 116 Kidney Transplantation

KIAN A. MODANLOU, MD • MICHAEL E. WACHS, MD •
IGAL KAM, MD • THOMAS E. BAK, MD

(A) The three most common causes of end-stage renal disease (ESRD) are diabetes mellitus, glomerulonephritis, and hypertensive nephrosclerosis. These account for about 60% of cases. Other important causes include polycystic kidney disease, Alport's disease, IgA nephropathy, systemic lupus erythematosus (SLE), interstitial nephritis, chronic pyelonephritis, and obstructive nephropathy. The cause may determine the timing of the transplantation (e.g., SLE must be quiescent) or the risk of recurrence (e.g., Ig A nephropathy and diabetes).

(B) Besides transplantation, patients with ESRD must choose between hemodialysis or chronic ambulatory peritoneal dialysis for renal replacement therapy. Diabetics who require chronic hemodialysis have a survival of less than 20% at 5 years. Not only is the quality of life better with transplantation than dialysis, but current results show that survival is also superior.

(C) Candidacy is determined by a team effort including surgeons, nephrologists, anesthesiologists, nurses, social workers, and members of the community.

(D) Patients on dialysis, especially those with diabetes or hypertension, are at increased risk for cardiovascular disease. This possibility should be assessed before proceeding with candidacy.

(E) Indications for pretransplant nephrectomy are rare but include polycystic kidney disease complicated by bleeding, infection, pain, and excessive size. Other indications include uncontrollable renin-mediated hypertension, massive proteinuria, and persistent urinary tract infection. Any necessary urinary tract reconstructions (e.g., lysis of posterior urethral valves or transurethral resection of obstructing prostate) as well as bladder reconstruction, augmentation, or ileal conduit construction should also be carried out before transplantation.

(F) Compatibility for ABO blood groups is mandatory because they function as important histocompatibility antigens.

(G) Potential recipients are human leukocyte antigen (HLA)–typed for two different HLA-A, HLA-B, and HLA-DR alleles. Matching these alleles is the best means of prolonging graft survival. Significant survival benefits have been seen with six of six antigen matches.

(H) Panel-reactive antibody (PRA) is an estimate of the patient's serum antibody response to antigens in the general population. A high PRA (from a previous blood transfusion or transplant) is predictive of a positive cross-match. A negative cross-match is required for kidney transplantation in order to eliminate hyperacute rejection and graft loss.

(I) For patients whose first transplant has failed, the cause of the failure (e.g., noncompliance, chronic rejection, technical failure, or recurrent disease) must be evaluated before another transplantation is undertaken.

(J) Live donor evaluation (of a relative or emotionally connected individual) involves assessment of a person with two normal kidneys and no other health problems. The long-term outcome for living donor transplants far exceeds that for cadaveric organs. The operative mortality of the donor is reported at 0.05% and long-term complications are rare. Laparoscopic donor nephrectomy is the preferred method because it has resulted in shorter hospital stays, less pain, and earlier return to work for the donor. About 30% of all kidney transplants in the United States are from living donors.

(K) The optimal cadaveric donors are previously healthy subjects who have been declared brain dead. Contraindications to donation included generalized infections (including HIV, HBV, and HCV); high-risk individuals (e.g., intravenous drug users); malignancy; known renal disease; hypertension; and advanced arteriosclerosis. The kidney is usually transported in ice after being cooled by flushing with a buffered solution.

(L) The operation is most often performed by exposing the iliac vessels retroperitoneally through an oblique incision just above the inguinal ligament. The dissection is slightly easier on the right side, but either side may be used.

(M) Potential technical complications include arterial or venous thrombosis (less than 1%), ureteral leak or stenosis (less than 4%), and lymphocele resulting in hydroureter (less than 2%). Of these, only vascular thrombosis typically leads to graft loss unless early recognition and immediate reoperation take place.

(N) Immunosuppression begins immediately after transplantation. In patients with immediate graft function this includes a calcineurin inhibitor (e.g., cyclosporin or tacrolimus), most commonly used with an antimetabolite (e.g., mycophenolate mofetil or azithropurine) and tapering doses of steroids. Patients at high risk for rejection or with delayed graft function (acute tubular necrosis) usually receive either monoclonal (OKT3) or polyclonal (thymoglobulin) antibody induction therapy while calcineurin inhibitors (which are nephrotoxic) are withheld until kidney function improves.

(O) Hyperacute rejection and graft loss is obviated by a negative pretransplant cross-match. Acute cellular rejection typically occurs during the first 3 months and is usually reversible by either steroid or antilymphocyte antibody therapy. The typical course of chronic rejection is gradual, progressive loss of renal function. It is more often seen in patients who have had previous episodes of acute rejection.

Chronic rejection is irreversible and can develop without previously diagnosed acute rejection.

(P) Because of the immunodepression caused by uremia and antirejection therapy, 30% to 60% of patients suffer some type of infection within the first year after transplantation. Early postoperative infections usually affect the urinary tract and are easily treatable. Late infections typically are opportunistic (viral or fungal) and can often be prevented with lower doses of immunosuppressives and chemoprophylaxis.

(Q) Patient and graft survival rates in cadaveric kidney transplantation have steadily improved: they are 98% and 90%, respectively, at 1 year; and 80% and 60%, respectively, at 5 years. The live donor transplant survival rates continue to be even better than these.

REFERENCES

Barker CF, Brayman KL, Markmann JF et al: Transplantation of Abdominal Organs. In Townsend CM, Beauchamp RD, Evers BM et al (eds): Sabiston Textbook of Surgery: The Biological Basis of Modern Surgical Practice, 16th ed. Philadelphia: WB Saunders, 2001.

Kam I, Chan L: Outcome and Complications of Renal Transplantation. In Schrier RW (ed): Diseases of the Kidney, 6th ed. Boston: Little, Brown, 1996.

Morris JP: Kidney Transplantation: Principles and Practice, 5th ed. Philadelphia: WB Saunders, 2001.

Novotny MJ: Laparoscopic live donor nephrectomy. Urol Clin N Am 28:127–135, 2001.

Pascual M, Theruvath T, Kawai T et al: Strategies to improve long-term outcomes after renal transplantation. N Engl J Med 346:580–590, 2002.

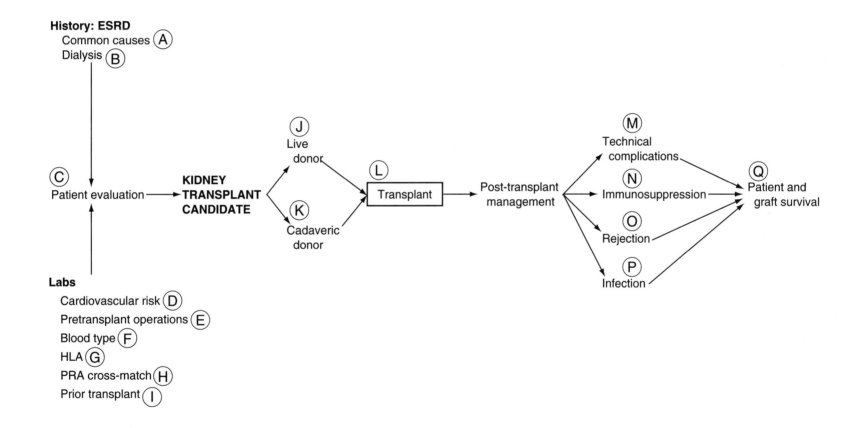

Chapter 117 *Pancreas Transplantation*

MARK D. STEGALL, MD

(A) Pancreas transplantation is performed in diabetic patients (Type 1 or 2) in three settings: (1) pancreas transplantation alone in a preuremic patient (PTA); (2) pancreas transplantation after successful kidney transplantation (PAK); or (3) simultaneous pancreas and kidney transplantation (SPK). Because graft survival in the last group is superior to that in either the PTA or the PAK group (approximately 90% 1-year graft survival vs. 79%), many centers restrict transplantation to patients who need both a kidney and a pancreas. With increasing waiting times for deceased donor kidneys, more patients are receiving a living donor kidney followed by a deceased donor pancreas, usually in two separate procedures.

(B) There are no strict age restrictions. Half of all pancreas transplant recipients are aged 30 to 40 years. Few are younger than 20 years or older than 50 years. Most patients have had diabetes for 10 to 20 years, but a third have had diabetes for less than 10 years.

(C) Pretransplant laboratory studies are identical to those for kidney transplantation—ABO blood group and human lymphocyte antigen (HLA) typing. Absolute prerequisites for transplantation are ABO compatibility and a negative cross-match.

(D) Recipient evaluation includes a thorough physical examination with special emphasis on neurologic, ophthalmic, and cardiac function. Transplantation should be done before the patient develops severe secondary complications such as disabling neuropathy, extensive vascular disease, and advanced retinopathy. Contraindications are a malignant process, active infection, advanced cardiovascular disease, a major amputation, and blindness.

(E) A potential cadaver donor should be aged 10 to 55 years and have no family history of diabetes, pancreatitis, or significant hypertension. The donor should be hemodynamically stable with minimal vasopressors and have no history of pancreatic trauma or peritoneal contamination.

Serum amylase may be elevated but the pancreas should look normal on visual examination.

(F) The ureters, abdominal vena cava, aorta, and major vascular branches are surgically dissected; then the liver and heart are removed. Finally, the pancreas and duodenum are harvested. Care is taken to identify vascular anomalies (particularly a right hepatic artery arising from the superior mesenteric artery) and to ensure that both pancreas and liver allografts have an adequate blood supply. A portal cannula may be inserted into the inferior mesenteric vein for liver precooling. The duodenum is irrigated with antibiotics through the nasogastric tube; then it is divided proximally and distally with a stapler knife. Heparin is administered. The abdominal organs are perfused and refrigerated by aortic cannula flush while the thoracic allografts are removed. After adequate cooling, the abdominal allografts are removed en bloc.

(G) The abdominal (but not the thoracic) allograft viscera are usually perfused with University of Wisconsin solution (Viaspan), using 2 to 3 L for the average adult. External cooling is effected with a sterile saline slush solution. After the pancreas and liver are removed, verapamil is added to the renal allograft perfusate to reduce vasospasm. The abdominal donor viscera are placed in sterile containers and can be held at 4°C for 24 hours or longer before transplantation.

(H) The abdomen is opened through a midline incision. Vascular anastomoses are created as follows: (1) between the donor splenic vein and the recipient common iliac vein or mesenteric vein; and (2) between the donor splenic artery (to which the donor's superior mesenteric artery has already been attached) and the recipient common iliac artery. In SPK transplantation, the kidney is usually placed on the left side of the abdomen and drained into the bladder. Recipients of PAK and PTA usually receive anticoagulation perioperatively to decrease the risk of graft thrombosis.

(I) Adequate pancreatic endocrine function can be provided by segmental transplantation of the body and tail. More often, the entire pancreas is transplanted because it provides more islet cells and allows monitoring of exocrine excretion in the urine after pancreaticocystostomy.

(J) Over the past few years, the majority of centers have switched from bladder drainage to enteric drainage of the pancreatic exocrine secretions, performing either a Roux-en-Y or a side-to-side anastomosis from the duodenal segment of the pancreas to an ileal loop. Enteric drainage prevents several of the complications of bladder drainage (e.g., dehydration, recurrent urinary tract infection, and urethral strictures) but carries an increased risk of early leakage.

(K) Simultaneous pancreas and kidney transplantation has the highest graft survival rate. The use of living donor kidney followed by PAK is being used increasingly; it allows patients to be transplanted before the need for dialysis and increases the living donor pool.

(L) With improved immunosuppression, acute rejection rates in SPK are now less than 10% in most centers. Most patients receive antibody induction therapy, either with anti-T cell antibody or with antibody against the interleukin-2 receptor. Maintenance immunosuppression includes tacrolimus, mycophenolate mofetil, and prednisone. Some centers have demonstrated good results in steroid-free immunosuppression.

(M) With simultaneous pancreas and kidney transplantation and bladder drainage, a drop in urine amylase usually accompanies allograft rejection, as do elevations of serum creatinine and blood urea nitrogen. In this case, needle biopsy of the kidney is used to determine rejection in combined kidney-pancreas transplantations. For solitary pancreas transplants, pancreas graft biopsies are performed in the first months after transplantation according to protocol.

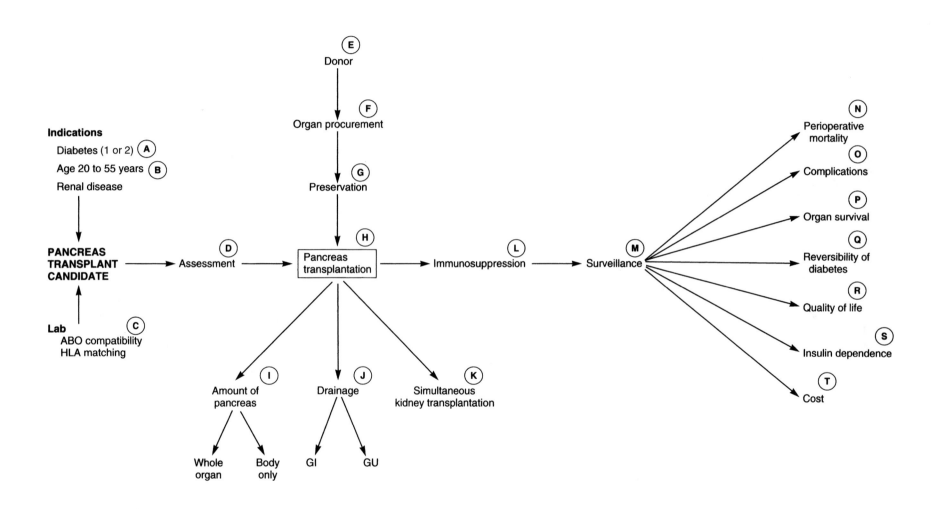

Indications

Diabetes (1 or 2) (A)

Age 20 to 55 years (B)

Renal disease

PANCREAS TRANSPLANT CANDIDATE

Lab (C)
ABO compatibility
HLA matching

(D) Assessment

(E) Donor

(F) Organ procurement

(G) Preservation

(H) Pancreas transplantation

(I) Amount of pancreas
Whole organ
Body only

(J) Drainage
GI
GU

(K) Simultaneous kidney transplantation

(L) Immunosuppression

(M) Surveillance

(N) Perioperative mortality

(O) Complications

(P) Organ survival

(Q) Reversibility of diabetes

(R) Quality of life

(S) Insulin dependence

(T) Cost

(N) Perioperative mortality is less than 1%. Occasionally, cardiovascular catastrophe or infection may cause death.

(O) Complications include accelerated rejection, primary pancreas graft nonfunction, early pancreatic venous thrombosis, infections (especially cytomegalovirus), hematuria, pancreatitis, and pancreatic fistula.

(P) One-year pancreas graft survival continues to improve: 90% for SPK and 79% for PAK. The leading cause of pancreas graft loss today is no longer rejection but rather graft thrombosis.

(Q) After successful transplantation, recipients' vision may stabilize and their neuropathy may improve or stabilize. The pancreas transplant can protect kidney allografts from diabetic neuropathic changes.

(R) Quality of life is much improved, especially for those who had unstable diabetes before transplantation and for those who have functioning eyes, limbs, and heart.

(S) Successful recipients are insulin independent within hours to days after transplantation and have normal glucose tolerance test results and glycosylated hemoglobin levels. Unstable diabetics become free of the dangers of insulin reactions and hyperglycemia. Transient hyperglycemia can occur with rejections and infections. Permanent hyperglycemia recurs if the allograft is rejected.

(T) The cost, about $85,000, does not include post-discharge care or medications. The cost of pancreas transplantation accompanying kidney transplantation is about $20,000, because much of the overhead is included in the cost of the kidney procedure.

REFERENCES

Drachenberg CB, Papadimitriou JC, Klassen DK et al: Evaluation of pancreas transplant needle biopsy: Reproducibility and revision of histologic grading system. Transplantation 63:1579–1586, 1997.

Gruessner AC, Sutherland DE, Dunn DL et al: Pancreas after kidney transplants in posturemic patients with type 1 diabetes mellitus. J Amer Soc Nephrol 12:2490–2499, 2001.

Philosophe B, Farney AC, Schweitzer EJ et al: Superiority of portal venous drainage over systemic venous drainage in pancreas transplantation: a retrospective study. Ann Surg 234:689–696, 2001.

Stegall MD, Kim DY, Prieto M et al: Thymoglobulin induction decreases rejection in solitary pancreas transplantation. Transplantation 72:1671–1675, 2001; www/optn.org.data for survival data.

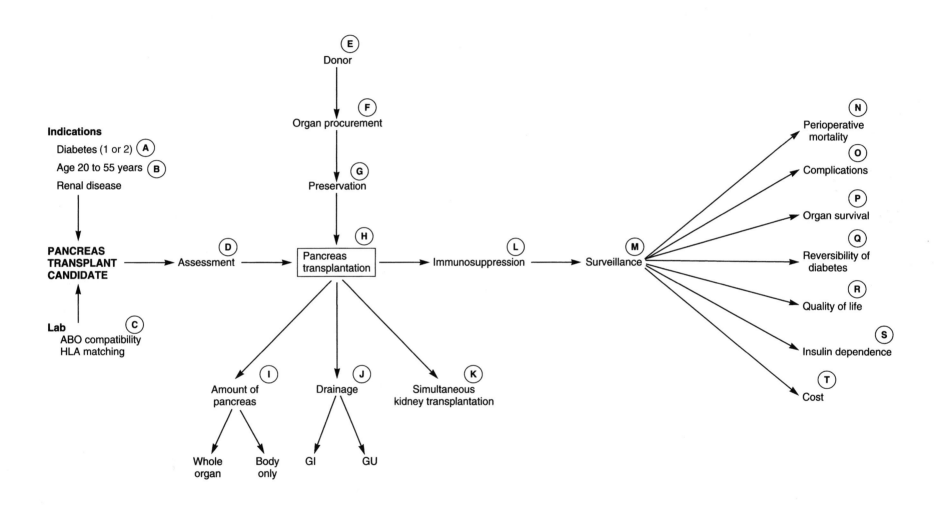

Chapter 118 *Liver Transplantation*

KIAN A. MODANLOU, MD ● MICHAEL E. WACHS, MD ●
IGAL KAM, MD ● THOMAS E. BAK, MD

(A) Liver transplantation is the procedure of choice for a wide range of diseases that result in end-stage liver disease (ESLD). In adults, common causes include noncholestatic disease (e.g., viral hepatitis B and C, alcoholic hepatitis, and cryptogenic cirrhosis); cholestatic disease (e.g., primary biliary cirrhosis and primary sclerosing cholangitis); and autoimmune disease. In children, common causes include biliary atresia, inborn errors of metabolism, cholestatic disease (e.g., primary sclerosing cholangitis and Alagille's syndrome); and autoimmune disease. Despite the different etiologies of these diseases, their pathophysiology leads to a common set of symptoms and signs of ESLD.

(B) Candidacy is determined by a team effort including surgeons, hepatologists, anesthesiologists, nurses, social workers, and members of the community.

(C) Symptoms or complications of ESLD that suggest a need for transplantation include variceal hemorrhage, worsening ascites, spontaneous bacterial peritonitis, and encephalopathy. The Child-Turcote-Pugh (CPT) score uses assessment of encephalopathy, ascites, total bilirubin, albumin, and prothrombin time (PT) to quantify the severity of liver failure. Computed tomography (CT) and ultrasonography (US) are both useful in assessing liver size, portal venous flow, the amount of ascites, and the presence or absence of tumor in the liver.

(D) All patients undergo physiologic evaluation to ensure that they will be able to tolerate the surgical procedure. Contraindications that preclude transplant include extrahepatic malignancy, irreversible brain damage, severe cardiac disease, severe pulmonary hypertension, and uncontrollable sepsis. Epstein-Barr virus (EBV) and cytomegalovirus (CMV) serologies are helpful in determining the risk of post-transplantation viral infection and the need for chemoprophylaxis. Those with alcoholic liver disease must document abstinence for at least 6 months and undergo psychosocial evaluation to assess the likelihood of recidivism.

(E) Hepatitis C (HCV) infection now accounts for 35% to 45% of all liver transplants. Virtually all patients with HCV will reinfect their grafts after transplant; this has led to the use of donors with positive serologies and no evidence of hepatic disease. Hepatitis B (HBV) reinfection can be prevented with proper post-transplant therapy. Approximately 10% to 25% of HCV-infected recipients of liver allografts will develop cirrhosis within 5 years of transplantation. Both HCV and HBV are risk factors for development of hepatocellular carcinoma (HCC). Reports show that 30% of liver explants obtained at the time of transplantation had incidental HCC despite appropriate screening protocol before transplant.

(F) Evaluation for HCC is necessary in determining both candidacy and position on the waiting list. Generally, transplant will benefit those with histologic grading of Grade 1 or 2, tumor size less than 5 cm, multifocally limited, and no evidence of extrahepatic metastases.

(G) For patients whose first transplant has failed, the cause of the failure (e.g., noncompliance, chronic rejection, technical failure, or recurrent disease) must be evaluated before another transplantation is undertaken.

(H) Position on the waiting list is determined by the Model for End-Stage Liver Disease (MELD). The score is a reliable estimate of 1-year survival over a wide range of liver disease severity and diverse etiology. The MELD score is calculated using serum bilirubin and creatinine levels, international normalized ratio (INR) for prothrombin time, and etiology of liver disease. Extra points are given for documented evidence of HCC.

(I) More than 95% of liver transplants are livers from donors whose blood type is compatible with that of the recipient. In critical situations, ABO-incompatible transplantation is performed, leading to varied results.

(J) The vast majority of liver transplants are cadaver organs from heart-beating, brain dead donors without evidence of systemic infection, malignancy, or alcohol abuse. Liver enzyme values and synthetic functions are indicative of the degree of liver injury and predict the potential for recovery. Acceptable results can be obtained if steatosis is mild to moderate (10% to 30%). Marginal grafts are sometimes used in patients with relative contraindications to transplant. After cold preservation, most organs are transplanted within 8 to 12 hours.

(K) Organ shortage has also led to the use of adult-to-pediatric and adult-to-adult live donor transplants. Advantages include decreased waiting time, optimization of recipient health status, ideal graft quality, and decreased cold-ischemia time. Disadvantages include the potential risks to the donor, smaller hepatic mass, and increased complications in the recipient (e.g., bile leak from the cut surface). Results are best from specialized centers with extensive experience in the procedure.

(L) After administration of preoperative antibiotics, placement of invasive monitoring lines, and acquisition of adequate venous access, the recipient operation begins. Hepatectomy is followed by caval anastomosis in an end-to-end or piggyback fashion. Portal vein and hepatic arterial anastomoses are next. The biliary system is then connected in a duct-to-duct fashion or by Roux-en-Y choledochojejunostomy.

(M) In order to maximize the limited number of available organs, a cadaveric graft can be split into a right trisegmentectomy and a left lateral lobe for transplant into two size-matched recipients. The left lateral segment is often used in pediatric patients. The lobe is transplanted in a piggyback fashion, and biliary anastomosis is most often via

410

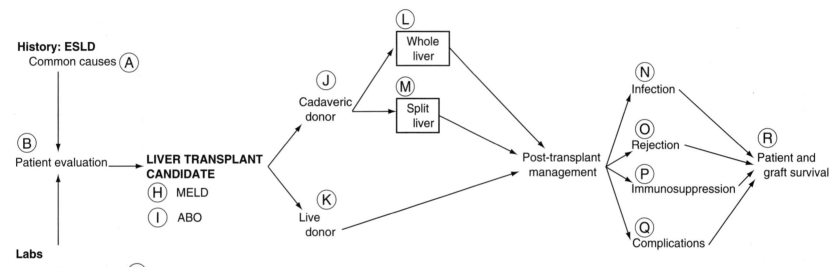

hepaticojejunostomy. These patients are at increased risk for technical complications.

(N) Infections are the most significant complications in liver transplantation and account for most of the mortalities in the early postoperative period. Most bacterial infections are aggressively treated with broad-spectrum antibiotics. Fungal infection remains a potential lethal complication of immunosuppression.

(O) Acute cellular rejection occurs in approximately 25% of cases during the first 6 months and is characterized by fever, abdominal pain, and elevated enzymes and bilirubin. Most episodes are responsive to therapy with high-dose steroids. Antithymocyte therapy (OKT3 or thymoglobulin) is used in recalcitrant cases. Chronic rejection is seen months or years after transplantation and is manifested by poor synthetic liver function and

hyperbilirubinemia. As long as the patient adheres to the immunosuppressive protocol, chronic rejection should not be a problem.

(P) Immunosuppression begins immediately after transplantation. Current protocols use a calcineurin inhibitor (e.g., cyclosporin or tacrolimus); steroids; and an antimetabolite. Rapid weaning from steroids has been shown in long-term follow-up to decrease metabolic complications without subjecting grafts to increased incidence of rejection. Steroid-free protocols are also being used.

(Q) Surgical complications include bleeding, bile leak, primary nonfunction, and hepatic artery thrombosis. The first two are usually amenable to reoperation, whereas the latter two, although rare, often require retransplantation.

(R) Survival after liver transplantation has improved dramatically over the past 10 years (from 60% to 90% at 1 year and from 50% to 80% at 5 years). The majority of these patients return to fully functional status.

REFERENCES

Barker CF, Brayman KL, Markmann JF et al: Transplantation of Abdominal Organs. In Towsend CM, Beauchamp RD, Evers BM et al (eds): Sabiston Textbook of Surgery: The Biological Basis of Modern Surgical Practice, 16th ed. Philadelphia: WB Saunders, 2001.

Busuttil RW, Klintmalm GB: Transplantation of the Liver. Philadelphia: WB Saunders, 1996.

Kamath PS, Wiesner RH, Malinchoc M et al: A model to predict survival in patients with end-stage liver disease. Hepatology 33:464–470, 2001.

Lok ASF, Villamil FG, McDiarmid SV (eds): Liver transplantation for viral hepatitis. Liver Transplantation 8:supplement 1, 2002.

Trotter JF, Wachs M, Everson GT et al: Adult-to-adult transplantation of the right hepatic lobe from a living donor. N Engl J Med 346:1074–1082, 2002.

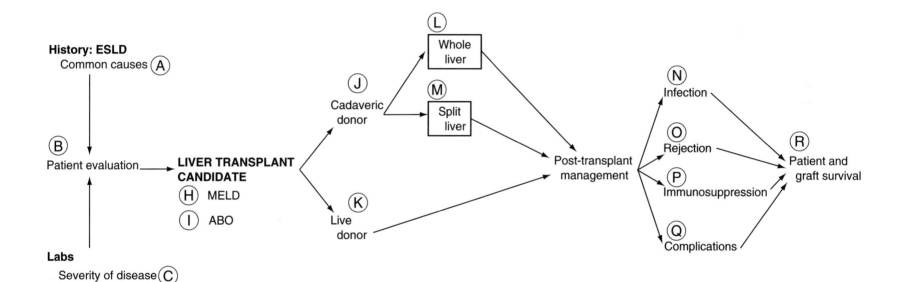

History: ESLD
Common causes (A)

(B)
Patient evaluation → **LIVER TRANSPLANT CANDIDATE**

(H) MELD

(I) ABO

Labs
Severity of disease (C)
Comorbidities (D)
Hepatitis serologies (E)
Tumor evaluation (F)
Prior transplant (G)

(J)
Cadaveric donor

(L)
Whole liver

(M)
Split liver

(K)
Live donor

Post-transplant management

(N) Infection

(O) Rejection

(P) Immunosuppression

(Q) Complications

(R) Patient and graft survival

Chapter 119 Lung Transplantation

JOHN D. MITCHELL, MD

(A) Tobacco abuse, congenital malformations, genetic diseases, and idiopathic systemic illnesses may lead to pulmonary failure necessitating lung transplantation. Patients are considered for transplantation when they are found to be in the "transplantation window" (i.e., ill enough to warrant transplantation, yet not so ill that they would likely die while on the transplantation waiting list). The timing of the window varies according to the underlying disease.

(B) Many of the same studies used to characterize the nature of the pulmonary failure are employed during the transplantation evaluation. Occasionally these preliminary studies will reveal findings (e.g., an occult thoracic malignancy) that will make transplantation referral untenable.

(C) Patients with cystic fibrosis and an FEV1 less than 30% have a 2-year survival of 55%. In addition, the presence of a rapidly falling FEV1 (even if greater than 30%), recurrent hospitalizations, significant hemoptysis, a PaO_2 less than 55 mm Hg, or a $PaCO_2$ greater than 55 mm Hg are all factors associated with a poor outcome. Any of these findings in a patient with cystic fibrosis should prompt referral for transplantation. Symptomatic liver disease and uncontrolled super-infection/colonization with certain organisms (e.g., *Burkholderia cepacia*) may present contraindications to transplantation. Patients with other types of suppurative lung disease (e.g., severe chronic bronchiectasis) should be referred according to the guidelines for cystic fibrosis patients.

(D) Severe pulmonary hypertension may be primary pulmonary hypertension (PPH), secondary to thromboembolic disease or systemic collagen vascular disease, or may be caused by underlying congenital heart disease (i.e., Eisenmenger's syndrome). Successful use of intravenous epoprostenol (Flolan) has changed the timing of referral for transplantation in many patients with pulmonary hypertension. In addition, some patients may be candidates for pulmonary thromboendarterectomy.

In general, patients should be referred when NYHA class III or IV heart failure exists despite optimal medical or surgical therapy. Hemodynamic parameters for referral include a cardiac index less than $2\,L/min/m^2$, a right atrial pressure greater than 15 mm Hg, and a mean pulmonary artery pressure greater than 55 mm Hg. Patients with Eisenmenger's syndrome often function better than suggested by these parameters, and in this group of patients the presence of progressive symptoms is the most important factor for referral.

(E) Only a minority of patients with restrictive lung disease (e.g., idiopathic pulmonary fibrosis) respond to medical therapy. A forced vital capacity less than 60% to 70% of predicted and a DLCO less than 50% to 60% of predicted are correlated with poor survival and should trigger referral for transplantation. These patients can suffer abrupt declines in clinical status, and late referral to transplant centers remains a significant problem. Frequent reassessment is therefore crucial for appropriate timing. The high mortality associated with pulmonary fibrosis has led the United Network for Organ Sharing (UNOS) to permit these patients a 90-day waitlist "bonus" when listed for transplant.

(F) Patients with chronic obstructive pulmonary disease (COPD), most commonly tobacco-associated emphysema, are usually referred for transplantation evaluation when the FEV1 remains less than 25% of predicted despite optimal bronchodilator therapy, the $PaCO_2$ is greater than 55 mm Hg, and/or pulmonary hypertension is present. Progressive clinical deterioration, even if these factors are not met, merits referral. Although most COPD patients experience improved quality of life after lung transplantation, the procedure does not confer a survival benefit. For some of these patients, lung volume reduction surgery (LVRS) may be preferred as an alternative procedure.

(G) Data from the National Emphysema Treatment Trial (NETT) revealed that an FEV1 less than 20% of predicted, combined with either a DLCO less than 20% of predicted or a homogeneous pattern of emphysema as noted in radiologic studies, is predictive of a poor outcome following LVRS. These patients may be considered for transplantation but should not be referred for LVRS.

(H) It is important to determine whether best possible medical therapy has been instituted in patients referred for lung transplantation. Occasionally significant clinical improvements can be realized, particularly in the COPD population, when the medical regimen is optimized. The age limit of 65 years is a guideline only. Many transplantation centers will consider otherwise healthy patients older than 65 years, principally in disease processes such as interstitial pulmonary fibrosis (IPF) where successful medical therapy is uncommon.

(I) An exhaustive evaluation is performed for patients thought to be within the window for transplantation. Along with laboratory, pulmonary function, and exercise testing, patients are evaluated for the presence of occult malignancy and cardiac disease. Additional comorbidities are evaluated when indicated. An intensive psychosocial evaluation is a key part of the process, including assessment of the social support system in place and available for the transplant patient.

(J) The NETT study suggested that in patients with upper-lobe predominant emphysema and low exercise capacity, an improvement in survival and exercise capacity (and presumably, quality of life) could be anticipated with LVRS. In patients with upper-lobe disease and high exercise capacity, and in those with non–upper-lobe disease and low exercise capacity, an improvement in exercise capacity but not survival was seen with LVRS. These three subgroups of emphysema patients, excluding those who meet the criteria listed in G, may be considered for LVRS. Finally, those with non–upper-lobe disease and a high exercise capacity did not benefit from LVRS, according to the NETT findings, but they may be considered for transplantation.

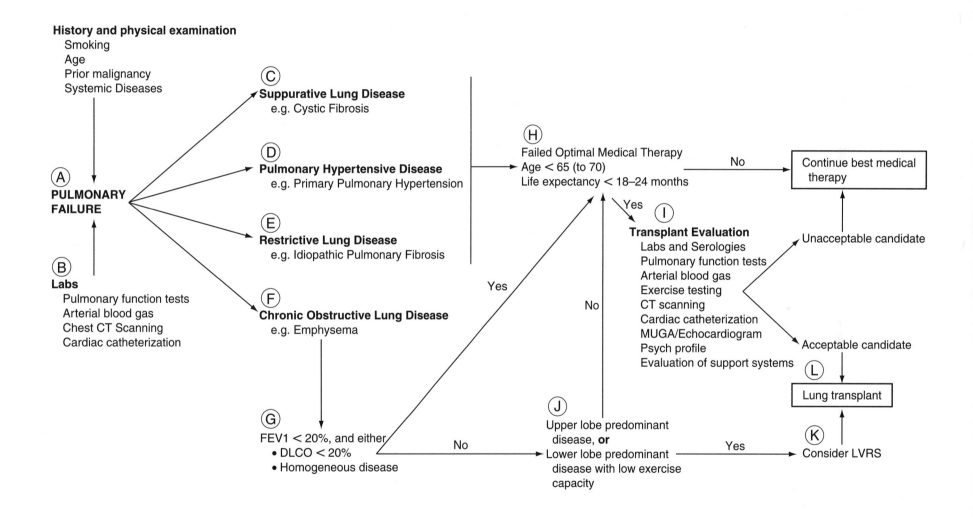

History and physical examination
Smoking
Age
Prior malignancy
Systemic Diseases

(A)
**PULMONARY
FAILURE**

(B)
Labs
Pulmonary function tests
Arterial blood gas
Chest CT Scanning
Cardiac catheterization

(C)
Suppurative Lung Disease
e.g. Cystic Fibrosis

(D)
Pulmonary Hypertensive Disease
e.g. Primary Pulmonary Hypertension

(E)
Restrictive Lung Disease
e.g. Idiopathic Pulmonary Fibrosis

(F)
Chronic Obstructive Lung Disease
e.g. Emphysema

(G)
FEV1 < 20%, and either
• DLCO < 20%
• Homogeneous disease

(H)
Failed Optimal Medical Therapy
Age < 65 (to 70)
Life expectancy < 18–24 months

No → Continue best medical therapy

Yes

(I)
Transplant Evaluation
Labs and Serologies
Pulmonary function tests
Arterial blood gas
Exercise testing
CT scanning
Cardiac catheterization
MUGA/Echocardiogram
Psych profile
Evaluation of support systems

Unacceptable candidate → Continue best medical therapy

Acceptable candidate

(L)
Lung transplant

(J)
Upper lobe predominant disease, **or**
Lower lobe predominant disease with low exercise capacity

No

Yes

(K)
Consider LVRS

Yes

No

Ⓚ Factors other than those previously listed (e.g., severe pulmonary hypertension) may exclude a patient from LVRS consideration. LVRS may be used as a bridge to subsequent lung transplantation.

Ⓛ The average time for patients on the waitlist can approach or exceed 2 years in many transplant centers. The 1-year survival rate after transplantation is approximately 80% to 85%, and 5-year survival rates are in the 40% to 55% range. Overall survival rate varies with the underlying indication for transplantation. The development of obliterative bronchiolitis remains the biggest obstacle to long-term success. Patients with suppurative lung disease or pulmonary hypertension undergo bilateral lung transplantation, whereas most patients with restrictive lung disease receive single lung transplants. Younger individuals (less than 55 years)

with COPD, or those COPD patients with alpha-1 antitrypsin deficiency, typically undergo a bilateral procedure, whereas older emphysema patients receive a single graft. Although most COPD patients undergo single lung transplantation, some centers routinely perform bilateral procedures in all COPD patients, feeling it provides a superior outcome.

REFERENCES

Aris RM, Gilligan PH, Neuringer IP et al: The effect of panresistant bacteria in cystic fibrosis patients on lung transplant outcome. Am J Respir Crit Care Med 155:1699–1704, 1997.

Cassivi SD, Meyers BF, Battafarano RJ et al: Thirteen-year experience in lung transplantation for emphysema. Ann Thorac Surg 74:1663–1670, 2002.

Grover FL, Fullerton DA, Zamora MR et al: The past, present, and future of lung transplantation. Am J Surg 173:523–533, 1997.

Heng D, Sharples LD, McNeil K et al: Bronchiolitis obliterans syndrome: Incidence, natural history, prognosis, and risk factors. J Heart Lung Transplant 17:1255–1263, 1998.

Hosenpud JD, Bennett LE, Keck BM et al: Effect of diagnosis on survival benefit of lung transplantation for end-stage lung disease. Lancet 351:24–27, 1998.

Kerem E, Reisman J, Corey M et al: Prediction of mortality in patients with cystic fibrosis. N Engl J Med 326:1187–1191, 1992.

Maurer JR, Frost AE, Estenne M et al: International guidelines for the selection of lung transplant candidates. J Heart Lung Transplant 17:703–709, 1998.

National Emphysema Treatment Trial Research Group: Patients at High Risk of Death after Lung-Volume–Reduction Surgery. N Engl J Med 345:1075–1083, 2001.

National Emphysema Treatment Trial Research Group: A Randomized Trial Comparing Lung-Volume–Reduction Surgery with Medical Therapy for Severe Emphysema. N Engl J Med 348:2059–2073, 2003.

Schwartz DA, Helmers RA, Galvin JR et al: Determinants of survival in idiopathic pulmonary fibrosis. Am J Respir Crit Care Med 149:450–454, 1994.

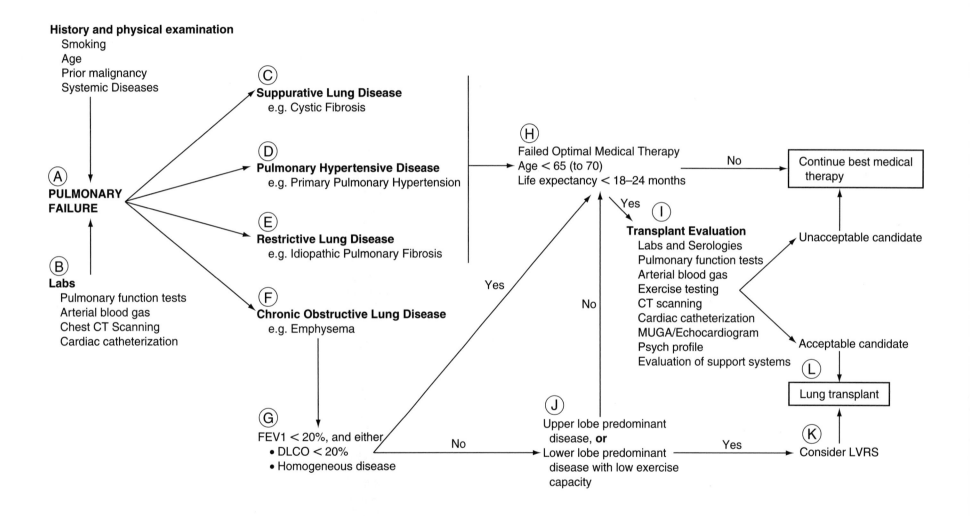

History and physical examination
Smoking
Age
Prior malignancy
Systemic Diseases

Ⓒ **Suppurative Lung Disease**
e.g. Cystic Fibrosis

Ⓓ **Pulmonary Hypertensive Disease**
e.g. Primary Pulmonary Hypertension

Ⓔ **Restrictive Lung Disease**
e.g. Idiopathic Pulmonary Fibrosis

Ⓐ **PULMONARY FAILURE**

Ⓑ **Labs**
Pulmonary function tests
Arterial blood gas
Chest CT Scanning
Cardiac catheterization

Ⓕ **Chronic Obstructive Lung Disease**
e.g. Emphysema

Ⓖ FEV1 < 20%, and either
• DLCO < 20%
• Homogeneous disease

Ⓗ Failed Optimal Medical Therapy
Age < 65 (to 70)
Life expectancy < 18–24 months

No → Continue best medical therapy

Yes

Ⓘ **Transplant Evaluation**
Labs and Serologies
Pulmonary function tests
Arterial blood gas
Exercise testing
CT scanning
Cardiac catheterization
MUGA/Echocardiogram
Psych profile
Evaluation of support systems

Unacceptable candidate

Acceptable candidate

Ⓛ Lung transplant

Yes

No

Ⓙ Upper lobe predominant disease, **or**
Lower lobe predominant disease with low exercise capacity

No

Yes

Ⓚ Consider LVRS

Chapter 120 *Heart Transplantation*

PETER A. SEIRAFI, MD • DAVID N. CAMPBELL, MD

(A) Myocardial failure refractory to optimal medical therapy is the primary indication for adult heart transplantation. Typical candidates have Class III or IV heart failure, restricted physical activity, and are receiving maximal pharmacologic treatment. These end-stage heart failure patients have disease not amenable to optimal medical or surgical therapy. The most common preoperative diagnoses worldwide are ischemic cardiomyopathy (45%) and idiopathic cardiomyopathy (45%). Congenital heart disease is the most common indication in the pediatric age group. Although the number of heart transplants performed in the United States has remained relatively stable over the past decade (2000 to 2300 per year), the number of patients on the waiting list has nearly doubled (2160 in 1991 vs. 4100 in 2001). Ventricular assist devices have been used successfully as a bridge to transplant and continue to be evaluated as an alternative to heart transplantation. Although the role of the total artificial heart is still to be defined, continued improvements in design and function in ventricular assist devices, as well as the artificial heart, provide hope for the increasing number of patients awaiting heart transplantation.

(B) Right-side heart catheterization determines the reactivity of the pulmonary vasculature. Fixed pulmonary vascular resistance greater than 6 to 8 Wood units; or a transpulmonary gradient greater than 17 mm Hg that is unresponsive to milrinone, nitroprusside, and/or nitric oxide (+ dipyridamole) are absolute contraindications for heart transplantation. Heart-lung transplantation should be considered for this group.

(C) Irreversible disease in other vital organs is usually a contraindication to heart transplantation alone. In some cases, liver or kidney transplantation can be carried out at the same time. Relative contraindications include obstructive or restrictive lung disease, neurologic impairment, and poor patient and family support structure. Absolute contraindications include conditions worsened by immunosuppression (i.e., active infections and malignancies).

(D) A panel-reactive antibody (PRA) level measures potential reactivity to donor human leukocyte antigens (HLA). Most commonly, PRA levels greater than 10% are considered elevated. PRA thresholds for initiating therapy to reduce the degree of sensitization before transplantation vary widely. Treatment regimens most commonly include one or more of the following: immunoglobulin, plasmapheresis, cyclophosphamide, and mycophenylate mofetil.

(E) Screening for reactivity to Epstein-Barr nuclear antigen, cytomegalovirus, and toxoplasmosis helps guide postoperative therapy.

(F) Hemodynamic deterioration before transplantation may necessitate a pharmacologic or mechanical bridge to transplantation. These patients are accorded top priority (Status I). Initial management includes admission to the ICU and inotropic agents such as dopamine, dobutamine, and milrinone. If drug therapy fails, an intra-aortic balloon pump is placed. Continued cardiogenic shock requires use of a left ventricular assist device. Twenty percent of patients also require a right ventricular assist device. Ventricular arrhythmias may require an automatic implantable cardiac defibrillator (AICD). Sudden cardiac death caused by ventricular arrhythmia is the most common cause of death in patients awaiting cardiac transplantation.

(G) Consent from the donor's next of kin is mandatory. A donor must be brain dead, have a relatively normal heart, and have a compatible blood type. Preoperative HLA crossmatching is necessary only when the PRA is greater than 10% to 15%. The ideal donor characteristics are: age less than 45 years; no known heart disease; size match +20%; and no prolonged hypotension or cardiac arrest, trauma to the heart, significant cardiotonic or vasopressor requirement, systemic infection, or history of long-term alcohol or cocaine abuse. Echocardiography is necessary to confirm normal cardiac anatomy and function. Donors aged more than 45 years or with risk factors for coronary artery disease should be studied with coronary angiography.

Pediatric donors should be two or three times as large as the recipient. The final assessment of the donor heart is made at the time of procurement.

(H) Procuring multiple organs from a single donor is common: kidneys, livers, hearts, and lungs are harvested in that order of frequency. The viability of other organs depends on preservation of cardiac function until the final, swift isolation and removal of the heart. The heart is arrested with cold cardioplegia, excised, and put in cold saline-filled bags and transported in an ice cooler.

(I) Operation is fairly standard; however, many centers have changed to bicaval anastomosis because of reported decreased incidence of conduction disturbances, atrial dysrhythmias, and tricuspid valve incompetence. The donor heart requires "payback" unloaded perfusion for 20 to 30 minutes. Pharmacologic support is necessary for several days. Isuprel is used for its β-adrenergic effect, and dopamine is usually given in "renal doses." Vasodilators such as nitroglycerin and nitroprusside are helpful, and phosphodiesterase inhibitors like milrinone are particularly helpful in patients with elevated pulmonary artery pressures. Nitric oxide may also be useful as a pulmonary vasodilator. Heterotopic implantation is rarely indicated.

(J) Heart-lung transplantation is used for severe pulmonary hypertension or disease of both heart and lungs. Some 48 heart-lung transplants were performed in the United States in 2000, and congenital heart disease and primary pulmonary hypertension were the most common preoperative diagnoses. The 1- and 5-year survival rates for these diagnoses were 60% and 50%, respectively.

(K) Induction therapy with rabbit antithymocyte globulin, equine antilymphocytic globulin, or OKT3 may be used selectively to lower the T-cell count. More often, maintenance immunosuppression consists of azathioprine or mycophenolic acid, cyclosporine or FK506, and low-dose steriods. Antithymocyte globulin can replace cyclosporine in the early postoperative period if renal failure occurs.

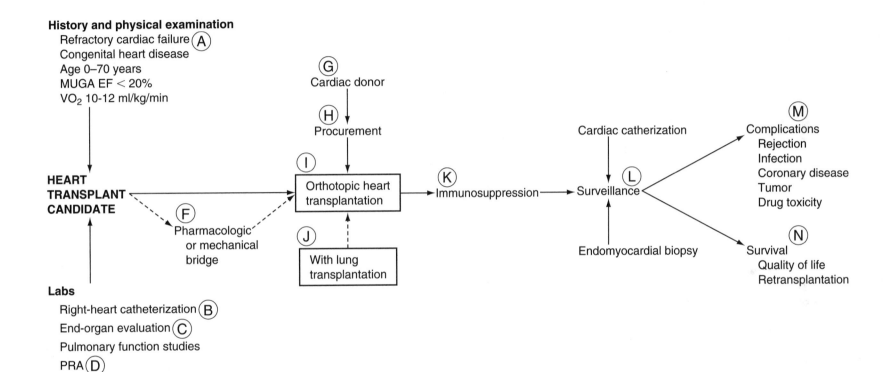

History and physical examination
Refractory cardiac failure (A)
Congenital heart disease
Age 0–70 years
MUGA EF < 20%
VO$_2$ 10-12 ml/kg/min

(G)
Cardiac donor

(H)
Procurement

(M)
Complications
Rejection
Infection
Coronary disease
Tumor
Drug toxicity

Cardiac catherization

(I)

(L)

**HEART
TRANSPLANT
CANDIDATE**

(F)
Pharmacologic
or mechanical
bridge

Orthotopic heart
transplantation

(K)
Immunosuppression

Surveillance

(J)
With lung
transplantation

Endomyocardial biopsy

(N)
Survival
Quality of life
Retransplantation

Labs
Right-heart catheterization (B)
End-organ evaluation (C)
Pulmonary function studies
PRA (D)
Blood group
Absence of infection (E)

(L) Endomyocardial biopsy is performed weekly and then at less frequent intervals during the first year. Drug doses are adjusted to combat renal toxicity and the reciprocal problems of infection and rejection. Annual reevaluations look for lymphoproliferative disease and for fungal, viral, and parasitic infections and nephrotoxicity from immunosuppressive agents. Cardiac catheterization is used to monitor atherosclerosis of the coronary arteries, which develops in 8% of patients at 1 year and in 35% to 40% of patients at 5 years. Intravascular ultrasound has been used to better assess intimal thickening in the coronary arteries.

(M) Rejection occurs when immunosuppression is inadequate; it is inversely related to infection, which is secondary to overzealous immunosuppression. The majority of cases of acute rejection occur within 3 months after transplant, and usually are successfully treated with corticosteriods.

Renal dysfunction and hypertension are chiefly caused by toxicity from cyclosporine. Some 95% of patients at 5 years post-transplant will have hypertension. Diabetes mellitus (32% at 5 years) and osteoporosis can result from overuse of corticosteroids. Because of chronic immunosuppression and infection with the Epstein-Barr virus, there is a 16% incidence of skin malignancy and 4.4% incidence of lymphoma at 7 years post-transplant.

(N) Perioperative mortality is 5% to 7%. It is higher in children, in the elderly, in women, and in those whose transplantations are more urgent. Infection and rejection are the leading causes of mortality during the first year following transplantation, with allograft coronary artery disease being the leading cause thereafter. The 1- and 5-year survival rates are 85% and 70%, respectively. Although the functional status of long-term survivors is excellent, with more than 90% reporting no activity limitations at 5 years after transplant, one area of interest is that fewer than 40% have returned to full- or part-time employment.

REFERENCES

Betkowski AS, Graff R, Chen JJ et al: Panel-reactive antibody screening practices prior to heart transplantation. J Heart Lung Transplant 21:644–650, 2002.

Brann WM, Bennett LE, Keck BM et al: Morbidity, functional status, and immunosuppressive therapy after heart transplantation. An analysis of the Joint International Society for Heart and Lung Transplantation/ United Network for Organ Sharing Thoracic Registry. J Heart Lung Transplant 17:374–381, 1998.

Hertz MI, Taylor DO, Trulock EP et al: The registry of the International Society for Heart and Lung Transplantation: Nineteenth official report 2002. J Heart Lung Transplant 21:950–970, 2002.

Shumway S, Shumway N: Thoracic Transplantation. Cambridge: Blackwell Scientific, 1995.

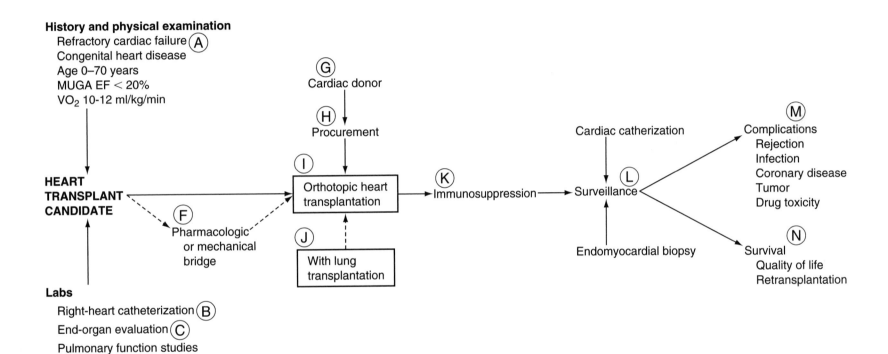

History and physical examination
  Refractory cardiac failure (A)
  Congenital heart disease
  Age 0–70 years
  MUGA EF < 20%
  VO₂ 10-12 ml/kg/min

(G)
Cardiac donor

(H)
Procurement

(I)
Orthotopic heart transplantation

HEART TRANSPLANT CANDIDATE

(F)
Pharmacologic or mechanical bridge

(J)
With lung transplantation

(K)
Immunosuppression

Cardiac catherization

(L)
Surveillance

Endomyocardial biopsy

(M)
Complications
  Rejection
  Infection
  Coronary disease
  Tumor
  Drug toxicity

(N)
Survival
  Quality of life
  Retransplantation

Labs
  Right-heart catheterization (B)
  End-organ evaluation (C)
  Pulmonary function studies
  PRA (D)
  Blood group
  Absence of infection (E)

Chapter 121 *Organ Donation*

BRIAN D. SHAMES, MD • JONATHAN LEWIS, RN, BSN, CPTC •
ANTHONY M. D'ALESSANDRO, MD

(A) A potential nonliving organ donor is any patient who has sustained a severe neurologic injury secondary to trauma, cerebrovascular accident, cardiac arrest, or anoxia. According to the United Network for Organ Sharing (UNOS), intracranial hemorrhage/stoke, blunt injury, and gunshot wounds are the leading mechanisms of death leading to organ donation.

(B) The President's Commission on Death Determination supports two separate, complementary sets of death criteria, one based on the absence of circulation and respiration, the other based on the irreversible absence of whole brain function. Either is satisfactory for the determination of death before organ donation. Brain death is defined as the total and irreversible cessation of cerebral function as manifested by apnea, unresponsiveness to all stimuli, and lack of cranial nerve reflexes in the absence of either hypothermia or drug intoxication. Objective evidence of brain death includes the absence of cerebral flow on nuclear perfusion study; and silence on electroencephalography.

(C) Some patients will not progress to brain death; however, they will have irreversible neurologic injury. If withdrawal of life support is planned, these patients may be considered for donation after cardiac death (DCD). DCD occurs when death is determined by the absence of circulation and respiration. Controlled DCD occurs after the planned withdrawal of life-sustaining therapy. Uncontrolled DCD refers to organ procurement occurring after unexpected circulatory arrest and unsuccessful cardiopulmonary resuscitation. The majority of DCDs in the United States are controlled. Evaluation of a potential DCD donor includes assessing the patient's hemodynamic stability and respiratory drive (i.e., negative inspiratory force [NIF], tidal volume, respiratory rate, and oxygen saturation on room air) in conjunction with his or her age, past medical history, and mechanism of injury.

(D) Federal regulations enacted in 1998 require hospitals to report all deaths and imminent deaths to their federally designated organ procurement organization (OPO). The definition of imminent death is mutually agreed upon by a hospital and its OPO and may be defined by parameters such as any mechanically ventilated patient with a Glasgow Coma Score of 5 or less who is going to be withdrawn from life support. Contacting the OPO allows a procurement coordinator to evaluate the potential donor for suitability before approaching a family for consent.

(E) Consent for organ donation is typically obtained from the patient's next of kin, (e.g., spouse, adult child, or parent). Some countries have "presumed consent" that gives automatic consent for organ donation unless the patient specifically indicated no wish to be an organ donor. In the United States several mechanisms have been established to indicate the patient's donation wishes; these include a signed driver's license, durable power of attorney for health care, living wills, and donor registries. Federal regulations require that any individual requesting organ donation must have completed a training course approved by a federally designated OPO. These "designated requestors" approach the family and offer the option of donation. Studies demonstrate that the request for donation should be decoupled from the notification of death. In other words, the family should be given time to grieve before being offered the option of donation.

(F) The evaluation of a cadaveric organ donor includes a medical history, physical examination, and laboratory studies. The main goals are first to exclude donors with diseases that can be transmitted to the recipient; and second to exclude organs that may have compromised function. Absolute contraindications to donation include positive HIV serologies, systemic infection, and widespread malignancy. Possible heart and lung donors should undergo an echocardiogram and bronchoscopy.

(G) Because of a continuing shortage of organ donors, the use of extended or marginal donors has become more common. The presence of vascular abnormalities, arterial hypertension, prolonged cold ischemia, extremes of age, hepatitis B or C, and mild renal diseases have previously been considered absolute contraindications to organ donation. Most transplant centers will now utilize these organ donors and accept a higher incidence of delayed graft function. However, long-term function of these grafts appears to be equivalent to other donors.

(H) Management of the potential multi-organ donor involves keeping the body in a homeostatic state until organ procurement can occur. Severe brain injury and brain death will often lead to multiple physiologic alterations. Hemodynamic instability is common because of the lack of circulating catecholamines and hypovolemia. Maintaining blood pressure through volume replacement and/or vasopressor support is necessary to adequately perfuse all organs. Hormone replacement with thyroxine or vasopressin has been shown to help stabilize labile blood pressures presumably caused by endocrine dysfunction associated with brain death. Hypothermia is common secondary to injury of the hypothalamus and may lead to cardiac instability, pulmonary edema, and/or coagulopathy. All potential organ donors are maintained on mechanical ventilation and must be continually monitored for adequate oxygenation. Aspiration, atelectasis, and neurogenic pulmonary edema are common problems in pulmonary management and require aggressive treatment. Diabetes insipidus (DI) from lack of endogenous antidiuretic hormone results in excessive urinary output and may further compromise donor stability becaue of hypovolemia and electrolyte imbalance. DI is typically treated with volume replacement and the use of desmopressin (DDAVP).

(I) Multi-organ procurement after neurologic death occurs in the operating room under controlled conditions. A combined median laparotomy and median sternotomy is the preferred approach regardless if the heart and lungs are to be procured. Critical dissection is preformed before cross clamping the aorta and perfusing the organs with preservation solution. The organs are removed and the final preparation is done on the back table. Procurement of DCD, or non–heart-beating donors, occurs after the withdrawal of life support by the primary team caring for the patient. Most centers will wait 1 to 2 hours after withdrawal of life support for death to occur; beyond that there is excessive ischemic damage to the organs. Death is pronounced based on cessation of circulation and respiration by a physician not involved with organ transplantation. Current guidelines recommend that a 5-minute period be observed after the cessation of circulation and respiration and before beginning organ recovery. Once the patient has been pronounced the abdomen and chest are rapidly

opened and the distal aorta cannulated. The organs are perfused with preservation solution and then removed en bloc.

(J) After evaluating each organ for suitability, the local OPO will register the potential organ donor with the United Network for Organ Sharing (UNOS). UNOS will then generate a recipient list for each organ being considered for transplantation. Each potential recipient listed for an organ is compared to the donor's parameters and receives a numerical score indicating degree of match. Points may be awarded for matching blood type, size, length of time waiting, prognosis, age, HLA typing, prior donation, and antibody sensitivity. The lists ranks individuals by point total first within the local transplant center(s), then at centers within the region, and finally with transplant centers nationwide. The organ is then allocated to the individual who is closest and best matches the donor. Each organ is allocated according to a specific algorithm.

For example, if an identical HLA match is found for a kidney, the potential recipient's transplant center will be offered that organ first regardless of geographical location.

REFERENCES

Alexander JW, Zola JC: Expanding the donor pool: Use of marginal donors for solid organ transplantation. Clin Transplant 10:1–19, 1996.

Delmuncio FJ: Cadaver Donor Management. In Norman DJ, Turka LA (eds): Primer on Transplantation, 2nd ed. Mt. Laurel, NJ: American Society of Transplantation, 2001.

Non–heart-beating organ transplantation: Practice and protocols. Committee on non–heart-beating transplantation IIL: The scientific and ethical basis for practice and protocols. Division of Health Care Services, Institute of Medicine, Washington, DC: National Academy Press, 1999.

Pratschke J, Wilhelm MJ, Kusaka M et al: Brain death and its influence on donor organ quality and outcome after transplantation. Transplantation 67(3):343–348, 1999.

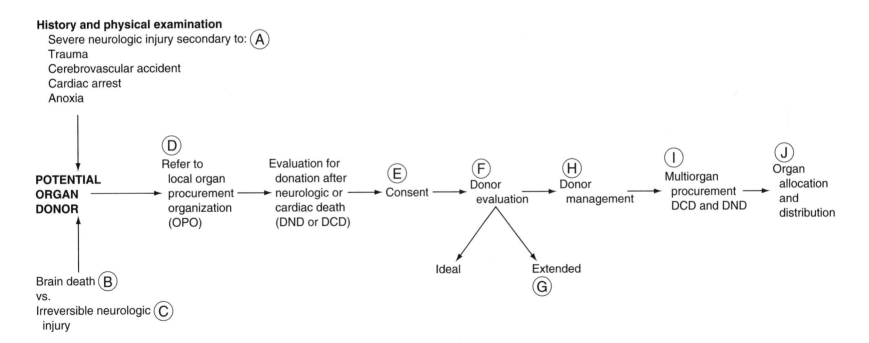

UROLOGY

Chapter 122 *Ureteral and Renal Calculi*

RANDALL B. MEACHAM, MD • ALEX J. VANNI, MD

A Patients with ureteral stones often present with severe renal colic secondary to obstruction of urinary flow. The pain is often intense, and typically it "crescendoes." Fever is a sign of urinary sepsis and must be treated as a medical emergency.

B Provided the patient is adequately hydrated, 80% of ureteral stones smaller than 5 mm in greatest diameter pass spontaneously, whereas only 10% of stones larger than 10 mm do. If at any time during this period the patient becomes febrile, ureteral obstruction must be relieved by one of several means to avoid life-threatening septic shock. If the patient is vomiting and cannot be hydrated, or if the pain is intractable, obstruction should also be relieved by operation.

C Some 10% of stones are radiolucent; such stones are typically composed of uric acid. Individuals with uric acid stones generally maintain urinary pH below 6.0, and these stones can be dissolved via urinary alkalinization. Alkalinization is best achieved by oral medication such as sodium bicarbonate or potassium citrate.

D The proximal ureter extends from the kidney to the superior aspect of the bony pelvis. The midureter extends from there to the inferior margin of the bony pelvis. The distal segment extends to the trigone.

E Stones in the proximal ureter are best treated with extracorporeal shockwave lithotripsy (ESWL).

F Patients who present with fever and ureteral stones should be hospitalized. They can then be vigorously hydrated; closely monitored; and, after obtaining urine and blood culture, treated with broad-spectrum antimicrobials that should cover both anaerobes and aerobes.

G Lower pole stones 1 cm or less in diameter; and upper pole, middle calyx, and renal pelvic stones 2 cm or less in diameter respond well to ESWL.

H Lower pole stones larger than 1 cm and all stones larger than 2 cm in diameter are usually treated with percutaneous nephrolithotripsy.

I Patients without calyceal stenosis, diverticula, or severe obstruction can be treated with ESWL. Multiple treatments are usually necessary.

J Very large staghorn stones and those with calyceal scarring are usually treated by open surgical stone removal.

K Staghorn stones associated with very poor function (i.e., creatinine clearance less than 15 ml/min) often require nephrectomy.

L Although stones in the distal ureter can be treated using ESWL, stones overlying the bony pelvis may be difficult to visualize and target, and thus may require ureteroscopic removal.

M Percutaneous nephrostomy under radiographic guidance may be necessary to provide drainage. If that approach is unsuccessful, cystoscopy with retrograde placement of a ureteral stent past the obstruction is required.

N Patients with stones larger than 2 cm in diameter may require a combination of ESWL and percutaneous nephrolithotripsy.

O Staghorn stones can also be treated with percutaneous stone extraction, but this may involve multiple procedures. This may be combined with ESWL.

P A perinephric fluid collection should be drained percutaneously under radiographic guidance.

Q If fever persists despite a ureteral stent, position and adequacy of drainage by the stent or the percutaneous nephrostomy should be checked by ultrasound.

REFERENCES

Dawson C, Whitfield H: ABC of urology: Urinary stone disease (review). Br Med J 312:1219–1221, 1996.

Eisenberger F, Schmidt A: ESWL and the future of stone management (review). Wld J Urol 11:2–6, 1993.

Gleeson MJ, Griffith DP: Struvite calculi (review). Br J Urol 71:503–511, 1993.

Lingeman JE, Preminger GM (eds): New Developments in the Management of Urolithiasis. New York: Igaku-Shoin, 1996.

Pardalidis NP, Kosmaoglon EV, Kapotis CG: Endoscopy vs. extracorporeal shockwave lithotripsy in the treatment of distal ureteral stones: Ten years experience. J Endourol 12:161–164, 1999.

Politis G, Griffith DP: ESWL: Stone-free efficacy based upon stone size and location. Wld J Urol 5:255, 1987.

Sorensen CM, Chandhoke PS: Is lower pole calyceal anatomy predictive of initial treatment or retreatment success for extracorporeal shockwave lithotripsy of primary lower pole kidney stones? 3 Urol 168:2377–2382, 2002.

Wickham JE: Treatment of urinary tract stones (review). Br Med J 307:1414–1417, 1993.

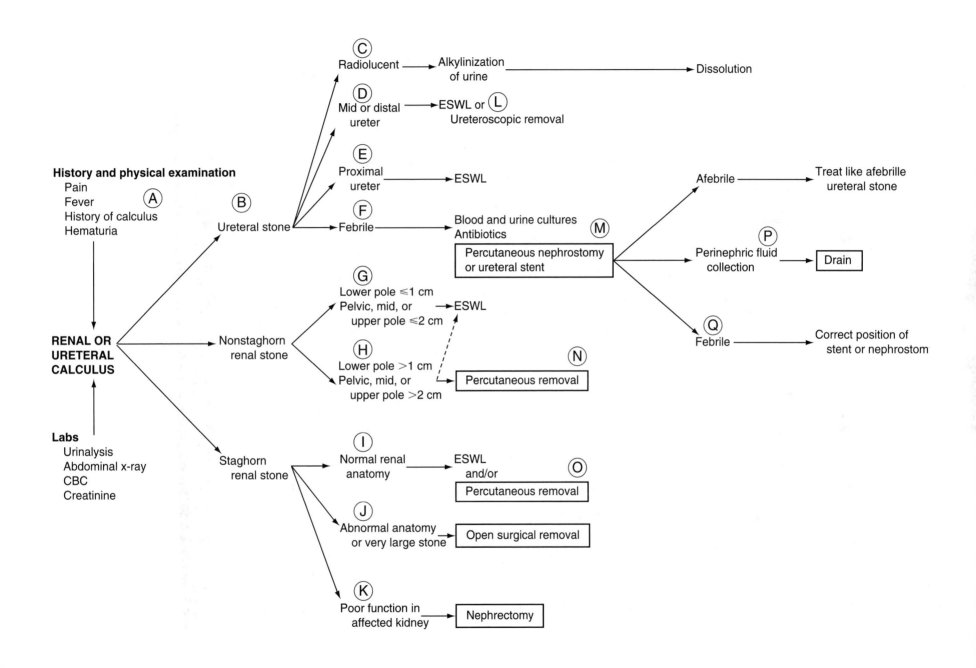

Chapter 123 *Renal Mass*

ROBERT C. FLANIGAN, MD

(A) A renal mass is usually detected by intravenous pyelography (IVP), renal ultrasound (US), abdominal computed tomography (CT) scan, or magnetic resonance imaging (MRI). Masses can generally be divided into solid and cystic varieties.

(B) Special caution should be used when using iodinated contrast media in patients with impaired renal function. In such situations, renal US, transesophageal US (to assess vena caval involvement), and MRI may be indicated.

(C) The radiographic tests most often used to evaluate a renal mass include IVP, US, and CT. Typically, a patient with hematuria or urinary tract infection is evaluated with an IVP and cystoscopy. If the IVP suggests a renal cystic lesion, abdominal US should be used to confirm the "simple" character of the cyst. If on IVP the mass appears solid or equivocal, CT examination of the abdomen should be undertaken.

(D) A simple renal cyst is the most common renal mass. When such a cyst has a smooth, thin wall, is filled with fluid, and does not contain septa or calcifications, it is nearly always benign. A simple cyst can grow very large and cause symptoms. A cystic renal mass can also be a parapelvic cyst, a multilobulated cyst, or cystic renal cell cancer.

(E) A solid renal mass must be considered carcinoma until proven otherwise. Other solid renal masses are angiomyolipomas, oncocytomas, lobar nephromas, xanthogranulometric pyelonephritis, hypertrophic columns of Bertin, and renal abscesses. Renal cell carcinoma (RCC) is the most common renal malignancy, but transitional cell cancer (TCC) of the renal pelvis and calyces is also common. The distinction between these lesions is important because the surgical treatment of each

is different. Both RCC and TCC can present with hematuria or flank pain. Factors in the history or physical examination that increase the suspicion of RCC are family history of RCC, tuberous sclerosis, a new varicocele, erythrocytosis, hypercalcemia, and calcification within the mass. Other malignant solid renal masses include leukemia, lymphoma, and metastatic lesions (most often secondary to lung or breast cancer).

(F) Under special circumstances, evaluation of a renal mass may involve needle biopsy or percutaneous drainage of the mass. A cyst that does not meet the criteria of a simple cyst or one that produces symptoms can be percutaneously aspirated, the fluid being sent for cell count, cytology, and culture. A suspected renal abscess should be drained percutaneously and the fluid sent for culture and Gram stain.

(G) Several solid renal masses display characteristic radiologic appearances that are helpful in diagnosis. Angiomyolipomas have a characteristic fat density on CT. This finding may make further evaluation unnecessary. Oncocytomas often display a characteristic central necrosis with a "spoke-wheel" appearance but, in general, this finding is not sufficient to rule out renal cancer. Xanthogranulomatous pyelonephritis is suggested by the presence of a solid renal mass with abscess formation and an associated renal collecting system calculus.

(H) If an RCC is suspected on CT, the renal vein and inferior vena cava must be delineated to rule out venous tumor thrombus. If CT is inconclusive, MRI or inferior venacavography should be done. Renal angiography, once a mainstay for evaluating solid renal masses, is seldom required today.

Occasionally this invasive and expensive technique is required to study an indeterminate mass, to identify tumor neovascularity, to delineate vascular distribution before nephron-sparing renal surgery, or in conjunction with preoperative arterial embolization of very large renal cancers. However, CT angiography or magnetic resonance angiography are typically able to provide the same information without the need for invasive access to the vascular system. Percutaneous renal biopsy should not be performed on solid renal masses unless it is necessary to resolve a diagnostic dilemma. Such biopsies can cause bleeding and occasionally tumor spillage.

(I) If a renal TCC is suspected, additional evaluation, including retrograde pyelography, brush biopsy, or ureteroscopy (with or without biopsy), may be helpful. Because the treatment for RCC (radical nephrectomy) differs from that for TCC (nephroureterectomy), this distinction is very important.

(J) The treatment of a solid renal mass suggestive of RCC is radical nephrectomy. Nephron-sparing surgery is an option in small (less than 5 cm), peripheral, or polar lesions that on CT appear to be confined to the kidney and not to extend beyond the renal capsule or to regional lymph nodes.

REFERENCES

Balfe DM, McClennan BL, Stanley RJ et al: Evaluation of renal masses considered indeterminate on computed tomography. Radiology 142:421–428, 1982.

Bosniak M: The current radiological approach to renal cysts. Radiology 158:1–10, 1986.

Radford MG Jr., Donadio JV Jr., Holley KE et al: Renal biopsy in clinical practice. Mayo Clin Proc 69:983–984, 1994.

Van Baal JG, Smits NJ, Keeman JN et al: The evolution of renal angiomyolipomas in patients with tuberous sclerosis. J Urol 152:35–38, 1994.

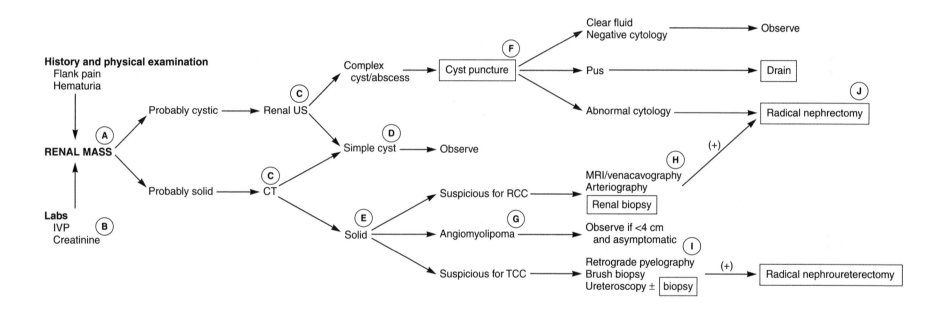

History and physical examination
Flank pain
Hematuria

RENAL MASS Ⓐ

Probably cystic ⟶ Renal US Ⓒ

Probably solid ⟶ CT Ⓒ

Labs Ⓑ
IVP
Creatinine

Complex cyst/abscess ⟶ Cyst puncture Ⓕ

Clear fluid
Negative cytology ⟶ Observe

Pus ⟶ Drain

Abnormal cytology ⟶ Radical nephrectomy Ⓙ

Simple cyst Ⓓ ⟶ Observe

Solid Ⓔ

Suspicious for RCC ⟶ MRI/venacavography
Arteriography Ⓗ
Renal biopsy

(+) ⟶ Radical nephrectomy

Angiomyolipoma Ⓖ ⟶ Observe if <4 cm
and asymptomatic Ⓘ

Suspicious for TCC ⟶ Retrograde pyelography
Brush biopsy
Ureteroscopy ± biopsy

(+) ⟶ Radical nephroureterectomy

Chapter 124 *Bladder Tumor*

GARY D. GROSSFELD, MD • PETER R. CARROLL, MD

(A) The most common presenting symptom of bladder cancer is gross, painless hematuria. Patients may also present with symptoms of bladder irritability (e.g., urinary frequency, urgency, and dysuria); microscopic hematuria; flank pain from ureteral obstruction; a pelvic mass; or symptoms of advanced disease, including weight loss and bone pain. Physical examination should include a complete abdominal examination, digital rectal examination, and bimanual pelvic examination.

(B) Approximately 56,500 new cases of bladder cancer will be diagnosed every year. It is the fifth most common noncutaneous malignancy, and second most common genitourinary tract malignancy in the United States. Bladder cancer is more common in men and is diagnosed more often in whites than in African Americans. Risk factors include cigarette smoking, industrial exposure to arylamines, heavy use of analgesics, and previous treatment with cyclophosphamide or pelvic radiation.

(C) Evaluation for all patients with gross hematuria should include urinalysis and culture, urine cytology, and radiographic imaging of the upper urinary tracts. Upper tract tumors occur in 2% to 4% of patients with bladder cancer. Hydronephrosis may be indicative of a muscle-invasive bladder tumor. Ultrasound is less invasive and less costly than intravenous pyelography (IVP), but the collecting system and ureter are better visualized with IVP. Computed tomography (CT) can also evaluate the kidneys and collecting system. The sensitivity of urine cytology varies between 40% and 70%, depending upon the grade of the tumor (i.e., increased sensitivity with higher-grade disease).

(D) Cystoscopy is used for the diagnosis of bladder cancer. Initial treatment is transurethral (cystoscopic) resection of bladder tumor (TURBT). All visible tumor should be resected. Resection continues to the base of the tumor, where a portion of the muscularis propria of the bladder wall should be resected to determine depth of invasion. Random biopsy specimens of grossly uninvolved bladder mucosa are also taken, because carcinoma in situ or dysplasia in sites adjacent to or distant from the primary tumor can predict increased likelihood of tumor recurrence. A bimanual examination should be performed with the patient under anesthesia to determine the extent and mobility of any pelvic mass.

(E) Bladder tumors are staged according to the TNM system as follows:

T0	No tumor in the specimen
Tis	Carcinoma in situ
Ta	Non-invasive papillary tumor (limited to the epithelial lining of the bladder)
T1	Tumor invasion into the lamina propria
T2a	Tumor invades superficial muscle
T2b	Tumor invades deep muscle
T3a	Microscopic invasion of perivesical tissue
T3b	Macroscopic invasion of perivesical tissue
T4a	Invasion of contiguous organ(s) (e.g., prostate, vagina, uterus)
T4b	Tumor invades pelvic wall, abdominal wall
N0	No regional lymph node metastases
N1-3	Involvement of lymph nodes
M0	No distant metastasis
M1	Distant metastasis

(F) Approximately 80% of patients with bladder cancer have superficial disease (i.e., stages Tis, Ta, or T1). The risk of distant disease is low in such patients. Tumor recurs in 50% to 70% of patients with superficial bladder cancer, whereas progression to a higher stage of disease occurs in 10% to 15%. Risk factors for recurrence and progression include tumor grade, tumor stage (Ta versus T1), the number of tumors at presentation, atypia or carcinoma in situ adjacent to the primary tumor or on random biopsy, and the presence of tumor at the first follow-up cystoscopy (3 months).

(G) Superficial papillary tumors should be treated by complete transurethral resection. In very rare cases the tumor may not be amenable to TURBT because of size or location, and partial cystectomy is appropriate. When partial cystectomy is performed, the remainder of the bladder must be free of both carcinoma in situ and additional tumors, and clear surgical margins must be obtained.

(H) Patients with muscle-invasive bladder cancer should undergo a complete staging evaluation including a CT scan of the abdomen and pelvis, chest x-ray, and bone scan. The most common sites of metastasis for invasive bladder cancer include regional lymph nodes, liver, lung, and bone.

(I) Patients with superficial disease who are at a low risk for tumor recurrence require no additional treatment after complete TURBT. These patients should be monitored closely. In patients with superficial disease who are at moderate or high risk for tumor recurrence or progression, intravesical chemotherapy or immunotherapy is warranted. Chemotherapeutic agents commonly used in the United States include thiotepa, doxorubicin, and mitomycin-C. There is no compelling evidence to suggest that one of these drugs is significantly better than the others. Recent studies have examined the utility of a single perioperative dose of intravesical chemotherapy at the time of TURBT because of concern that tumor cell implantation at the time of endoscopic resection may contribute to recurrence.

Intravesical immunotherapy with bacillus Calmette-Guérin (BCG) decreases the rate of recurrence and progression for patients with superficial bladder cancer. Intravesical BCG is currently the

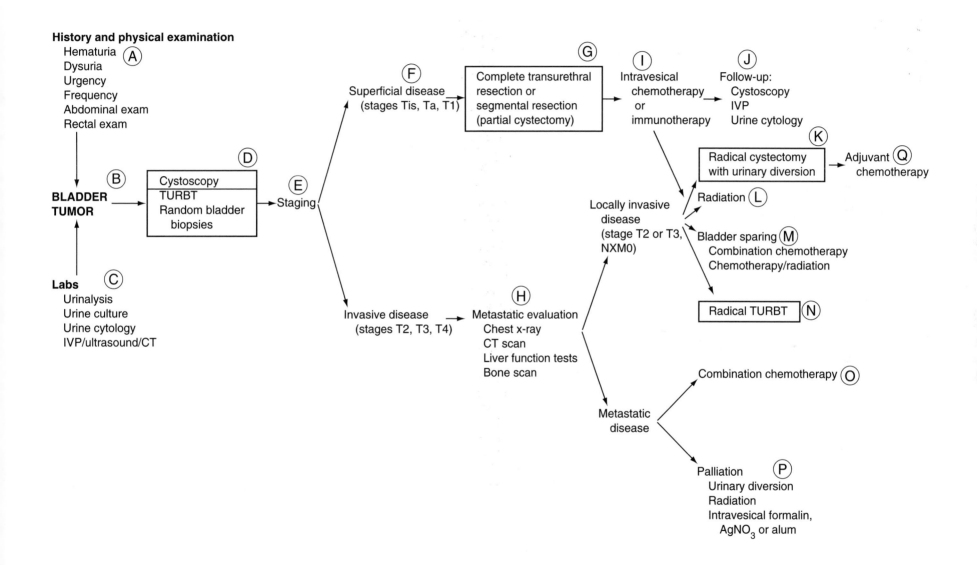

History and physical examination
Hematuria (A)
Dysuria
Urgency
Frequency
Abdominal exam
Rectal exam

BLADDER TUMOR (B)

Labs (C)
Urinalysis
Urine culture
Urine cytology
IVP/ultrasound/CT

Cystoscopy (D)
TURBT
Random bladder
biopsies

Staging (E)

Superficial disease (F)
(stages Tis, Ta, T1)

Complete transurethral (G)
resection or
segmental resection
(partial cystectomy)

Intravesical (I)
chemotherapy
or
immunotherapy

Follow-up: (J)
Cystoscopy
IVP
Urine cytology

Radical cystectomy (K)
with urinary diversion

Adjuvant (Q)
chemotherapy

Locally invasive
disease
(stage T2 or T3,
NXM0)

Radiation (L)

Bladder sparing (M)
Combination chemotherapy
Chemotherapy/radiation

Radical TURBT (N)

Invasive disease
(stages T2, T3, T4)

Metastatic evaluation (H)
Chest x-ray
CT scan
Liver function tests
Bone scan

Metastatic
disease

Combination chemotherapy (O)

Palliation (P)
Urinary diversion
Radiation
Intravesical formalin,
    $AgNO_3$ or alum

treatment of choice for patients with carcinoma in situ of the bladder, with complete response rates in excess of 70%. Therefore a trial of intravesical BCG is appropriate for patients with a high risk of disease progression, including those with carcinoma in situ or high-grade, stage T1 disease.

Ⓙ Following TURBT, patients with superficial bladder cancer should undergo surveillance cystoscopy every 3 months for 2 years, every 6 months for 2 years, and then yearly for life. Annual or biannual screening of the upper tracts has also been recommended.

Ⓚ Radical cystectomy with pelvic lymph node dissection (to include complete excision of the bladder, prostate, and seminal vesicles in men and complete excision of the bladder, uterus, ovaries, and fallopian tubes in women) remains the gold standard for treatment of patients with muscle-invasive bladder cancer. Five-year recurrence-free survival is 80% to 90% for stage p1 to p2N0, 60% to 80% for stage p3N0, and 50% for stage p4N0 disease. Lymph node metastases are found in 20% to 35% of patients undergoing radical cystectomy, with 5-year disease-free survival ranging from 10% to 35%, depending upon the extent of lymph node involvement and T-stage of the primary tumor.

The type of urinary diversion performed following radical cystectomy depends upon patient preference and the ability to preserve the urethra at surgery. Urethrectomy is recommended for male patients with tumor involving the prostatic stroma or anterior urethra, and for female patients with tumor involving either the anterior vaginal wall or urethra. If the urethra can be preserved, bladder replacement using a continent intestinal reservoir is preferred by most patients. If a urethrectomy is necessary, or if the patient is not a good candidate for bladder replacement, a cutaneous diversion should be performed.

Ⓛ Radiation (6000 to 7000 cGY) has been used as a single modality treatment for patients who are poor surgical candidates because of advanced age or concurrent medical problems. Five-year survival rates for stages T2 through T4

disease range from 16% to 41%. Local recurrence is common, occurring in 33% to 68% of patients.

Ⓜ Several groups have reported on a bladder-sparing treatment approach for selected patients with muscle-invasive bladder cancer. After complete TURBT, patients are given combination chemotherapy followed by concomitant chemotherapy and radiation. Early cystectomy is offered to patients who do not tolerate chemotherapy or radiation and to those in whom a complete response is not achieved. Complete response is seen in 50% to 70% of patients, but local recurrence exceeds 50%. Five-year overall survival rates are approximately 50% to 60%, with 18% to 44% of patients alive with an intact bladder at 5 years.

Ⓝ A select group of patients with minimally invasive bladder cancer may benefit from "radical" TURBT performed by an experienced urologist. This treatment is appropriate only for a highly selected patient population.

Ⓞ Approximately 15% of patients with bladder cancer have regional or distant metastases at presentation. Combination chemotherapy with MVAC (methotrexate, vinblastine, Adriamycin, and cisplatin) has proven to be the most effective treatment for these patients, with overall response rates of 60% to 70% and complete response rates as high as 35%. However, there is significant toxicity, and a sustained response is seen in only 10% of patients. Gemcitabine and cisplatin may have equivalent efficacy with significantly less toxicity than MVAC.

Ⓟ Patients with disseminated bladder cancer may suffer with persistent gross hematuria, dysuria, urinary urgency, bone pain, and bladder or pelvic pain. Palliative radiation may control local bladder symptoms or bone pain from metastases. Intravesical alum, silver nitrate, or formalin may be given to control hematuria. In rare situations, a palliative urinary diversion (with or without cystectomy) may be performed to alleviate refractory local symptoms.

Ⓠ Chemotherapy may be given before or after radical cystectomy in an attempt to improve

progression-free and overall survival. Neoadjuvant chemotherapy before surgery may improve outcomes when compared with surgery alone for patients with invasive bladder cancer. Chemotherapy may also be given after surgery to patients with extravesical disease extension (i.e., stages P3, P4, and N+). Because there have been no prospective randomized trials addressing this issue, strict recommendations regarding the use of adjuvant chemotherapy cannot be made.

REFERENCES

Cookson MS, Herr HW, Zhang ZF et al: The treated natural history of high-risk superficial bladder cancer: 15-year outcome. J Urol 158:62–67, 1997.

Grossfeld GD, Litwin MS, Wolf JS et al: Evaluation of asymptomatic microscopic hematuria in adults: The American Urological Association best practice policy-part I: Definition, detection, prevalence and etiology. Urology 57:599–603, 2001.

Grossfeld GD, Litwin MS, Wolf JS et al: Evaluation of asymptomatic microscopic hematuria in adults: The American Urological Association best practice policy-part II: Patient evaluation, cytology, voided markers, imaging, cystoscopy, nephrology evaluation and follow-up. Urology 57:604–610, 2001.

Herr HW: Tumor progression and survival of patients with high grade, noninvasive papillary (TaG3) bladder tumors: 15-year outcome. J Urol 163:60–61, 2000.

Kachnic LA, Kaufman DS, Heney NM et al: Bladder preservation by combined modality therapy for invasive bladder cancer. J Clin Oncol 15:1022–1029, 1997.

Natale RB, Grossman HB, Blumenstein BA et al: SWOG 8710 (INT-0080): Randomized phase III trial of neoadjuvant MVAC+cystectomy versus cystectomy alone in patients with locally advanced bladder cancer. Proc Amer Soc Clin Oncol 20:2a (abstract), 2001.

Stein JP, Lieskovsky G, Cote R et al: Radical cystectomy in the treatment of invasive bladder cancer: Long-term results in 1054 patients. J Clin Oncol 19:666–675, 2001.

Stockle M, Meyenburg W, Wellek S et al: Adjuvant polychemotherapy of nonorgan-confined bladder cancer after radical cystectomy revisited: Long-term results of a controlled prospective study and further clinical experience. J Urol 153:47–52, 1995.

Von der Maase H, Hansen SW, Roberts JT et al: Gemcitabine and cisplatin versus methotrexate, vinblastine, doxorubicin, and cisplatin in advanced or metastatic bladder cancer: Results of a large, randomized, multinational, multicenter phase III study. J Clin Oncol 17:3068–3077, 2000.

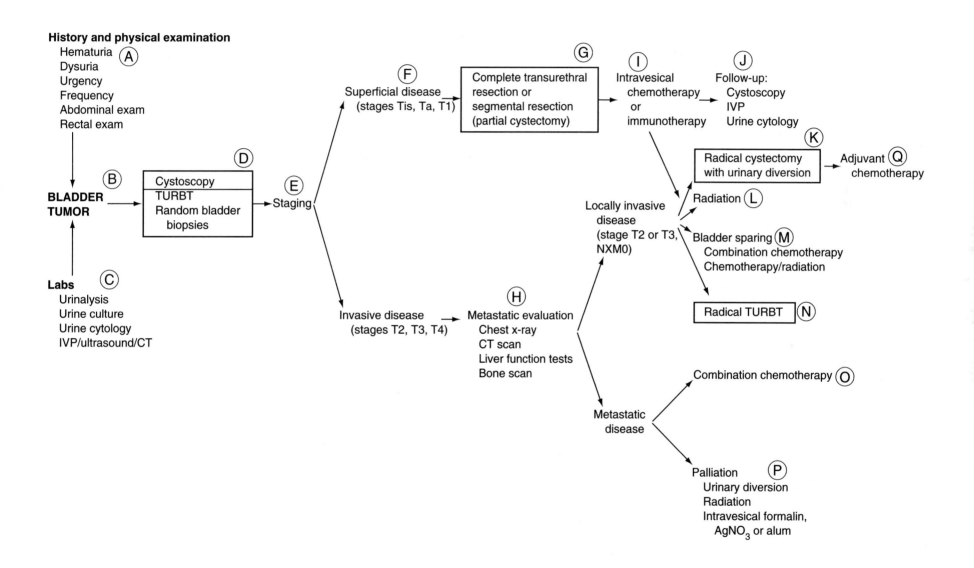

History and physical examination
Hematuria (A)
Dysuria
Urgency
Frequency
Abdominal exam
Rectal exam

(B)
BLADDER TUMOR

(D)
Cystoscopy
TURBT
Random bladder
 biopsies

Labs (C)
Urinalysis
Urine culture
Urine cytology
IVP/ultrasound/CT

(E)
Staging

Superficial disease (F)
(stages Tis, Ta, T1)

Invasive disease
(stages T2, T3, T4)

(G)
Complete transurethral
resection or
segmental resection
(partial cystectomy)

Intravesical (I)
chemotherapy
 or
immunotherapy

Follow-up: (J)
Cystoscopy
IVP
Urine cytology

(H)
Metastatic evaluation
Chest x-ray
CT scan
Liver function tests
Bone scan

Locally invasive
disease
(stage T2 or T3,
NXM0)

Radical cystectomy (K)
with urinary diversion

Adjuvant (Q)
chemotherapy

Radiation (L)

Bladder sparing (M)
Combination chemotherapy
Chemotherapy/radiation

Radical TURBT (N)

Metastatic
disease

Combination chemotherapy (O)

Palliation (P)
Urinary diversion
Radiation
Intravesical formalin,
 $AgNO_3$ or alum

Chapter 125 *Prostatism*

JOHN A. WHITESEL, MD

(A) "Prostatism" refers to symptoms secondary to prostatic hyperplasia: urinary frequency and urgency, decreased size and force of urine stream, nocturia, and incontinence. Bladder outlet obstruction can lead to voiding dysfunction including retention, infection, and azotemia.

(B) A prostatic nodule or induration may indicate cancer and should be investigated.

(C) Irritative symptoms (dysuria) plus obstructive symptoms may be caused by prostatitis or by a combination of hyperplasia and prostatitis (bladder tumor, stone, and prostatic carcinoma would be differential).

(D) Biopsy of the prostate is usually done transrectally with a core needle device under ultrasound (US) guidance. It can also be done transperineally, guided by a finger in the rectum; or transurethrally, using a resectoscope. In the US, cancer is commonly hypoechoic, but it can be hyper- or isoechoic. Repeat biopsies are necessary if the first biopsy is negative. The first biopsy finds 75% of prostate cancers, the second finds 20%, and the third usually finds the remaining 5%.

(E) Prostatic hyperplasia causing symptoms without significant obstruction can be managed with α-adrenergic blockers. The 5-α-reductase inhibitors can shrink large prostates by 20% to 30% and thus increase urinary flow rate. Very little shrinkage is obtained with small fibrotic prostates having less glandular structure. Antiandrogens and luteinizing hormone–releasing hormone (LHRH) agonists can also reduce prostate size and increase urinary flow rate in many cases, but impotence and decreased libido are common complications. Hyperthermia (in various techniques), lasers (several types), and cryotherapy are evolving techniques currently being utilized to relieve significant bladder outlet obstruction. The principal methods of controlling urinary tract infection from prostatic hyperplasia remain open simple prostatectomy (e.g., retropubic, suprapubic, or perineal); transurethral resection of the prostate (TURP); and transurethral

incision of the prostate (TUIP). Urethral stents may be useful for debilitated patients, but they must be further refined. Balloon dilation of the prostatic urethra has fallen into disuse because the technique gives only temporary or minimal results.

(F) Median bar obstruction of the bladder outlet results from fibromuscular hypertrophy of the posterior bladder neck–prostate junction. It can develop at any age and is often the cause of bladder obstruction in younger men. Relief of symptoms and some increase in urine flow rates can be achieved with α-adrenergic blockers. Success delays surgery in younger men and preserves fertility by avoiding retrograde ejaculation. Definitive treatment involves TURP or TUIP of the median bar. The former is associated with greater flow rates, but the majority of patients have retrograde ejaculation. After TUIP, the majority of patients have antegrade ejaculation, so the anatomic mechanism of fertility is preserved. Hyperthermia, lasers, and cryotherapy treat prostatic hyperplasia more effectively than they treat median bar obstruction.

(G) Bacterial prostatitis is best treated with pathogen-specific antibiotics directed by the results of urine cultures or expressed prostatic secretions. Nonbacterial prostatitis (NBP) is treated symptomatically with sitz baths; avoidance of alcohol and caffeine; and, after the acute stage, massage. NBP is commonly resistant to cure and is prone to recur if a specific cause is not identified. Chlamydia infection and trichomoniasis should be considered and treated if identified in recurrent prostatitis.

(H) Urethral stricture is always a possibility with lower urinary tract obstruction. It can be diagnosed via instrumentation, retrograde urethrography, or cystourethroscopy.

(I) Staging carcinoma of the prostate with digital rectal exam, prostate-specific antigen, serum enzymatic acid phosphatase, bone scan, skeletal x-rays, chest x-ray, and computed tomography (CT) or spiral CT determines further treatment. Transrectal US and transrectal coil CT plus magnetic resonance

imaging (MRI) provide some additional information for staging.

(J) Persistent debilitating prostatitis can be ameliorated by removing infected, inflamed tissue and abscesses.

(K) Neurologic causes of urologic symptoms are evaluated using urodynamic studies of cystometrics and a basic neurologic examination. Electromyography (EMG) and biothesiometry and uroflow may also be utilized.

(L) Urethral strictures are treated by judicious urethral dilation or direct-vision internal urethrotomy. Complicated or persistent strictures often require various types of urethroplasties. Urethral stents may be helpful, depending on the nature of the stricture and the patient's condition.

(M) Metastatic carcinoma of the prostate is treated to control symptoms, to limit progression, and to prevent complications. Therapy may include androgen ablation with estrogen, LHRH agonists, antiandrogens, or orchiectomy. Local radiation or systemic radioisotopes for pain control are used for short-term palliation. Hormone manipulation can help to relieve urethral obstruction caused by progressive prostatic carcinoma. If that is not successful, TURP is necessary.

(N) Pharmacologic treatment of outlet obstruction includes α-adrenergic blockers, diazepam, and possibly baclofen. An atonic neurogenic bladder can be helped with bethanechol chloride; but clean, intermittent, self-catheterization is best for severe cases. Reduction of outlet resistance by standard surgical techniques can improve emptying of a partially neurogenic bladder.

(O) Surgical treatment of prostatic obstruction is accomplished transurethrally or by open techniques (i.e., retropubic, suprapubic, or perineal), depending on the surgeon's experience and the size of the prostate. For larger glands or for intercurrent disease processes (e.g., stones or diverticula), an open technique is usually used. Cancer confined to the prostate currently is treated by radical retropubic

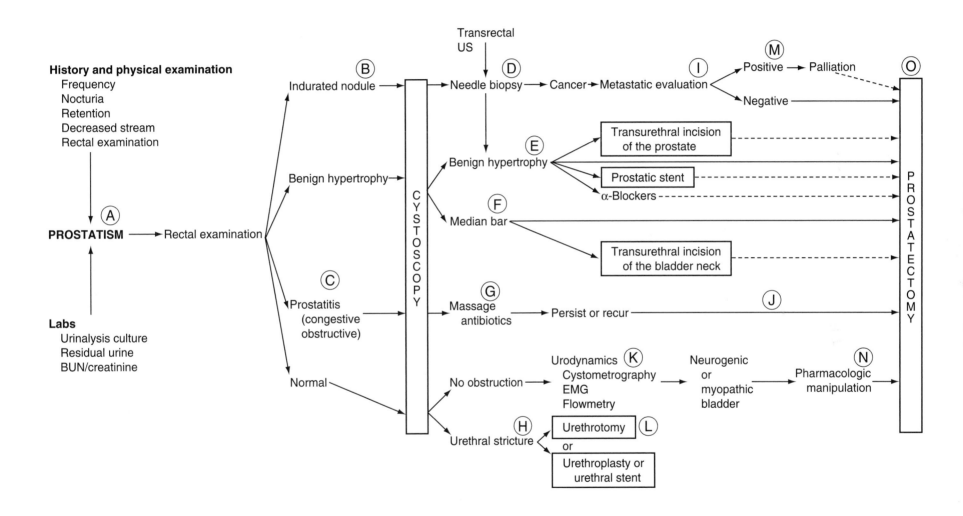

History and physical examination
Frequency
Nocturia
Retention
Decreased stream
Rectal examination

Ⓐ
PROSTATISM → Rectal examination

Labs
Urinalysis culture
Residual urine
BUN/creatinine

Ⓑ Indurated nodule →

Benign hypertrophy →

Ⓒ Prostatitis (congestive obstructive)

Normal

CYSTOSCOPY

Transrectal US
Ⓓ Needle biopsy → Cancer → Metastatic evaluation Ⓘ
Positive Ⓜ → Palliation
Negative →

Ⓔ Benign hypertrophy
Transurethral incision of the prostate
Prostatic stent
α-Blockers

Ⓕ Median bar
Transurethral incision of the bladder neck

Ⓖ Massage antibiotics → Persist or recur Ⓙ

No obstruction → Urodynamics Ⓚ Cystometrography EMG Flowmetry → Neurogenic or myopathic bladder → Pharmacologic manipulation Ⓝ

Ⓗ Urethral stricture
Urethrotomy Ⓛ
or
Urethroplasty or urethral stent

PROSTATECTOMY Ⓞ

or perineal prostatectomy, radiation therapy, or observation depending on patient's physical condition and preference. Cryotherapy and thermal therapy are evolving processes.

REFERENCES

Abrams P, Blaivas J, Griffiths D et al: The Objective Evaluation of Bladder Outlet Obstruction (Urodynamics). In The Second International Consultation of Benign Prostatic Hyperplasia (BPH). Channel Islands: Scientific Communications International, 1993.

Ball AJ, Feneley RCL, Abrams PH: The natural history of untreated prostatism. Br J Urol 53:613, 1981.

Barry MJ: Epidemiology and Natural History of Benign Prostatic Hyperplasia. AUA Update Series, Vol. XII, Lesson 2. Houston: American Urologic Association, Office of Education, 1993.

Kapoor DA, Randy PK: Surgical Alternatives to TURP in the Management of BPH. AUA Update Series, Vol. III, Lesson 3. Houston: American Urologic Association, Office of Education, 1993.

McConnell J, Barry M, Bruskewitz R et al: Benign Prostatic Hyperplasia: Diagnosis and Treatment Clinical Practice Guidelines. No. 8. AHCPR Publications No. 94-0582. Rockville, MD: Agency for Health Care Policy and Research, Public Health Service, U.S. Department of Health and Human Services, 1994.

Roehl KA, Antenor AV, Catalona WJ: Serial biopsy in prostate cancer screening study. J Urol 167:2435–2439, 2002.

Vaughan ED Jr., Lepor H: Medical Management of BPH, Part I. AUA Update Series, Vol. XV, Lesson 3 and 4. Houston: American Urologic Association, Office of Education, 1996.

Whitesel JA, Donohue RE, Mani JH, et al: Acid phosphatase: Its influence on the management of carcinoma of the prostate. J Urol 131:70, 1984.

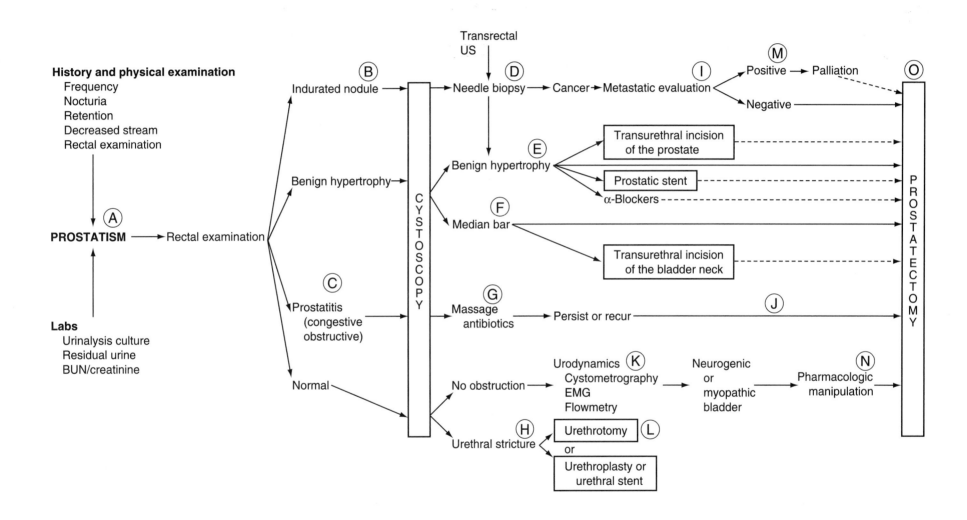

Chapter 126 Staging and Management of Prostate Cancer

BADRINATH R. KONETY, MD, MBA • RICHARD D. WILLIAMS, MD

(A) Prostate cancer is the most common malignancy affecting men in the United States, with an estimated 189,000 cases and 30,200 deaths resulting from it in 2002. The incidence of prostate cancer peaked in the early 1990s after the advent of widespread serum prostate specific antigen (PSA) based screening and diagnosis. The management paradigm usually accepted as standard of care for prostate cancer relies heavily on serum PSA, digital rectal examination (DRE), and biopsy Gleason sum assessments. A management approach of watchful waiting (noncurative intent) is a viable option in elderly men or those with substantial comorbidity who have low Gleason prostate cancer because disease progression and consequent mortality can be extremely low in these men. These individuals are more likely to succumb to intercurrent illness rather than prostate cancer, thereby rendering attempts at curative therapy, which harbor an inherent risk of side effects that may impact long-term quality of life, very unattractive. Men with metastatic disease can be managed with noncurative androgen deprivation therapy.

(B) The cornerstones of prostate cancer screening are serum PSA and DRE. Serum PSA using a normal cutoff of 4 ng/ml has a higher positive predictive value compared with DRE (33% vs. 20%).

(C) A patient with an abnormal serum PSA or an abnormal DRE should have a prostate needle biopsy performed using transrectal ultrasound (TRUS) guidance to establish a histologic diagnosis of prostate cancer. The standard is to obtain systematic sextant biopsies from the right and left sides of the prostate directed at the lateral portions of the peripheral zone. Prostate cancer is most commonly an adenocarcinoma and is graded according to the Gleason grading system (grade 1–5). Prostate cancer is a multifocal disease and different foci can be of different grades. A grade is assigned to the predominant and second most common pattern and

these are combined to yield a Gleason sum or score. Higher scores imply less differentiated cancers with poor prognosis. Prostate cancer is staged using the TNM staging system, with stages T1 (nonpalpable) and T2 (palpable nodule) indicating disease confined to the prostate and stage T3 indicating locally extensive disease outside the prostate or extending into the seminal vesicles. Stage T4 disease indicates spread to adjacent organs/structures. N0 indicates no nodal metastases, whereas N1 indicates presence of nodal metastases. M0 indicates absence of distant metastases, whereas M1 indicates the presence of metastases, most commonly to bones.

(D) Patients with clinical stage T1 or T2 disease who have a serum PSA less than 10 ng/ml and biopsy Gleason sum of 7 or less do not routinely require additional staging evaluation because the likelihood of radiographically detectable metastases is extremely low in this group.

(E) Patients with clinical T3 disease may benefit from an endorectal MRI to verify locally extensive disease and a laparoscopic/mini-lap pelvic lymphadenectomy to evaluate nodal disease status. They can then be offered external beam radiation therapy (EBRT) along with androgen ablation prior to and for an extended period after external beam radiation therapy.

(F) Patients who present with metastatic disease to the bones or soft tissue are primarily managed with androgen ablation therapy that, if instituted at the time of diagnosis, may improve survival.

(G) Patients with a biopsy Gleason sum of 8 to 10 or a serum PSA greater than 10 ng/ml will require a bone scan to rule out the presence of osteoblastic metastases from prostate cancer.

(H) Patients with a biopsy Gleason sum of 8 to 10, a PSA of greater than 20 ng/ml, or a palpable tumor outside the prostate (stage T3) may also benefit from a CT scan of the abdomen and pelvis to rule out regional nodal metastases. The use of endorectal

MRI, which is a very sensitive test, can yield useful information regarding local extent of disease, but the results have to be interpreted with caution because of a high false positive rate.

(I) Patients with clinical stage T1 or T2 disease who have a life expectancy of less than 10 years or severe comorbid illness can be managed with watchful waiting (serial follow-up with PSA and DRE). Healthy patients with clinical stage T1 or T2 disease who have a small volume, low Gleason score tumor (6 or less) and do not wish to be treated can be managed with watchful waiting as well.

(J) Stage T1 or T2 patients with a life expectancy greater than 10 years (and in particular, those that are healthy) are managed primarily with curative intent. They are candidates for radical prostatectomy performed by the retropubic, perineal, robotic, or laparoscopic approaches; or interstitial seed implantation (brachytherapy) and EBRT.

Brachytherapy performed using I^{125}, Pd^{103}, or Ir^{192} is typically used as a single modality approach in patients with serum PSA less than 10 ng/ml, biopsy tumor with Gleason score of 6 or less, and a prostate gland volume of 50 cc or less.

EBRT can be delivered using conformal 3-dimensional technique or intensity modulated approaches with a total dose of around 70 Gy. Higher doses result in increased toxicity (e.g., radiation cystitis and radiation proctitis but may improve cancer control rates).

Radical prostatectomy is performed with a bilateral nerve-sparing approach, especially in patients who are potent and have no palpable tumor. The main complications with a bilateral nerve sparing approach are incontinence (less than 5% of patients) and impotence (30% to 35%).

(K) Stage T1 or T2 patients with a serum PSA greater than 10 ng/ml or a biopsy showing

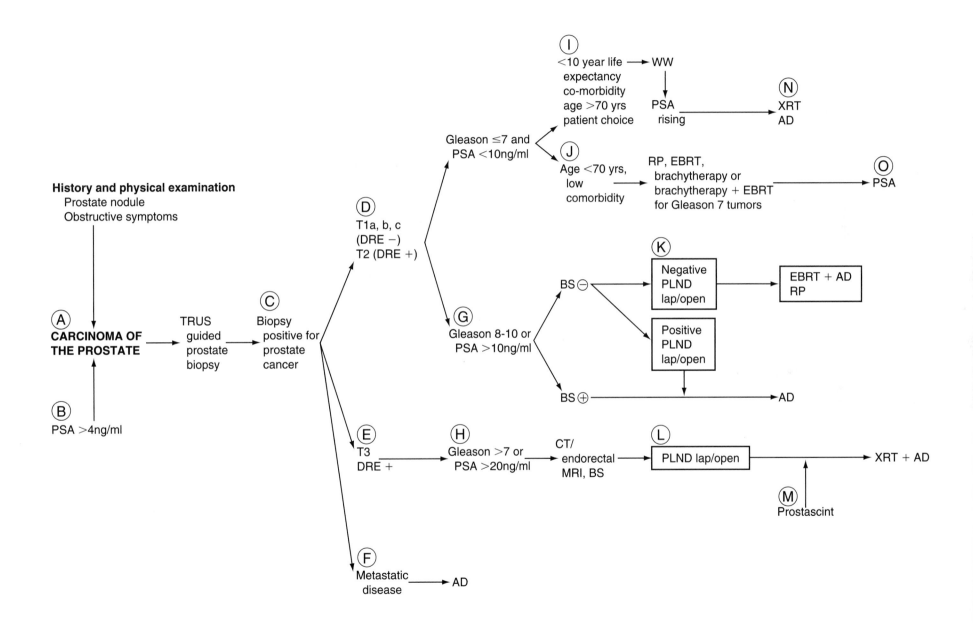

tumor with Gleason score of 8 to 10 will require a bone scan to rule out metastatic disease; they can be offered radical prostatectomy with pelvic lymphadenectomy or EBRT. Those who undergo EBRT will benefit from concomitant androgen ablation therapy for 1 to 2 months prior to and during radiation therapy.

(L) In patients who are found to have enlarged pelvic lymph nodes (i.e., greater than 1 cm by imaging criteria), a reasonable option is percutaneous needle biopsy of the enlarged lymph node to detect metastases. Alternatively, a pelvic lymph node dissection can be performed either through a mini-laparotomy incision or laparoscopically to evaluate the nodes for metastatic disease.

(M) In some situations where there is a high index of suspicion, a Prostascint scan, which uses a monoclonal antibody directed against the intracellular epitope of the prostate specific membrane antigen (PSMA), can be utilized to evaluate metastases to the lymph nodes and soft tissue.

(N) Patients who choose or are offered watchful waiting may benefit from close observation with annual DRE and PSA and offered intervention in the form of surgery (only for those younger than 70 years and with life expectancy greater than 10 years) or radiation if there is a palpable change or a PSA rise. Androgen deprivation (AD) therapy can be instituted in these patients by means of leutinizing hormone releasing hormone (LHRH) agonists (Lupron or Zoladex) or surgical castration if they develop evidence of metastatic disease or rapidly rising serum PSA.

(O) Serum PSA remains the mainstay for the follow-up of patients once diagnosed with prostate cancer. Undetectable levels (less than 0.03 ng/ml depending on the lower limit of sensitivity of the assay) are expected after radical prostatectomy. A nadir serum PSA less than 0.5 ng/ml after radiation therapy is associated with lower likelihood of biochemical recurrence. Cryotherapy of the prostate remains an option in patients who have local failure from radiation therapy, and as primary therapy in select individuals with clinically localized disease who are not candidates for the other modes of therapy.

REFERENCES

Bolla M, Collette L, Blank L et al: Long-term results with immediate androgen suppression and external irradiation in patients with locally advanced prostate cancer (an EORTC study): A phase III randomised trial. Lancet 360:103–106, 2002.

Critz FA, Levinson AK, Williams WH et al: The PSA nadir that indicates potential cure after radiotherapy for prostate cancer. Urology 49:322–326, 1997.

Jemal A, Thomas A, Murray T et al: Cancer statistics, 2002. CA Cancer J Clin 52:23-47, 2002.

Messing EM, Manola J, Sarosdy M et al: Immediate hormonal therapy compared with observation after radical prostatectomy and pelvic lymphadenectomy in men with node-positive prostate cancer. N Engl J Med 341:1781–1788, 1999.

Rabbani F, Stapleton AM, Kattan MW et al: Factors predicting recovery of erections after radical prostatectomy. J Urol 164:1929–1934, 2000.

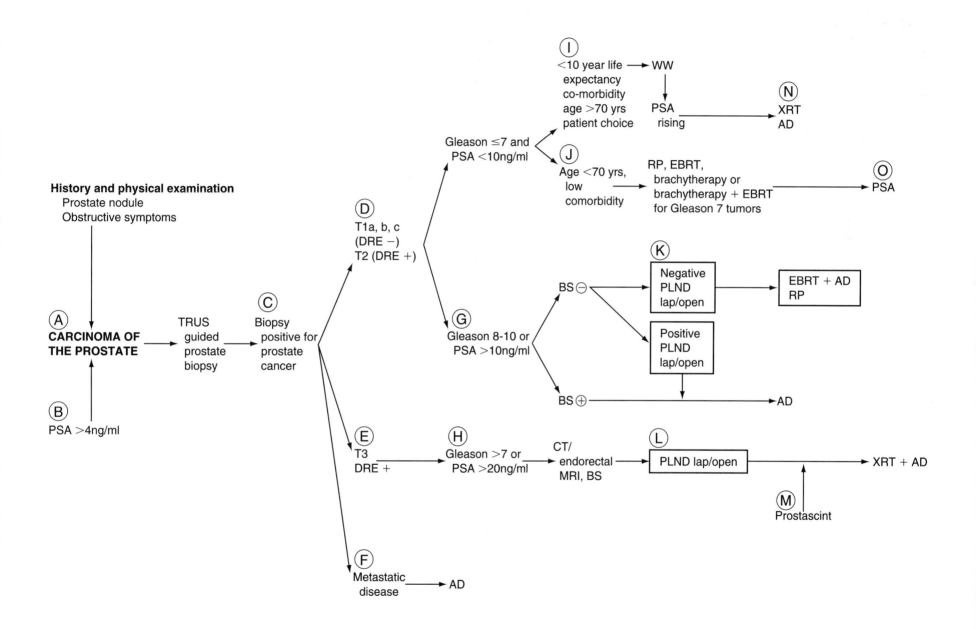

Chapter 127 *Scrotal Mass*

ROBERT E. DONOHUE, MD

(A) History, physical examination, and transillumination detect and diagnose most scrotal masses. Urinalysis is useful to differentiate spermatic cord torsion from acute epididymitis.

(B) Five structures in the scrotum can be associated with scrotal masses: testis, epididymis, vas deferens, veins, paratesticular tissue, and the potential space between the visceral and parietal layers of the tunica albuginea.

(C) Ultrasonography (US) of the scrotum is an accurate ancillary imaging study and is useful for determining the cause of a scrotal mass, except in the presence of spermatocele, giant spermatocele, postvasectomy enlargement of the epididymis, and a postvasectomy mass in the vas (sperm granuloma).

(D) The space between the visceral and parietal layers of the tunica vaginalis can be occupied by hydrocele fluid or peritoneal fluid, blood, omentum, or small or large bowel. The latter three are associated with an indirect inguinal hernia. Intermittent scrotal swelling is similar to a patent processus vaginalis in a pediatric patient. US establishes the diagnosis with certainty.

(E) Tunica albuginea cyst and plaque can be diagnosed by US and observed without excision.

(F) Varicocele, usually left-sided, occurs in 8% to 15% of males. US is used to determine whether the affected testis is smaller than the contralateral one in a preteenage or teenage male. If testicular volume is decreased, ligation of the varicocele encourages normal growth of the testis.

(G) A definite palpable intratesticular mass is a tumor, and inguinal orchiectomy should be done. With palpable mass, questionable cyst, or low suspicion of malignancy, the mass can be biopsied with ultrasound guidance. A mass within the parenchyma of the testis is considered to be a germ cell tumor. The mass is removed with US guidance, or orchiectomy is performed.

(H) Torsion of the spermatic cord caused by a cremasteric reflex in a testis not properly attached to the dartos causes intense pain that peaks instantly, nausea, vomiting, and scrotal swelling. The patient is usually awakened from sleep, and he may have experienced previous episodes. Examination reveals a transverse lie to the opposite testis and no evidence of urethritis, meatal reddening, or urethral discharge. Urinalysis is normal. US reveals a swollen testis and epididymis. Doppler flow studies show no perfusion.

(I) Torsion of the testicular appendage, a müllerian remnant present in 99% of males, can be observed or operated on with excision of the appendage. Torsion of an epididymal appendage, a wolffian remnant present in 69% of males, can also be observed or treated surgically. Testicular fixation is not necessary for either lesion if operation is performed.

(J) Acute epididymitis (caused by *Neisseria gonorrhoeae* or *Chlamydia trachomatis* in younger males and *Escherichia coli* or other gram-negative bacteria or enterococci in older men) usually presents as pain and swelling that gradually peaks after several days. It is associated with urethral discharge or cystitis. Fever can occur. Examination reveals a mass in the lower pole of the epididymis. A hydrocele may have formed that obscures the epididymis. The urethral meatus may be reddened. Analysis of the first few drops of urine shows white blood cells. Midstream urine is positive in cystitis. US may demonstrate focal lower pole diffuse enlargement of the epididymis or an abscess. Doppler US can show increased blood flow. Bedrest, scrotal elevation, antibiotics, and NSAIDs help to eliminate pain, but the mass may persist for months.

(K) Trauma to the scrotum requires US imaging to rule out rupture of the tunica albuginea. If rupture is confirmed, the scrotum should be explored and testicular reconstruction or orchiectomy performed. Sensitivity is low, however, and exploration may be undertaken based on clinical presentation.

(L) Rotating the testis laterally to undo the torsion can be successful if attempted within 6 hours. Bilateral orchidopexy should then be performed electively. If the testis is not viable, orchiectomy is unavoidable.

REFERENCES

Batata M, Chu F, Whitmore WF et al: Testicular cancer in cryptorchids. Cancer 49:1023–1030, 1982.

Berger R, Alexander R, Harnash J et al: Etiology, manifestations and therapy of acute epididymitis: A prospective study of 50 cases. J Urol 121:750–754, 1979.

Casella R, Leibundgut B, Lehmann K et al: Mumps orchitis: Report of a miniepidemic. J Urol 158:2158–2161, 1997.

Coolsaet B: The varicocele syndrome: Venography determining the optimum level for surgical management. J Urol 124: 833–839, 1980.

Donohue E, Fauver HE: Unilateral absence of the vas deferens: A useful clinical sign. JAMA 261:1180–1182, 1989.

Donohue R, Utley WEB: Torsion of the spermatic cord. Urology 11:33–36, 1978.

Meacham R, Mata J, Espada R, et al: Testicular metastases as the first manifestation of colon carcinoma. J Urol 140:621–622, 1988.

Richie J, Steele G: Neoplasms of the Testis. In Walsh PC, Retik A, Vaughan D, et al (eds): Campbell's Urology, 6th ed. Philadelphia: WB Saunders, 1992.

Shapeero L, Vordermark J: Epidermoid cyst of the testis and the role of sonography. Urology 41:75–79, 1993.

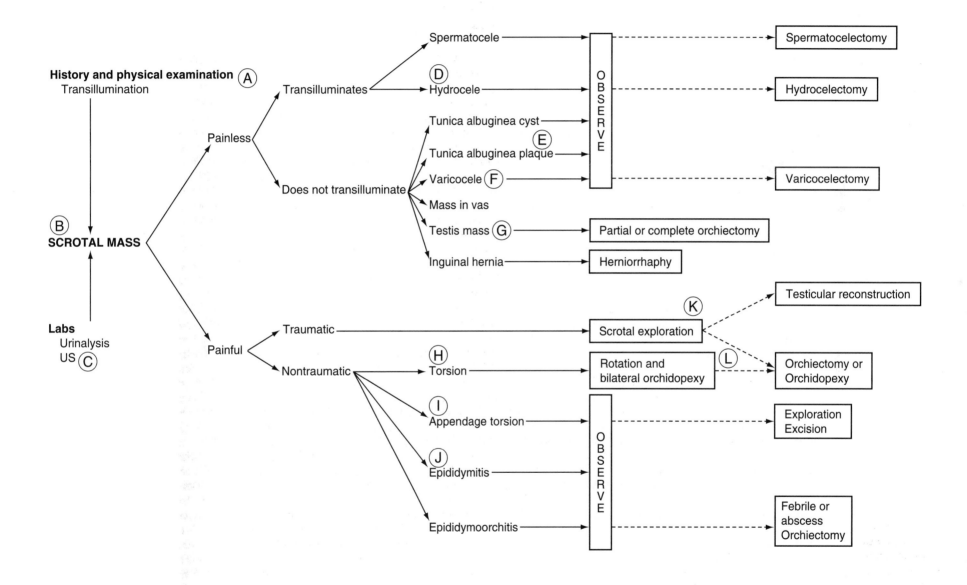

Chapter 128 *Testis Tumor*

SIAM OOTTAMASATHIEN, MD • E. DAVID CRAWFORD, MD

Ⓐ The classic description is a lump, swelling, or hardness of the testicle. In approximately 50% of patients the mass is painless; 30% to 40% may complain of a dull ache or a heavy sensation in the lower abdomen, anal area, or scrotum; and in 10% of patients, acute pain is the presenting symptom. There is often a delay in diagnosis while patients are treated for presumed epididymitis. Acute onset of pain is rare unless there is an associated epididymitis or bleeding within the tumor. Physical examination should proceed as follows:

1. Testicle-bimanual; start with the normal testicle; appreciate size, contour, and consistency; any firm, hard, or fixed area within the substance of the tunica albuginea is suspicious. Also examine the cord, scrotal investments, and skin.
2. Metastatic sites (approximately 10% of patients) include neck mass (supraclavicular lymph node metastasis); respiratory symptoms (pulmonary metastasis); bone and lumbar back pain (skeletal metastasis); gynecomastia (5% of patients from endocrine effects); CNS and PNS symptoms (neural metastasis); and lower extremity swelling (venous thrombosis or obstruction).

Ⓑ With any suspect testicular mass, an ultrasound (US) of the scrotum should be obtained. Serum markers for testis cancer should be drawn, including human chorionic gonadotropin (HCG), alpha-fetoprotein (AFP), and lactate dehydrogenase (LDH). HCG is produced by syncytiotrophoblast of choriocarcinoma and seminoma. AFP is produced by yolk sac cells in embryonal carcinoma and yolk sac cancers. AFP is *never* elevated in a seminoma. If abnormal, this signals a non-seminoma. Chest x-ray should be obtained as part of an initial metastatic work-up.

Ⓒ Testicular cancer, although rare, represents the most common malignancy in males in the 15- to 35-year-old age group. They are one of the most curable genitourinary malignancies, with 5-year survival rates for all stages being greater than 90% to 95%.

Ⓓ All testicular tumors require surgery: radical inguinal orchiectomy. This is the definitive treatment for a large percentage of patients. Control of the spermatic cord during orchiectomy minimizes tumor spread and local recurrence. Rarely, extensive metastasis and pulmonary compromise necessitate immediate treatment with chemotherapy and a delay in orchiectomy. Primary testicular tumors include germ cell (90% to 95%) and non–germ cell tumors (5% to 10%). Only 1% of testis tumors are benign. Germ cell tumors are categorized as seminoma and nonseminoma (e.g., teratoma, embryonal, yolk sac, choriocarcinoma, teratocarcinoma, and mixed). Non–germ cell tumors include Leydig cell, Sertoli cell, and gonadoblastoma. Secondary (metastatic) testicular tumors occur, most commonly lymphoma. Sperm banking should be considered prior to surgery.

Ⓔ Clinical stage is determined by imaging and surgery. A CT scan cannot differentiate tumor, teratoma, necrosis, or fibrosis. Abdominal CT has a 25% to 30% false negative rate; therefore staging is accurate in approximately 75% of patients. If the CT scan of the abdomen shows nodal metastases, a chest CT should be obtained. Surgical staging by retroperitoneal lymph node dissection (RPLND) can be done transabdominally.

STAGE DESCRIPTION

Royal Marsden Hospital Staging System

I	Tumor confined to testis
IIA	Minimal nodal metastasis to retroperitoneum
IIB	Moderate nodal metastasis to retroperitoneum
IIC	Bulky nodal metastasis to retroperitoneum
III	Nodal metastatsis to retroperitoneum and other nodes
IV	Visceral metastasis

TNM Staging System

T0	No evidence of primary tumor
Tis	Carcinoma in situ
T1	Limited to testis, may be into but not beyond the tunica albuginea
T2	Tumor invades beyond tunica albuginea or into epididymis
T3	Tumor invades spermatic cord
T4	Tumor invades scrotum
N0	No lymph node metastasis
N1	Metastasis to a single node <2 cm in greatest dimension
N2	Metastasis to node(s) 2-5 cm in greatest dimension
N3	Metastasis to node(s) >5 cm in greatest dimension
M0	No distant metastasis
M1	Distant metastasis

Ⓕ Non–germ cell testis tumors are rare (5% to 10%). These include Leydig cell, Sertoli cell, gonadoblastoma, and secondary metastasis such as lymphoma. Both Leydig cell and Sertoli cell tumor types are rare and benign, but in a very small percentage of each (5% to 10%) they have a malignant potential. Surveillance is therefore warranted after the initial work-up and radical orchiectomy. Gonadoblastoma is also rare, but in many cases mixed germinal elements can be present; treatment is guided by which elements are present (see F and G). The treatment for lymphoma (average age at presentation is more than 50 years) is the appropriate chemotherapeutic regimen.

Ⓖ Seminoma accounts for approximately 65% of germ cell tumors, with a peak age around 35 to 40 years (spermatocytic is an exception, with average age at presentation of more than 50 years). Classic seminoma accounts for about 85% of

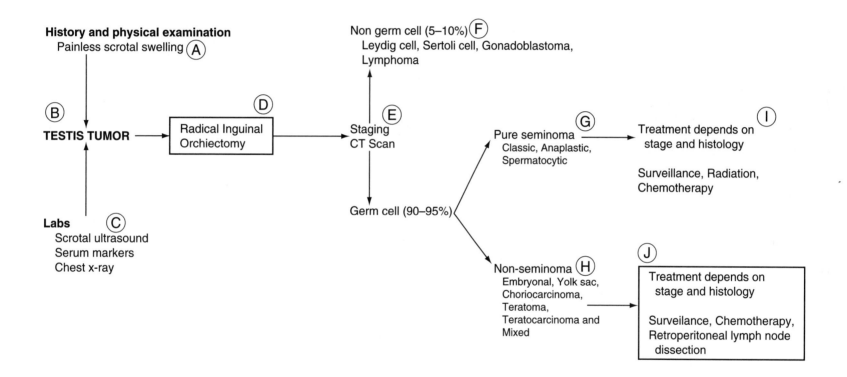

History and physical examination
Painless scrotal swelling (A)

(B)

TESTIS TUMOR

Radical Inguinal
Orchiectomy (D)

Labs (C)
Scrotal ultrasound
Serum markers
Chest x-ray

Non germ cell (5–10%) (F)
Leydig cell, Sertoli cell, Gonadoblastoma,
Lymphoma

Staging
CT Scan (E)

Germ cell (90–95%)

Pure seminoma (G)
Classic, Anaplastic,
Spermatocytic

Treatment depends on
stage and histology (I)

Surveillance, Radiation,
Chemotherapy

Non-seminoma (H)
Embryonal, Yolk sac,
Choriocarcinoma,
Teratoma,
Teratocarcinoma and
Mixed

(J)
Treatment depends on
stage and histology

Surveilance, Chemotherapy,
Retroperitoneal lymph node
dissection

seminomas; anaplastic seminoma accounts for around 10%; and spermatocytic seminoma accounts for around 5%. Spermatocytic seminoma has a low metastatic potential. Pure seminoma never secretes AFP, and a low percentage of these tumors (up to 10%) secrete HCG.

(H) Nonseminoma tumor types account for approximately 35% of germ cell tumors. Embryonal cell has a peak age of 25 to 35 years, and can secrete both AFP and HCG. Yolk sac tumor is the most common testis cancer in infants and children, with a characteristic histology of embryoid (Schiller-Duvall) bodies. They may secrete both AFP and HCG, with hematogenous spread as the most common route for metastasis. Choriocarcinoma portends the worst prognosis of all testis tumors, with a peak age range of 20 to 30 years. Pure choriocarcinoma is rare. Histologically, choriocarcinoma has both syncytiotrophoblasts and cytotrophoblasts, and never secretes AFP but always secretes HCG. Teratoma can have more than one germ cell layer present (e.g., endoderm, mesoderm, and ectoderm elements) and has a peak age range of 25 to 35 years. Pure teratomas should not secrete AFP or HCG. Teratocarcinoma is a mixture of both embryonal cell and teratoma. Mixed tumors are a combination of seminoma and/or nonseminoma, and are more common than pure tumors.

(I) In clinical stage I disease, if the postorchiectomy tumor markers normalize and if the histology is a pure spermatocytic seminoma, observation is indicated. In stage I, if postsurgical markers normalize but it is not a pure spermatocytic seminoma, surveillance or abdominal XRT is indicated. If in stage I and the postsurgical markers remain elevated, chemotherapy or XRT is recommended. In stage IIA patients, abdominal XRT is recommended; if relapse occurs, chemotherapy is instituted. In stage IIB and IIC, chemotherapy is the first line treatment after orchiectomy, then further treatment is mandated based on the level of residual disease (postchemotherapy markers and abdominal CT). In stage III and IV, chemotherapy is the initial treatment, with salvage chemotherapy if progression occurs. Rarely is removal of residual disease necessary.

(J) In clinical stage I nonseminoma disease, if postorchiectomy tumor markers normalize, then either surveillance (with chemotherapy for relapse) vs. RPLND is recommended. If RPLND is performed and complete tumor resection is obtained, observation is recommended for pathologic stage I patients; however, adjuvant chemotherapy is instituted for pathologic stage IIA and IIB. If an incomplete resection is performed, then chemotherapy is recommended. In clinical stage IIA, RPLND is recommended with or without chemotherapy. In clinical stage IIB and IIC, chemotherapy is the first line treatment and either observation, RPLND, or salvage chemotherapy is instituted depending on postchemotherapy markers and abdominal CT scan. In clinical stage III and IV, chemotherapy is recommended and, if progression occurs, salvage chemotherapy is instituted.

REFERENCES

Brandes SB: Surgical management of recurrent genitourinary malignancies. AUA Update Series. Volume XV, Lesson 31:246, 1996.

Foster RS: Early stage testis cancer. Curr Treat Options Oncol 2(5):413–419, 2001.

Klein EA: Tumor markers in testis cancer. Urol Clin North Am 20:67–73, 1993.

Malkowicz SB, Wein AJ: Adult Genitourinary Cancer. In Hanno PM, Wein AJ (eds): Clinical Manual of Urology, 2nd ed. New York: McGraw-Hill, 1994.

NCCN Practice guidelines for testicular cancer. Oncology 12:417–462, 1998.

Nichols CR: Testicular cancer. Curr Probl Cancer 22:187–274, 1998.

Rowland RG, Foster RS, Donohue FP: Scrotum and Testis. In Gillenwater JY, Grayhack JT, Howards SS et al (eds): Adult and Pediatric Urology, 3rd ed. Saint Louis: Mosby-Year Book, 1996.

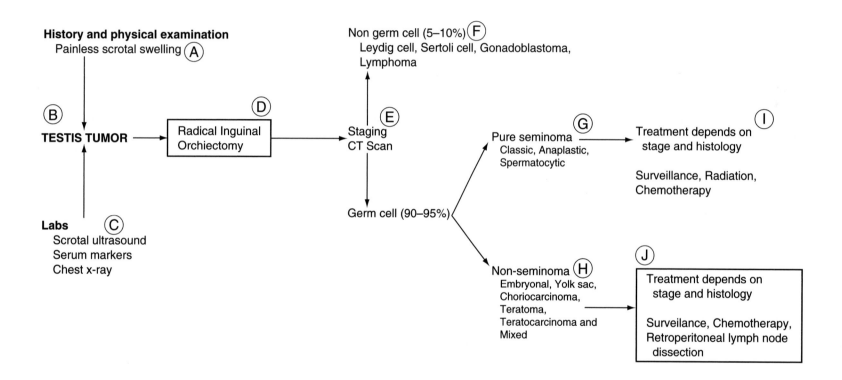

History and physical examination
Painless scrotal swelling (A)

(B)

TESTIS TUMOR

Labs (C)
Scrotal ultrasound
Serum markers
Chest x-ray

(D)
Radical Inguinal
Orchiectomy

Non germ cell (5–10%) (F)
Leydig cell, Sertoli cell, Gonadoblastoma,
Lymphoma

Staging (E)
CT Scan

Germ cell (90–95%)

Pure seminoma (G)
Classic, Anaplastic,
Spermatocytic

Treatment depends on (I)
stage and histology

Surveilance, Radiation,
Chemotherapy

Non-seminoma (H)
Embryonal, Yolk sac,
Choriocarcinoma,
Teratoma,
Teratocarcinoma and
Mixed

(J)
Treatment depends on
stage and histology

Surveilance, Chemotherapy,
Retroperitoneal lymph node
dissection

Chapter 129 *Ureteral Injuries*

DAN ROSENSTEIN, MD • JACK W. MCANINCH, MD

(A) Ureteral injuries caused by external trauma are uncommon. Approximately 80% of ureteral injuries are caused by iatrogenic causes, with the remaining 20% related to external trauma. Because of the ureter's protected position in the retroperitoneum adjacent to the spine and major muscle groups, it is unlikely to be injured unless directly penetrated or ligated. Most ureteral injuries caused by external violence result from penetrating trauma, with gunshot injury occurring more commonly than stab wounds. The ureter may be damaged secondarily and display delayed necrosis and stricture or fistula as a result of "blast effect." High velocity missiles have a higher complication rate and are associated with delayed presentation. Ureteral injuries caused by blunt trauma are rare. Rapid deceleration may cause disruption or avulsion at the ureteropelvic junction; these injuries are usually associated with multiple organ injuries.

(B) The American Association for the Surgery of Trauma has graded ureteral injuries according to severity as follows:

Grade 1: Contusion or hematoma without devascularizion

Grade 2: Laceration with less than 50% transection

Grade 3: Laceration with more than 50% transection

Grade 4: Laceration with complete transection and less than 2 cm devascularization

Grade 5: Laceration with avulsion and more than 2 cm devascularization

(C) Gynecologic surgery is the most common setting for iatrogenic ureteral injury. The ureter is typically injured as it passes through the broad ligament beneath the uterine artery. It may be clamped or ligated during transection of the lower uterine pedicle. General surgical procedures involving the rectosigmoid colon, where inflammation or malignancy

surrounds the ureter, may place it at increased risk for injury. Vascular reconstructive procedures involving aortic or iliac aneurysms may also predispose to ureteral injury. Prompt recognition and repair of ureteral injuries in the setting of a freshly placed vascular graft is of paramount importance. Urologic procedures that have been associated with ureteral injury include salvage radical prostatectomy, retroperitoneal lymph node dissection, and ureteroscopy and ureteral stone manipulation. Most ureteroscopic injuries (excluding avulsion) may be successfully managed with ureteral stenting. Laparoscopic ureteral injuries have also been described and are usually managed by immediate open repair.

(D) Hematuria is not a reliable indicator for ureteral injury. The surgeon must maintain a high index of suspicion for this injury. Absence of hematuria therefore does not rule out ureteral injury. Delayed signs of ureteral injury include increasing drain output, flank pain, fever, urinoma formation, ileus, and sepsis.

(E) Intravenous pyelography may be diagnostic of ureteral injury. Radiographic indicators may include extravasation of radiographic contrast, ureteral dilation, and incomplete visualization or nonvisualization of the ureter. Any of these findings should prompt further investigation.

(F) Retrograde pyelography is highly sensitive for the detection of ureteral injuries. It may clearly define the presence, location, and degree of injury. It has limited utility in the trauma setting because it is impractical to perform acutely. This study has more utility in the evaluation and treatment of a ureteral injury that is detected in a delayed fashion.

(G) Abdominal CT scan with intravenous contrast may also demonstrate extravasation, urinoma, or hydronephrosis, as well as injuries to associated organs. With the advent of rapid helical CT scanning, contrast may not have reached the collecting system and ureter by the time of scan completion.

Ureteral injuries may only be seen with delayed images after contrast has reached the bladder. CT may be combined with a delayed plain abdominal film (KUB) for maximal information regarding the collecting system.

(H) Early/intraoperative detection and treatment of ureteral injury significantly reduces later morbidity. Direct visual inspection reliably assesses ureteral integrity. Methylene blue or indigo carmine dye injected through the ureter with a 25-gauge needle, or through a ureteral catheter inserted via a cystotomy, serves as a useful adjunct in localizing the site of injury. In the trauma setting, the ureter should be carefully evaluated for discoloration, extravasation, and viability of the transected segment.

(I) Most (60% to 70%) iatrogenic injuries to the ureter are diagnosed postoperatively. Delayed diagnosis typically presents with renal obstruction or fistula. If the diagnosis is made within 7 to 10 days beyond the initial injury, the ureter should be repaired primarily. Repair beyond 10 days of leakage is hazardous because of ureteral inflammation. Nephrostomy tube placement followed by delayed reconstruction at 3 months postinjury is best in this setting.

(J) In the setting of an unstable (e.g., acidemic, coagulopathic, or hypotensive) patient with multiple other life-threatening injuries, a temporary cutaneous ureterostomy is the safest option. Alternatively, ureteral ligation and percutaneous nephrostomy tube placement may be performed. The patient may then undergo planned reconstruction when clinically feasible.

(K) If imaging studies suggest that ureteral continuity is still present postinjury, an attempt to pass an indwelling ureteral stent is warranted. If successful, stenting for approximately 6 weeks may permit low-pressure drainage and healing such that no further treatment may be necessary. Retrograde pyelography should be performed at the time of

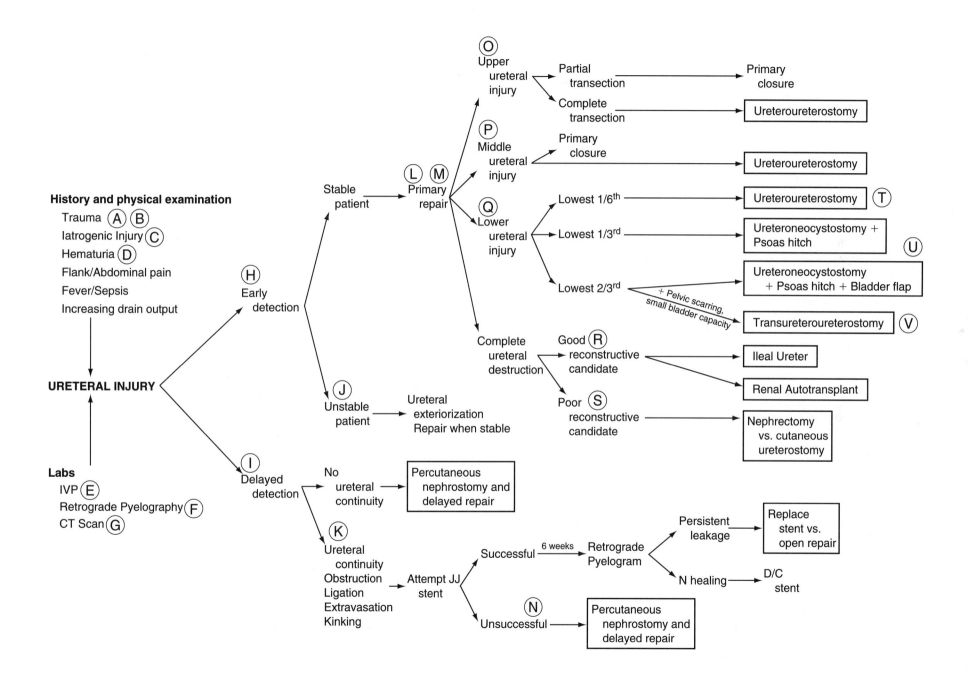

History and physical examination

Trauma Ⓐ Ⓑ
Iatrogenic Injury Ⓒ
Hematuria Ⓓ
Flank/Abdominal pain
Fever/Sepsis
Increasing drain output

URETERAL INJURY

Labs

IVP Ⓔ
Retrograde Pyelography Ⓕ
CT Scan Ⓖ

Ⓗ Early detection

Ⓘ Delayed detection

Stable patient

Ⓛ Ⓜ Primary repair

Ⓙ Unstable patient → Ureteral exteriorization Repair when stable

Ⓞ Upper ureteral injury
→ Partial transection ──── Primary closure
→ Complete transection ──── Ureteroureterostomy

Ⓟ Middle ureteral injury
→ Primary closure
Ureteroureterostomy

Ⓠ Lower ureteral injury
→ Lowest 1/6th ──── Ureteroureterostomy Ⓣ
→ Lowest 1/3rd ──── Ureteroneocystostomy + Psoas hitch Ⓤ
→ Lowest 2/3rd ──── Ureteroneocystostomy + Psoas hitch + Bladder flap
   + Pelvic scarring, small bladder capacity ──── Transureteroureterostomy Ⓥ

Complete ureteral destruction
→ Good Ⓡ reconstructive candidate
   Ileal Ureter
   Renal Autotransplant
→ Poor Ⓢ reconstructive candidate
   Nephrectomy vs. cutaneous ureterostomy

No ureteral continuity → Percutaneous nephrostomy and delayed repair

Ⓚ Ureteral continuity
Obstruction
Ligation
Extravasation
Kinking
→ Attempt JJ stent
→ Successful ── 6 weeks ── Retrograde Pyelogram
   → Persistent leakage → Replace stent vs. open repair
   → N healing → D/C stent
→ Unsuccessful → Ⓝ Percutaneous nephrostomy and delayed repair

stent removal so that complete resolution of the injury can be documented. A short residual stricture may then be treated by endourologic incision and repeat stenting. Longer strictures will require open reconstruction.

(L) Primary repair of ureteral injuries upon recognition results in the best long-term outcome. General principles of ureteral repair include the following:

Adequate ureteral debridement and mobilization
Precise, tension-free mucosal approximation
Spatulated anastomosis over ureteral stent
Isolation of repair from associated injuries (especially in cases of simultaneous bowel or vascular injuries).
Retroperitoneal drainage

(M) The type of repair employed for the injured ureter depends upon the length and location of the injury. The ureter may be divided into three segments: (1) the upper ureter, extending from the ureteropelvic junction to the sacrum; (2) the mid-ureter, overlying the sacrum; and (3) the lower (pelvic) ureter, extending from the lower margin of the sacrum to the ureterovesical junction.

(N) If stent passage is impossible because of complete ligation and/or lack of ureteral wall continuity, a percutaneous nephrostomy tube should be placed in the affected kidney with planned ureteral reconstruction following a 3-month delay.

(O) Upper ureteral injuries are routinely managed by ureteroureterostomy. This involves mobilization and debridement of the ureteral stumps back to vital, bleeding tissue. The spatulated anastomosis should be performed with fine absorbable sutures. An internal ureteral stent should be placed for a minimum of 6 weeks. If the two ends cannot be re-anastomosed without tension, a few centimeters may be successfully gained by downward

nephropexy. This involves mobilizing the kidney downwards and fixing its capsule to the quadratus lumborum muscle. Partial ureteral transections can usually be managed by primary closure.

(P) Midureteral injuries are managed by ureteroureterostomy or primary repair, as described above.

(Q) Injuries to the distal ureter may jeopardize the blood supply of the distal segment and thus are rarely amenable to primary anastomotic repair. Direct re-implant of the proximal segment into the bladder (ureteroneocystostomy) is usually feasible if only the distal part of the pelvic ureter is injured. The ureter is re-implanted in the posterior bladder wall just medial to the original hiatus.

(R) Destruction of the entire ureter may be managed with ileal interposition or renal autotransplantation. Ileal interposition requires appropriate bowel preparation and is only appropriate in patients with relatively normal renal function (i.e., serum creatinine below 2.5). A 25-cm segment of ileum is typically anastomosed proximally to the renal pelvis and distally directly into the bladder. This technique is associated with a high success rate. Complications may include bacteriuria, mucusuria, and metabolic acidosis. Renal autotransplantation into the iliac fossa requires comfort with vascular surgery because the renal vessels are anastomosed to the iliac vessels. Urinary continuity may then be restored by pyelovesicostomy.

(S) Patients who are unfit for an extensive reconstructive procedure with a normal contralateral kidney are best managed by nephrectomy. Alternatively, these patients may be managed with percutaneous nephrostomy tubes or cutaneous ureterostomies, but these are often associated with considerable long-term morbidity.

(T) If the entire pelvic ureter is injured, ureteroneocystostomy may be combined with the

psoas hitch technique in order to repair this longer defect. The psoas hitch requires bladder mobilization off the peritoneal reflection and ligation of the contralateral superior vesical pedicle. These maneuvers allow for the bladder to be anchored to the psoas tendon on the injured side. The ureter is then re-implanted as previously described.

(U) Injuries to the entire lower two thirds of the ureter may be repaired by combining a psoas hitch and ureteroneocystostomy with an anterior bladder wall (Boari) flap. This flap is then tubularized with the proximal ureter re-implanted into the tip. Defects of as much as 15 cm may be bridged using this technique.

(V) A transureteroureterostomy may be employed in the setting of long lower ureteral defects with insufficient bladder capacity for bladder flaps, or for severe pelvic scarring that renders bladder mobilization impossible. This technique involves mobilization of the injured ureter to the contralateral side through a retroperitoneal window. The injured ureter is then anastomosed end-to-side to the recipient ureter. This procedure potentially endangers the normal contralateral ureter and should be employed selectively.

REFERENCES

Armenakas N: Current methods of diagnosis and management of ureteral injuries. World J Urol 17:78–83, 1999.
Armenakas N: Ureteral trauma: Surgical repair. Atlas Urol Clin N Amer 6:71–84, 1998.
Brandes SB, McAninch JW: Reconstructive surgery for trauma of the upper urinary tract. Urol Clin N Amer 26:183–199, 1999.
Matthews R, Marshall FF: Management of extensive ureteral defects. AUA Update Series 20:177–184, 2001.
Png JCD, Chapple CR: Principles of ureteric reconstruction. Curr Opin Urol 10:207–212, 2000.
Presti JC, Carroll PR: Ureteral and Renal Pelvic Trauma: Diagnosis and Management. In McAninch JW, Jordan GH, Carroll PR (eds): Traumatic and Reconstructive Urology. Philadelphia, WB Saunders, 1996.

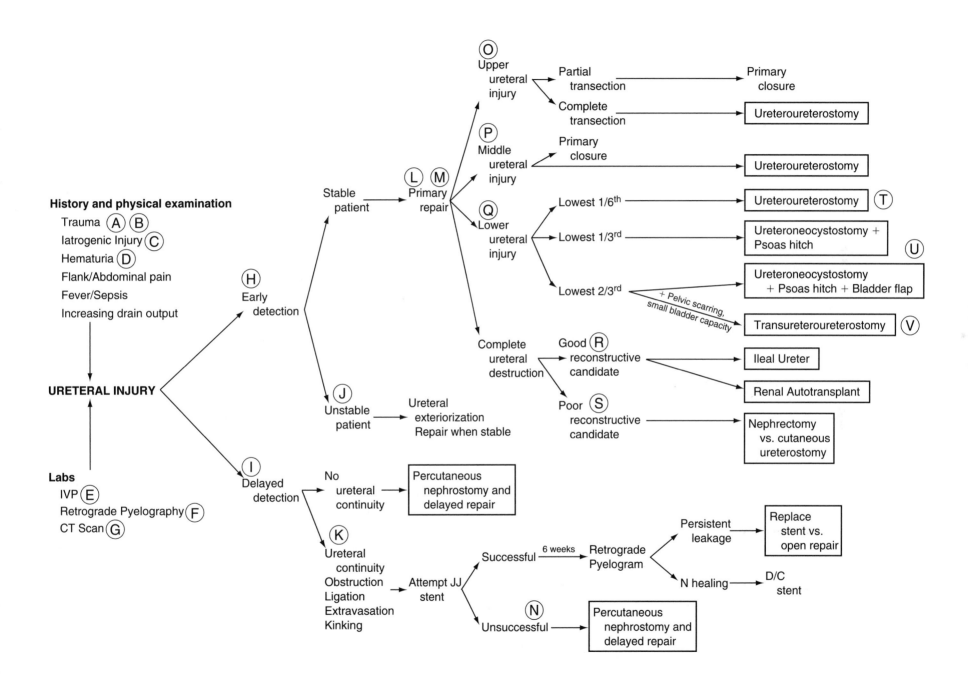

History and physical examination

Trauma (A) (B)
Iatrogenic Injury (C)
Hematuria (D)
Flank/Abdominal pain
Fever/Sepsis
Increasing drain output

URETERAL INJURY

Labs

IVP (E)
Retrograde Pyelography (F)
CT Scan (G)

(H) Early detection

(I) Delayed detection

(J) Unstable patient → Ureteral exteriorization Repair when stable

Stable patient → (L) (M) Primary repair

(O) Upper ureteral injury → Partial transection → Primary closure

Complete transection → Ureteroureterostomy

(P) Middle ureteral injury → Primary closure

Ureteroureterostomy

(Q) Lower ureteral injury → Lowest 1/6th → Ureteroureterostomy (T)

Lowest 1/3rd → Ureteroneocystostomy + Psoas hitch (U)

Lowest 2/3rd → Ureteroneocystostomy + Psoas hitch + Bladder flap

+ Pelvic scarring, small bladder capacity → Transureteroureterostomy (V)

Complete ureteral destruction → Good (R) reconstructive candidate → Ileal Ureter

Renal Autotransplant

Poor (S) reconstructive candidate → Nephrectomy vs. cutaneous ureterostomy

No ureteral continuity → Percutaneous nephrostomy and delayed repair

(K) Ureteral continuity
Obstruction
Ligation
Extravasation
Kinking

Attempt JJ stent → Successful → 6 weeks → Retrograde Pyelogram → Persistent leakage → Replace stent vs. open repair

N healing → D/C stent

Unsuccessful → (N) → Percutaneous nephrostomy and delayed repair

Chapter 130 *Urinary Diversion*

SOREN N. CARLSEN, MD ● BRIAN J. FLYNN, MD

(A) There are a multitude of indications for both temporary and permanent urinary diversion based upon the patient's history, physical examination, and imaging results.

(B) Some patients may benefit from presumed diagnosis and empiric treatment (e.g., Foley catheterization for urinary retention in an elderly male with presumed benign prostatic hypertrophy), whereas others may need further evaluation by imaging. Evaluation of obstruction is necessary to define the level and etiology of the obstruction and thereby direct temporary relief of the obstruction. Contrast-enhanced imaging is often contraindicated because of renal insufficiency; therefore imaging customarily occurs by unenhanced computer tomography, ultrasound, retrograde urography, or renal scintigraphy.

(C) The most common indication for cystectomy with urinary diversion is urothelial carcinoma involving the lower urinary tract (i.e., bladder, prostate, or urethra). Urinary diversion with or without cystectomy may also be indicated in severe cases of cystitis (e.g., caused by radiation, hemorrhage, or infection); fistula; or neurogenic dysfunction, when bladder preservation is not feasible. The urinary diversion should not compromise the extirpative procedure and should store or expel urine under low pressure. Urinary diversions, either a simple conduit (incontinent diversion) or the more elaborate continent diversion, may be constructed from any portion of the gastrointestinal tract (e.g., stomach, jejunum, ileum, colon, or rectum).

(D) Acute obstruction of the urinary tract can occur at any level from the kidneys to urethral meatus and may cause pain, infection, loss of renal function, and even renal failure. The decision to perform temporary urinary drainage may be brought about by concurrent infection, trauma, pain, or other factors.

(E) Adequate renal function is needed to prevent metabolic disturbances caused by urine storage in an absorptive reservoir. In general the serum creatinine must be less than 2.5 mg/dl for a continent diversion unless a renal transplantation is planned.

(F) Signs of gastrointestinal blood loss (e.g., bright red blood per rectum or melena) or a personal or family history of gastrointestinal (GI) neoplasms or inflammatory diseases necessitate further evaluation to rule out disease in the proposed segment.

(G) Lower urinary tract obstruction may be caused by any process from the bladder neck to the urethra meatus (e.g., bladder neck contracture, benign prostatic hypertrophy, prostate or urethral cancer, foreign bodies, or urethral stricture or disruption).

(H) Upper urinary tract obstruction (i.e., between the kidney and bladder) may be caused by ureteropelvic junction (UPJ) obstruction; intrinsic ureteral obstruction (e.g., calculi, stricture, malignancy, blood clot, polyp, or sloughed papilla); or extrinsic compression by malignant or benign processes in adjacent organs (e.g., colon, prostate, bladder, cervix, uterus, or ovary) or the retroperitoneum (e.g., fibrosis or aneurysm).

(I) Each segment of the GI tract has its own advantages and disadvantages for use in creating a urinary diversion. A wedged segment of stomach has the advantage of being less permeable, producing less mucus, and having a lower infection rate. In addition, the stomach will excrete H+ ions and is therefore useful in patients with metabolic acidosis. However, use of the stomach may cause hypochloremic hypokalemic metabolic alkalosis, contribute to ulcer disease (because of high gastrin levels), result in hematuria-dysuria syndrome, and is limited by its size and location. Therefore it is used primarily for bladder augmentation, not diversion. Jejunum has the largest diameter and mesentery of the small intestine; however, the severe electrolyte abnormalities that commonly occur following diversion preclude its use in most instances. The ileum is mobile, has a constant blood supply, and the ileocecal valve can be incorporated for prevention of ureteral reflux. Common problems associated with the use of ileum include a higher incidence (10%) of postoperative bowel obstruction because of its small diameter, and B_{12} deficiency and diarrhea secondary to bile salt and fat malabsorption. In addition, hyperchloremic metabolic acidosis is common when either ileum or colon is utilized. The colon has the distinct advantage of a large diameter, allowing the creation of a large reservoir, and a low incidence (4%) of postoperative bowel obstruction. Because of its location, it is usually preserved in patients with prior abdominal or pelvic irradiation. If the ileocecal valve is disrupted, diarrhea, excessive bacterial colonization, malabsorption, and fluid and bicarbonate loss can ensue in as many as 15% of patients. The most commonly used GI segments are the ileum and colon, whereas continent diversions often use both (ileocolic).

(J) Urethral and bladder outlet obstruction can often be temporarily relieved by an indwelling urethral catheter or clean intermittent catheterization (CIC). If there is any resistance or difficulty in passing the catheter (especially in cases of pelvic or perineal trauma), a urologist should be consulted for catheter placement because a partial urethral injury may be converted to a complete disruption by an imprudent attempt at catheter placement.

(K) Percutaneous nephrostomy or, when feasible, ureteral stenting may be used to temporarily relieve upper tract obstruction and preserve renal function while awaiting more definitive treatment.

(L) Patients with multiple comorbidities, advanced disease, or a short life expectancy in general do not benefit from continent diversion; they therefore should undergo a conduit diversion because of its simplicity, shorter operative time, and reduced morbidity and convalescence.

(M) The most important requirement for continent diversion is the patient's ability to care

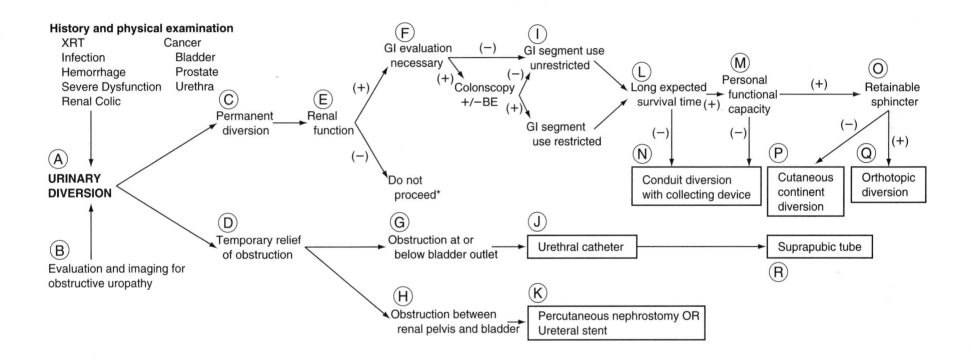

History and physical examination

XRT	Cancer
Infection	Bladder
Hemorrhage	Prostate
Severe Dysfunction	Urethra
Renal Colic	

Ⓐ **URINARY DIVERSION**

Ⓑ Evaluation and imaging for obstructive uropathy

Ⓒ Permanent diversion

Ⓓ Temporary relief of obstruction

Ⓔ Renal function

Ⓕ GI evaluation necessary

Colonscopy +/−BE

GI segment use unrestricted

GI segment use restricted

Do not proceed*

Ⓘ GI segment use unrestricted

Ⓛ Long expected survival time

Ⓜ Personal functional capacity

Ⓞ Retainable sphincter

Ⓝ Conduit diversion with collecting device

Ⓟ Cutaneous continent diversion

Ⓠ Orthotopic diversion

Ⓖ Obstruction at or below bladder outlet

Ⓙ Urethral catheter

Suprapubic tube

Ⓡ

Ⓗ Obstruction between renal pelvis and bladder

Ⓚ Percutaneous nephrostomy OR Ureteral stent

*unless patient is considered for renal transplant

for the diversion and perform CIC. Poor eye-hand coordination or limited mental or physical capacity may preclude continent diversion.

(N) Conduits are composed of a short segment of bowel (primarily ileum or colon) that passively drains urine from the ureters to an abdominal wall collection device. The stoma should be sited before surgery by the surgeon or an enterostomal therapist in an area that is unaffected by skin creases and is easily accessed by the patient (customarily in the right lower quadrant). These stomas should protrude (rosebud) to allow an adequately fitted appliance and to prevent skin breakdown.

(O) If the urinary sphincter is uninvolved in the primary disease process and is competent, an orthotopic neobladder may be planned. However, a number of intraoperative findings (e.g., positive margins, advanced disease, or persistent hemodynamic instability) may preclude orthotopic diversion, and therefore all patients should also be consented for a conduit diversion.

(P) Continent cutaneous diversions are reservoirs composed of ileum and/or colon. These reservoirs rely on a valve mechanism to store urine internally. The valve mechanism may be a reinforced ileocecal valve (e.g., Indiana pouch or right colon pouch); embedded appendix (Mitrofanoff principle); or tapered, tunneled ileum (Monti). The reservoir ideally holds 500 ml and is periodically (4 or 5 times a day) emptied by CIC. The abdominal stoma should be in an accessible location and provide a direct route to the reservoir, thereby permitting a simple and efficient means of catheterization.

(Q) An orthotopic neobladder (continent diversion) is created from a segment of bowel and anastamosed to the intact urinary sphincter. Voiding occurs by urethral relaxation and Valsalva's maneuver. If emptying is insufficient, CIC can be performed per urethra to empty the neobladder. If significant intrinsic sphincter deficiency persists beyond the sixth postoperative month, an artificial urinary sphincter can be performed.

(R) When urethral catheterization fails, a suprapubic catheter may be placed to temporarily drain the bladder.

REFERENCES

Fichtner J: Follow-up after urinary diversion. Urol Int 63:40–45, 1999.

Hobisch A, Tosun K, Kinzl J et al: Life after cystectomy and orthotopic neobladder versus ileal conduit urinary diversion. Semin Urol Oncol 19:18–23, 2001.

Holmes DG, Thrasher JB, Park GY et al: Long-term complications related to the modified Indiana pouch. Urology 60:603–606, 2002.

Madersbacher S, Schmidt J, Eberle JM et al: Long-term outcome of ileal conduit diversion. J Urol 169:985–990, 2003.

Mansson A, Davidsson T, Hunt S et al: The quality of life in men after radical cystectomy with a continent cutaneous diversion or orthotopic bladder substitution: Is there a difference? BJU Int 90:386–390, 2002.

Saika T, Suyama B, Murata T et al: Orthotopic neobladder reconstruction in elderly bladder cancer patients. Int J Urol 8:533–538, 2001.

Walsh PC, Retik AB, Vaughn ED, Wein AJ: Campbell's Urology, 8th ed. Philadelphia, Saunders, 2002.

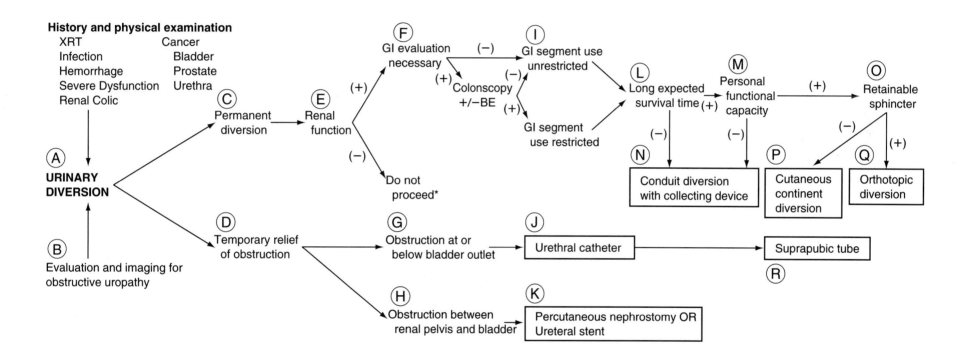

History and physical examination

XRT   Cancer
Infection   Bladder
Hemorrhage   Prostate
Severe Dysfunction Urethra
Renal Colic

Ⓐ **URINARY DIVERSION**

Ⓑ Evaluation and imaging for obstructive uropathy

Ⓒ Permanent diversion

Ⓓ Temporary relief of obstruction

Ⓔ Renal function

(+) Ⓕ GI evaluation necessary

(−) Do not proceed*

(+) Colonscopy +/−BE

(−) Ⓘ GI segment use unrestricted

(+) GI segment use restricted

Ⓛ Long expected survival time

Ⓜ Personal functional capacity

(+) Ⓞ Retainable sphincter

(−) Ⓝ Conduit diversion with collecting device

(−) Ⓟ Cutaneous continent diversion

(−) Ⓠ Orthotopic diversion

(+)

Ⓖ Obstruction at or below bladder outlet

Ⓙ Urethral catheter

Suprapubic tube

Ⓡ

Ⓗ Obstruction between renal pelvis and bladder

Ⓚ Percutaneous nephrostomy OR Ureteral stent

*unless patient is considered for renal transplant

GYNECOLOGY

Chapter 131 *Vaginal Bleeding in Reproductive Years*

KARLOTTA M. DAVIS, MD, MPH

(A) Normal menstruation occurs as a universal, synchronous endometrial event following the withdrawal of ovarian hormones (estrogen and progesterone) subsequent to a normal ovulatory cycle. Normal mean flow quantity is 30 ml of menstrual blood, with greater than 80 ml of menstrual blood loss per cycle defined as menorrhagia. Bleeding 60 to 80 ml per month is associated with iron deficiency anemia. Average duration of flow is from 2 to 7 days. Quantitating the amount of bleeding is difficult, and deviation from normal flow as well as number of sanitary products used, episodes of flooding, and frequency of changing sanitary products are useful historical clues to determine blood loss. Determining whether cycles are ovulatory or anovulatory is key to successful treatment of abnormal vaginal bleeding. Duration of menstrual flow, length of cycle, and molimenal symptoms such as bloating, cramping, and breast tenderness suggest ovulatory cycles. Oral contraceptive pills (OCPs) are most typically associated with irregular spotting, whereas intrauterine devices cause increased menstrual bleeding. In the context of a recent pregnancy, bleeding suggests retained placental fragments. A history of infertility, prior ectopic pregnancy, prior tubal ligation, or tubal disease raises the possibility of ectopic pregnancy. Persistent regular heavy menstrual bleeding in adolescents is suggestive of a coagulopathy.

(B) Important findings of the speculum examination include the amount and nature of vaginal bleeding, presence of cervical discharge, and evidence of pregnancy such as the bluish discoloration of the cervix seen in pregnancy. Bimanual examination will determine cervical motion tenderness, uterine tenderness or mass, and adnexal tenderness or masses. Cervical motion tenderness is the sign elicited when the cervix is cradled between the two examining vaginal fingers and gently moved to one side; a lesion in the contralateral side will be stretched, causing significant pain if cervical motion tenderness is present. A rectovaginal examination completes the pelvic examination and confirms the findings on bimanual examination as well as assessing for uterosacral nodularity, cul de sac of Douglas masses, and rectal masses.

(C) Pregnancy *must* be ruled out in any reproductive age woman who presents with abnormal bleeding. Urine pregnancy tests are positive as early as the expected time of menses (14 days after ovulation).

(D) If bleeding is secondary to abortion, the uterine cavity must be emptied.

(E) A closed cervical os with a positive β-hCG suggests pregnancy. The location of the pregnancy (intrauterine or extrauterine) must be determined.

(F) The curetted specimen is examined for products of conception. Fluid-filled vesicles indicate hydropic villi of a hydatidiform mole. With this finding, follow-up quantitative measurement of β-human chorionic gonadotropin (β-hCG) is necessary because of the possibility of malignant transformation of trophoblastic tissue.

(G) If fetal Doppler echocardiography does not detect heart tones and the cervical os is closed, ultrasound (US) is obtained urgently. Intrauterine pregnancy is detectable as an intrauterine double sac when β-hCG levels reach 1500 mIU/ml. Endovaginal US can also show a corpus luteum cyst or ectopic pregnancy. Heterotopic pregnancy is rare, occurring in approximately 1 in 30,000 pregnancies, and may be seen on US.

(H) Bleeding from an inflamed cervix is usually scant; however, cervical determination of infection with *Chlamydia trachomatis* or *Neisseria gonorrhea* should be performed if inflammatory exudate ("mucopus") from the cervix is seen.

(I) Cervical polyps bleed irregularly or postcoitally. A narrow-based cervical polyp can easily be removed by twisting the polyp on its stalk and sending the tissue for pathologic evaluation. Endocervical curettage should follow to remove any remaining fragment of the stalk. Broad-based polyps may bleed profusely with removal, and therefore access to electrocautery and surgical facilities are essential. Cervical cancer presenting as a protruding cervical polyp is rare.

(J) Any visible cervical lesion *must* be biopsied because it may represent a cervical cancer. Postcoital spotting may be the presenting symptom of cervical cancer.

(K) Hysterosonography or fluid-contrast US involves instillation of saline into the uterine cavity via a catheter with concomitant performance of an endovaginal ultrasound. This technique will outline endometrial polyps and intracavitary or submucosal myomata because these lesions are echogenic against the dark fluid background. Polyps may actually seem to float in the intracavitary fluid. Evaluation of endometrial thickness and endometrial heterogeneity should be evaluated on ultrasound because a thickened endometrial "stripe" with significant heterogeneity is suggestive of endometrial hyperplasia, an endometrial polyp, or adenocarcinoma. Endometrial stripe thickness varies throughout the menstrual cycle and must be interpreted with respect to the onset of the menstrual bleeding. Ideally, an endometrial stripe evaluation performed within 5 days of the onset of bleeding will be thin.

(L) A granulosa-cell tumor can cause irregular bleeding because of excessive endogenous estrogen production. Tubo-ovarian abscess (end-stage pelvic inflammatory disease) may be associated with irregular spotting secondary to endometritis. Drainage by laparoscopy, or more commonly by exploratory laparotomy and abdominal hysterectomy bilateral salpingo-oophorectomy, may be required if intravenous antibiotic therapy fails to resolve the symptoms of pain and the signs of infection.

(M) Irregular bleeding from uterine myomata may be controlled by oral contraceptive pills (OCPs). In addition, uterine artery embolization is available for women who do not desire future

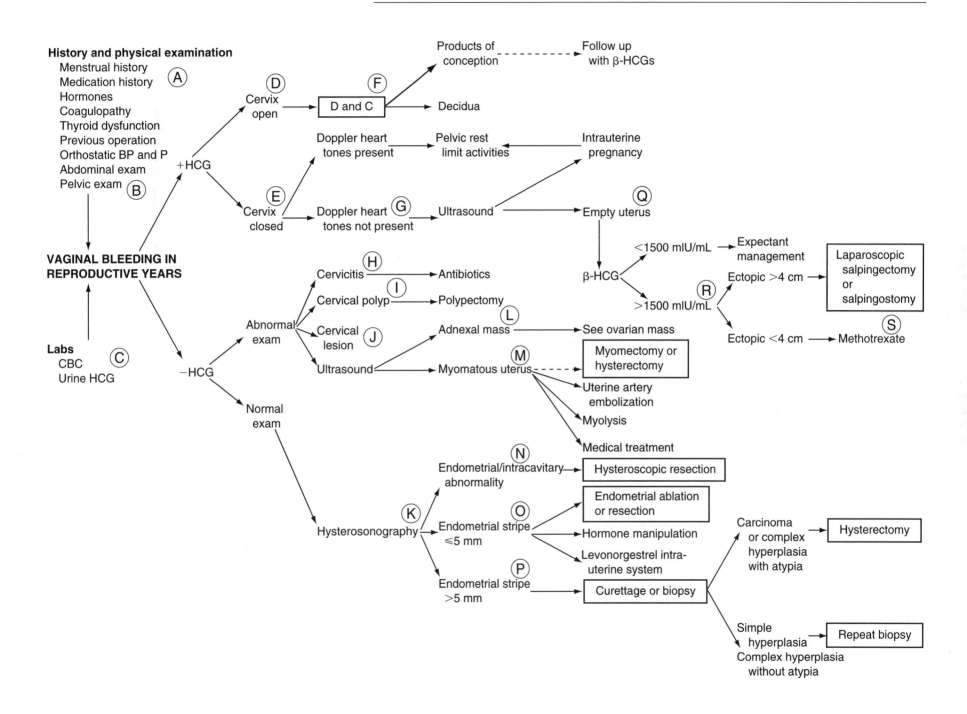

childbearing and are willing to accept the possibility of declining ovarian function secondary to the injected material occluding the ovarian blood vessels. Coagulative necrosis may be induced within individual myomata using cold therapy ("cryomyolysis"), electrical current ("electromyolysis"), or interstitial thermotherapy probes placed inside the individual myoma. Visualization by laparoscopy or hysteroscopy is required. Nonsteroidal anti-inflammatory drugs can alleviate heavy bleeding by inhibiting deposition of prostaglandins. Gonadotropin-releasing hormone agonists (GnRH-a) such as leuprolide can control bleeding by inhibiting the hypothalamic-pituitary-ovarian axis and inducing a hypoestrogenic state.

(N) Endometrial polyps, submucosal myomata, and intracavitary myomata can be resected hysteroscopically.

(O) Denuded atrophic endometrium (with an endometrial stripe less than 5 mm) can be treated with monophasic OCPs. Hysteroscopic endometrial resection (HER) or endometrial thermal ablation (ETA) may be performed in patients who have completed childbearing and who are unable to tolerate OCPs. HER is performed after suppressing the endometrium with GnRH-a medication and involves removing the endometrium in strips with a resectoscope (a large hysteroscope) placed through the cervix. Ablation of the endometrium may be performed under direct hysteroscopic visualization using an electrosurgical ball, which is rolled across the endometrium and destroys the tissue. ETA is performed by passing a silicon balloon with a heating element into the uterine cavity. As the heat is distributed throughout the uterine cavity, the endometrium is destroyed. Patient satisfaction with these techniques is high; however, they should be avoided in patients with a high risk of endometrial hyperplasia or carcinoma because endometrial glands could potentially be buried in the myometrium and be inaccessible to sampling. The levonorgestrel intrauterine system (Mirena®) delivers high dose progestin to the endometrium and decreases menstrual blood loss by 90% but may be expelled in patients with leiomyomata. Thyroid dysfunction, a common cause of anovulatory bleeding, should be ruled out.

(P) Curettage can lessen bleeding associated with chronic anovulation (stripe greater than 5 mm). Endometrial hyperplasia or neoplasia is diagnosed by endometrial biopsy. Hysterectomy is indicated for hyperplasia with cytologic atypia. Simple hyperplasia or complex hyperplasia without cytologic atypia is treated with progestin. Repeat endometrial biopsy after treatment with progestin is necessary to ensure regression of the hyperplasia.

(Q) An empty uterus requires follow-up by both hCG titers and US. In pregnant women, hCG titers should double every 48 hours. A lesser rise may indicate a nonviable pregnancy; however, repeat hCG titers are recommended in 48 hours if the pregnancy is desired. If bleeding is not heavy and the patient is clinically stable, most nonviable pregnancies are reabsorbed or pass spontaneously and do not require a dilation and curettage.

(R) β-hCG titers greater than 1500 mIU/ml and endovaginal US findings that do not show an intrauterine gestational sac suggest ectopic pregnancy. Laparoscopic management is usually the first line treatment when the adnexal mass suggestive of ectopic pregnancy is greater than 4 cm or when cardiac activity is seen in the mass. Laparoscopic salpingectomy is indicated for women who no longer wish to become pregnant, for those who have uncontrolled bleeding, and for patients who have a second ectopic pregnancy in the same tube. Salpingostomy without closure is used for others.

(S) Methotrexate is appropriate treatment when the ectopic pregnancy is less than 4 cm in diameter, the patient is hemodynamically stable, and the patient has the ability to follow up for repeat blood work. Endometrial biopsy should confirm the absence of chorionic villi but is not necessary before giving methotrexate.

REFERENCES

Berek JS (ed): Novak's Gynecology, 13th ed. Baltimore: Williams & Wilkins, 2002.

Broder MS, Goodwin S, Chen G et al: Comparison of long-term outcomes of myomectomy and uterine artery embolization. Obstet Gynecol 100:864–868, 2002.

Falcone T, Bedaiwy MA: Minimally invasive management of uterine fibroids. Current Opin Obstet Gynecol 14:401–407, 2002.

Ikomi A, Pepra EF: Efficacy of the levonorgestrel intrauterine system in treating menorrhagia: Actualities and ambiguities. J Fam Plan Reproductive Health Care 28:99–100, 2002.

Livingstone M, Fraser IS: Mechanisms of abnormal uterine bleeding. Human Reproduction Update 8:60–67, 2002.

Pellicano M, Guida M, Acunzo G et al: Hysteroscopic transcervical endometrial resection versus thermal destruction for menorrhagia: A prospective randomized trial on satisfaction rate. Am J Obstet Gynecol 187:545–550, 2002.

Stenchever MA, Droegemueller W, Herbst AL et al (eds): Comprehensive Gynecology, 4th ed. St. Louis: Mosby, 2001.

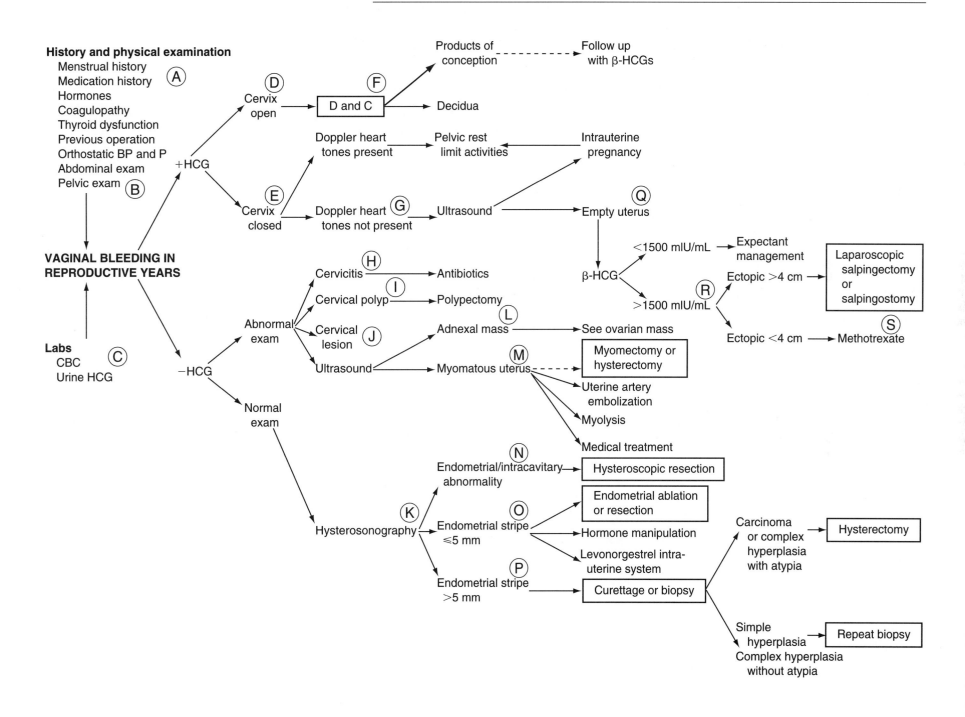

Chapter 132 *Postmenopausal Vaginal Bleeding*

KARLOTTA M. DAVIS, MD, MPH

(A) Medication history may reveal that anticoagulant therapy is a cause of abnormal uterine bleeding. More commonly, breakthrough bleeding from estrogen replacement therapy (ERT) is implicated. Although the recent results of the Women's Health Initiative have resulted in a stampede away from patient continuance or acceptance of postmenopausal ERT, symptomatic relief from the troublesome symptoms of the menopause is best accomplished with estrogen treatment. Estrogen must be given with progestin in women with uteri to prevent endometrial hyperplasia. The addition of daily progestin with estrogen, while necessary, causes bleeding in most postmenopausal women. Bleeding ceases in 80% of women who continue ERT for 1 year. Increasing the dose of medroxyprogesterone acetate (MPA) from the usual 2.5 mg per day to 5.0 mg per day stops the bleeding in another 10% of women. Cyclic addition of progestin is an option for women who cannot tolerate the unpredictable bleeding associated with continuous daily estrogen and progestin therapy and may be used for 14 days every 3 months in a dosage of MPA 5 mg per day for 14 days. Withdrawal bleeding may follow. Micronized progesterone 100 mg per day is associated with less bleeding than MPA. Tamoxifen therapy is associated with increased incidences of endometrial polyps, endometrial hyperplasia, and adenocarcinoma. All patients who take tamoxifen and experience bleeding must undergo evaluation of the endometrium to rule out these lesions. Hysterosonography is the first step in evaluation of bleeding in a tamoxifen-treated patient with bleeding. If no polyps are found, then an endometrial biopsy should be performed. If polyps are found on hysterosonography, resection under hysteroscopy guidance is indicated. The endometrial effect of tamoxifen is unpredictable: 40% of patients exhibit proliferative effects; 40% exhibit atrophic changes; and 20% exhibit a mixed effect.

(B) Vaginal atrophy is common in postmenopausal women who are not receiving estrogen. The signs of urogenital atrophy are a pale vaginal mucosa; loss of vaginal rugations; and a thin, watery discharge. Bleeding from the atrophic vaginal epithelium may occur, especially with minor trauma from a speculum examination or from coitus.

(C) Cessation of menses (onset of menopause) occurs on average at age 51 years. Estrogen production declines during perimenopause, and abnormal bleeding, usually anovulatory in nature, is common. Hot flushes, sleep abnormalities, and mood lability are common seconday to the characteristic hypoestrogenism. Ovulation can occur despite declining levels of endogenous estrogen but occurs with greater inefficiency than in a younger woman. Bleeding may be controlled by suppression of ovulation with oral contraceptive pills (OCPs) in nonsmoking, perimenopausal women. An added benefit of estrogen replacement is almost immediate improvement in the troublesome symptoms of hot flushes, sleep disturbances, fatigue, labile mood, and memory disturbances. The 7-day pill-free period prescribed for reproductive age women using OCPs for birth control may be adjusted in the perimenopausal woman to suit her symptoms. Some women will experience hot flushes within 1 or 2 days of not taking the OCP. In these women the pill-free period may be eliminated, and the active estrogen and progesterone pill may be taken continuously.

(D) Patients with impaired liver function may not metabolize estrogen efficiently, and the result may be a relative excess of estrogen and bleeding.

(E) Any cervical abnormality may represent a cervical carcinoma and should be biopsied to rule out neoplasia. A cervical polyp can be twisted off its stalk and sent for pathologic evaluation. Endocervical curettage should be performed to remove any fragments of the polyp stalk; these also should be sent to pathology for evaluation.

(F) Hysterosonography or fluid-contrast ultrasound (US) may delineate an intracavitary abnormality such as a polyp or a submucosal fibroid. Endometrial thickness or stripes may be determined by routine standard ultrasound. Stripes greater than 5 mm and irregular or heterogeneous echo texture are associated with endometrial adenomatous hyperplasia or adenocarcinoma. Endometrial polyps not seen on standard US are delineated with accuracy by hysterosonography as the dark intrauterine fluid outlines the echogenic polyps, which appear to float in the saline. Submucous myomata are seen to protrude into the intrauterine cavity and distort the endometrium. Why submucous myomata cause bleeding is not known. Perhaps increased bleeding occurs because of increased endometrial surface area, or because the endometrium is atrophied over a myoma. Each myoma is supplied by a single artery, and the supply of estrogen or progesterone is lower to the endometrium overlying the myoma, leading to irregular shedding of the endometrium.

(G) An endometrial stripe less than 5 mm is not associated with hyperplasia, and endometrial sampling is not necessary. Initial adjustment of the ERT dose may include slightly increasing estrogen, increasing progestin, or considering a cyclic regimen of daily estrogen with 14 days of progestin so that the patient experiences predictable withdrawal bleeding episodes.

(H) Endometrial abnormalities such as polyps or myomata can be resected hysteroscopically in conjunction with dilation and curettage (D&C). Hysterectomy may be considered if the bleeding is refractory to medical treatment. Myomata tend to shrink at the time of the menopause, so expectant management is another treatment option.

(I) Endometrial sampling can be performed with a plastic suction catheter device (Pipelle®), a rigid suction catheter (Novak curette), or in the operating room via traditional fractional dilation and curettage. A patient with a stenotic cervix may require IV sedation or a paracervical block for pain control during cervical dilation. Pretreatment with vaginal misoprostol pills softens the cervix and

History and physical examination
Menses cessation
Medications (A)
Medical history
Vaginal atrophy (B)
Cervical lesion
Uterine enlargement

POSTMENOPAUSAL (C)
VAGINAL BLEEDING

Labs
CBC (D)
Liver function tests
Chest x-ray (for
   endometrial cancer)

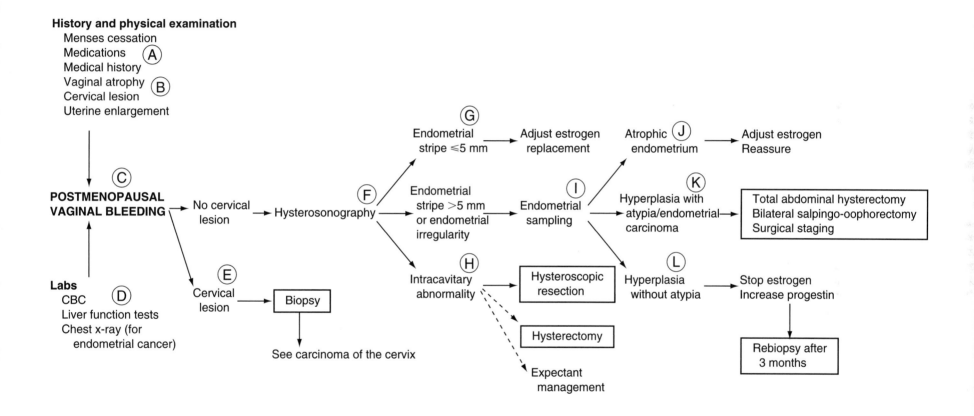

No cervical
lesion → Hysterosonography (F)

Cervical (E)
lesion → Biopsy

See carcinoma of the cervix

Endometrial (G)
stripe ≤5 mm → Adjust estrogen
replacement

Endometrial
stripe >5 mm
or endometrial
irregularity → Endometrial (I)
sampling

Intracavitary (H)
abnormality → Hysteroscopic
resection

Hysterectomy

Expectant
management

Atrophic (J)
endometrium → Adjust estrogen
Reassure

Hyperplasia with (K)
atypia/endometrial
carcinoma → Total abdominal hysterectomy
Bilateral salpingo-oophorectomy
Surgical staging

Hyperplasia (L)
without atypia → Stop estrogen
Increase progestin → Rebiopsy after
3 months

allows for easier passage of an endometrial curette or a hysteroscope.

(J) If atrophic endometrium is returned, the patient may be reassured. Increasing the estrogen component of ERT may control the bleeding.

(K) Complex endometrial hyperplasia with cytologic atypia and adenocarcinoma of the endometrium are treated with total abdominal hysterectomy and bilateral salpingo-oophorectomy. Frozen-section pathologic examination should be routine for all patients with hyperplasia with cytologic atypia because adenocarcinoma may coexist with hyperplasia. Surgical staging (i.e., pelvic and periaortic lymph node biopsies and peritoneal washings) is required when the histologic grade of the adenocarcinoma is poorly differentiated or when the tumor has invaded more than half of the myometrium. Vaginal hysterectomy may be considered for patients who have a well-differentiated carcinoma and are poor surgical candidates.

(L) Endometrial hyperplasia indicates a relative estrogen excess. For simple hyperplasia or complex endometrial hyperplasia without cytologic atypia, progestin doses must be increased (medroxyprogesterone acetate, 30 mg/day for 30 days followed by 10 mg/day for 2 months; or norethindrone acetate 10 mg/day for 30 days, 5 mg/day for 2 months), and estrogen should be stopped. When repeat biopsy detects resolution of the hyperplasia, consideration may be given to restarting the estrogen. Cyclic ERT (conjugated equine estrogens, 0.625 mg/day PO; and medroxyprogesterone acetate, 5 mg PO for days 1 to 14 each month) may cause regular sloughing of the endometrium in these patients.

REFERENCES

Berek JS (ed): Novak's Gynecology, 13th ed. Baltimore: Williams & Wilkins, 2002.

Clark TJ, Voit D, Gupta JK et al: Accurary of hysteroscopy in the diagnosis of endometrial cancer and hyperplasia. JAMA 288:1610–1621, 2002.

Lindenfeld EA, Langer RD: Bleeding patterns of the hormone replacement therapies in the postmenopausal estrogen and progestin interventions trial. Obstet Gynecol 100:853–863, 2002.

Shau WY, Hsieh CC, Hsieh TT et al: Factors associated with endometrial bleeding in continuous hormone replacement therapy. Menopause 9:188–194, 2002.

Stenchever MA, Droegemueller W, Herbst AL et al (eds): Comprehensive Gynecology, 4th ed. St. Louis: Mosby, 2001.

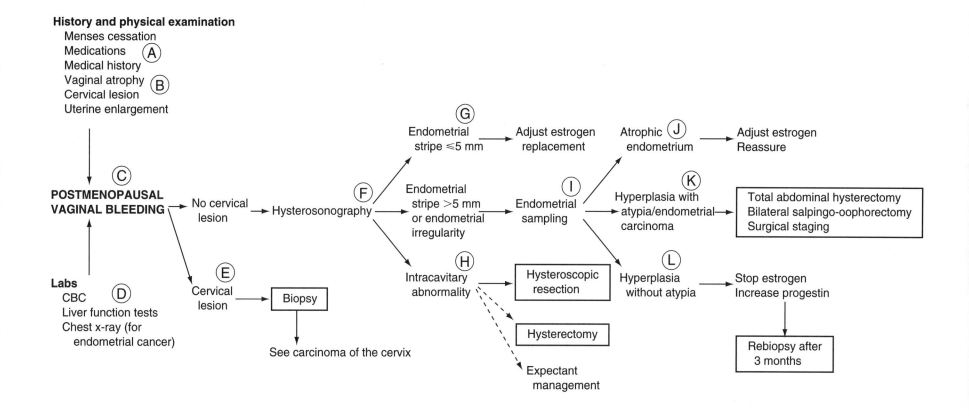

History and physical examination
Menses cessation
Medications (A)
Medical history
Vaginal atrophy (B)
Cervical lesion
Uterine enlargement

(C)
POSTMENOPAUSAL VAGINAL BLEEDING → No cervical lesion → Hysterosonography (F)

Labs
CBC (D)
Liver function tests
Chest x-ray (for endometrial cancer)

(E)
Cervical lesion → Biopsy → See carcinoma of the cervix

(G) Endometrial stripe ≤5 mm → Adjust estrogen replacement

Endometrial stripe >5 mm or endometrial irregularity → Endometrial sampling (I)

(H) Intracavitary abnormality → Hysteroscopic resection
→ Hysterectomy
→ Expectant management

(J) Atrophic endometrium → Adjust estrogen Reassure

Hyperplasia with atypia/endometrial carcinoma (K) → Total abdominal hysterectomy / Bilateral salpingo-oophorectomy / Surgical staging

(L) Hyperplasia without atypia → Stop estrogen Increase progestin → Rebiopsy after 3 months

Chapter 133 *Pelvic Inflammatory Disease*

HAROLD C. WIESENFELD, MD, CM ● R. PHILLIP HEINE, MD

(A) Variables that increase the incidence of pelvic inflammatory disease (PID) include teenage years; multiple sexual partners; a history of PID; intrauterine devices (IUD), when PID develops during the first 2 months after insertion; and uterine instrumentation. Use of mechanical or oral contraceptives decreases the incidence of symptomatic upper tract pelvic infections.

(B) The clinical diagnosis of acute PID is often imprecise. Laparoscopic evaluation shows that a third of patients hospitalized for the disease do not have it. Pain (99%) and pelvic tenderness (95%) are common. Only a third of women have a temperature greater than 38° C. A pelvic mass or swelling is palpable in 48% of patients; vaginal discharge is found in 80%. Many women with PID have subtle symptoms or signs of upper genital tract infection. Clinicians therefore need to have a high index of suspicion, particularly in women at risk for PID. It is prudent to treat suspected disease because tubal obstruction follows an initial episode of PID in approximately 11% of cases.

(C) PID is a major health concern in the United States. More than 1 million new cases occur annually, at a cost exceeding $4 billion.

(D) Laboratory testing sometimes aids in diagnosis. Fewer than 50% of patients have a white blood cell (WBC) count greater than 10,000/mm³. Only 30% and 25%, respectively, have positive cultures for *Chlamydia trachomatis* or *Neisseria gonorrhoeae*. Because PID is a polymicrobial infection involving endogenous aerobes and anaerobes as well as sexually transmitted pathogens, endocervical testing for sexually transmitted diseases (STDs) has limited value in selecting antibiotic therapy. STD testing should be performed nonetheless because STDs are a public health concern and must be reported. In addition, partner notification and treatment are warranted. Vaginal fluid should be collected for pH measurement and microscopic examination for bacterial vaginosis and *Trichomonas vaginalis*.

Syphilis serology status is also determined. HIV and hepatitis B screening tests are offered routinely. Women diagnosed with PID should be counseled on safe-sex practices.

(E) If the results of pelvic examination are inconclusive, ultrasonography is helpful to establish the presence or absence of a pelvic abscess.

(F) An important therapeutic decision is the choice between outpatient treatment and hospitalization. If outpatient treatment is used, it is important to reexamine the patient after 48 to 72 hours. If response is suboptimal, the patient must be hospitalized and IV antibiotic therapy instituted. In general, women with HIV may be treated similarly to HIV-negative women but may be more likely to have tubo-ovarian abscesses.

(G) All sexual partners of women diagnosed with PID should be treated empirically for gonorrhea and chlamydia regardless of the infected woman's STD test results.

(H) Indications for hospitalization include known or suspected tubo-ovarian complex or abscess, uncertain diagnosis, high fever, significant GI symptoms, immunocompromise, and pregnancy.

(I) Because hepatitis B is a sexually transmitted infection, serious consideration should be given to initiating the hepatitis B vaccine series.

(J) There are two CDC-recommended regimens for outpatient therapy of PID. One regimen includes a single dose of a parenteral cephalosporin administered intramuscularly (ceftriaxone, 250 mg, cefoxitin 2 g IM with probenecid, 1 g PO, or other third-generation cephalosporins) with a 14-day course of doxycycline, 100 mg PO twice daily. Many experts enhance anaerobic coverage by adding metronidazole 500 mg PO twice daily for 14 days. The other CDC-recommended outpatient regimen consists of ofloxacin, 400 mg PO, or levofloxacin 500 mg PO once daily each for 14 days. Many experts add metronidazole, 500 mg PO twice daily, each for 14 days.

(K) The CDC recommends several broad-spectrum antibiotic regimens for parenteral treatment of acute PID. Regimen A consists of a second-generation cephalosporin (cefotetan 2 g IV every 12 hours or cefoxitin 2 g IV every 6 hours) with doxycycline 100 mg PO or IV every 12 hours. Regimen B includes both clindamycin 900 mg IV every 8 hours with gentamicin 2 mg/kg IV or IM loading dose followed by a maintenance dose of 1.5 mg/kg every 8 hours. Single daily dosing of gentamicin may be substituted. Many experts prefer regimen B if a tubo-ovarian abscess is present because of its enhanced anaerobic activity. Alternative parenteral regimens (on which there is limited data compared with regimens A and B) include ofloxacin 400 mg IV every 12 hours or levofloxacin 500 mg IV once daily (with or without the addition of metronidazole 500 mg IV every 8 hours); and ampicillin/sulbactam 3 g IV every 6 hours with doxycycline 100 mg PO or IV every 12 hours. Parenteral therapy in many cases may be switched to oral therapy within 24 hours of clinical improvement. Women with tubo-ovarian abscesses generally require longer duration of parenteral therapy. When parenteral treatment is discontinued, oral therapy with either doxycycline 100 mg PO twice daily or clindamycin 450 mg PO four times a day (especially for tubo-ovarian abscess) is continued to complete a 14-day course.

(L) Laparoscopy is indicated when the diagnosis of PID is in doubt or when the patient is not responding to medical therapy.

(M) Complications of PID include ectopic pregnancy (prevalence is 6 to 10 times normal); infertility (rate increases proportionally to the number of episodes of acute PID: one episode, 11%; two episodes, 23%; three episodes, 54%); chronic pelvic pain (about 20%); and recurrent PID (about 25%).

(N) Approximately 10% of patients with the diagnosis of PID have a documented tubo-ovarian abscess. With appropriate antibiotics, most abscesses regress and do not require operative drainage. Patients who do not respond to antibiotic therapy may be candidates for abscess drainage via laparoscopy, or a percutaneous catheter placed under ultrasound or computed tomography guidance. If surgery becomes necessary, conservatism is appropriate to protect childbearing potential and continued hormonal function.

REFERENCES

Centers for Disease Control and Prevention: Sexually transmitted diseases treatment guidelines 2002. MMWR 51:48–52, 2002.

Kahn JG, Walker CK, Washington E et al: Diagnosing pelvic inflammatory disease: Comprehensive analysis and considerations for developing a new model. JAMA 266:2594–2604, 1991.

McCormack WM: Pelvic inflammatory disease. N Engl J Med 330:115–119, 1994.

Scholles D, Stergachis A, Heidrich FE et al: Prevention of pelvic inflammatory disease by screening for cervical chlamydial infection. N Engl J Med 334:1362–1366, 1996.

Westrom L: Incidence, prevalence, and trends of acute pelvic inflammatory disease and its consequences in industrialized countries. Am J Obstet Gynecol 138:880–892, 1980.

Wiesenfeld HC, Hillier SL, Krohn MA et al: Lower genital tract infection and endometritis: Insight into subclinical pelvic inflammatory disease. Obstet Gynecol 100:456–463, 2002.

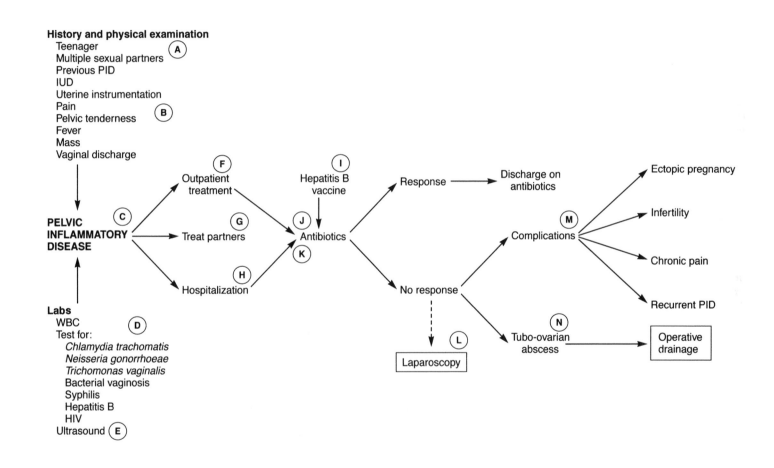

Chapter 134 *Endometriosis*

RUBEN J. ALVERO, MD ● JANI R. JENSEN, MD

(A) Endometriosis, the presence of endometrial glands and stroma outside of the uterus, is estimated to affect up to 10% of reproductive age women. The etiology is uncertain and theories include retrograde menstruation and metaplasia; variable immunologic susceptibility among women is also possible. Endometriosis may present as chronic pelvic pain, dysmenorrhea, dyspareunia, infertility, or a combination of these. For women who are symptomatic, the disorder is a chronic disease for which there is no cure but whose manifestations can be controlled to ensure a good quality of life. Endometriosis can be identified in up to 40% of infertile women.

(B) Physical examination findings may include uterosacral nodularity and tenderness, generalized pelvic or uterine tenderness, fixation of the pelvic organs, retroversion of the uterus, and adnexal masses.

(C) Evaluation should be performed to rule out other causes of chronic pelvic pain (e.g., gastrointestinal, genitourinary, musculoskeletal, or psychiatric disorders). Patients who do not desire fertility may benefit from a trial of oral contraceptives and nonsteroidal anti-inflammatory drugs (NSAIDs). More aggressive intervention may be required if symptoms worsen or do not improve after 3 months of combined oral contraceptive and NSAID therapy.

(D) Definitive diagnosis relies on direct visualization of endometriotic implants by laparoscopy. Laboratory tests such as measurement of CA-125 currently have little role in diagnosing endometriosis. Disease stage is classified by lesion size, depth of penetration, status of the posterior cul-de-sac, presence and size of ovarian endometriomas, and presence and nature of pelvic adhesions.

(E) Characteristic lesions are described as having a powder burn appearance surrounded by a stellate scar, but endometriosis may appear as clear vesicles; puckered pigmented lesions; white plaques; petechiae; or raised red, blue, or brown discolorations. Fresh implants are often red and contain glands and stroma. Biopsies of suspicious areas should be performed if the diagnosis is uncertain. Endosalpingiosis, aberrantly located tubal mucosa without stroma, is the most common false positive histologic finding.

(F) Treatment of endometriosis depends on whether or not the patient desires current or future fertility. Expectant management may be reasonable when infertility is the major complaint and endometriosis is minimal or mild. Some 50% to 70% of these patients conceive. One multicenter randomized clinical trial reported that surgically-treated women with minimal or mild endometriosis had an enhanced fecundity rate compared with untreated women with a similar extent of disease. Patients who fail to conceive after a period of observation may elect to undergo ovarian hyperstimulation with intrauterine insemination or in vitro fertilization to maximize fertility.

(G) Medical therapy is effective for patients who have moderate to severe pain, but it delays fertility because therapy usually requires 6 months. Treatment includes gonadotropin-releasing hormone (GnRH) analogs, danazol, and progestational agents. GnRH analogs create a hypoestrogenic state and cause atrophy of endometriosis implants by down-regulation of pituitary GnRH receptors. Side effects include hot flashes, vaginal dryness, insomnia, decreased libido, depression, headache, and fatigue. Trabecular bone loss may occur but does not appear to be severe with a 6-month regimen. Add-back therapy with estrogens or progestins minimizes hypoestrogenic side effects while maintaining therapeutic efficacy. Danazol, a synthetic testosterone derivative, directly inhibits steroid production from the ovary, endometrial proliferation, growth of endometriosis implants, and pituitary gonadotropin secretion. Danazol also decreases the concentration of sex hormone–binding globulin, resulting in elevated free testosterone levels. Androgenic side effects are common and may limit its use. Side effects include weight gain, acne, muscle cramps, edema, and vaginal spotting. Because of the significant side-effect profile, danazol is rarely the indicated choice for therapy. Progestational agents such as medroxyprogesterone acetate inhibit the growth of endometriosis implants by causing their decidualization and subsequent atrophy. Side effects include breakthrough bleeding, weight gain, nausea, fluid retention, headache, and depression. Amenorrhea may occur. Decreased pain symptoms (75% to 90%) are comparable with all of these agents. Recurrence rates are high after discontinuation of any therapy and pregnancy rates are not improved following medical treatment.

Laparoscopic surgery is advised for moderate to severe endometriosis associated with infertility or pain, or for patients who fail medical management. Endometriomas can usually be removed laparoscopically, depending on the size of the lesion and the skill of the surgeon. Excision of deep endometriosis is technically difficult and requires considerable expertise. Laparoscopic uterosacral nerve ablation may be performed for pain relief, although no controlled prospective studies have been done to show long-term benefit. Following laparoscopic surgery, 60% to 80% of patients report improvement in pain symptoms. Up to 82% of patients with moderate to severe endometriosis become pregnant within 3 years after surgery.

(H) In vitro fertilization is recommended for persistent infertility.

(I) Abdominal conservative surgery is recommended for endometriosis with severe anatomic distortion associated with infertility or pain. A presacral neurectomy provides effective relief of severe midline dysmenorrhea in 85% of women. The goal of conservative surgery is the removal of all visible endometriosis and restoration of normal pelvic anatomy. Some 75% to 90% of patients experience significant pain relief after

History and physical examination
Pelvic pain (A)
Dysmenorrhea
Dyspareunia
Infertility
Uterosacral nodularity (B)
Adnexal mass
Uterine tenderness

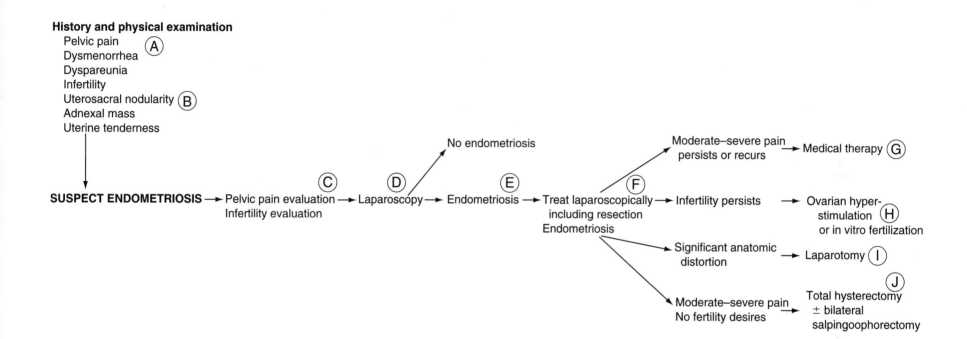

SUSPECT ENDOMETRIOSIS → Pelvic pain evaluation (C) → Laparoscopy (D) → Endometriosis (E) → Treat laparoscopically (F)
Infertility evaluation   including resection
                                  Endometriosis

No endometriosis

Moderate–severe pain → Medical therapy (G)
persists or recurs

Infertility persists → Ovarian hyper-
stimulation (H)
or in vitro fertilization

Significant anatomic → Laparotomy (I)
distortion

Moderate–severe pain → Total hysterectomy (J)
No fertility desires   ± bilateral
                        salpingoophorectomy

conservative surgery, and 50% to 60% of infertile women conceive but disease recurrence is common. Whether this represents true recurrence or progression of incompletely resected disease is unknown. The timeline is dependent on the severity of the disease as well as the thoroughness of the primary resection.

(J)   Total abdominal hysterectomy with bilateral salpingo-oophorectomy is recommended for moderate to severe pain when fertility is no longer desired. Laparoscopically assisted vaginal hysterectomy with bilateral salpingo-oophorectomy is another option. Ovarian conservation may be attempted for patients remote from menopause, but recurrent pain occurs in almost 60% of these women. Over 90% of patients can expect relief after total abdominal hysterectomy with bilateral salpingo-oophorectomy. Estrogen therapy is usually recommended to treat the effects of surgical castration and there is no evidence that giving this treatment immediately after the surgery is associated with increased pain caused by stimulation of endometriotic foci. Additionally, reports exist of malignant transformation of endometriosis in postmenopausal women under the influence of either estrogen or selective estrogen receptor modulators such as tamoxifen. Some clinicians recommend cotreatment with progesterone to prevent this occurrence.

REFERENCES

American Society for Reproductive Medicine: Revised American Society for Reproductive Medicine classification of endometriosis: 1996. Fertil Steril 817–821, 1997.

Hickman TN, Namnoum AB, Hinton EL et al: Timing of estrogen replacement therapy following hysterectomy with oophorectomy for endometriosis. Obstet Gynecol 91:673–677, 1998.

Ling FW: Randomized controlled trial of depot leuprolide in patients with chronic pelvic pain and clinically suspected endometriosis. Pelvic Pain Study Group. Obstet Gynecol 93:51–58, 1999.

Marcoux S, Maheux R, Berube S et al: Laparoscopic surgery in infertile women with minimal or mild endometriosis. N Engl J Med 337:217–222, 1997.

Mol BW, Bayram N, Lijmer JG et al: The performance of CA-125 measurement in the detection of endometriosis: A meta-analysis. Fertil Steril 70:1101–1108, 1998.

Morales AJ, Murphy AA: Endoscopic treatment for endometriosis. Obstet Gynecol Clin North Am 26:121–133, 1999.

Okugawa K, Hirakawa T, Ogawa S et al: Ovarian endometrioid adenocarcinoma arising from an endometriotic cyst in a postmenopausal woman under tamoxifen therapy for breast cancer. Gynecol Oncology 87:231–234, 2002.

Prentice A, Deary AJ, Goldbeck-Wood S et al: Gonadotrophin-releasing hormone analogues for pain associated with endometriosis (Cochrane Review). In: The Cochrane Library, Issue 4, 2002. Oxford: Update Software.

Selak V, Farquhar C, Prentice A et al: Danazol for pelvic pain associated with endometriosis (Cochrane Review). In: The Cochrane Library, Issue 4, 2002. Oxford: Update Software.

Walter AJ, Hentz JG, Magtibay PM et al: Endometriosis: Correlation between histologic and visual findings at laparoscopy. Am J Obstet Gynecol 184:1407–1413, 2001.

History and physical examination
- Pelvic pain   Ⓐ
- Dysmenorrhea
- Dyspareunia
- Infertility
- Uterosacral nodularity Ⓑ
- Adnexal mass
- Uterine tenderness

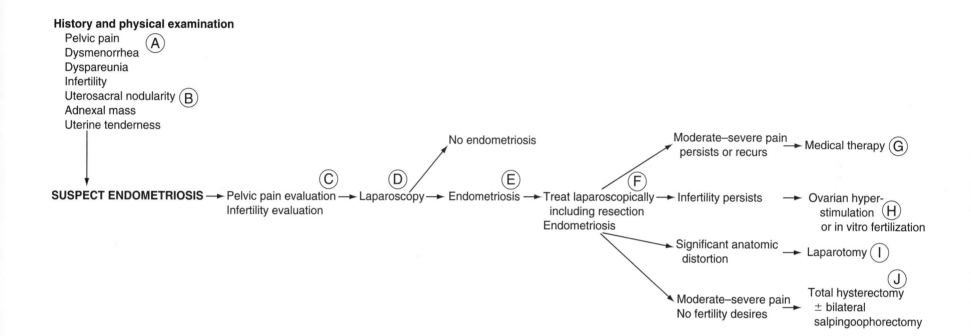

SUSPECT ENDOMETRIOSIS → Pelvic pain evaluation → Laparoscopy → Endometriosis → Treat laparoscopically →
Infertility evaluation (Ⓒ) (Ⓓ) (Ⓔ) including resection (Ⓕ)
Endometriosis

No endometriosis

Moderate–severe pain persists or recurs → Medical therapy Ⓖ

Infertility persists → Ovarian hyper-stimulation Ⓗ or in vitro fertilization

Significant anatomic distortion → Laparotomy Ⓘ

Moderate–severe pain No fertility desires → Total hysterectomy ± bilateral salpingoophorectomy Ⓙ

Chapter 135 *Carcinoma of the Cervix*

SUSAN A. DAVIDSON, MD

(A) Risk factors for carcinoma of the cervix include coital activity, human papillomavirus, smoking, and failure to have regular Pap tests.

(B) Squamous intraepithelial lesions on Pap smear require tissue diagnosis. Colposcopy-directed biopsies and endocervical curettage are required if no gross lesion is seen. Cone biopsy of the cervix may be necessary.

(C) Staging is clinical and may require examination under anesthesia, cystoscopy, and proctosigmoidoscopy. These procedures are part of the staging and are usually indicated for lesions larger than stage IB1. Ureteral evaluation (usually computed tomography [CT] with IV contrast) and chest radiography are required.

(D) Stage I disease is confined strictly to the cervix. Stage IA is identified only microscopically and requires cone biopsy for diagnosis. Stage IA1 is invasion 3 mm or less in depth and 7 mm or less in width (5-year survival, 99%). Stage IA2 is invasion 3.1 to 5 mm in depth and 7 mm or less in width (5-year survival, 90% to 95%). Stage IB1 is clinical disease 4 cm or less in diameter or preclinical and greater than 5 mm in depth or greater than 7 mm in width (5-year survival, 85%). Stage IB2 is gross disease greater than 4 cm in diameter (5-year survival, 67%).

(E) Stage IIA disease extends to the upper two thirds of the vagina without parametrial involvement (5-year survival, 68%). Stage IIB is disease with obvious parametrial involvement but not to the pelvic side walls (5-year survival, 60% to 65%).

(F) In stage III disease the tumor extends to the pelvic wall, involves the lower third of the vagina, or causes hydronephrosis (5-year survival, 25% to 48%). Stage IIIA disease affects the lower third of the vagina without pelvic wall extension or hydronephrosis. Stage IIIB is disease to the pelvic wall or hydronephrosis, or both.

(G) Stage IVA is disease extension to the mucosa of the bladder or rectum (5-year survival, 18%). Stage IVB disease is spread to distant organs (5-year survival, less than 5%).

(H) Radical hysterectomy with pelvic and low para-aortic lymphadenectomy is applicable as primary treatment only for stage I and small stage IIA lesions. In these cases, surgery and radiation give comparable survival rates. Surgery is usually selected for younger patients who are good surgical candidates because the ovaries can be preserved. Coital activity is more satisfactory after surgery than after radiation.

(I) Stage IB2 is synonymous with "barrel-shaped" cervix. Preoperative radiation treatment options include extrafascial hysterectomy, radical hysterectomy and lymphadenectomy followed by postoperative radiation, or radical radiation therapy.

(J) Radical radiation therapy consists of whole pelvis teletherapy plus brachytherapy. It is used for advanced disease or for patients who have operative risks. The complication rate is about 5% with either radical surgery (acute complications) or radical radiation (chronic complications to bladder and bowel) for early stage disease.

Interstitial brachytherapy is occasionally used for bulky parametrial disease. Chemotherapy, usually cisplatin, is commonly used as a radiation sensitizer.

(K) Palliative radiation may or may not require brachytherapy or other modifications. Patients usually die from uremia or sepsis.

(L) Recurrence limited to the pelvis is potentially curable (5-year survival, 25% to 50%). Radiation may be used if it has not been used before. Patients with central recurrence after radiation are candidates for pelvic exenteration.

REFERENCES

Green JA, Kirwan JM, Tierney JF et al: Survival and recurrence after concomitant chemotherapy and radiotherapy for cancer of the uterine cervix: A systematic review and meta-analysis. Lancet 358:781, 2001.

Grigsby PW, Herzog TJ: Current management of patients with invasive cervical carcinoma. Clin Obstet Gynecol 44:531, 2001.

Hopkins MP, Morley GW: Radical hysterectomy versus radiation therapy for stage IB squamous cell cancer of the cervix. Cancer 68:272, 1991.

Im SS, Monk BJ: New developments in the treatment of invasive cervical cancer. Obstet Gynecol Clin North Am 29:659, 2002.

Janicek MF, Averette HE: Cervical cancer: Prevention, diagnosis, and therapeutics. CA Cancer J Clin 51:92, 2001.

Keys H, Gibbons SK: Optimal management of locally advanced cervical carcinoma. J Natl Cancer Inst Monogr 21:89, 1996.

Morley GW, Hopkins MP, Lindenauer SM et al: Pelvic exenteration. University of Michigan: 100 patients at 5 years. Obstet Gynecol 74:934, 1989.

Rose PG: Chemoradiotherapy for cervical cancer. Eur J Cancer 38:270, 2002.

Sawaya GF, Brown AD, Washington AE: Current approaches to cervical cancer screening. N Engl J Med 344:1603, 2001.

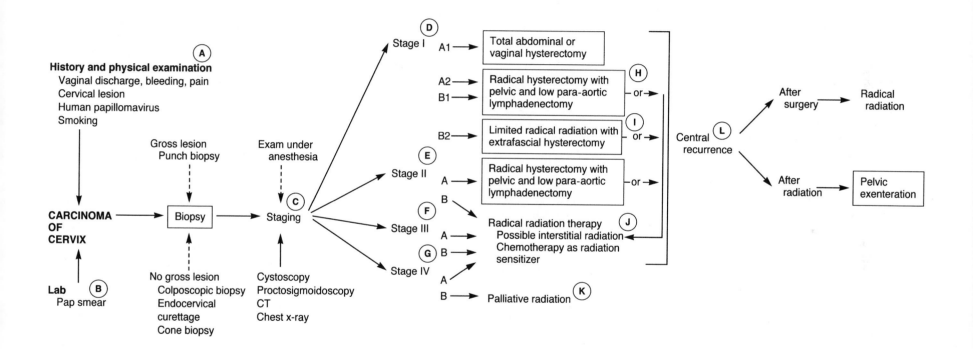

History and physical examination (A)
 Vaginal discharge, bleeding, pain
 Cervical lesion
 Human papillomavirus
 Smoking

Gross lesion
Punch biopsy

Exam under
anesthesia

CARCINOMA
OF
CERVIX → Biopsy → Staging (C)

No gross lesion
 Colposcopic biopsy
 Endocervical
 curettage
 Cone biopsy

Cystoscopy
Proctosigmoidoscopy
CT
Chest x-ray

Lab (B)
 Pap smear

Stage I (D)
 A1 → Total abdominal or
 vaginal hysterectomy
 A2 → Radical hysterectomy with
 B1 → pelvic and low para-aortic
 lymphadenectomy (H) — or →
 B2 → Limited radical radiation with
 extrafascial hysterectomy (I) — or →

Stage II (E)
 A → Radical hysterectomy with
 pelvic and low para-aortic
 lymphadenectomy — or →
 B →

Stage III (F)
 A → Radical radiation therapy (J)
 B → Possible interstitial radiation
 Chemotherapy as radiation
 sensitizer

Stage IV (G)
 A →
 B → Palliative radiation (K)

Central
recurrence (L)
 After surgery → Radical radiation
 After radiation → Pelvic exenteration

Chapter 136 Endometrial Carcinoma

HOWARD M. GOODMAN, MD • ROSS S. BERKOWITZ, MD

(A) Risk factors for endometrial carcinoma include hyperestrogen states (e.g., obesity, estrogen-secreting tumors, and use of exogenous unopposed estrogen); reproductive history (e.g., low parity, late menopause, and anovulatory states); intercurrent illness (e.g., diabetes mellitus and hypertension); heredity (e.g., family risk); and atypical endometrial hyperplasia (progresses to frank cancer in 25% to 30% of patients). A major symptom is abnormal vaginal bleeding (first symptom in 90% of women with endometrial carcinoma, usually postmenopausal).

(B) The pelvic examination is usually negative in early disease. Cervical involvement, adnexal enlargement, and parametrial spread are indicative of advanced disease. Ascites is seen rarely.

(C) Endometrial carcinoma is the most common gynecologic malignancy (40,000 new cases per year). There is currently no satisfactory screening technique for endometrial carcinoma.

(D) Office biopsy is the initial diagnostic procedure. Accuracy approaches that of formal dilation and curettage (D&C).

(E) Formal fractional D&C remains the standard against which other diagnostic tests are measured. This procedure is usually performed in the operating room with either general or regional anesthesia. Although it is slightly more accurate than office biopsy, the need for hospitalization, anesthesia, and a higher complication rate and cost relegate it to situations when an office procedure cannot be performed or when an inadequate specimen is obtained, or when symptoms persist after office biopsy has negative findings.

(F) Preoperative evaluation should include general medical history and physical examination, pelvic examination to assess resectability and evidence of extracorporal spread, chest radiography, liver and renal blood testing, and routine hematologic testing.

(G) The International Federation of Gynecology and Obstetrics (FIGO) adopted a surgical staging system in 1990. Surgical staging entails exploratory laparotomy with complete assessment of the intra-abdominal contents; peritoneal washings; total abdominal hysterectomy and bilateral salpingo-oophorectomy with estimation of grade and depth of myometrial invasion; lymphadenectomy based on these two factors; omental biopsy and biopsy of suspicious areas; and, when possible, resection of areas of disseminated disease. Assignment of FIGO stage is based on histopathologic findings.

(H) Stage I disease is confined to the uterine corpus and is stratified by depth of invasion (e.g., IA, IB, or IC) and further by tumor grade (e.g., 1, 2, or 3). The probability of regional metastases depends on histologic subtype, grade, and depth of invasion. There is a 10% risk of nodal spread with G3 inner, G2 middle, and G1 outer myometrial invasion. Patients with these or deeper levels of invasion may be treated 4 to 6 weeks after hysterectomy with pelvic radiation therapy. Patients with deep myometrial invasion who undergo complete pelvic lymphadenectomy may expect a 90% 5-year survival without external beam pelvic irradiation. Patients with disease confined to the endometrium are at little risk for recurrence and require no adjuvant treatment. Patients with evidence of myometrial invasion less extensive than that noted above are at low risk for pelvic nodal spread but have a risk for vaginal apex recurrence. They may be considered for vaginal radiation postoperatively, which reduces their risk level to 2% or less. Reported 5-year survival for more than 10,000 patients with stage I endometrial carcinoma was 75%. Studies suggest 5-year survival is greater than 90%, with the likelihood of cure approaching 100% in low-risk patients; and 60% to 70% in higher-risk patients, as defined by grade and depth of myometrial invasion.

(I) Stage II is defined as disease confined to corpus and cervix and is stratified by grades 1 to 3, and involvement of cervical glands (IIA) or cervical stroma (IIB). These patients are at high risk for pelvic nodal involvement (35% to 40%). Radical hysterectomy offers improved survival versus simple hysterectomy and irradiation in patients who can tolerate extensive surgery. Five-year survival ranges from 80% to 90%.

(J) Stage III is stratified into IIIA (serosa, adnexa, positive washings); IIIB (vagina); and IIIC (retroperitoneal nodes) and is further stratified by grades 1 to 3. Current treatment is exploratory laparotomy, cytoreduction, and staging followed by tailored radiation therapy. Survival approaches 50%. Patients with metastases to the retroperitoneal nodes are usually treated with radiation therapy. Survival rates of 40% to 50% have been achieved with extended-field para-aortic irradiation.

(K) Stage IV is divided into IVA (bladder and rectum) and IVB (distal disease) and stratified by grades 1 to 3. Treatment is individualized. Patients with IVA disease may be considered for radiation therapy or supraradical surgery. Women with stage IVB disease are usually treated with systemic agents, either hormonal (usually progesterone) or cytotoxic chemotherapy. Recurrent disease confined to the pelvis can be treated with radiation therapy if overlapping fields are avoided. Patients not eligible for radiation therapy are usually managed with hormones or cytotoxic chemotherapy. The probability of response to progestational agents is related to grade and receptor status. The response rates in patients with well-differentiated tumors range from 30% to 50%. The response rate with high-grade tumors is less than 10%. Cytotoxic chemotherapy has a role in the management of women with advanced recurrent disease. Adriamycin, Cytoxan, and cisplatin have considerable activity and are commonly used in combination.

REFERENCES

Aalders J, Abeler V, Kolstad P et al: Postoperative external irradiation and prognostic parameters in Stage I endometrial carcinoma. Obstet Gynecol 56:419–426, 1980.

Cornielson T, Trimble E, Kosary C: SEER data, corpus uteri cancer: Treatment trends versus survival for FIGO Stage II, 1988-1994. Gynecol Oncol 74:350–355, 1999.

Creasman WT, Morrow CP, Bundy BN et al: Surgical pathologic spread patterns of endometrial cancer. Cancer 60:2035–2041, 1987.

Feldman S, Berkowitz RS, Tosteson ANA: Cost effectiveness of strategies to evaluate postmenopausal bleeding. Obstet Gynecol 81:968–975, 1993.

Irvin W, Rice L: Advances in the management of endometrial adenocarcinoma. J Reprod Med 47:173–190, 2002.

Larson DM, Broste SK, Krawisz BR: Surgery without radiotherapy for primary treatment of endometrial cancer. Obstet Gynecol 91:355–359, 1998.

Mohan DS, Samuels MA, Selim MA et al: Long-term outcomes of therapeutic pelvic lymphadenectomy for Stage I endometrial adenocarcinoma. Gynecol Oncol 70:165–171, 1998.

Orr JW: Surgical staging of endometrial cancer: Does the patient benefit? Gynecol Oncol 71:335–339, 1998.

Rose PG: Endometrial carcinoma. N Engl J Med 335:640–649, 1996.

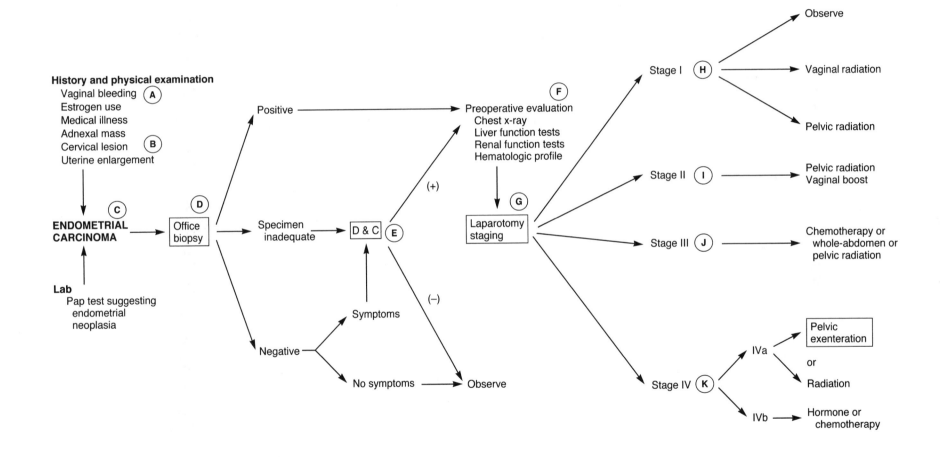

Chapter 137 **Adnexal Mass**

KARLOTTA M. DAVIS, MD, MPH

(A) Important historical elements in the evaluation of a patient found to have an adnexal mass are regularity of menses (potentially indicating regular ovulation), use of contraceptive measures, gastrointestinal symptoms, genitourinary symptoms, the presence of pain, and the age of the patient. A change in bowel habits, early satiety, and increasing abdominal girth are symptoms that commonly occur in patients who have ovarian carcinoma. Only 5% of ovarian carcinomas are diagnosed in children and adolescents, and most of those are germ cell in origin.

(B) Abdominal examination may reveal an abdominal mass arising from the pelvis. Vaginal discharge originating from the cervix accompanies pelvic infection, which occurs with tubo-ovarian complexes or abscesses. Cervical motion tenderness is found in patients with inflammatory masses or when a simple ovarian cyst is placed on stretch by the examining hand. Rectal examination determines rectal involvement by a mass and is essential in sizing an adnexal mass as well as determining extension into the cul de sac of Douglas and uterosacral nodularity.

(C) A pregnancy test must be performed in all women of reproductive age. The CA-125 level is elevated in 80% of women with advanced ovarian carcinoma. In premenopausal women, it may be elevated secondary to nonmalignant conditions such as endometriosis and is of very limited utility as a screening test for ovarian carcinoma.

(D) Pelvic ultrasound must be obtained when a pelvic mass is found on examination. Ultrasonography delineates the origin of the mass and determines whether it is cystic, solid, or a combination of the two. Septations, loculations, papillations, and increased bloodflow within an ovarian mass are very suggestive of malignancy. Fluid in the pouch of Douglas is seen with ruptured simple or functional ovarian cysts or may represent ascites consistent with a malignant process. A massive hemoperitoneum may result when a functional cyst ruptures in a patient with a coagulopathy or in a patient on Coumadin. Doppler flow studies revealing normal bloodflow to the adnexa can exclude the diagnosis of ovarian torsion.

(E) Simple ("functional") ovarian cysts require no therapy unless they are large or symptomatic. Oral contraceptive pills (OCPs) prevent development of new functional cysts by preventing ovulation and are therefore appropriate therapy; however, they do not cause regression of existing funtional cysts.

(F) Ectopic pregnancy must be considered in patients who have a positive pregnancy test and an adnexal mass. Ultrasound aids in the diagnosis by locating the site of the pregnancy and delineating the adnexa. Corpus luteum cysts are functional cysts that produce progesterone,which is essential for the continuation of pregnancies and should be managed expectantly. If a mass is discovered early in pregnancy and is suspicious for a malignant neoplasm, exploratory laparotomy should be delayed until 16 to 20 weeks' gestation, when the risks of anesthesia and of miscarriage are minimized.

(G) Tubo-ovarian complexes, usually preceded by salpingitis, are pockets of purulent, inflammatory material bounded by the adnexa, bowel, pelvic sidewalls, and uterus. Triple antibiotic therapy is essential before surgical extirpation of the infected tissue. A "cooling off" period of 6 weeks after the acute infectious phase is desirable; however, if clinical improvement within 48 to 72 hours of initiation of intravenous antibiotic therapy does not occur, surgical intervention is necessary. Bowel injury is more common when surgery is performed during acute infection. If antibiotic therapy fails, unilateral salpingo-oophorectomy (USO) may be undertaken to preserve fertility, but usually total abdominal hysterectomy with bilateral salpingo-oophorectomy (TAHBSO) is necessary.

(H) A complex ovarian mass in a patient with dysmenorrhea, dyspareunia, and dyschezia suggests endometriosis. Medical therapy with danocrine or gonadotropin-releasing hormone analogs can resolve large "chocolate cysts" of the ovary occasionally; however, ovarian cystectomy with reconstruction of the ovary may be required. Preservation of the ovarian cortex with conservation of hormonal production must be attempted if fertility is desired.

(I) Complex adnexal masses containing both cystic and solid components in women aged more than 40 years must be considered malignant until proven otherwise. Exploratory laparotomy, TAHBSO, peritoneal cytology, omentectomy, and periaortic lymph node sampling are indicated for patients with ovarian carcinoma. Epithelial ovarian cancer spreads over peritoneal surfaces, and all peritoneal sites from the diaphragm to the pelvic must be evaluated to complete surgical staging. Palpation of the entire bowel is essential as well. Removal of all malignant or potentially malignant implants (cytoreductive surgery) is essential before chemotherapy is instituted.

(J) Pedunculated fibroids may present as adnexal masses and need treatment only when symptomatic.

(K) Sudden onset of colicky lower abdominal pain with nausea, vomiting, and mild leukocytosis accompanying an ultrasonographic picture of increased ovarian volume and decreased Doppler bloodflow to the ovary must be considered an ovarian torsion until proven otherwise. Untwisting the adnexa to preserve the ovary is now standard therapy. Even the most dusky, swollen,

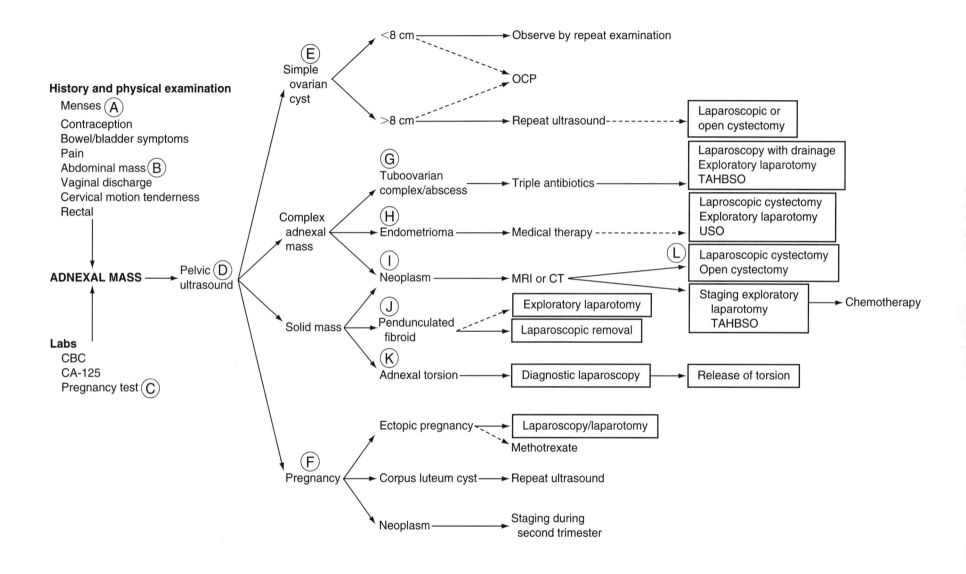

History and physical examination
Menses (A)
Contraception
Bowel/bladder symptoms
Pain
Abdominal mass (B)
Vaginal discharge
Cervical motion tenderness
Rectal

ADNEXAL MASS → Pelvic (D) ultrasound

Labs
CBC
CA-125
Pregnancy test (C)

(E) Simple ovarian cyst

<8 cm ──→ Observe by repeat examination

──→ OCP

>8 cm ──→ Repeat ultrasound ----→ Laparoscopic or open cystectomy

Complex adnexal mass

(G) Tuboovarian complex/abscess ──→ Triple antibiotics ──→ Laparoscopy with drainage / Exploratory laparotomy / TAHBSO

(H) Endometrioma ──→ Medical therapy ----→ Laproscopic cystectomy / Exploratory laparotomy / USO

(I) Neoplasm ──→ MRI or CT

(L) Laparoscopic cystectomy / Open cystectomy

Staging exploratory laparotomy / TAHBSO ──→ Chemotherapy

Solid mass

(J) Pendunculated fibroid ----→ Exploratory laparotomy / Laparoscopic removal

(K) Adnexal torsion ──→ Diagnostic laparoscopy ──→ Release of torsion

(F) Pregnancy

Ectopic pregnancy ──→ Laparoscopy/laparotomy ----→ Methotrexate

Corpus luteum cyst ──→ Repeat ultrasound

Neoplasm ──→ Staging during second trimester

nonviable-appearing ovary regains normal blood supply when untwisted. Normal production of ovarian hormones after untwisting is expected. Release of a blood clot from the veins draining a torsed ovary, although feared as a complication of untwisting, has never been reported. Torsion is more common in pregnancy as the uterus is rapidly enlarging or after pregnancy as the uterus is rapidly involuting. Fallopian tubes or paratubal cysts may torse and present similarly to ovarian torsion. Bloodflow to the ovary will occur on Doppler imaging, however the extraordinary degree of pain the patient experiences requires surgical intervention. Cystectomy of an ovarian cyst accompanying the torsion and oophoropexy is recommended in order to prevent a recurrence of the torsion.

Ⓛ Benign ovarian tumors such as dermoid tumors or Brenner tumors may be removed laparoscopically. Reconstruction of the ovary after removal of the tumor is ideal because the ovarian cortex contains the ovarian follicles. If the dead space can be eliminated with access of the fallopian tubes to the ovarian cortex, fertility may be preserved.

REFERENCES

Berek JS (ed): Novak's Gynecology, 13th ed. Baltimore: Williams & Wilkins, 2002.

Canis M, Ravishing B, Houlle C et al: Laparoscopic management of adnexal masses: A gold standard. Curr Opin Obstet Gynecol 14:423–428, 2002.

Funt SA, Hann LE: Detection and characterization of adnexal masses. Radiol Clin N Am 40:591–608, 2002.

Jung SE, Lee FM, Rha SE et al: CT and MR imaging of ovarian tumors with emphasis on differential diagnosis. Radio Graphics 22:1305–1325, 2002.

Stenchever MA, Droegemueller W, Herbst AL et al (eds): Comprehensive Gynecology, 4th ed. St. Louis: Mosby, 2001.

History and physical examination

Menses (A)

Contraception
Bowel/bladder symptoms
Pain
Abdominal mass (B)
Vaginal discharge
Cervical motion tenderness
Rectal

ADNEXAL MASS → Pelvic (D) ultrasound

Labs

CBC
CA-125
Pregnancy test (C)

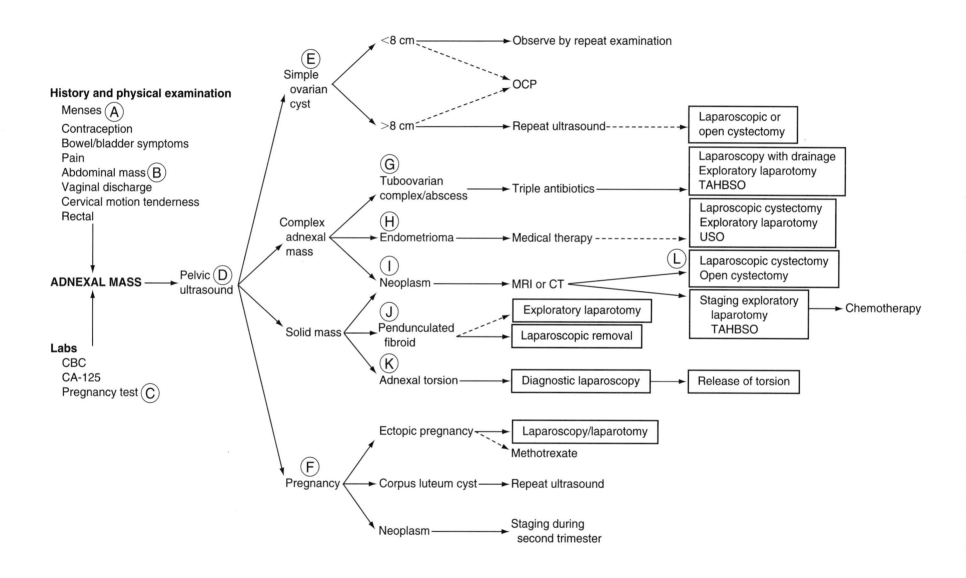

(E) Simple ovarian cyst
- <8 cm ──→ Observe by repeat examination
- <8 cm ----→ OCP
- >8 cm ----→ OCP
- >8 cm ──→ Repeat ultrasound ----→ Laparoscopic or open cystectomy

Complex adnexal mass
- (G) Tuboovarian complex/abscess ──→ Triple antibiotics ──→ Laparoscopy with drainage / Exploratory laparotomy / TAHBSO
- (H) Endometrioma ──→ Medical therapy ----→ Laproscopic cystectomy / Exploratory laparotomy / USO
- (I) Neoplasm ──→ MRI or CT ──→ (L) Laparoscopic cystectomy / Open cystectomy
  - ──→ Staging exploratory laparotomy / TAHBSO ──→ Chemotherapy

Solid mass
- (J) Pendunculated fibroid ----→ Exploratory laparotomy / Laparoscopic removal
- (K) Adnexal torsion ──→ Diagnostic laparoscopy ──→ Release of torsion

(F) Pregnancy
- Ectopic pregnancy → Laparoscopy/laparotomy / Methotrexate
- Corpus luteum cyst ──→ Repeat ultrasound
- Neoplasm ──→ Staging during second trimester

Chapter 138 Ovarian Mass

KIAN BEHBAKHT, MD

(A) Simple ovarian masses are more likely to be functional than complex or solid ovarian masses. Size by itself is not predictive of malignancy. All complex or solid masses in postmenopausal women need to be removed.

(B) Pelvic examination is mandatory. It can exclude pelvic inflammatory disease, pregnancy, cervical cancer, and uterine myomas. It can confirm the presence of a pelvic mass. Depending on the nature of the mass, it may not be possible to define it as ovarian vs. other etiology.

(C) Ultrasound distinguishes cystic from solid and unilocular (cystic) vs. multilocular (complex) masses and delineates the relationship of a mass to the uterus. Color flow Doppler can help distinguish benign from malignant masses. A resistive index less than 0.4 is worrisome for malignancy.

(D) The blood tumor marker CA-125 is elevated (greater than 35 mIU/ml) in 70% of serous malignancies. It is often normal in mucinous malignancies. It is elevated in many diverse diagnoses (e.g., pregnancy, uterine myomas, pancreatitis, and endometriosis). It has no value in the screening or diagnosis of ovarian cancer.

(E) If laboratory and radiographic evidence suggests a malignancy, laparotomy should be performed for diagnosis, resection, and staging.

(F) Laparoscopy is valuable if, after other work-up, there is still a question about the nature of the mass. Biopsy of suspicious implants can be performed. A cystic/solid ovarian mass cannot be adequately biopsied using laparoscopy because there is a risk of rupture with dissemination of the cancer cells. Furthermore, the worst histologic area may be missed. An ovarian mass should never be intentionally ruptured in the abdominal cavity. Ovaries can be removed intact with laparoscopy, drained in a bag, removed and sent for frozen section. If a malignancy is found, patient should undergo laparotomy and subsequent treatment within a week so that port site metastases can be minimized.

(G) The age of the patient is the most important variable. All specimens from cystectomy or oophorectomy should be sent for frozen section, if available. Subsequent treatment depends on findings. Treatment should be as conservative as possible in all prereproductive and reproductive age women. Masses in pregnant women are best removed in the second trimester of pregnancy.

(H) Other diagnoses are possible at the time of laparotomy for a suspected ovarian mass. These possibilities should be discussed with the patient preoperatively. In patients with prior surgery, periovarian adhesions and fluid can mimic the appearance of a complex mass.

(I) Germ cell tumors and stromal tumors occur in the prepubertal age group; they are often solid and unilateral. All solid masses in this age group should be investigated. These tumors are treated with conservative surgery and subsequent chemotherapy. Cystic masses are unusual in this age group because ovulation has not yet begun. They can be observed.

(J) The majority of masses in this group are related to ovulation, and these are benign. The risk of malignancy is about 10%. CA-125 is commonly elevated in benign diagnoses and is not helpful. Masses less than 5 cm can be observed, with repeat ultrasound in 6 weeks. Persistent or enlarging masses must be removed and sent for pathologic evaluation. Masses greater than 5 cm have a risk for torsion and rupture and should be removed. Treatment should be conservative if the patient desires childbearing. When childbearing is complete, TAH/BSO may be appropriate for benign diagnoses. Cancers are most likely epithelial and bilateral. Suspected tumors clinically confined to the ovary should be staged with omentectomy, peritoneal washings, random peritoneal biopsies, and pelvic and para-aortic lymph node sampling. Tumors spread in the peritoneal cavity should be debulked. Borderline tumors of the ovary are staged similar to a malignancy but have a much better prognosis.

(K) Simple cystic masses less than 5 cm may be observed. All other masses must be removed. Risk of malignancy in complex masses exceeds 50%. CA-125 elevations are more likely related to malignancy.

(L) All suspicious masses should be evaluated by frozen section if available. Malignant masses should undergo staging. If frozen section is not available, the mass should be removed and further management deferred until final pathology. There is no visual appearance of the ovary that is diagnostic for a malignancy. Survival of a patient with ovarian cancer depends primarily on correct surgical staging and maximal tumor debulking.

(M) Pelvic inflammatory disease not responsive to antibiotics and drainage should be treated with total abdominal hysterectomy and bilateral salpingo-oophorectomy (TAH/BSO).

(N) Use of methotrexate or salpingostomy may preserve fertility.

REFERENCES

Disaia PJ, Creasman WT: Clinical Gynecologic Oncology. St. Louis: Mosby-Year Book, 1997.

Gershenson DM: Contemporary treatment of borderline ovarian tumors. Cancer Investigation 17:206–210, 1999.

Buchsbaum HJ, Brady MF, Delgado G et al: Surgical staging of ovarian carcinoma: A gynecologic oncology group study. Surg Gynecol Obstet 169:226–232, 1989.

Canis M, Rabischong B, Botchorishvili R et al: Risk of spread of ovarian cancer after laparoscopic surgery. Curr Opin Obstet Gynecol 13:9–14, 2001.

Chapman WB: Developments in the pathology of ovarian tumors. Curr Opin Obstet Gynecol 13:53–59, 2001.

Doret M, Raudrant D: Functional ovarian cysts and the need to remove them. Eur J Obstet Gynecol 100:1–4, 2001.

History and physical examination

Menses

Bleeding

Mass (A)

Pelvic examination (B)

Rectal examination

Fever

OVARIAN MASS

(suspected)

Laparotomy (E)

Laparoscopy (F)

Labs

CBC

Cervical culture

Ultrasound (C)

Pregnancy test

CA-125 (D)

Appendicitis, Diverticulitis

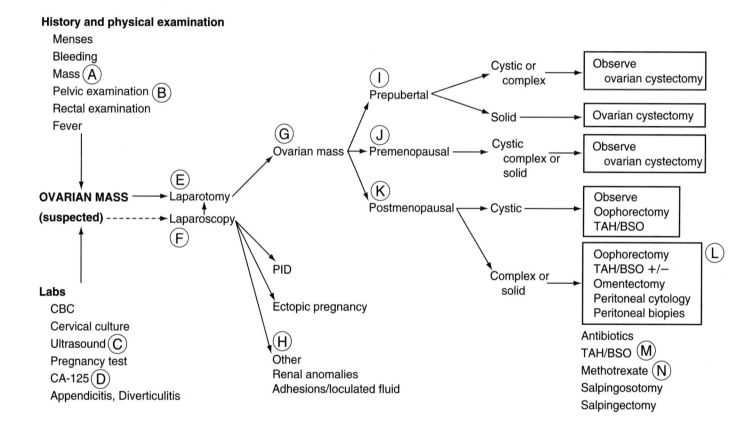

(G) Ovarian mass

PID

Ectopic pregnancy

(H) Other

Renal anomalies

Adhesions/loculated fluid

(I) Prepubertal

Cystic or complex → Observe / ovarian cystectomy

Solid → Ovarian cystectomy

(J) Premenopausal

Cystic complex or solid → Observe / ovarian cystectomy

(K) Postmenopausal

Cystic → Observe / Oophorectomy / TAH/BSO

Complex or solid → Oophorectomy / TAH/BSO +/− / Omentectomy / Peritoneal cytology / Peritoneal biopies (L)

Antibiotics

TAH/BSO (M)

Methotrexate (N)

Salpingosotomy

Salpingectomy

Chapter 139 *Prepubertal Vaginal Bleeding*

STEPHEN M. SCOTT, MD

(A) Uterine bleeding caused by waning maternal estrogen levels may normally occur within the first 2 months of life. Genital bleeding that occurs between the ages of 3 months and 10 years should be investigated. Questions to address during the history include hygienic routines; vaginal discharge or odor, which may accompany bacterial vaginal infections and foreign body placement; sexual and nonsexual trauma; and any exogenous hormonal ingestion.

(B) It is important to recognize evidence of estrogen stimulation on physical examination leading to a diagnosis of precocious puberty. An anatomical cause of genital bleeding is assumed when no estrogen stimulation is present. Signs of estrogen stimulation include breast development, axillary and pubic hair growth, visual signs of estrogen stimulation of the vulva, and a predominance of mature vaginal epithelium on a microscopic wet prep. Traumatic lesions should be carefully assessed and correlated with historical events. Straddle injuries tend to occur lateral to the labia majora, whereas penetrating sexual injuries tend to cause midline lacerations to the posterior hymen, perineum, and/or rectum.

(C) LH and FSH levels will determine central versus peripheral precocious puberty. Elevated gonadotropins suggest central stimulation of GnRH from the hypothalamus. Central precocious puberty may be idiopathic, but the etiology may stem from a hypothalamic or pituitary tumor. Brain imaging is recommended. Pedunculated lesions may be amenable to surgical removal, but embedded tumors usually require medical therapy. GnRH agonists shut down the pituitary's release of LH and FSH and the ovaries' hormonal production. Therapy should be instituted as soon as possible to prevent growth plate closure and reduced final height. If a lesion is present, other pituitary hormones (e.g., growth hormone) should be monitored and replaced as indicated. Suppressed LH and FSH levels suggest estrogen production independent from pituitary stimulation. If no evidence exists for exogenous estrogen consumption, imaging studies to rule out an ovarian or adrenal tumor are indicated. Estrogen-producing ovarian tumors (e.g., granulosa-theca cell tumors and teratomas) should be removed by cystectomy, if possible, to preserve the surrounding normal ovarian tissue.

(D) When no sign of estrogen stimulation is present, nonhormonal etiologies of genital bleeding should be pursued. Vulvovaginitis may irritate thin, unestrogenized mucosa to the point of bleeding. Almost all prepubertal infections are caused by enteric bacteria and should be treated in the short term with appropriate antibiotics; and, in the long term, with sitz baths three times a day and topical skin emollients. Yeast is almost never found before puberty and should raise concern for immunocompromise if found. Recurrent or persistent vaginal discharge and odor may indicate the presence of a foreign body. Copious vaginal washings using saline through a pediatric feeding tube and a large syringe will often dislodge the foreign body if it is not visible at the introitus. No antibiotics are required once a foreign body is retrieved. Dermatologic disorders of the vulva may create enough irritation to cause bleeding. Lichen sclerosis is a hypertrophic skin condition in which thickened white plaques form a "figure of eight" around the vulva and rectum. Dysuria, pruritis, and skin breakdown are common. A skin biopsy showing loss of rete pegs and hyalinization is diagnostic but is discouraged in children. Treatment includes sitz baths and low- to medium-potency topical steroids weaned to the least frequent dose possible.

(E) Urethral prolapse is associated with high intra-abdominal pressures. It is often preceded by periods of coughing with URIs or asthma, or by Valsalva maneuvers during times of constipation. The everted mucosa may appear normal or edematous and dusky. Diagnosis is aided by visualization of a normal hymen and vaginal canal posterior to the mass. Treatment should begin medically with sitz baths to reduce edema, and topical estrogens to promote inversion of the mucosa. If prolapse persists, excision of the mucosa and reapproximation of its edges using interrupted sutures is recommended.

(F) Every effort should be made to rule out the possibility of sexual abuse given evidence of trauma to the genital area. Any suspicion should prompt law enforcement and social services notification.

(G) If no obvious etiology for genital bleeding is evident, complete visualization of the vaginal canal and cervix is required. To avoid discomfort and achieve optimal visualization, a vaginoscopy (using a 3-mm hysteroscope or 7 French cystoscope under conscious sedation or general anesthesia) is preferred over an office speculum examination. Biopsy of suspicious tissue in the vagina is recommended. Embryonal carcinoma and sarcoma botryoides, a vaginal rhabdomyosarcoma, are the most common vaginal tumors seen in childhood. Preoperative chemotherapy has allowed vaginectomy and hysterectomy to replace exenteration as the preferred surgery. Adenocarcinoma of the vagina or cervix may also present with genital bleeding. GU and GI etiologies should be pursued if visualization of the entire vagina fails to find a cause for bleeding.

REFERENCES

Imai A, Horibe S, Tamaya T: Genital bleeding in premenarcheal children. Int J Gynaecol Obstet 49:41–45, 1995.

Merritt DF: Evaluation of vaginal bleeding in the preadolescent child. Semin Pediatr Surg 7:35–42, 1998.

Muram D: Vaginal bleeding in childhood and adolescence. Obstet Gynecol Clin N Am 17:389–408, 1990.

Sanfilippo JS, Wakim NG: Bleeding and vulvovaginitis in the pediatric age group. Clin Obstet Gynecol 30:653–661, 1987.

History and physical examination
 Nature of bleeding
 Hormones
 Foreign body (A)
 Sexual assault
 Trauma
 Hygiene
 External vulva
 Secondary sexual characteristics

PREPUBERTAL VAGINAL BLEEDING → Pelvic examination under anesthesia

(B) Estrogen stimulation ⟶ (C) Central vs peripheral precocious puberty

(D) Foreign body ⟶ Remove
 Vaginal lavage

Vaginitis ⟶ Wet preparation of vaginal discharge
 Culture for bacteria, gonococci,
  Chlamydia trachomatis
 Sitz baths and antibiotics

Vulvar disorders

(E) Urethral prolapse ⟶ Sitz baths
 Estrogen application
 Excision

Trauma ⟶ Straddle injury ⟶ Repair lacerations

(F) Sexual abuse ⟶ Repair lacerations
 Culture for sexually transmitted diseases,
  VDRL, HIV
 Report to child welfare
 Counseling for patient and family

(G) Genital tumor ⟶ Vaginoscopy and biopsy ⟶ Chemotherapy and/or surgery

GI or GU source

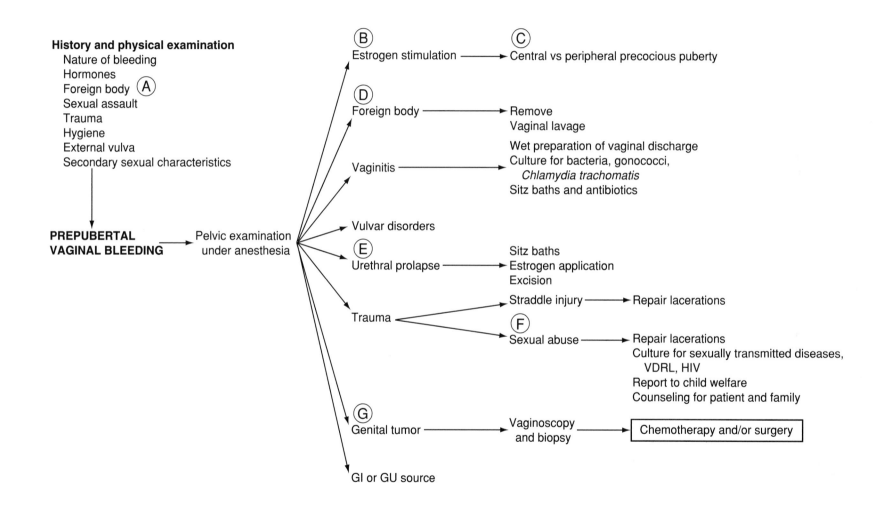

TRAUMA

Chapter 140 *Airway Management*

RICHARD E. WOLFE, MD

(A) It is important to be able to recognize the indications for airway management: lack of normal upper airway protection from gastric aspiration because of altered mental status, loss of patency from an obstructive lesion or an upper airway hematoma, inadequate oxygenation or ventilation, need for ventilatory control because of elevated ICP, and the need to deeply sedate a patient for diagnostic or therapeutic procedures. Predicting the patient's swelling also represents an important indication because it is better to act before the patient deteriorates.

(B) Pulse oximetry is a useful guide in indicating intubation because of falling oxygen saturation and in monitoring the patient during intubation. Generally, the decision to intubate is made on the clinical presentation and only rarely on the results of the arterial blood gas.

(C) Attempts should be made to identify a difficult airway before paralyzing a patient. Techniques used include Mallampati criteria where a difficult airway is found with a class IV (only the hard palate can be visualized when the patient opens his or her mouth). The rule of 3, 3, 2 suggests a difficult airway if the mouth opens less than 3 fingerbreadths, the horizontal length of mandible more than 3 fingerbreadths, or the thyromental distance less than 2 fingerbreadths. Congenital syndromes, goiter, morbid obesity, acromegaly, and cervical arthritis also predispose to a difficult airway. Acquired conditions that cause a loss of patency (e.g., epiglottitis, supraglottitis, intraoral or retropharyngeal abscesses, or Ludwig's angina) lead to great difficulties in visualizing the glottis. Finally, certain traumatic injuries (e.g., facial injury, blunt and penetrating neck trauma, and airway burns) also cause a difficult airway.

(D) When time permits, imaging studies may provide information that will modify the approach to the airway. A pneumothorax, discovered on the chest radiograph, should be vented before intubating because it may be converted to a tension pneumothorax by positive pressure ventilation. Detection of a cervical spine fracture or an intracranial bleed requires varying the approach to prevent long-term sequelae. However, one must still take the needed precautions when there is not enough time to exclude these injuries.

(E) Airway assessment is used to determine both the need for intubation and the technique to be used to control the airway. Before initiating airway management, one must ensure that all the needed equipment is functional, that the patient's heart rate and oxygen saturation are monitored, and that at least one functional intravenous line is present. Simple omissions (e.g., failing to position the patient correctly, removing dentures, or misplacing the suction device) can seriously hamper the performance of the procedure.

(F) Although it does not provide protection against aspiration, bag-valve-mask ventilation bolsters the patient's ventilatory effort and may provide critical temporary support to an apneic patient until a more definitive intervention can be performed. However, it may be ineffective in certain patients indicating an earlier need for a surgical airway. Risk factors for failed bag-valve-mask ventilation include edentulousness, obesity, a beard, anatomically abnormal facies, facial/neck trauma, obstructive airways disease, and patients in the third trimester of pregnancy.

(G) When preintubation evaluation has identified a potentially difficult airway, paralyzing agents should not be administered unless the operator believes that intubation is likely to be successful and the patient can be ventilated with bag-valve-mask.

Alternatives to rapid sequence intubation include blind nasotracheal intubation and awake intubation. In this context, "awake" means that the patient continues to breathe and is able to respond to or interact with caregivers. Usually the technique involves sedation and topical anesthesia. As described later, these awake techniques include direct laryngoscopy, fiberoptic intubation, and the intubating laryngeal mask airway.

(H) RSI is the simultaneous administration of a potent induction agent (e.g., etomidate or thiopental) and a neuromuscular blocking agent (usually succinylcholine 1.5 mg/kg). This approach provides optimal intubating conditions while minimizing the risk of aspiration of gastric contents.

(I) When ICP is elevated, maintenance of cerebral perfusion pressure (CPP) and avoidance of further increases in ICP are desirable. Control the reflex hemodynamic stimulation from intubation with fentanyl, (3 μg/kg) 3 minutes before intubation. IV lidocaine (1.5 mg/kg) given at the same time as fentanyl blunts the ICP response to laryngoscopy. Prior administration of a defasciculating dose of a competitive neuromuscular blocking agent blocks the ICP rise attributed to succinylcholine. Etomidate (0.3 mg/kg) probably is the best choice for an induction agent for patients with elevated ICP, although thiopental also is a good alternative when hypotension is not present. Nasotracheal intubation should be avoided in patients with elevated ICP.

(J) In-line stabilization during intubation limits the risk of cervical spine movement. It also improves the laryngoscopic view of the larynx compared with conventional cervical immobilization. Fiberoptic intubation or use of the Bullard laryngoscope further reduces the amount of cervical spine movement during oral intubation and should be used when time permits.

(K) Confirm correct tube placement in the trachea using end-tidal CO_2 devices. A postintubation chest radiograph should be obtained to ensure that the tip of the tube is not in the right main stem bronchus. Chest auscultation, gastric auscultation, bag resistance, and visualization of condensation within the ET tube are all prone to failure.

(L) A failed airway is defined by three failed attempts. Other noninvasive techniques may be tried when the patient is stable and can be ventilated. Presently the intubating laryngeal mask airway and bougie-guided orotracheal intubation are the rescue techniques of choice.

(M) In the setting of a failed airway, if endotracheal intubation was undertaken to sedate a patient for a procedure, the patient should be bag-mask-valve ventilated until the medication can wear off and the patient can be revived.

(N) Cricothyrotomy is the surgical airway of choice for failed and emergency surgical airways. It is relatively contraindicated by distorted neck anatomy, pre-existing infection, and coagulopathy.

It should be avoided in children under the age of 10 years because anatomic considerations make it exceedingly difficult in small children.

REFERENCES

Atkins RF: Simple method of tracking patients with difficult or failed intubation. Anesthesiology 83:1373–1374, 1995.

Brimacombe JR, Berry AM: Cricoid pressure. Can J Anaesth 44:414–425, 1997.

Campbell TP, Stewart RD, Kaplan RM et al: Oxygen enrichment of bag-valve-mask units during positive-pressure ventilation: A comparison of various techniques. Ann Emerg Med 17:232–235, 1988.

Criswell JC, Parr MJ, Nolan JP: Emergency airway management in patients with cervical spine injuries. Anaesthesia 49:900–903, 1994.

Lev R, Rosen P: Prophylactic lidocaine use preintubation: A review. J Emerg Med 12:499–506, 1994.

Walls RM: Airway management. Emerg Med Clin N Am 11:53–60, 1993.

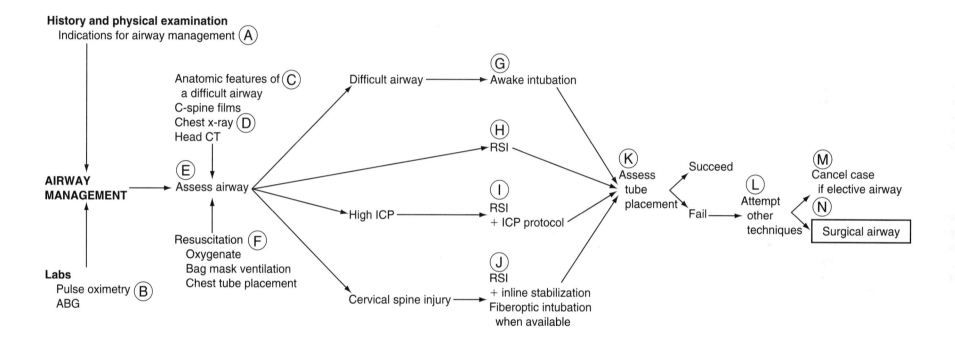

Chapter 141 **Penetrating Neck Injury**

L.D. BRITT, MD, MPH

(A) The essential principles of the initial assessment in the Advanced Trauma Life Support (ATLS) are just as applicable with neck trauma as with any other injury. The ATLS-directed primary survey, with its mandatory emphasis on the ABCs (*airway, breathing, circulation*), resuscitative efforts, and secondary survey, are all imperative in the optimal management of major injuries of the neck. Traditionally, wounds to the neck have been grouped into three anatomic zones of the neck. With a trend toward more nonoperative management of patients with penetrating injuries to the neck, the distinction regarding the zones is less important unless there are "hard" signs.

(B) In addition to an anteroposterior (AP) and lateral neck x-ray, a chest x-ray should be performed because pleural space entry is a possibility with a penetrating neck injury, depending on the object and the trajectory of the object or missile.

(C) Zone I is that horizontal area between the clavicle and the cricoid cartilage that encompasses the thoracic outlet vasculature, along with the vertebral and proximal carotid arteries, the lung, trachea, esophagus, spinal cord, thoracic duct, and major cervical nerve trunks. Injuries in this area requiring mandatory exploration should only be done when the patient presents in refractory shock. Such expeditious operative intervention might necessitate resection of the proximal clavicle or a median sternotomy.

(D) Zone II is the central neck area between the cricoid cartilage and the angle of the mandible. The jugular veins, vertebral and common carotid arteries, and the external and internal branches of the carotid are located in this zone. The

trachea, esophagus, spinal cord, and larynx traverse this area. Irrespective of the mechanism of injury, positive signs/symptoms including airway compromise, subcutaneous emphysema, expanding or pulsatile hematoma, hoarseness, hematemesis, hemoptysis, and leakage of saliva through the wound should prompt surgical intervention. In addition to a patient in refractory shock, any high velocity injury (HVI greater than 2500 ft/sec) is an indication for exploration. Also, some surgeons use a transcervical missile injury is an indication for surgical exploration even in the absence of signs/symptoms.

(E) Zone III, the most cephalad area, lies between the angle of the mandible and the base of the skull. The pharynx is located in this zone, along with the jugular veins, vertebral arteries, and the distal internal carotid arteries. As with the other two anatomic zones, exploration is required for any penetrating injury resulting in refractory shock.

(F) Hemodynamically stable patients with positive signs or symptoms (S/S) should undergo selective management, which includes aortography of the aortic arch and great vessels, tracheobronchoscopy, and esophagoscopy/contrast swallow.

(G) Although still controversial, there are some advocates for expectant management (i.e., observation only) in the presence of Zone II injuries without any hard or overt finding of a major injury.

(H) Selective management is indicated for patients who are hemodynamically stable with or without signs or symptoms.

(I) Depending on the specific injury, a positive finding might necessitate exploration.

(J) If the selective work-up is negative, the patient should undergo observation with

plans for an early discharge, provided the patient has no other injuries or problems that would warrant further management.

(K) This management approach includes the following:

Aortic arch/great vessel aortography
Laryngoscopy/tracheoscopy
Esophagoscopy/contrast swallow

REFERENCES

Britt L, Peyser M: Penetrating and blunt neck trauma. Trauma 20:437–449, 2000.

Cozzi S, Gemma M, DeVitis A et al: Difficult diagnosis of laryngeal blunt trauma. J Trauma 40:845–846, 1996.

Demetriades D, Theodorou D, Cornwell E et al: Penetrating injuries of the neck in patients in stable condition. Arch Surg 130:971–975, 1995.

Demetriades D, Theodorou D, Cornwell E et al: Evaluation of penetrating injuries of the neck: Prospective study of 233 patients. World J Surg 21:41–47, 1997.

Feliciano D, Bitondo C, Mattox K et al: Combined tracheoesophageal injuries. Am J Surg 150:710–714, 1985.

Hirshberg A, Wall M, Johnston R et al: Transcervical gunshot injuries. Am J Surg 167:309–312, 1994.

Mathisen D, Grillo H: Laryngotracheal trauma. Ann Thoracic Surg 43:254–262, 1987.

McConnell D, Trunkey D: Management of penetrating trauma to the neck. Adv Surg 27:97–127, 1994.

Noyes L, McSwain N, Markowitz I: Panendoscopy with arteriography versus mandatory exploration of penetrating wounds of the neck. Ann Surg 204:21–31, 1986.

Ordog G: Penetrating neck trauma. J Trauma 27:543–554, 1987.

Sofianos C, Degiannis E, Van den Aardweg M et al: Selective surgical management of zone II gunshot injuries of the neck: A prospective study. Surgery 120:785–788, 1996.

Velmahos G, Souter I, Degiannis E et al: Selective surgical management in penetrating neck injuries. JCC 37:487–490, 1994.

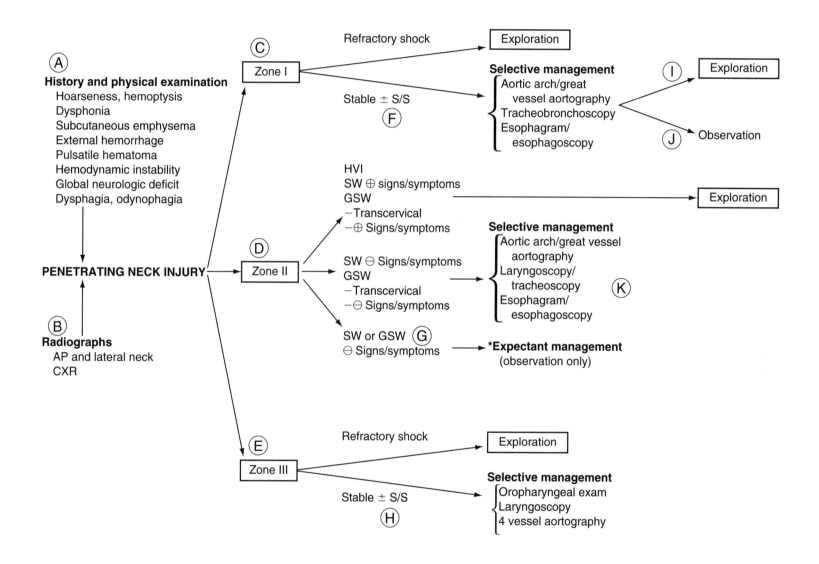

Chapter 142 Chest Injury

JEFFREY L. JOHNSON, MD • ERNEST EUGENE MOORE, MD

PENETRATING CHEST INJURY

(A) The initial approach to the patient with penetrating chest injury should follow the Advanced Trauma Life Support guidelines: airway, breathing, circulation, disability, and exposure (ABCDE). Copious hemoptysis, depressed level of consciousness, or audible evidence of airway compromise should prompt immediate orotracheal intubation. Absence of breath sounds may represent tension pneumothorax or massive hemothorax. Intravenous access is secured and warm crystalloid is begun. Distended neck veins can indicate either pericardial tamponade or tension pneumothorax. Presence of subcutaneous emphysema indicates violation of the airways, lung, or pleural space.

(B) A chest radiograph and the FAST ultrasound examination are pivotal adjuncts to the initial evaluation. These studies should be considered part of the primary survey in penetrating chest injuries because they can rapidly identify life-threatening problems. Although extensive laboratory tests may be sent, the only two that are likely to contribute significantly to the care of the patient are an arterial blood gas and a clot for the blood bank.

(C) Tube thoracostomy is the only intervention required in most penetrating thoracic injuries. In an unstable patient with a possible tension pneumothorax or massive hemothorax, placement of a pleural tube should proceed before radiographic assessment. For hemothorax, insert a large-bore (36 French) chest tube in the midaxillary line at the level of the nipple and guide it posteriorly and superiorly. For simple pneumothoraces, smaller catheters including "pigtail–type" catheters are acceptable. When in doubt, use a large tube.

(D) Persistent hemodynamic instability after tube thoracostomy is an indication for emergent operation. Before operation, the surgeon should recheck the ABCs, repeat the FAST examination, and initiate transfusion of packed red cells.

(E) Cardiac arrest from penetrating thoracic wounds is associated with significant survivability (approximately 25%) if it occurs within 15 minutes of arrival and the initial cardiac rhythm is something other than asystole. This warrants an aggressive approach to resuscitative thoracotomy in this group of patients. After opening the pericardium, the heart is assessed for wounds; stapling devices can provide rapid control of simple lacerations. The pulmonary hilum on the injured side is assessed, and a clamp is applied if needed to control major hemorrhage and/or air leak. Twisting of the hilum on its bronchovascular pedicle has also been described as a damage-control procedure. Application of an aortic crossclamp has a limited role outside of exsanguinating injuries below the diaphragm because of the detrimental effects of increased left ventricular afterload in the presence of penetrating cardiopulmonary injuries.

(F) Assessing for Beck's triad (i.e., distended neck veins, muffled heart tones, and hypotension), although warranted, is not reliable in the emergency department setting. Pericardial ultrasound is highly sensitive and specific for pericardial fluid and is the test of choice. In the persistently unstable patient, ultrasound should be repeated because the initial examination of a patient arriving soon after injury may be negative. Presence of fluid in the pericardium after a precordial penetrating injury indicates a cardiac wound until proven otherwise. Patients may be deceptively stable; immediate pericardial drainage should be pursued, followed by definitive repair.

(G) In the stable patient, pleural tube output can be used as a guide for planning operative intervention. For penetrating injuries, an initial output greater than 1 liter, or ongoing output greater than 200 cc/hour for 3 hours, generally warrants operation.

(H) Persistent pneumothorax after tube thoracostomy with a substantial air leak ("dropped lung") may indicate an operative injury to the proximal airways. A second pleural tube should be placed and bronchoscopy promptly performed. Proximal airway injuries greater than one-third the circumference of the bronchus should be operatively repaired.

(I) Persistent hemothorax after initial tube thoracostomy ("caked hemothorax") may indicate rapid hemorrhage that is not accurately measured by chest tube output. A second tube should be placed; at that point, failure to clear the pleural space warrants urgent operative intervention.

(J) Stable patients with gunshots that appear (by surface wounds) to cross the mediastinum need evaluation of the airway, esophagus, and great vessels. Computed tomography of the chest allows the surgeon to more accurately assess trajectory of the missile and selectively apply esophagoscopy, bronchoscopy, and angiography. It should be noted that the sensitivity of either esophagoscopy or contrast esophogram alone approximates 80%; for this reason, both studies are recommended when there is clinical suspicion of esophageal injury.

(K) Injuries below a line drawn from the nipple to the tip of the scapula deserve consideration of diaphragmatic and/or intraperitoneal injuries. If the patient is hemodynamically stable, and FAST is negative for intraperitoneal fluid, a diagnostic peritoneal lavage is indicated. Red blood cell counts of more than 5000/mm^3 indicate potential diaphragmatic injury; thoracoscopy is the procedure of choice.

(L) Injury to pulmonary vessels close to the hilum presents a significant challenge. The preferred technique for gaining access to these vessels within the lung parenchyma is tractotomy: rapid division of the parenchyma peripheral to the wound tract between surgical staplers. This permits oversewing of bleeding vessels and segmental bronchi in the depth of the lung. Although anatomic resection may seem tempting as an alternative, it is associated with significant mortality in the emergent setting.

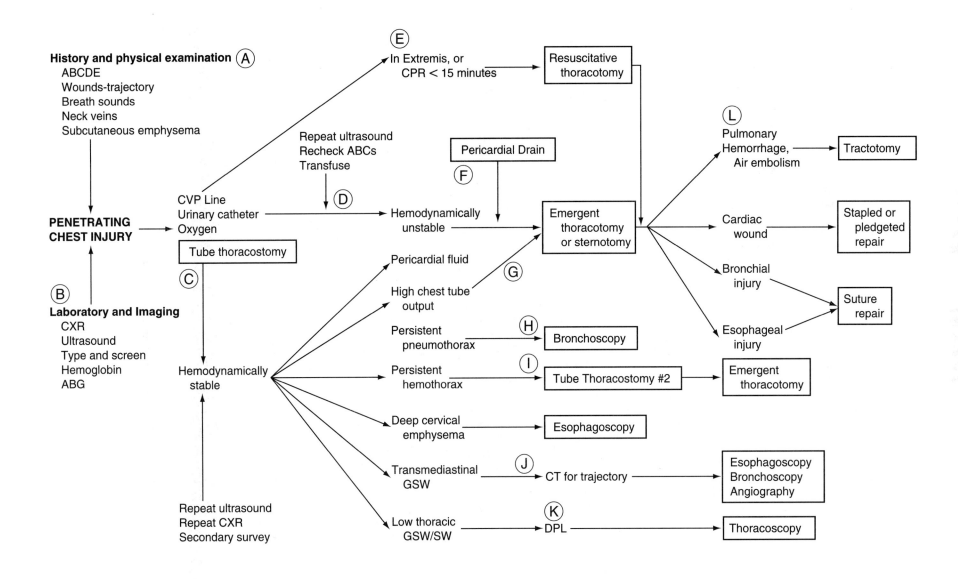

History and physical examination (A)
ABCDE
Wounds-trajectory
Breath sounds
Neck veins
Subcutaneous emphysema

PENETRATING CHEST INJURY

(B)
Laboratory and Imaging
CXR
Ultrasound
Type and screen
Hemoglobin
ABG

CVP Line
Urinary catheter
Oxygen

Tube thoracostomy
(C)

Repeat ultrasound
Repeat CXR
Secondary survey

Repeat ultrasound
Recheck ABCs
Transfuse
(D)

(E)
In Extremis, or
CPR < 15 minutes

Hemodynamically
unstable

Pericardial Drain
(F)

Hemodynamically
stable

Pericardial fluid

High chest tube
output
(G)

Persistent
pneumothorax
(H)

Persistent
hemothorax
(I)

Deep cervical
emphysema

Transmediastinal
GSW
(J)

Low thoracic
GSW/SW
(K)

Resuscitative
thoracotomy

Emergent
thoracotomy
or sternotomy

Bronchoscopy

Tube Thoracostomy #2

Esophagoscopy

CT for trajectory

DPL

(L)
Pulmonary
Hemorrhage,
Air embolism

Cardiac
wound

Bronchial
injury

Esophageal
injury

Tractotomy

Stapled or
pledgeted
repair

Suture
repair

Emergent
thoracotomy

Esophagoscopy
Bronchoscopy
Angiography

Thoracoscopy

BLUNT CHEST INJURY

(A)   The initial approach to the patient with blunt chest injury should follow the Advanced Trauma Life Support guidelines: airway, breathing, circulation, disablity, and exposure. Absence of breath sounds may represent tension pneumothorax or massive hemothorax. Intravenous access is secured and warm crystalloid is begun. Distended neck veins can indicate either pericardial tamponade or tension pneumothorax. Presence of subcutaneous emphysema indicates violation of the airways, lung, or pleural space. Paradoxical movement of the chest during the respiratory cycle ("flail chest") indicates an area of bony thorax that has lost continuity with the rest of the chest. The most important determinant of outcome after flail chest is not the degree of bony injury but the severity of the underlying pulmonary contusion.

(B)   A chest radiograph and the FAST ultrasound examination are pivotal adjuncts in the initial evaluation. These studies should be considered part of the primary survey because they can rapidly identify life-threatening problems. In addition to a clot for the blood bank, a hemoglobin, and an arterial blood gas, tests relevant to coagulation (e.g., platelet count and PT/PTT) are warranted in the patient with multiple blunt injuries. An electrocardiogram (ECG) should be obtained; a completely normal study indicates a very low likelihood of arrhythmia from blunt cardiac injury. Patients with abnormal ECGs should be monitored for 24 to 48 hours.

(C)   Tube thoracostomy is the only intervention required in most blunt thoracic injuries. In an unstable patient with a possible tension pneumothorax or massive hemothorax, placement of a pleural tube should proceed before radiographic assessment. For hemothorax, insert a large bore (36 French) chest tube in the midaxillary line at the level of the nipple and guide it posteriorly and superiorly. For simple pneumothoraces, smaller catheters including "pigtail-type" catheters are acceptable. When in doubt, use a large tube.

(D)   Persistent hemodynamic instability after tube thoracostomy is an indication for emergent operation. Before operation, the surgeon should recheck the ABCs, repeat the FAST examination, and initiate transfusion of packed red cells.

(E)   Neurologically intact survival after cardiac arrest from blunt injury is vanishingly rare (less than 1%). This warrants a limited approach to resuscitative thoracotomy in this group of patients unless the patient arrests after arrival. The pericardium is opened, the thoracic aorta is cross-clamped, and open cardiac massage is initiated. The pulmonary hilae are assessed and a clamp applied if needed to control major hemorrhage and/or air leak. If a sustained systolic blood pressure of 70 mm Hg cannot be achieved within 45 minutes of aortic crossclamping, the patient is considered unsalvageable.

(F)   In the stable patient, pleural tube output can be used as a guide for planning operative intervention. For blunt injuries, an initial output greater than 1.5 liters, or ongoing output greater than 250 cc/hour for 3 hours generally warrants operation. This represents a higher threshold for operation than penetrating injuries because most blunt chest injuries with hemodynamic stability are nonoperative lacerations of lung and chest wall. Initial attention should be directed towards correction of hypothermia, acidosis, and coagulopathy. Interventional radiology can be considered for moderate ongoing bleeding.

(G)   Patients injured during rapid deceleration are at risk for a tear of the thoracic aorta. The most common mechanism is motor vehicle crash, with side impact accounting for almost one-third of injuries. For those patients arriving alive in the hospital, the vast majority of these tears (95%) are located in the proximal descending thoracic aorta. Although some CXR signs may be suggestive (e.g., wide mediastinum and indistinct aortic knob), plain radiographs are not adequate. Beta blockade should be initiated when there is a high clinical suspicion or confirmed injury. The screening test of choice is dynamic helical CT, followed by angiography if necessary to define the lesion. Repair in concert with left-heart or full cardiopulmonary bypass is associated with the lowest rates of paraplegia.

(H)   Persistent pneumothorax after tube thoracostomy with a substantial air leak ("dropped lung") may indicate an operative injury to the proximal airways. A second pleural tube should be placed, and prompt bronchoscopy performed. Proximal airway injuries greater than one-third the circumference of the bronchus should be operatively addressed. The vast majority of these injuries after a blunt mechanism occur within 3 cm of the carina.

(I)   Persistent hemothorax after initial tube thoracostomy ("caked hemothorax") may indicate rapid hemorrhage that is not accurately measured by chest tube output. A second tube should be placed; failure to clear the pleural space at that point warrants urgent operative intervention.

(J)   Although blunt injuries to the esophagus are rare (less than 1% of all chest injuries), a patient with deep cervical emphysema should be evaluated. It should be noted that the sensitivity of either esophagoscopy or contrast esophogram alone approximates 80%; for this reason, both studies are recommended when there is clinical suspicion of esophageal injury.

(K)   Major chest wall injuries impair ventilation, cough, and mobility of the patient. The greater the number of fractures, and the greater the age of the patient, the more likely a progression to pneumonia, pulmonary failure, and a prolonged hospital

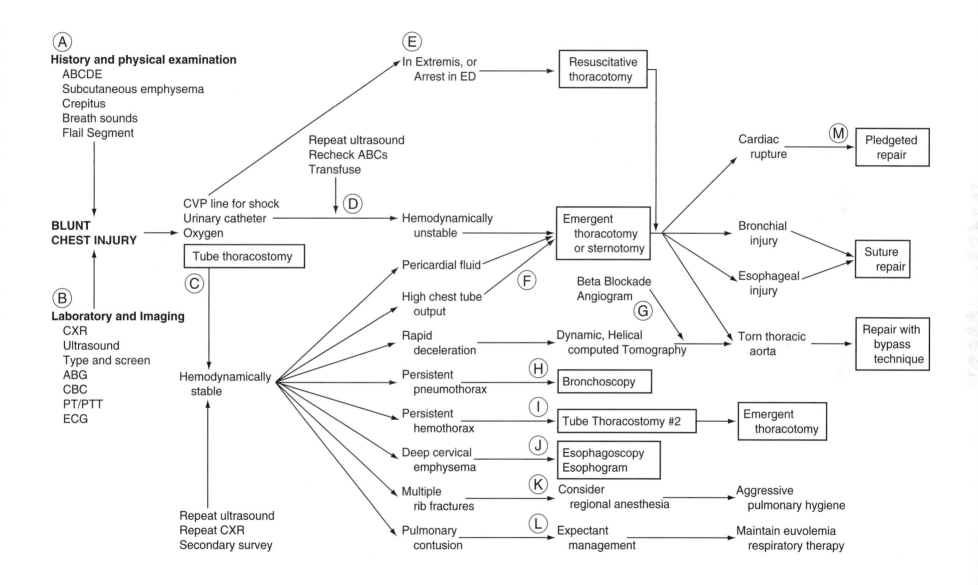

(A)
History and physical examination
- ABCDE
- Subcutaneous emphysema
- Crepitus
- Breath sounds
- Flail Segment

BLUNT CHEST INJURY

(B)
Laboratory and Imaging
- CXR
- Ultrasound
- Type and screen
- ABG
- CBC
- PT/PTT
- ECG

CVP line for shock
Urinary catheter
Oxygen

Tube thoracostomy

(C)

Repeat ultrasound
Repeat CXR
Secondary survey

(E) In Extremis, or Arrest in ED → Resuscitative thoracotomy

Repeat ultrasound
Recheck ABCs
Transfuse

(D) Hemodynamically unstable → Emergent thoracotomy or sternotomy

Hemodynamically stable

- Pericardial fluid
- High chest tube output
- Rapid deceleration → Dynamic, Helical computed Tomography
- (H) Persistent pneumothorax → Bronchoscopy
- (I) Persistent hemothorax → Tube Thoracostomy #2 → Emergent thoracotomy
- (J) Deep cervical emphysema → Esophagoscopy Esophogram
- (K) Multiple rib fractures → Consider regional anesthesia → Aggressive pulmonary hygiene
- (L) Pulmonary contusion → Expectant management → Maintain euvolemia respiratory therapy

(F)

Beta Blockade Angiogram

(G)

Cardiac rupture → (M) Pledgeted repair

Bronchial injury → Suture repair

Esophageal injury → Suture repair

Torn thoracic aorta → Repair with bypass technique

course will ensue. Regional anesthesia with an epidural catheter is often the most effective way to both provide excellent analgesia and avoid the adverse effects of parenteral narcotics.

Ⓛ Pulmonary contusion can be expected to worsen in the first 24 to 48 hours. Radiographic changes often lag behind the clinical course of the patient, so a high degree of vigilance is required. Euvolemia should be maintained (diuresis is not helpful) and aggressive respiratory therapy initiated.

Ⓜ Occasionally, a patient with blunt rupture of the heart (usually a low pressure chamber, with pericardium intact) will arrive alive in the emergency department. Prompt pericardial drainage and cardiac repair can result in salvage of some patients.

REFERENCES

Allen GS, Coates NE: Pulmonary contusion: A collective review. Am Surgeon 62:895–900, 1996.

Branney SW, Moore EE, Feldhaus KM et al: Critical analysis of two decades of experience with postinjury emergency department thoracotomy in a regional trauma center. J Trauma 45:87–94, 1998.

Bulger EM, Arneson MA, Mock CN et al: Rib fractures in the elderly. J Trauma 48:1040–1046, 2000.

Cothren C, Moore EE, Biffl WL et al: Lung-sparing techniques are associated with improved outcome compared with anatomic resection for severe lung injuries. J Trauma 53:483–487, 2002.

Durham RM, Zuckerman D, Wolverson M et al: Computed tomography as a screening exam in patients with suspected blunt aortic injury. Ann Surg 220:699–704, 1994.

Fabian TC, Richardson JD, Croce MA et al: Prospective study of blunt aortic injury: Multicenter trial of the American Association for the Surgery of Trauma. J Trauma 42:374–380, 1997.

Hoff SJ, Shotts SD, Eddy VA et al: Outcome of isolated pulmonary contusion in blunt trauma patients. Am Surgeon 60:138–142, 1994.

Mackersie RC, Karagianes TG, Hoyt DB et al: Prospective evaluation of epidural and intravenous administration of fentanyl for pain control and restoration of ventilatory function following multiple rib fractures. J Trauma 31:443–451, 1991.

Mansour MA, Moore EE, Moore FA et al: Exigent postinjury thoracotomy: Analysis of blunt versus penetrating trauma. Surg Gynecol Obstet 175:97–101, 1992.

Nagy KK, Lohmann C, Kim DO et al: Role of echocardiography in the diagnosis of occult penetrating cardiac injury. J Trauma 38:859–862, 1995.

Stassen NA, Lukan JK, Spain DA et al: Reevaluation of diagnostic procedures for transmediastinal gunshot wounds. J Trauma 53:635–638, 2002.

Wall MJ, Hirshberg A, Mattox KL: Pulmonary tractotomy with selective vascular ligation for penetrating injuries to the lung. Am J Surg 168:665–669, 1994.

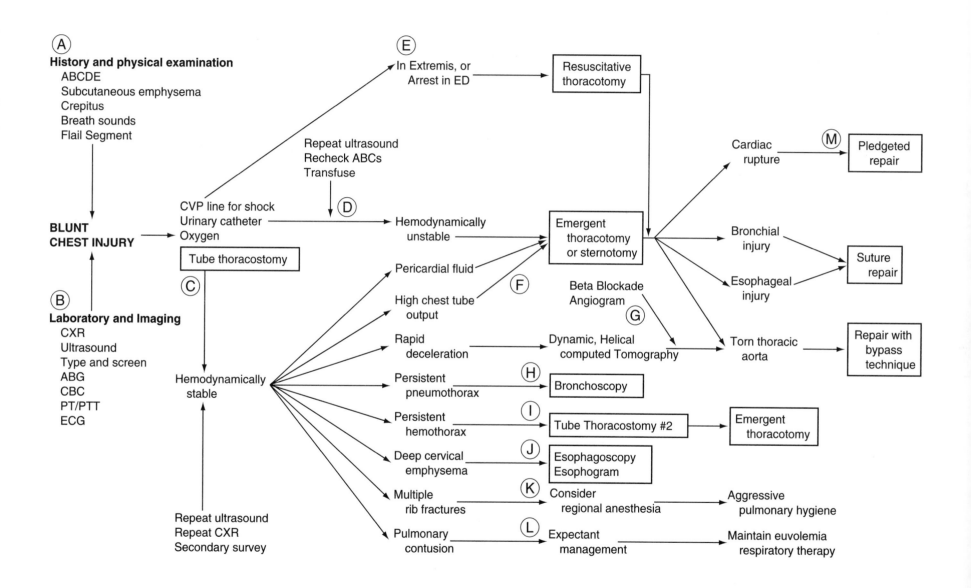

A
History and physical examination
ABCDE
Subcutaneous emphysema
Crepitus
Breath sounds
Flail Segment

BLUNT CHEST INJURY

B
Laboratory and Imaging
CXR
Ultrasound
Type and screen
ABG
CBC
PT/PTT
ECG

CVP line for shock
Urinary catheter
Oxygen

Tube thoracostomy

C

Repeat ultrasound
Repeat CXR
Secondary survey

E
In Extremis, or
Arrest in ED

Resuscitative
thoracotomy

Repeat ultrasound
Recheck ABCs
Transfuse

D
Hemodynamically
unstable

Hemodynamically
stable

Pericardial fluid

High chest tube
output

Rapid
deceleration

Persistent
pneumothorax

Persistent
hemothorax

Deep cervical
emphysema

Multiple
rib fractures

Pulmonary
contusion

Emergent
thoracotomy
or sternotomy

F

Beta Blockade
Angiogram

G

Dynamic, Helical
computed Tomography

H
Bronchoscopy

I
Tube Thoracostomy #2

J
Esophagoscopy
Esophogram

K
Consider
regional anesthesia

L
Expectant
management

Cardiac
rupture

M
Pledgeted
repair

Bronchial
injury

Esophageal
injury

Suture
repair

Torn thoracic
aorta

Repair with
bypass
technique

Emergent
thoracotomy

Aggressive
pulmonary hygiene

Maintain euvolemia
respiratory therapy

Chapter 143 *Thoracic Aorta Injury*

JON M. BURCH, MD • ERNEST E. MOORE, MD

(A) Blunt tears of the descending thoracic aorta are a common cause of death in high-energy injuries. Motor vehicle collisions are a common mechanism, especially those that involve frontal or side impact. Patients who do not die immediately often reach the hospital alive and may survive, provided the diagnosis is made promptly.

(B) A widened mediastinum on A-P chest x-ray is present in approximately 85% of patients with these injuries. Other findings on chest x-ray include, in decreasing order of incidence, left apical cap, blurring of the aortic knob, obliteration of the aortic pulmonary window, and deviation of the nasogastric tube (esophagus).

(C) It is well established that 5% to 7% of patients with torn thoracic aortas will have an entirely normal chest x-ray. For this reason further diagnostic evaluation is essential based on high-energy transfer mechanism.

(D) Beta blockade has been successfully used to prevent in-hospital rupture in patients with other serious injuries requiring immediate attention. In some instances, repair has been delayed for several days.

(E) Spiral CT has been documented to be the screening test of choice. It can localize injuries so precisely that angiography can be eliminated in most cases.

(F) Aortic repair requires several hours of uninterrupted attention. Patients with active hemorrhage from other sources (e.g., liver, spleen, or pelvic fracture) must have those injuries treated first. Also, patients with severe pulmonary contusions may not tolerate single lung ventilation in the right lateral decubitus position. In this instance, repair may have to be delayed for several days. Beta blockade may help to prevent rupture in either case.

(G) The author prefers to repair all injuries using partial left heart bypass because it virtually eliminates the risk of paraplegia. Partial left heart bypass is accomplished by cannulation of the left superior pulmonary vein and left femoral artery. A centrifugal pump is used to pump oxygenated blood from the pulmonary vein to the femoral artery.

REFERENCES

Dyer DS, Moore EE, Ilke DN et al: Thoracic aortic injury: How predictive is mechanism and is chest computed tomography a reliable screening tool? A prospective study of 1561 patients. J Trauma 48:673–682, 2000.

Fabian TC, Richardson JD, Croce MA et al: Prospective study of blunt aortic injury: Multicenter trial of the American Association for the Surgery of Trauma. J Trauma 42:374–380, 1997.

Kepros J, Angood P, Jaffe CC et al: Aortic intimal injuries from blunt trauma: Resolution profile in nonoperative management. J Trauma 52:475–478, 2002.

Kim FJ, Moore EE, Moore FA et al: Trauma surgeons can render definitive surgical care for major thoracic injuries. J Trauma 36:871–875, 1994.

Malhotra AK, Fabian TC, Croce MA et al: Minimal aortic injury: A lesion associated with advancing diagnostic techniques. J Trauma 51:1042–1048, 2001.

Marty-Ane CH, Berthet JP, Branchereau P et al: Endovascular repair for acute traumatic rupture of the thoracic aorta. Ann Thorac Surg 75:1803–1807, 2003.

Moore EE, Burch JM, Moore JB: Repair of the torn descending thoracic aorta using the centrifugal pump for partial left heart bypass. Ann Surg, In press.

Nagy K, Fabian T, Rodman G et al: Guidelines for the diagnosis and management of blunt aortic injury: An EAST practice management guidelines work group. J Trauma 48:1128–1143, 2000.

Santaniello JM, Miller PR, Croce MA et al: Blunt aortic injury with concomitant intra-abdominal solid organ injury: Treatment priorities revisited. J Trauma 53:442–445, 2002.

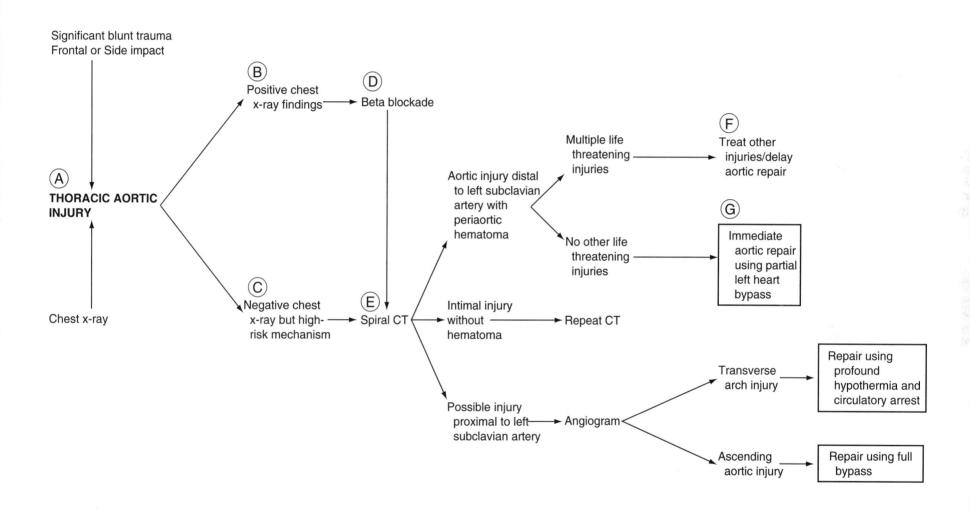

Ⓐ **THORACIC AORTIC INJURY**

Significant blunt trauma
Frontal or Side impact

Chest x-ray

Ⓑ Positive chest x-ray findings

Ⓒ Negative chest x-ray but high-risk mechanism

Ⓓ Beta blockade

Ⓔ Spiral CT

Aortic injury distal to left subclavian artery with periaortic hematoma

Multiple life threatening injuries

Ⓕ Treat other injuries/delay aortic repair

No other life threatening injuries

Ⓖ Immediate aortic repair using partial left heart bypass

Intimal injury without hematoma

Repeat CT

Possible injury proximal to left subclavian artery

Angiogram

Transverse arch injury

Repair using profound hypothermia and circulatory arrest

Ascending aortic injury

Repair using full bypass

Chapter 144 *Blunt Abdominal Trauma*

SARAH D. MAJERCIK, MD • WALTER L. BIFFL, MD

(A) Blunt abdominal trauma is a source of significant morbidity and of preventable deaths.

(B) In the primary survey, sequential treatment priorities are based on assessment of the patient's *airway*, *breathing*, and *circulation* (ABCs). Disability is assessed, and the patient is exposed while resuscitation is performed.

(C) The secondary survey consists of systemic reassessment and detailed physical examination literally from head to toe. The major objective is to identify all potentially significant occult injuries.

(D) It is important to know the injury mechanism to anticipate injury patterns and to raise the index of suspicion for occult injuries. An AMPLE medical history includes *allergies*, *medications*, *past illnesses and operations*, *last meal*, and *events* preceding the injury. Relevant information from the scene (e.g., restraint use, vehicular damage, blood loss, or deaths at scene), including prehospital vital signs and findings, should be obtained. Obvious evidence of major thoracic and/or pelvic trauma should heighten suspicion for intra-abdominal injury.

(E) Physical examination is notoriously unreliable because symptoms and signs are often masked by head trauma, distracting injuries, or intoxication. Moreover, free intraperitoneal blood does not produce acute abdominal pain or tenderness. Abdominal wall ecchymosis ("seat belt sign") should be noted because it is a significant predictor of injury.

(F) Although admission laboratory values are rarely helpful, they serve as a basis for comparison with later values. For most patients, a hematocrit and urinalysis are adequate. A white blood cell count is added for those at high risk for intra-abdominal injuries. Toxicology screening may help to explain changes in mental status.

For patients in shock, blood should be typed and cross-matched. Additional laboratory tests may be required based on preexisting conditions (e.g., cardiac, respiratory, hepatic, or renal disease; or use of anticoagulants).

(G) Chest, pelvis, and lateral cervical spine x-rays are obtained for all patients with potential multisystem trauma.

(H) Diffuse peritoneal irritation warrants prompt laparotomy.

(I) A trauma ultrasound (US) examination is a pivotal triage tool in the early management of blunt trauma. The US examination seeks fluid in (1) Morison's pouch, (2) the pelvis, (3) the left upper quadrant, and (4) the pericardial space.

(J) A midline incision is recommended because it can be done rapidly and extended for additional exposure. Control of hemorrhage is the first objective, followed by systematic evaluation of abdominal and retroperitoneal contents. Management of specific injuries is outlined elsewhere in this book.

(K) The vast majority of patients are hemodynamically stable and can tolerate a thorough systematic evaluation or secondary survey.

(L) Management of hemodynamic instability is based on US findings: confirmation of hemoperitoneum mandates emergent laparotomy, whereas an equivocal or negative (i.e., no free fluid) result should be followed by repeat US or diagnostic peritoneal lavage (DPL). Continued reassessment is critical in this setting. Although the sensitivity of abdominal US for free intraperitoneal fluid exceeds 98%, previous abdominal surgery, obesity, and excessive bowel gas may limit its accuracy.

(M) Stable patients with free peritoneal fluid on US should be further evaluated by CT if they are potential candidates for nonoperative

management, have cirrhosis, or present more than 12 hours after the injury; if otherwise, DPL is in order.

(N) DPL is a traditional technique used to rapidly exclude significant intraperitoneal hemorrhage. A catheter is inserted into the abdominal cavity below the umbilicus using local anesthesia. If initial aspiration does not return 10 ml of gross blood, 1 L of crystalloid is infused and then drained. A "positive lavage" in blunt trauma patients is defined as fluid that contains $100,000\,RBC/mm^3$. DPL is nearly 100% accurate in identifying intraperitoneal hemorrhage. In addition, it is useful for detecting occult hollow viscus injuries. Lavage fluid that contains bile or intestinal contents mandates operative exploration. An elevated lavage fluid WBC count (greater than $500/mm^3$) is no longer considered an absolute indication for laparotomy, although it is a relative indication. Elevated enzyme levels (greater than 20 IU/L amylase and greater than 3 IU/L alkaline phosphatase) warrant consideration for laparotomy. The false-negative rate for a DPL is 2%. Most often missed are injuries to the diaphragm, urinary bladder, small bowel, and pancreas.

(O) CT allows assessment of solid organ injury. It also evaluates the retroperitoneum and genitourinary tract, both of which are missed by DPL and poorly assessed by US.

(P) Hemodynamically stable patients with equivocal or negative US findings should be evaluated by abdominal computed tomography (CT) if they have GCS greater than 11, distracting injuries, major thoracic or pelvic injury, persistent localized abdominal tenderness, gross hematuria, or unexplained anemia. In the absence of these conditions, clinical observation is appropriate.

(Q) Observation involves repeated physical examinations; monitoring of vital signs; serial laboratory testing; and, possibly, repeat US.

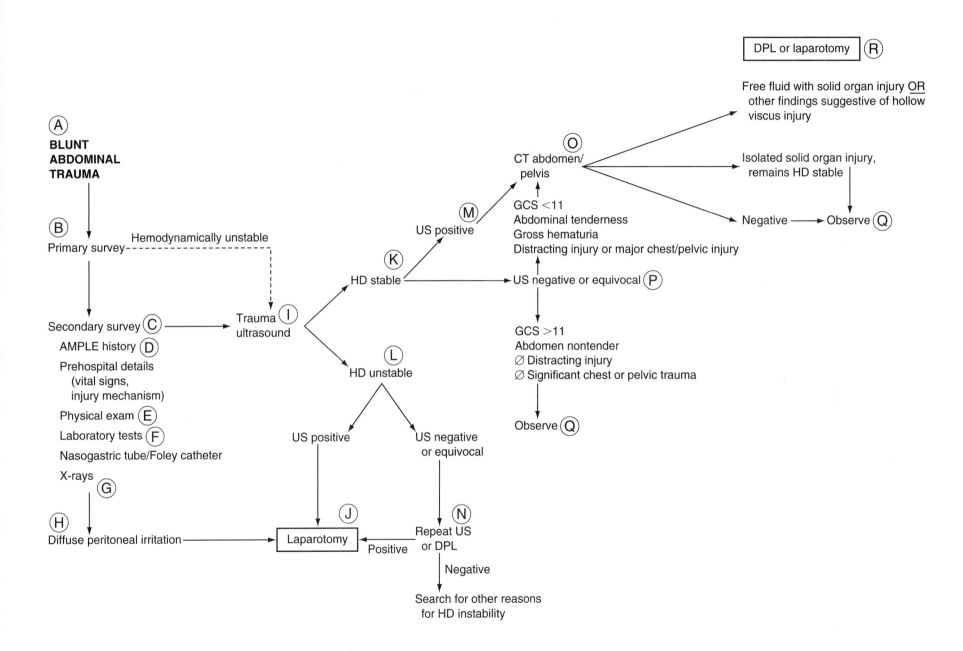

Ⓡ CT that demonstrates free fluid without solid organ injury is worrisome for small bowel injury. The alert patient can undergo close observation, whereas the comatose patient should undergo DPL. The criteria for laparotomy should be based upon a combination of clinical judgment, the patient's hemodynamics, and DPL results. Particular attention should be paid to the WBC count, or the ratio of WBC to RBC, as well as the presence of bile or enzymes. Less focus should be placed on the RBC count in this setting.

REFERENCES

American College of Surgeons Committee on Trauma: Advanced Trauma Life Support. Chicago: American College of Surgeons, 1997.

Branney SW, Moore EE, Cantrill SV et al: Ultrasound based key clinical pathway reduces the use of hospital resources for the evaluation of blunt abdominal trauma. J Trauma 42:1086–1090, 1997.

Henneman PL, Marx JA, Moore EE et al: Diagnostic peritoneal lavage: Accuracy in predicting necessary laparotomy following blunt and penetrating trauma. J Trauma 30:1345–1355, 1990.

Malhotra AK, Fabian TC, Katsis SB et al: Blunt bowel and mesenteric injuries: The role of screening computed tomography. J Trauma 48:991–1000, 2000.

Rozycki RA, Ballard RB, Feliciano DV et al: Surgeon-performed ultrasound for the assessment of truncal injuries: Lessons learned from 1540 patients. Ann Surg 228:557–567, 1998.

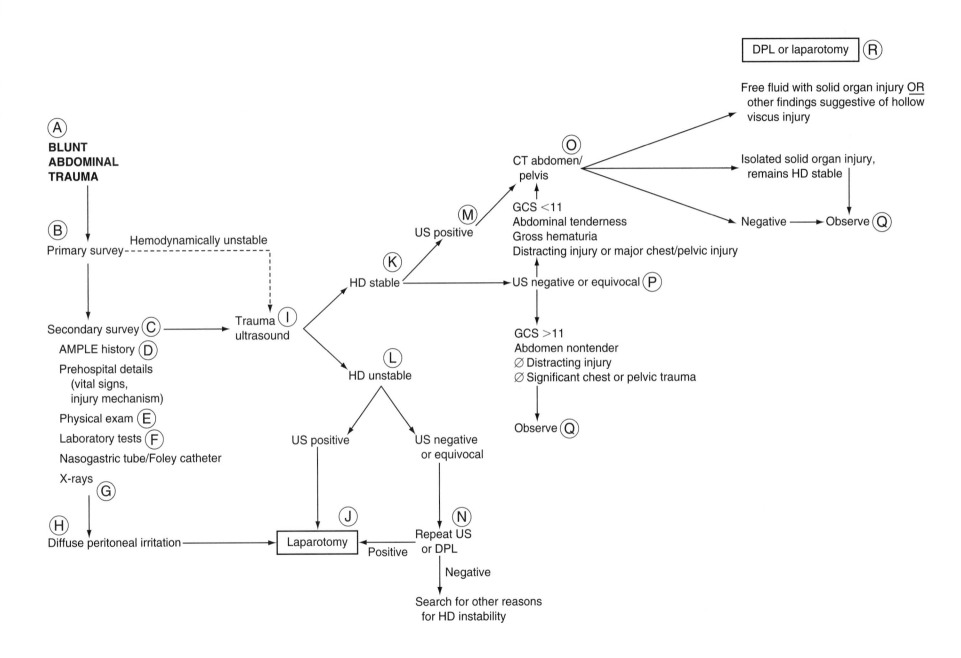

Chapter 145 *Penetrating Abdominal Injury*

DAVID V. FELICIANO, MD

(A) Evaluation of a patient who might possibly have a penetrating abdominal wound requires hemodynamic evaluation; physical examination; and, in some patients, further diagnostic studies. Signs of intra-abdominal injury mandating laparotomy are present immediately or eventually in 60% to 75% of stab wound patients and 70% to 95% of gunshot wound patients with peritoneal penetration. The assessment of need for advanced trauma life support (ATLS) can be summarized by the acronym AMPLE (allergies, medications, past medical history, last meal, events or description of the injury).

(B) A hypotensive patient (systolic BP less than 100 mm Hg) with clear-cut peritoneal penetration or traverse injury needs only venipuncture for type-specific blood, good intravenous access, and an identification bracelet before being moved to the OR. An agonal patient may need an emergency center or operating room thoracotomy to help maintain cardiac activity until control of abdominal hemorrhage is obtained.

(C) A hemodynamically stable patient who has clear-cut diffuse peritonitis after a penetrating abdominal wound should have an urgent laparotomy.

(D) There are hemodynamically stable patients in whom penetration of the peritoneal cavity or upper visceral/vascular retroperitoneum by a stab wound or gunshot wound is unclear. There are other patients in whom a penetrating wound may still not cause a visceral/vascular injury or, even if it does, no operative therapy is indicated. Patients in either of these groups will require further in-hospital evaluation.

(E) A possible penetrating thoracoabdominal stab wound or gunshot wound enters anteriorly between the costal margins or posteriorly below the tips of the scapulas.

(F) A possible penetrating stab wound of the anterior abdomen enters between the anterior axillary lines from the costal margins to the inguinal ligaments.

(G) A possible penetrating gunshot wound through-and-through the anterior abdomen or from the anterior abdomen to the flank (or vice versa) may be extraperitoneal or tangential in an obese or muscular patient.

(H) A possible penetrating wound of the flank (between anterior and posterior axillary lines) or back (posterior to posterior axillary lines) may be extraperitoneal or posterior to the visceral/vascular area of the retroperitoneum in an obese or muscular patient.

(I) In an injured patient with an initial body temperature of less than 35°C, arterial pH less than 7.2, or base deficit less than -15; or when the INR or PTT are more than 50% of normal, the patient has "metabolic failure" secondary to profound shock. A limited or "damage control" laparotomy should then be performed. This would include the following: packing of solid organ injuries; exclusion or excision of multiple GI perforations with a stapler; ligation of major venous injuries other than to the suprarenal inferior vena cava; insertion of temporary intraluminal shunts into the injured superior mesenteric, common iliac, or external iliac artery; and temporary silo coverage of the open abdomen.

(J) The management of possible thoracoabdominal wounds differs between the right and the left sides because the right upper quadrant is filled with the liver, and injuries there may be managed nonoperatively.

(K) A surgeon-performed ultrasound that is "positive" for intraperitoneal fluid (blood) after an anterior stab wound confirms peritoneal penetration. A "negative" ultrasound is not helpful because there may be little intraperitoneal blood despite the presence of a visceral injury.

(L) A surgeon-performed ultrasound after a gunshot wound is performed to document peritoneal penetration. If hematuria is present at the onset, a contrast-enhanced CT is used in some centers (local choice) to see if there is an isolated nonbleeding injury to the kidney.

(M) Diagnostic options are physical examinations over a 36 hour period or a CT scan using simultaneous double-contrast (IV and oral) or triple-contrast (add Gastrografin enema). Serial examinations result in a delayed therapeutic laparotomy rate of 2% to 2.5% and a nontherapeutic or negative laparotomy rate of 4%. Contrast CT with the occasional addition of an arteriogram rarely misses injuries and has a 4% nontherapeutic or negative laparotomy rate.

(N) If a possible right thoracoabdominal stab wound has occurred, serial physical examinations are performed for 24 hours to see if delayed peritonitis develops. Serial chest x-rays are performed to see if any herniation through the right hemidiaphragm occurs.

(O) If a possible right thoracoabdominal gunshot wound has occurred, a contrast abdominal CT is performed. Extravasation of IV contrast from or in the injured liver mandates therapeutic embolization. Without extravasation of IV contrast from the liver in the hemodynamically stable patient, nonoperative management is appropriate. A febrile state or toxicity secondary to a posttraumatic biliary leak is managed with evacuation and irrigation during delayed laparoscopy.

(P) A positive abdominal ultrasound documents injury to the left hemidiaphragm and, possibly, to the stomach or colon, and a laparotomy is performed.

(Q) An abnormal appearance of the left hemidiaphragm after evacuation of a left hemothorax mandates laparoscopy, at least.

(R) After a positive ultrasound in the asymptomatic patient (no peritonitis), serial physical examinations are performed for 24 hours. A laparotomy is performed if peritonitis develops.

(S) After a negative ultrasound, an exploration of the stab wound site (local wound exploration) is performed in the cooperative patient to document penetration of the posterior fascia or, if possible, peritoneum. Penetration mandates serial

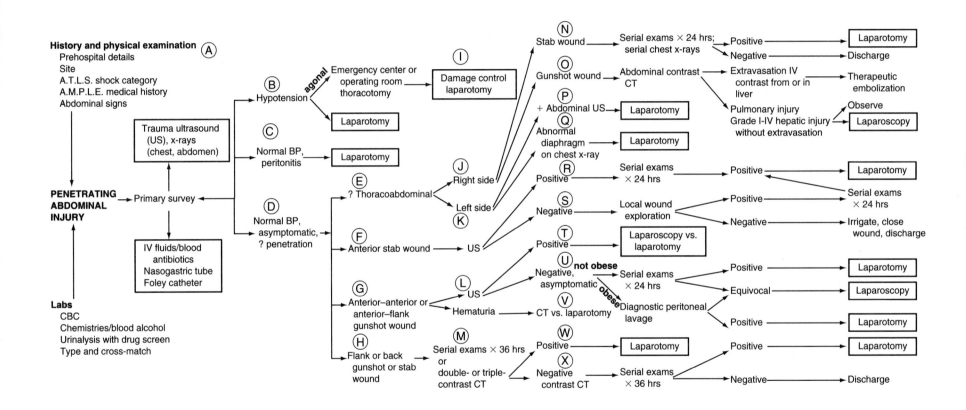

History and physical examination (A)
Prehospital details
Site
A.T.L.S. shock category
A.M.P.L.E. medical history
Abdominal signs

PENETRATING ABDOMINAL INJURY

Labs
CBC
Chemistries/blood alcohol
Urinalysis with drug screen
Type and cross-match

examinations, whereas the patient without penetration is discharged after closure of the wound.

(T) Peritoneal penetration is followed by laparoscopy versus laparotomy (local choice) because of the significantly greater risk of intra-abdominal injury with gunshot wounds as compared with stab wounds.

(U) Management after a negative ultrasound depends on the patient's size. Nonobese patients should undergo serial examinations for 24 hours, laparotomy if peritonitis develops, and laparoscopy if the examinations are equivocal. Obese patients should undergo a diagnostic peritoneal lavage; laparoscopy, if the results are equivocal (i.e., RBC less than 5000 to 10,000 RBC/mm^3); and laparotomy, if the study is positive.

(V) An isolated nonbleeding renal injury that does not involve the renal collecting system (grade I-III) is managed nonoperatively in some centers.

(W) The development of peritonitis, unexplained fever, or hypotension during serial examinations (36 hours because "retroperitonitis" may cause delayed symptoms) mandates laparotomy.

(X) Even with a "negative" double- or triple-contrast CT, serial examinations should be performed for 36 hours with the same indications for laparotomy as listed above.

REFERENCES

Boulanger BR, Kearney PA, Tsuei B et al: The routine use of sonography in penetrating torso injury is beneficial. J Trauma 51:320–325, 2001.

Chiu WC, Shanmuganathan K, Mirvis SE et al: Determining the need for laparotomy in penetrating torso trauma: A prospective study using triple-contrast enhanced abdominopelvic computed tomography. J Trauma 51: 860–869, 2001.

Demetriades D, Velmahos G, Cornwell E III et al: Selective nonoperative management of gunshot wounds of the anterior abdomen. Arch Surg 132:178–183, 1997.

Ferrada R, Birolini D: New concepts in the management of patients with penetrating abdominal wounds. Surg Clin North Am 79:1331–1356, 1999.

Gonzalez RP, Turk B, Falimirski ME et al: Abdominal stab wounds: Diagnostic peritoneal lavage criteria for emergency room discharge. J Trauma 51:939–943, 2001.

Kirton OC, Wint D, Thrasher B et al: Stab wounds to the back and flank in the hemodynamically stable patient: A decision algorithm based on contrast-enhanced computed tomography with colonic opacification. Am J Surg 173:189–193, 1997.

Nicholas JM, Rix EP, Easley KA et al: Changing patterns in the management of penetrating abdominal trauma: The more things change the more they stay the same. J Trauma 55:1095–1108, 2003.

Simon RJ, Rabin J, Kuhls D: Impact of increased use of laparoscopy on negative laparotomy rates after penetrating trauma. J Trauma 53:297–302, 2002.

Tremblay LN, Feliciano DV, Schmidt J et al: Skin only or silo closure in the critically ill patient with an open abdomen. Am J Surg 182:670–675, 2002.

Udobi KF, Rodriguez A, Chiu WC et al: Role of ultrasonography in penetrating abdominal trauma: A prospective clinical study. J Trauma 50:475–479, 2001.

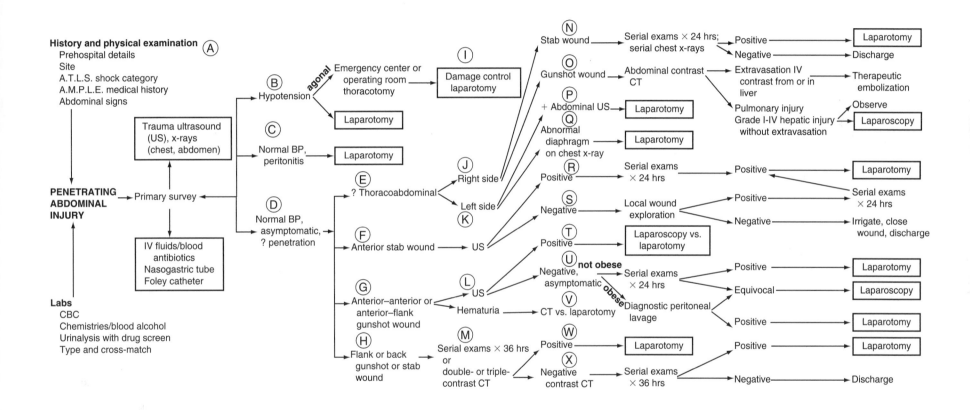

History and physical examination (A)
Prehospital details
Site
A.T.L.S. shock category
A.M.P.L.E. medical history
Abdominal signs

PENETRATING ABDOMINAL INJURY

Primary survey

Trauma ultrasound (US), x-rays (chest, abdomen)

IV fluids/blood
antibiotics
Nasogastric tube
Foley catheter

Labs
CBC
Chemistries/blood alcohol
Urinalysis with drug screen
Type and cross-match

(B) Hypotension

agonal → Emergency center or operating room thoracotomy → (I) Damage control laparotomy

→ Laparotomy

(C) Normal BP, peritonitis → Laparotomy

(D) Normal BP, asymptomatic, ? penetration

(E) ? Thoracoabdominal
(J) Right side
(K) Left side

(F) Anterior stab wound → US

(G) Anterior–anterior or anterior–flank gunshot wound
(L) US
Hematuria

(H) Flank or back gunshot or stab wound → (M) Serial exams × 36 hrs or double- or triple-contrast CT

(N) Stab wound → Serial exams × 24 hrs; serial chest x-rays → Positive → Laparotomy
→ Negative → Discharge

(O) Gunshot wound → Abdominal contrast CT → Extravasation IV contrast from or in liver → Therapeutic embolization
→ Pulmonary injury Grade I-IV hepatic injury without extravasation → Observe / Laparoscopy

(P) + Abdominal US → Laparotomy

(Q) Abnormal diaphragm on chest x-ray → Laparotomy

(R) Positive → Serial exams × 24 hrs → Positive → Laparotomy
→ Serial exams × 24 hrs

(S) Negative → Local wound exploration → Positive
→ Negative → Irrigate, close wound, discharge

(T) Positive → Laparoscopy vs. laparotomy

(U) Negative, asymptomatic **not obese** → Serial exams × 24 hrs → Positive → Laparotomy
→ Equivocal → Laparoscopy
obese → (V) Diagnostic peritoneal lavage → Positive → Laparotomy

(W) Positive → Laparotomy → Positive → Laparotomy

(X) Negative contrast CT → Serial exams × 36 hrs → Negative → Discharge

Chapter 146 *Abdominal Vascular Injury*

DAVID V. FELICIANO, MD

(A) Some 90% to 95% of patients who have injuries to named abdominal vessels have sustained penetrating trauma, especially gunshot wounds. In this latter group, 20% to 25% of patients undergoing a "therapeutic laparotomy" will require treatment for an abdominal vascular injury. The assessment of need for advanced trauma life support (ATLS) can be summarized by the acronym AMPLE (allergies, medications, past medical history, last meal, events or description of the injury).

(B) Whereas routine baseline studies are performed in all patients with suspected intra-abdominal injuries, only type and cross-match are absolutely necessary in those who are profoundly hypotensive. In more stable patients, a urinalysis positive for blood may be the first clue that there has been a renovascular or renal parenchymal injury.

(C) Patients with transabdominal or transpelvic gunshot wounds and overt signs of intra-abdominal injury (e.g., hypotension and/or peritonitis) need neither intubation nor insertion of a thoracostomy tube in the emergency center. Patients with multisystem blunt trauma and stable patients with truncal penetrating wounds that may be extracavitary may benefit from chest and abdominopelvic x-rays, surgeon-performed ultrasound of the pericardium and dependent peritoneal areas ("FAST"), and abdominopelvic CT. (The acronym FAST stands for *focused assessment with sonography examination of the trauma patient*.)

(D) Some 60% to 65% of patients with abdominal vascular injuries are hypotensive (systolic blood pressure less than 100 mm Hg) in the emergency center. In patients with multisystem blunt trauma, where injuries to other body areas might be responsible for hypotension, a positive surgeon-performed abdominal ultrasound or positive peritonitis on physical examination in the hypotensive patient confirms the abdominal cavity as the source.

(E) Gross hematuria may be transient or absent with renovascular injuries, but microscopic hematuria is always present. Further work-up is appropriate in all patients with this finding after blunt trauma, and in the highly selected group of patients with penetrating wounds to the flank or back but no hypotension or peritonitis.

(F) After a thoracic aortogram, it is worthwhile to have the angiographer perform a study of the abdominal aorta and its visceral and terminal branches before the transfemoral artery catheter is removed. Unsuspected intimal injuries and even occlusions of the proximal renal or superior mesenteric artery have been detected with this additional angiogram.

(G) Patients with blunt pelvic fractures and a continuing need for transfusion (4 to 6 units in the first 2 hours after admission) in the absence of other obvious sites of hemorrhage (negative ultrasound or diagnostic peritoneal lavage) need consultation with an orthopaedic surgeon and urgent pelvic arteriography with possible therapeutic embolization of bleeding sites.

(H) Active bleeding from one or more abdominal vessels is usually found at laparotomy in the group of patients who are hypotensive in the emergency center.

(I) A stable or expanding midline, perirenal, pelvic, portal, or retrohepatic hematoma is usually found at laparotomy in patients who were hemodynamically stable upon admission to the emergency center (systolic blood pressure greater than 100 mm Hg) or who had rapid (but often transient) reversal of modest or moderate hypotension with the infusion of 2 liters of crystalloid solutions.

(J) Renovascular lesions that may be noted on contrast-enhanced CT, or selective renal arteriography if the CT is unclear, include intimal flaps with intact distal flow or occlusion 2 to 3 cm from the abdominal aorta.

(K) Midline supramesocolic, midline inframesocolic, portal, perirenal, and pelvic hematomas are opened in patients with penetrating wounds because large named vessels may be injured underneath them. Perirenal and pelvic hematomas are not opened in patients with blunt trauma unless they are pulsatile, ruptured, or rapidly expanding. Retrohepatic hematomas are no longer opened after blunt or penetrating trauma unless, once again, they are pulsatile, ruptured, or rapidly expanding.

(L) An intimal flap in the renal artery with intact distal flow diagnosed on CT or on a selective renal arteriogram may be observed with administration of intravenous heparin in patients without other significant injuries. A follow-up renal arteriogram or isotope renogram is appropriate before discharge to document continuing flow to the kidney through the injured artery. In some centers with local expertise, an endovascular stent would be inserted with postprocedure heparinization. With blunt occlusion of the renal artery, the low yield of surgical revascularization in recent reports has prompted observation only if the contralateral kidney is intact on CT and the diagnosis has been made 6 hours after injury. If the contralateral kidney is absent or small, surgical revascularization is appropriate if the diagnosis has been made within 6 hours of injury. Some centers, however, would choose heparinization only in the hope that recanalization will occur. If the diagnosis is known and an early laparotomy for other injuries is performed, renal revascularization should be considered if only other minor injuries are present.

(M) Exposure for proximal control of the injured SMA is obtained by a left medial mobilization maneuver involving the left colon, left kidney, spleen and tail of the pancreas, and fundus of the stomach. On rare occasions, the pancreas may need to be transected between Glassman clamps at the level of the neck to obtain exposure of the artery (Fullen zone I). Many injuries occur beyond the pancreas at the base of the transverse mesocolon (Fullen zone II), and exposure is obtained by lifting the transverse colon anteriorly and opening the peritoneum at the base of the mesocolon in the midline. Lacerations are repaired in a transverse

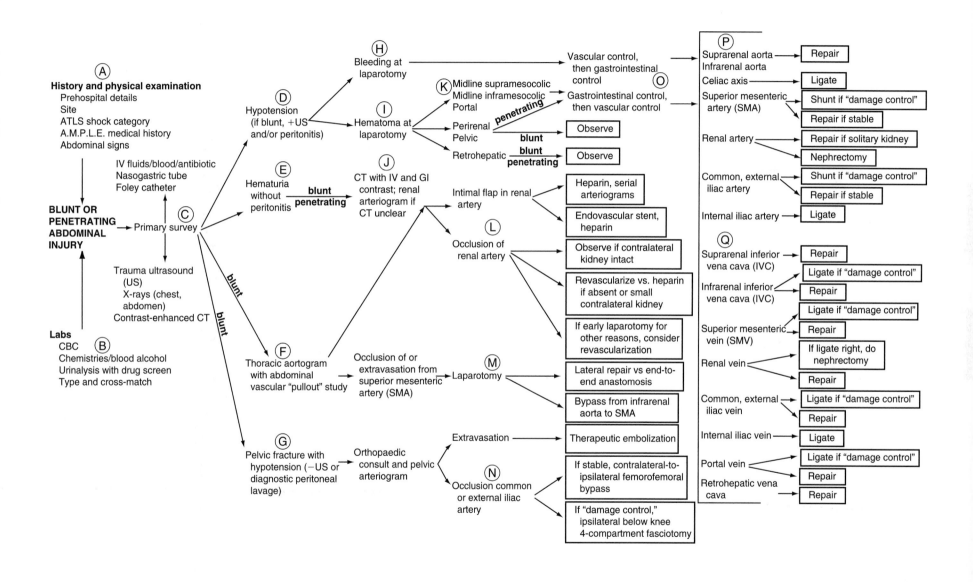

Ⓐ **History and physical examination**
Prehospital details
Site
ATLS shock category
A.M.P.L.E. medical history
Abdominal signs

IV fluids/blood/antibiotic
Nasogastric tube
Foley catheter

BLUNT OR PENETRATING ABDOMINAL INJURY

Ⓒ Primary survey

Trauma ultrasound (US)
X-rays (chest, abdomen)
Contrast-enhanced CT

Labs
Ⓑ CBC
Chemistries/blood alcohol
Urinalysis with drug screen
Type and cross-match

Ⓓ Hypotension (if blunt, +US and/or peritonitis)

Ⓔ Hematuria without peritonitis   **blunt**   **penetrating**

Ⓕ Thoracic aortogram with abdominal vascular "pullout" study

Ⓖ Pelvic fracture with hypotension (−US or diagnostic peritoneal lavage)

Ⓗ Bleeding at laparotomy

Ⓘ Hematoma at laparotomy

Ⓙ CT with IV and GI contrast; renal arteriogram if CT unclear

Ⓚ Midline supramesocolic
Midline inframesocolic
Portal
Perirenal   **penetrating**
Pelvic   **blunt**
Retrohepatic   **blunt**   **penetrating**

Vascular control, then gastrointestinal control

Ⓞ Gastrointestinal control, then vascular control

Observe
Observe

Intimal flap in renal artery
Occlusion of renal artery

Orthopaedic consult and pelvic arteriogram

Occlusion of or extravasation from superior mesenteric artery (SMA)

Extravasation

Ⓝ Occlusion common or external iliac artery

Ⓜ Laparotomy

Heparin, serial arteriograms
Endovascular stent, heparin
Observe if contralateral kidney intact
Revascularize vs. heparin if absent or small contralateral kidney
If early laparotomy for other reasons, consider revascularization
Lateral repair vs end-to-end anastomosis
Bypass from infrarenal aorta to SMA
Therapeutic embolization
If stable, contralateral-to-ipsilateral femorofemoral bypass
If "damage control," ipsilateral below knee 4-compartment fasciotomy

Ⓛ

Ⓟ
Suprarenal aorta → Repair
Infrarenal aorta
Celiac axis → Ligate
Superior mesenteric artery (SMA) → Shunt if "damage control"
→ Repair if stable
Renal artery → Repair if solitary kidney
→ Nephrectomy
Common, external iliac artery → Shunt if "damage control"
→ Repair if stable
Internal iliac artery → Ligate

Ⓠ
Suprarenal inferior vena cava (IVC) → Repair
→ Ligate if "damage control"
Infrarenal inferior vena cava (IVC) → Repair
Superior mesenteric vein (SMV) → Ligate if "damage control"
→ Repair
Renal vein → If ligate right, do nephrectomy
→ Repair
Common, external iliac vein → Ligate if "damage control"
→ Repair
Internal iliac vein → Ligate
Portal vein → Ligate if "damage control"
→ Repair
Retrohepatic vena cava → Repair

fashion or with resection and end-to-end anastomosis with polypropylene sutures. Because of the risk of a postoperative leak from injury to the adjacent pancreas, extensive proximal injuries are ligated and a reversed saphenous vein graft is inserted from the infrarenal abdominal aorta (end-to-side) to the distal SMA (end-to-end). Both anastomoses should be covered with mesenteric tissue or a mobilized flap of viable omentum.

(N) Extravasation from branches of the internal iliac artery is treated by selective therapeutic embolization. The very rare occlusion of the common or external iliac artery is treated with insertion of a contralateral-to-ipsilateral femorofemoral bypass graft using an 8-mm externally supported polytetrafluoroethylene graft. In a damage control situation, an ipsilateral below-knee 4-compartment fasciotomy will preserve the shank and foot for approximately 6 hours if a normal hemodynamic state is maintained. At this point, a crossover graft will have to be inserted.

(O) Control of active arterial bleeding is obtained by compression with a hand or laparotomy pad, grabbing the injured (iliac) artery with a hand, formal proximal and distal control, or insertion of a Fogarty or Foley balloon catheter into the defect. In addition to the techniques listed, venous bleeding can be controlled by grabbing the laceration with a series of Judd-Allis clamps or by proximal and distal compression with spongesticks. After bleeding has been controlled and before the arterial repair is started, extensive perforations in the gastrointestinal tract are closed with Allis, Babcock, Dennis, or Glassman clamps or a rapid continuous repair with polypropylene suture. Prior to opening any hematoma, complete gastrointestinal control is obtained using clamps or suture as above.

(P) Exposures and control of arteries listed:

Suprarenal aorta/celiac axis/SMA: Bleeding → cross-clamp aorta at diaphragm. Hematoma → left-sided medial mobilization

Infrarenal aorta: Bleeding or hematoma → Base of mesocolon

Renal artery: Bleeding → direct or medial mobilization. Hematoma → central control underneath left renal vein

Iliac artery: Bleeding → eviscerate midgut, grab artery. Hematoma → eviscerate midgut, proximal control at aortic bifurcation, distal control before inguinal ligament

(Q) Exposures and control of veins listed:

Suprarenal IVC: Bleeding or hematoma → Retract liver superiorly, right medial mobilization and Kocher maneuver, cross-clamp infrarenal IVC and loop or cross-clamp renal veins, apply Judd-Allis or Satinsky clamps vs. aortic-type cross-clamp on IVC at edge of liver. Will need cross-clamp on infrarenal aorta to preserve blood pressure if IVC completely clamped

Infrarenal IVC: Bleeding or hematoma → right medial mobilization and Kocher maneuver, apply Judd-Allis clamps or Satinsky clamp vs. aortic-type cross-clamps around perforation in IVC. Cross-clamp aorta as above

SMV: Bleeding or hematoma → divide neck of pancreas if needed; otherwise, open retroperitoneum at base of mesocolon

Renal vein: Left → base of mesocolon; right → right medial mobilization and Kocher maneuver

Iliac vein: Injury to proximal right common iliac vein may require temporary division of overlying right common iliac artery for exposure. Exposure of injured internal iliac vein may require division and ligation of internal iliac artery

Portal vein: Proximal Pringle, distal control with forceps, identify bile duct before repair

Retrohepatic vena cava: Direct lateral or transhepatic approach through laceration vs. atriocaval shunt with 36 French thoracostomy tube or No. 8 warmed endotracheal tube

REFERENCES

Asensio JA, Britt LD, Borzotta A et al: Multiinstitutional experience with the management of superior mesenteric artery injuries. J Am Coll Surg 193:354–366, 2001.

Asensio JA, Chahwan S, Hanpeter D et al: Operative management and outcome of 302 abdominal vascular injuries. Am J Surg 180:528–534, 2001.

Burch JM, Feliciano DV, Mattox KL et al: Injuries of the inferior vena cava. Am J Surg 156:548–552, 1988.

Burch JM, Richardson RJ, Martin RR et al: Penetrating iliac vascular injuries: Experience with 233 consecutive patients. J Trauma 30:1450–1459, 1990.

Davis TP, Feliciano DV, Rozycki GS et al: Results with abdominal vascular trauma in the modern era. Am Surg 67:565–571, 2001.

Feliciano DV: Abdominal Vascular Injury. In Moore EE, Mattox KL, Feliciano DV (eds): Trauma, 5th ed. New York: McGraw-Hill, 2004, pp. 755–777.

Feliciano DV: Injuries to the Great Vessels of the Abdomen. In Wilmore DW, Cheung LY, Harken AH et al (eds): ACS Surgery, Principles and Practice. New York: Web MD, 2002.

Haas CA, Dinchman KH, Nasrallah PF et al: Traumatic renal artery occlusion: A 15-year review. J Trauma 45:557–561, 1998.

Stone HH, Fabian TC, Turkleson ML: Wounds of the portal venous system. World J Surg 6:335–341, 1982.

Tyburski JG, Wilson RF, Dente C et al: Factors affecting mortality rates in patients with abdominal vascular injuries. J Trauma 50:1020–1026, 2001.

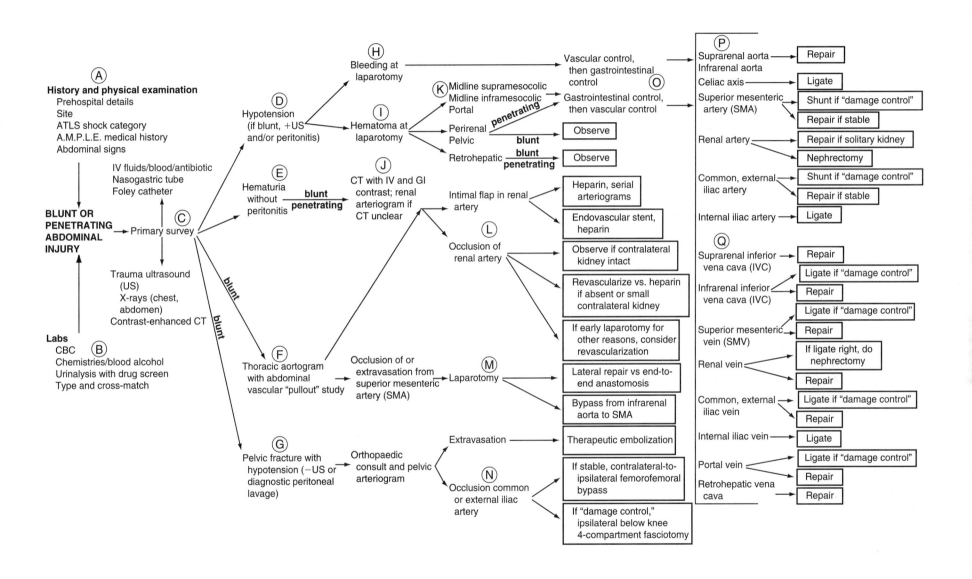

(A) **History and physical examination**
Prehospital details
Site
ATLS shock category
A.M.P.L.E. medical history
Abdominal signs

IV fluids/blood/antibiotic
Nasogastric tube
Foley catheter

BLUNT OR PENETRATING ABDOMINAL INJURY → (C) Primary survey

Trauma ultrasound (US)
X-rays (chest, abdomen)
Contrast-enhanced CT

Labs
CBC (B)
Chemistries/blood alcohol
Urinalysis with drug screen
Type and cross-match

(D) Hypotension (if blunt, +US and/or peritonitis)

(E) Hematuria without peritonitis — **blunt** / **penetrating** →

(F) Thoracic aortogram with abdominal vascular "pullout" study

(G) Pelvic fracture with hypotension (−US or diagnostic peritoneal lavage)

(H) Bleeding at laparotomy

(I) Hematoma at laparotomy

(J) CT with IV and GI contrast; renal arteriogram if CT unclear

(K) Midline supramesocolic
Midline inframesocolic
Portal — **penetrating**
Perirenal
Pelvic — **blunt** → Observe
Retrohepatic — **blunt** / **penetrating** → Observe

Vascular control, then gastrointestinal control

Gastrointestinal control, then vascular control (O)

Intimal flap in renal artery →
- Heparin, serial arteriograms
- Endovascular stent, heparin

(L) Occlusion of renal artery →
- Observe if contralateral kidney intact
- Revascularize vs. heparin if absent or small contralateral kidney
- If early laparotomy for other reasons, consider revascularization

Occlusion of or extravasation from superior mesenteric artery (SMA) → Laparotomy (M)
- Lateral repair vs end-to-end anastomosis
- Bypass from infrarenal aorta to SMA

Orthopaedic consult and pelvic arteriogram
- Extravasation → Therapeutic embolization
- Occlusion common or external iliac artery (N)
  - If stable, contralateral-to-ipsilateral femorofemoral bypass
  - If "damage control," ipsilateral below knee 4-compartment fasciotomy

(P)
Suprarenal aorta
Infrarenal aorta → Repair
Celiac axis → Ligate
Superior mesenteric artery (SMA) →
- Shunt if "damage control"
- Repair if stable
Renal artery →
- Repair if solitary kidney
- Nephrectomy
Common, external iliac artery →
- Shunt if "damage control"
- Repair if stable
Internal iliac artery → Ligate

(Q)
Suprarenal inferior vena cava (IVC) → Repair
Infrarenal inferior vena cava (IVC) →
- Ligate if "damage control"
- Repair
Superior mesenteric vein (SMV) →
- Ligate if "damage control"
- Repair
Renal vein →
- If ligate right, do nephrectomy
- Repair
Common, external iliac vein →
- Ligate if "damage control"
- Repair
Internal iliac vein → Ligate
Portal vein →
- Ligate if "damage control"
- Repair
Retrohepatic vena cava → Repair

Chapter 147 *Pancreatic Injury*

GREGORY J. JURKOVICH, MD

(A) Suspicion for a possible pancreatic injury is enhanced with high-energy direct blows to the epigastrium (e.g., kick, motor vehicle crash, or handlebar injury). Diagnostic delays are common and deadly.

(B) Serum amylase or isoamylase is unreliable early (first 4 hours); only 65% of patients with complete transection have elevated amylase. Rising amylase or early elevated amylase demands pancreatic imaging. Computed tomography (CT) is the most sensitive and specific imaging test, yet it misses about one-third of pancreatic injuries when performed in the first few hours after injury. Repeat CT with IV contrast can be valuable. Diagnostic peritoneal lavage is unreliable in retroperitoneal injuries, and ultrasound (FAST) is unproven in pancreatic trauma (Table 147-1).

(C) The vast majority of significant pancreatic injuries can be diagnosed by careful inspection of the gland. Wide exposure of the pancreas is required. Approach via the lesser sac because midbody injuries over the spine are most common. Kocherize the duodenum and take down the hepatic flexure of the colon to fully inspect the head. Unroof the retroperitoneum over any areas of contusion. All pancreatic injuries require drainage and debridement of devitalized tissue. In an unstable patient, hemostasis and drainage alone may be advisable even though a pancreatic fistula is anticipated. Most fistulas close spontaneously, and most reports suggest no benefit to the use of octreotide.

(D) Superficial contusions and lacerations should be unroofed, inspected carefully to confirm no duct injury, and drained.

(E) Moderate contusions and lacerations with no primary or secondary branch duct injury

TABLE 147-1
Pancreatic Organ Injury Severity (AAST Organ Injury Scaling Committee)

Grade	Injury	Description
I	Hematoma	Minor contusion without duct injury
	Laceration	Superficial laceration without duct injury
II	Hematoma	Major contusion without duct injury or tissue loss
	Laceration	Major laceration without duct injury or tissue loss
III	Laceration	Distal transection or parenchymal injury with duct
IV	Laceration	Proximal (to the right of the superior mesenteric vein) transection or parenchymal injury with duct injury
V	Laceration	Massive disruption of pancreaticoduodenal complex or devascularization of pancreas

should be managed with debridement and drainage alone.

(F) Distal transection or injury to the main pancreatic duct is best managed by distal pancreatectomy. Splenic salvage adds about 1 hour of time and should especially be considered in children. Proximal duct pancreatogram via the transected open proximal end should be done if blunt injury to the remaining pancreatic head is a concern. Drain and consider a feeding tube. Anticipate 10% to 20% fistula, nearly all closing spontaneously. Octreotide has no proven benefit in managing postoperative fistula following injury.

(G) Major injury to the head (right of mesenteric vessels) is rare but most challenging. In an unstable patient, hemostasis and drainage alone may be advisable, with postoperative ERCP recommended to define the anatomy of the main pancreatic duct and possibly to stent a duct injury. Alternatively, complete the transection and debride devitalized tissue, oversew proximal stump, and perform Roux-en-Y to the remaining distal segment (to avoid pancreatic endocrine and exocrine insufficiency).

(H) Pancreaticoduodenectomy, with its problematic anastomoses, is advisable only when the head of the pancreas, bile duct, and duodenum are extensively injured. If possible, injuries to the pancreas and duodenum should be treated separately.

(I) Pyloric exclusion is valuable in this setting to minimize pancreatic stimulation or if duodenal injury is present.

REFERENCES

Cogbill T, Moore E, Morris JJ et al: Distal pancreatectomy for trauma: A multicenter experience. J Trauma 31:1600–1606, 1991.

Jurkovich GJ: Duodenum and Pancreas. In Mattox KI, Feliciano DV, Moore EE (eds): Trauma, 4th ed. New York: McGraw-Hill, 2000.

Jurkovich GJ, Carrico CJ: Management of pancreatic injuries. Surg Clin North Am 70:575–593, 1990.

Moore EE, Cogbill TH, Malangoni MA et al: Organ injury scaling. Surg Clin North Am 75:293–303, 1995.

Nwariaku FE, Terracina A, Mileski WJ et al: Is octreotide beneficial following pancreatic injury? Am J Surg 170:582–585, 1995.

Patton JH, Lyden SP, Croce MA et al: Pancreatic trauma: A simplified management guideline. J Trauma 43:234–241, 1997.

Smego D, Richardson J, Flint L: Determinants of outcome in pancreatic trauma. J Trauma 24:771–776, 1985.

Takishima T, Hirata M, Kataoka Y et al: Pancreatographic classification of pancreatic ductal injuries caused by blunt injury to the pancreas. J Trauma 48(4):745–752, 2000.

Vaughn GD III, Frazier OH, Graham DY et al: The use of pyloric exclusion in the management of severe duodenal injuries. Am J Surg 134:785–790, 1977.

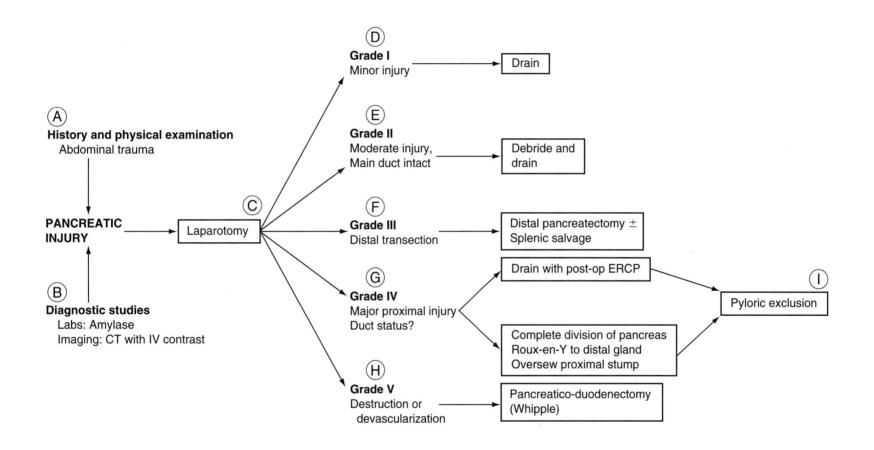

(A)

History and physical examination
Abdominal trauma

**PANCREATIC
INJURY**

(B)

Diagnostic studies
Labs: Amylase
Imaging: CT with IV contrast

(C)

Laparotomy

(D)

Grade I
Minor injury

Drain

(E)

Grade II
Moderate injury,
Main duct intact

Debride and
drain

(F)

Grade III
Distal transection

Distal pancreatectomy ±
Splenic salvage

(G)

Grade IV
Major proximal injury
Duct status?

Drain with post-op ERCP

Complete division of pancreas
Roux-en-Y to distal gland
Oversew proximal stump

(I)

Pyloric exclusion

(H)

Grade V
Destruction or
devascularization

Pancreatico-duodenectomy
(Whipple)

Chapter 148 *Duodenal Injury*

GREGORY J. JURKOVICH, MD

(A) Suspect duodenal injury with direct blows to epigastrium (e.g., handlebar injuries or kick to abdomen). Early preoperative diagnosis of duodenal injury is difficult because of the retroperitoneal position of the duodenum.

(B) Laboratory examination should include WBC and amylase.

(C) Abdominal radiographs occasionally show free air or a retroperitoneal stripe of air.

(D) Contrast studies occasionally show duodenal extravasation, but classic pathognomonic findings of duodenal rupture (e.g., air or contrast extravasation) are present in only a minority of cases. Computed tomography (CT) abdominal examination should include oral contrast. Diagnostic peritoneal lavage misses 50% of duodenal injuries. Abdominal ultrasound (FAST) is unproven in diagnosing duodenal injury.

(E) Thorough inspection of the duodenum is necessary when injury is suspected. This requires a Kocher maneuver, and sometimes requires takedown of the ligament of Treitz. Severity of duodenal injury influences management (Table 148-1).

(F) Primary closure should be attempted as the first option, with concomitant pyloric exclusion advised. If primary closure is technically compromised by tissue loss, narrowing, or tension, use a Roux-en-Y duodenojejunostomy to the proximal end of the duodenal injury with an oversew of the distal duodenum (injuries distal to the ampulla). "Sucker patch" buttressing (open mouth Roux-en-Y limb buttressing of primary repair) is *not* advised. Omentum for buttressing is preferred, although some also use serosal patching of a jejunal loop. Use of external closed suction drains is controversial, but the author prefers to use them for a few days.

(G) Injuries at the ampulla (Grade IV/V) are rare and complicate treatment greatly. Management

TABLE 148-1
Duodenal Injury Severity (AAST Organ Injury Scaling Committee)

Grade	Injury	Description
I	Hematoma	Single portion of duodenum
	Laceration	Partial thickness only
II	Hematoma	Involving more than one portion
	Laceration	Disruption <50% circumference
III	Laceration	Disruption 50%–75% circumference of D2
		Disruption 50%–100% circumference of D1, D3, D4
IV	Laceration	Disruption >75% circumference of D2
		Involving ampulla or distal common duct
V	Laceration	Massive disruption of duodenopancreatic complex or devascularization of duodenum

of the biliary injury can be done primarily at the time of the initial operation or in a delayed fashion. Bile duct injuries less than 50% of the diameter can be repaired primarily over a T-tube or with choledochojejunostomy. Primary repairs in an end-to-end fashion usually develop strictures and should not be done. In unstable patients with multiple injuries, the area is well drained and the injury is "fistulized" externally, and plans are made for delayed reconstruction. Management options include (1) pancreatoduodenectomy; (2) reimplantation of the ampulla or distal common bile duct into either the duodenum or a Roux-en-Y limb of the jejunum; (3) primary reconstruction using hepaticojejunostomies; or (4) delayed reconstruction. Grade V injuries mandate pancreaticoduodenectomy. External drainage is required and feeding tube placement is advised.

(H) Intramural hematoma seen at laparotomy requires evacuation to avoid obstruction and

to detect duodenal mucosal injury. Extramural (peri-duodenal) hematoma requires inspection to exclude pancreatic, duodenal, or vascular injuries.

(I) Duodenal obstruction from a hematoma can occur as late as 1 to 3 weeks after injury. The obstruction is relieved spontaneously in many patients during a period of observation. Support by nasogastric (NG) suction and total parenteral nutrition (TPN) is required. Obstruction by a hematoma should raise suspicion of associated injuries.

(J) Grade I or II simple laceration injuries account for 80% of duodenal injuries and most can be closed primarily. Debride any nonviable tissue. Single- or double-layer closure is performed. Pyloric exclusion or buttressing is unnecessary unless concomitant pancreatic injury is present.

(K) If there is greater than 50% injury to the first portion of the duodenum (Grade III D1), and primary repair is technically compromised, close the duodenal stump and perform antrectomy and gastrojejunostomy.

REFERENCES

Ballard RB, Badellino MM, Eynon A et al: Blunt duodenal rupture: A 6-year statewide experience. J Trauma 43: 229–233, 1997.

Cogbill T, Moore E, Feliciano D et al: Conservative management of duodenal trauma: A multicenter perspective. J Trauma 30:1469–1475, 1990.

Jurkovich GJ: Duodenum and Pancreas. In Mattox KI, Feliciano DV, Moore EE (eds): Trauma, 4th ed. New York: McGraw-Hill, 2000.

Martin TD, Feliciano DV, Mattox KL et al: Severe duodenal injuries. Arch Surg 118:631–635, 1983.

Moore EE, Cogbill TH, Malangoni MA et al: Organ injury scaling. Surg Clin North Am 75:293–303, 1995.

Snyder W, Weigelt J, Watkins W et al: The surgical management of duodenal trauma. Arch Surg 115:422–429, 1980.

Velmahos GC, Kamel E, Chan LS et al: Complex repair for the management of duodenal injuries. Am Surg 65: 972–975, 1999.

Carrillo EH, Richardson D, Miller FB: Evolution in the management of duodenal injuries. J Trauma 40:1037–1046, 1996.

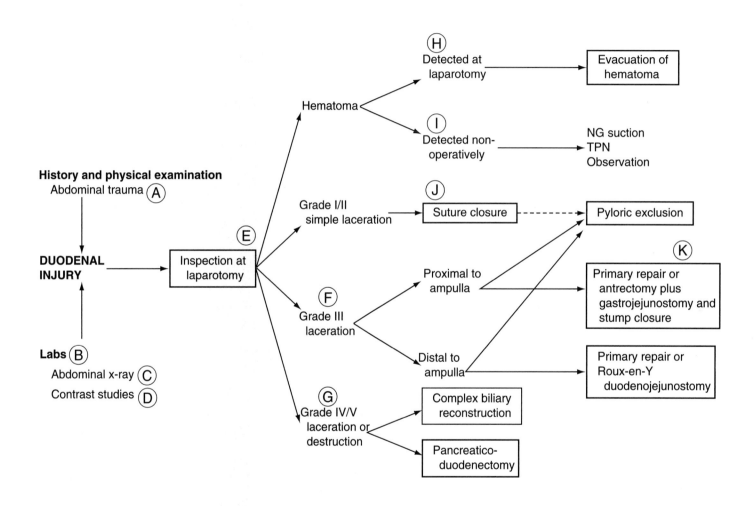

History and physical examination
Abdominal trauma (A)

DUODENAL
INJURY

Labs (B)
Abdominal x-ray (C)
Contrast studies (D)

Inspection at
laparotomy (E)

Hematoma
- Detected at
  laparotomy (H) → Evacuation of
  hematoma
- Detected non-
  operatively (I) → NG suction
  TPN
  Observation

Grade I/II
simple laceration → Suture closure (J) ----→ Pyloric exclusion

Grade III
laceration (F)
- Proximal to
  ampulla → Primary repair or
  antrectomy plus
  gastrojejunostomy and
  stump closure (K)
- Distal to
  ampulla → Primary repair or
  Roux-en-Y
  duodenojejunostomy

Grade IV/V
laceration or
destruction (G)
- Complex biliary
  reconstruction
- Pancreatico-
  duodenectomy

Chapter 149 *Penetrating Injury of the Colon*

REGINALD J. FRANCIOSE, MD • JON M. BURCH, MD

(A) The time and mechanism of injury and the patient's prehospital status are important determinants of operative management. Paramedics often provide this information. Fresh blood found on rectal examination or sigmoidoscopy is presumptive evidence of colon injury unless an alternative source of bleeding can be identified.

(B) The penalty for delay in treating colon injury is severe. Wounds near the retroperitoneal colon or rectum warrant laparotomy even in the absence of abdominal signs, unless diagnostic findings are unequivocally normal.

(C) Associated solid visceral or vascular injury is frequent with penetrating abdominal wounds and can be a source of major blood loss. If hypotension exists, blood is typed and cross-matched, and serial hematocrits (Hct) are obtained. Patients with stab wounds and signs of peritoneal irritation or shock should go directly to the operating room. Stable patients with abdominal stab wounds warrant local wound exploration followed by diagnostic peritoneal lavage (DPL) in patients where the fascia has been penetrated. Retroperitoneal colon injury must be considered with penetrating back or flank wounds. Triple-contrast computed tomography (CT) may detect such injury in asymptomatic patients.

(D) Gunshot wounds of the abdomen mandate laparotomy if the bullet violates the peritoneal cavity. Plain abdominal x-rays (anterior, posterior, and lateral views) are used to assess missile trajectory. A chest x-ray is obtained to rule out thoracic injury.

(E) Prophylactic antibiotics are given before the abdominal incision is made. The antibiotics should be active against anaerobic and aerobic bacteria. Broad-spectrum coverage with a single agent such as a second-generation cephalosporin or an extended-spectrum penicillin is effective. A midline abdominal incision provides rapid, wide exposure of the peritoneal cavity. Overt colon perforations are closed with intestinal clamps while vascular control is accomplished and exploration is completed.

(F) Critically injured patients who develop the triad of hypothermia (BT <35°C), acidosis (pH <7.2, lactate >5 mm/L, base deficit ≤15 mmol/l in patients <55 years or ≤6 mmol/l in patients >55 years of age), and coagulopathy (prothrombin time [PT] or partial thromboplastin time [PTT] >50% of normal) are at imminent risk of death and should undergo "damage control" or "abbreviated laparotomy." After vascular control has been achieved, no attempt at GI reconstruction should be made until the patient is adequately resuscitated.

(G) To prevent continued fecal soilage and septic complications, the colon is stapled on both sides of the injury. Alternatively, the colon is ligated by passing umbilical tapes through the mesentery on either side of the injury.

(H) The abdomen is rapidly, temporarily closed by placing a series of penetrating towel clamps on the skin edges to prevent further heat loss. Intraoperative shock resuscitation with IV fluid and blood products continues. An aggressive attempt is made to correct coagulopathy with fresh-frozen plasma, platelets, and cryoprecipitate when needed. All infusion fluids are warmed, room temperature is maximized, wet drapes and blankets are replaced, and all exposed body surfaces are covered. After 30–45 minutes, the towel clips are removed and the abdomen is reexplored while the patient's physiologic status is reassessed (vital signs, temperature, pH, lactate, base deficit, PT, PTT).

(I) If the patient is hemodynamically stable and no longer acidotic, hypothermic, and coagulopathic, the colon injury is addressed.

(J) If the patient is hemodynamically unstable and continues to be hypothermic, acidotic, and coagulopathic, the abdomen is briefly reexplored to ensure that no mechanical source of bleeding has been overlooked. The abdomen is towel clipped again, and the patient is transported to the ICU for resuscitation. Every attempt is made to fully resuscitate the patient for return to the OR and to effect definitive repair of all injuries within 24 hours.

(K) Severity of the colon injury can be graded anatomically with the American Association for the Surgery of Trauma (AAST) Colon Injury Scale:

Grade I. Contusion or hematoma without devascularization or partial-thickness laceration—no perforation
Grade II. Laceration <50% circumference
Grade III. Laceration >50% circumference
Grade IV. Transection of the colon
Grade V. Transection with segmental tissue loss

Lower-grade injuries are amenable to primary suture repair (with meticulous colon wound débridement), but more extensive wounds and higher-grade injuries usually require segmental colon resection. Multiple closely positioned perforations may be better managed by a single en bloc resection.

(L) Ideally, significant injuries below the peritoneal reflection (rectal injuries) should undergo débridement and repair with fecal diversion. This is not always possible with low injuries. Colostomy and presacral drainage are recommended under these conditions to prevent pelvic sepsis. Associated urologic trauma is frequent, and a traumatic urinary fistula increases the risk of pelvic sepsis. In rare instances, high-energy, widely destructive wounds of the pelvis necessitate abdominoperineal resection. Distal rectal wash out has historically been the fourth component of the treatments of rectal injuries (débride, divert, drain, decontaminate) due to the military experience where combatants are often constipated at the time of injury. This has been challenged in the civilian setting and should

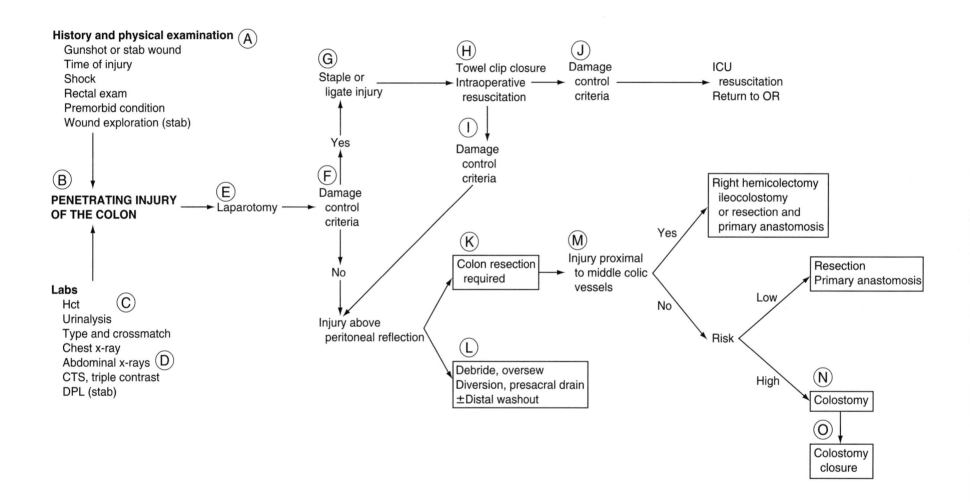

History and physical examination (A)
  Gunshot or stab wound
  Time of injury
  Shock
  Rectal exam
  Premorbid condition
  Wound exploration (stab)

(B)
PENETRATING INJURY
OF THE COLON

(E) Laparotomy

Labs
  Hct   (C)
  Urinalysis
  Type and crossmatch
  Chest x-ray
  Abdominal x-rays (D)
  CTS, triple contrast
  DPL (stab)

(G) Staple or
  ligate injury

Yes

(F) Damage
  control
  criteria

No

Injury above
peritoneal reflection

(H) Towel clip closure
  Intraoperative
  resuscitation

(I) Damage
  control
  criteria

(J) Damage
  control
  criteria

ICU
  resuscitation
  Return to OR

(K) Colon resection
  required

(L) Debride, oversew
  Diversion, presacral drain
  ±Distal washout

(M) Injury proximal
  to middle colic
  vessels

Yes

Right hemicolectomy
ileocolostomy
or resection and
primary anastomosis

No

Risk

Low

Resection
Primary anastomosis

High

(N) Colostomy

(O) Colostomy
  closure

be tailored to the individual patient based on the fecal load present at the time of injury.

(M) Ileocolostomy is believed to be a safer anastomosis than colocolostomy under emergency conditions. When injuries proximal to the middle colic vessels require resection, the right colon is resected and an ileocolostomy is constructed. Injuries distal to the middle colic vessels (left colon) frequently require colostomy with or without resection. Alternatively resection and primary anastomosis may be performed. Injuries distal to the middle colic vessels (left colon) will require resection with primary repair or infrequently colostomy.

(N) Primary repair (suture repair, ileocolostomy, or colocolostomy) is possible in 70% to 90% of patients with colon injuries. There are no absolute indications for colostomy or contraindications to colocolostomy. A small subset of patients at high risk for a poor outcome should undergo colostomy for left-sided colon injuries. Particular attention should be given to the patient who has undergone damage control laparotomy with massive volume resuscitation and has not resolved their bowel edema on return to the operating room. Other identified risk factors include advanced age, serious associated medical conditions, massive hemorrhage, multiple associated injuries, significant fecal contamination, and operation >6 hours after injury. However, these risk factors portend a worse outcome regardless of the type of treatment chosen.

(O) Low-risk patients should be considered for early colostomy closure. All patients undergoing colostomy closure should receive mechanical and oral antibiotic bowel preparation as well as preoperative IV antibiotics.

REFERENCES

Burch JM: Injury to the colon and rectum. In Moore EE, Feliciano DV, Mattox KL (eds.) Trauma, 5th ed. New York: McGraw-Hill, 2000: 735–753.

Demetraides D, Murray J et al: Penetrating colon injuries requiring resection: diversion of primary amastomasis: an AAST prospective multicenter study. J Trauma 50:765–775, 2001.

Feliciano DV, Moore EE, Mattox KL: Damage control in trauma. In Moore EE, Feliciano DV, Mattox KL (eds): Trauma, 5th ed. New York: McGraw-Hill, 2000: 877–899.

Gonzales RP, Falimirski ME, Holevar MR. The role of presacral drainage in the management of penetrating rectal injuries. J Trauma 45:656–661, 1998.

Miller PR, Fabian TC, Croce MA et al: Improving outcomes following penetrating colon wounds: application of a clinical pathway. Ann Surg 235:775–781, 2002.

Moore EE, Cogbill TH, Malagoni MA et al: Organ injury scaling II—pancreas, duodenum, small bowel, colon and rectum. J Trauma 30:1427–1429, 1990.

Stewart RM, Fabian TC, Croce MA et al: Is resection with primary anastomosis following destructive colon wounds always safe? Am J Surg 169:316–319, 1994.

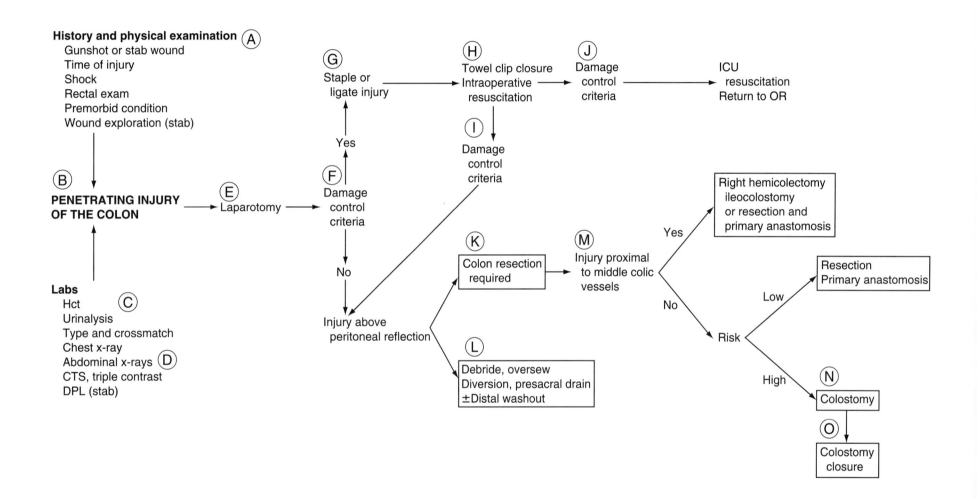

History and physical examination (A)
    Gunshot or stab wound
    Time of injury
    Shock
    Rectal exam
    Premorbid condition
    Wound exploration (stab)

(B)
PENETRATING INJURY OF THE COLON

Labs
    Hct
    Urinalysis (C)
    Type and crossmatch
    Chest x-ray
    Abdominal x-rays (D)
    CTS, triple contrast
    DPL (stab)

(E) Laparotomy

(G) Staple or ligate injury

Yes

(F) Damage control criteria

No

Injury above peritoneal reflection

(H) Towel clip closure Intraoperative resuscitation

(I) Damage control criteria

(J) Damage control criteria

ICU resuscitation Return to OR

(K) Colon resection required

(L) Debride, oversew Diversion, presacral drain ±Distal washout

(M) Injury proximal to middle colic vessels

Yes — Right hemicolectomy ileocolostomy or resection and primary anastomosis

No — Risk

Low — Resection Primary anastomosis

High — (N) Colostomy

(O) Colostomy closure

Chapter 150 *Damage Control Laparotomy/Abdominal Compartment Syndrome*

REGINALD J. FRANCIOSE, MD

(A) Damage control laparotomy is performed on injured patients with profound shock and metabolic failure; it is performed to control hemorrhage, minimize contamination, and allow for resuscitation before lengthy procedures or to minimize procedures in patients with multiple trauma that requires multiple interventions. In addition, trauma surgeons use damage control principles when dealing with thoracic, cervical, extremity, and neurosurgical injuries. Damage control principles are also applicable to complications of elective surgical procedures.

(B) Critically injured patients who develop metabolic failure are at imminent risk of death and should undergo "damage control" or "abbreviated laparotomy." "The bloody vicious triad" is characterized by the following: (1) hypothermia (body temperature less than 35° C); (2) acidosis (pH less than 7.2, lactate greater than 5 mmol/L, base deficit less than -15 mmol/L in patient younger than 55 years or less than -6 mmol/L in patient older than 55 years); and (3) coagulopathy (prothrombin time [PT] or partial thromboplastin time [PPT] greater than 50% above normal). Other indications for abbreviated laparotomy in multiple trauma patients include liver packing; gastrointestinal injury requiring time-consuming or complex reconstruction (e.g., trauma Whipple); mesenteric vascular injury requiring second-look operation for intestinal viability (e.g., ligation of the superior mesenteric vein); a need for nonoperative intervention (e.g., angioembolization of pelvis fracture); a need to proceed to other life-threatening surgical interventions (e.g., ruptured descending thoracic aorta); and an inability to perform definitive closure of abdomen because of bowel edema or impending abdominal compartment syndrome.

(C) Hemorrhage control is rapidly achieved using packs, ligation, suture control, and shunts when necessary. Gastrointestinal injuries are stapled,

ligated with umbilical tapes, or whip stitched. No attempt is made at a definitive repair.

(D) The abdomen is rapidly, temporarily closed by placing a series of penetrating towel clamps on the skin edges to prevent further heat loss. Intraoperative shock resuscitation with IV fluid and blood products continues. An aggressive attempt is made to correct coagulopathy with fresh-frozen plasma, platelets, and cryoprecipitate when needed. All infusion fluids are warmed, room temperature is maximized, wet drapes and blankets are replaced, and all exposed body surfaces are covered. After 30 to 45 minutes, the towel clips are removed and the abdomen is re-explored while the patient's physiologic status is reassessed (e.g., vital signs, temperature, pH, lactate, base deficit, PT, and PTT).

(E) If the patient is hemodynamically unstable and continues to be hypothermic, acidotic, and coagulopathic, the abdomen is briefly re-explored to ensure that no mechanical source of bleeding has been overlooked.

(F) Depending on the circumstances, several techniques are available for temporary abdominal closure. Two easily performed methods include towel clip or segmental suture of skin only. Towel clips will interfere with visualization if the patient is to undergo angiography. A "Bogata bag" temporary closure uses a sterile 3-liter irrigation bag cut open on three sides and sewn to the skin edges. A variety of improvised and commercial vacuum devices use towels or perforated plastic sheets placed over the bowel and under the fascial edges. An impervious material (e.g., Ioban sheet) is placed over the abdomen and suction is applied between the layers to remove pooling fluids and decrease visceral edema.

(G) Aggressive resuscitation continues in the ICU. Every attempt is make to fully resuscitate the patient for return to the OR and to effect definitive repair of all injuries within 24 hours.

(H) Abdominal compartment syndrome (ACS) is a potentially lethal complication of massive resuscitation. Swelling and edema cause intra-abdominal pressure to rise, producing adverse effects on the cardiopulmonary, renal, and neurologic systems. A manometer attached to the Foley catheter is used to measure and grade intra-abdominal pressure and direct therapy.

> GR I: 10 to 15 mm Hg, maintain normovolemia
> GR II: 16 to 25 mm Hg, hypervolemic resuscitation
> GR III: 26 to 35 mm Hg, decompression
> GR IV: greater than 35 mm Hg, decompression and re-exploration

Physiologic indicators of ACS include hypotension, tachycardia, hypoxemia, hypercarbia, high peak airway pressures, oliguria, and cardiac index less than 3.0 despite apparent adequate central venous pressure (CVP) and pulmonary capillary wedge pressure (PCWP). Increased intra-abdominal pressure falsely elevates the CVP and PCWP.

(I) Symptoms of ACS can often be relieved at the bedside by maneuvers that decrease abdominal pressure (e.g., removing central towel clips, removing central segments of suture skin closure, or expanding a Bogata bag). If successful at relieving ACS, resuscitation continues in the ICU.

(J) Ideally the patient is completely resuscitated on return to the OR and undergoes a definitive operation. Often this cannot be achieved and the patient undergoes cycles of resuscitation and operative intervention.

(K) At each operation an assessment is made about whether it is possible to close the abdomen. Commonly, the abdomen cannot be closed until the visceral edema resolves, something that may take several days. Patients with an open abdomen for more than 7 to 10 days often cannot undergo fascial closure secondary to abdominal wall retraction. This small subset of patients will have skin only closure; or in the extreme, skin grafting is done on the omentum or bowel once it has a bed of granulation tissue. These patients undergo repair of their large ventral hernia in a delayed (i.e., in 6 to 12 months) fashion.

REFERENCES

Etrel W, Oberholzer A, Platz A et al: Incidence and clinical pattern of the abdominal compartment syndrome after "damage control" laparotomy in 311 patients with severe abdominal and /or pelvic trauma. Crit Care Med 28: 1747–1753, 2000.

Feliciano DV, Moore EE, Mattox KL: Trauma Damage Control. In Moore EE, Feliciano DV, Mattox KL (eds): Trauma, 5th ed. New York: McGraw Hill, 2000.

Garner GB, Ware DN, Conanour CS et al: Vacuum-assisted wound closure provides early fascial reapproximation in trauma patients with open abdomens. Am J Surg 182:630–638, 2001.

Johnson JW, Gracias VH, Schwab CW et al: Evolution in damage control for exsanguinating penetrating abdominal injury. J Trauma 51:261–271, 2001.

Moore EE, Burch JM, Franciose RJ et al: Staged physiologic restoration and damage control surgery. World J Surg 22:1184–1190, 1998.

Raeburn CD, Moore EE, Biffl WL et al: The abdominal compartment syndrome is a morbid complication of post-injury damage control surgery. Am J Surg 182:542–546, 2001.

Rotondo MF, Schwab CW, McGonigal MD et al: Damage control and approach for improved survival in exsanguinating penetrating abdominal trauma. J Trauma 35:375–382, 1993.

Shapiro MB, Jenkins DH, Schwab CW et al: Damage control: Collective review. J Trauma 49: 969–978, 2000.

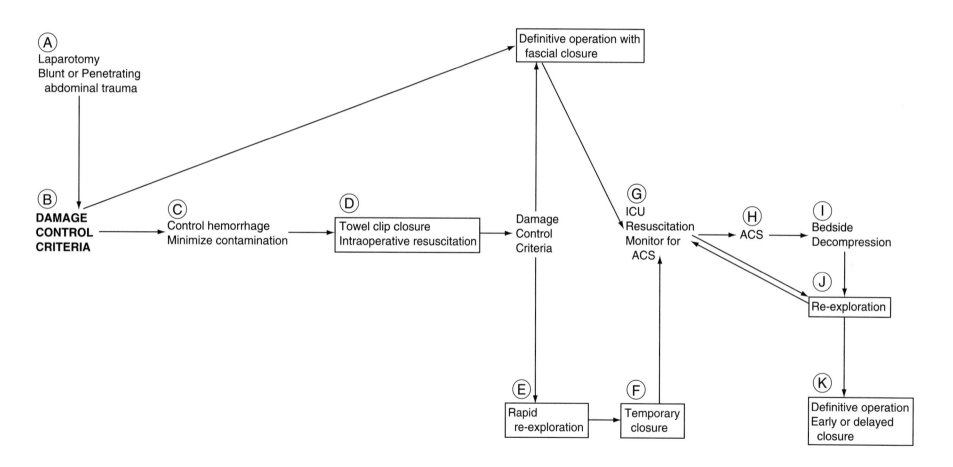

Chapter 151 *Traumatic Hematuria*

FERNANDO J. KIM, MD

(A) Gross or microscopic hematuria after trauma warrants investigation and can result from blunt, penetrating, or even iatrogenic injuries. The mechanism of injury and the associated injured organs will indicate the site of maximum trauma (e.g., abdomen and/or pelvis). Trauma patients with both upper and lower urinary tract involvement have higher mortality rates than with single organ injury. As a general guideline, surgical decision-making should focus on signs of clinical stability, grade of injury, and the presence of associated injuries.

(B) In blunt trauma, the diagnostic precept is to perform imaging from the bottom up. Assuming stability, a retrograde urethrogram is performed when urethral injury is suspected to avoid aggravating an injury. Catheterization can be performed safely in the absence of urethral injury, and a voiding cystogram (both full and postvoid images) or CT cystogram is performed. Major renal injury is rarely seen in patients with microscopic hematuria in the absence of shock after blunt trauma. However, patients with multisystem trauma with a major mechanism (e.g., deceleration injuries) should undergo urgent renal imaging to rule out renal injury (e.g., parenchymal or vascular) even when there is no gross or microscopic hematuria. Penetrating trauma to the urinary tract is almost always discovered at surgical exploration because of associated injuries (e.g., to the liver, small bowel, stomach, colon, or spleen). Patients with any degree of hematuria after penetrating trauma should undergo imaging, but absence of hematuria does not rule out renal injury. One should be aware of blast-effect injuries that may present days after the trauma occurred (e.g., ureteral injury caused by the blast effect secondary to a gunshot wound), delaying the diagnosis.

(C) Single shot IVP (150 ml of IV) contrast is performed in cases of urgent laparotomy.

(D) CT scan is considered a faster study when compared with IVP; therefore, excretory phase (5 minutes) delayed films should be obtained to ascertain collecting system integrity. Intravenous contrast helps define the integrity of the kidney and ureters.

(E) Management of solitary kidney trauma should be focused on preservation of renal function. Most blunt injuries can be managed without operation because the fascial coverings of the kidney tamponade bleeding. Upon exploration for hemodynamic instability and expanding hematoma, the surgeon should evaluate the viability of renal tissue and perform a nephrectomy, partial nephrectomy, with debridement of devitalized tissue or vascular repair, including auto-transplantation. Stents, drains, or nephrostomy tubes can be utilized as indicated.

(F) Perirenal extravasation is not an absolute indication for operation. Extravasation without any contrast in the ureter indicates a possible complete disruption of the collecting system at the ureteropelvic junction. Ureteral injury from blunt trauma is rare; however, if total disruption occurs, surgical repair is warranted. Ureteral injuries with a significant delay in diagnosis or in an unstable patient are best managed initially by percutaneous nephrostomy drainage.

(G) The failure of the kidney to excrete any contrast material suggests an arterial injury. Surgical revascularization rarely results in successful outcome. Recently, successful use of endovascular stent to treat post-trauma renal arterial occlusion (intimal flap) has been reported. Hypertension is uncommon; when it occurs, however, it usually becomes established within 3 to 6 months of injury.

(H) Presence of intravesical contrast with urethral injury translates into a partial urethral avulsion that requires urinary diversion; this is usually accomplished by suprapubic diversion.

(I) Intraperitoneal bladder injury is traditionally managed by surgical repair, but urethral catheterization may promote healing if the injury is small. Evaluation must rule out bowel and mesentery injury.

(J) Extraperitoneal bladder injury is successfully managed with urethral catheterization (1 to 2 weeks).

(K) Primary alignment may facilitate final surgical repair in 3 to 6 months.

REFERENCES

Feliciano DV, Mattox KL, Moore EE (eds): Trauma. Norwalk, CT: Appleton & Lange, 2000.

Iverson AJ, Morey AF: Radiographic evaluation of suspected bladder rupture following blunt trauma: Critical review. World J Surg 25:1588–1591, 2001.

Kim FJ: Urologic Trauma. In Moore EE, Feliciano DV, Mattox KL (eds): Trauma Companion Handbook, 4th ed. New York: McGraw-Hill, 2002.

Knudson MM, Harrison PB, Hoyt DB et al: Outcome after major renovascular injuries: A Western Trauma Association multi-center report. J Trauma 49:1116–1122, 2000.

McAninch JW: Traumatic and Reconstructive Urology. Philadelphia: WB Saunders, 1996.

Moore EE, Cogvill TH, Jurkovich GJ et al: Organ injury scaling, III: Chest wall, abdominal vascular, ureter, bladder, and urethra. J Trauma 33:337–339, 1992.

Santucci RA, McAninch JW, Safir M et al: Validation of the American Association for the Surgery of Trauma organ injury severity scale for the kidney. J Trauma 50:195–200, 2001.

Wessells H, Suh D, Porter JR et al: Renal injury and operative management in the United States: Results of a population-based study. J Trauma 54:423–430, 2003.

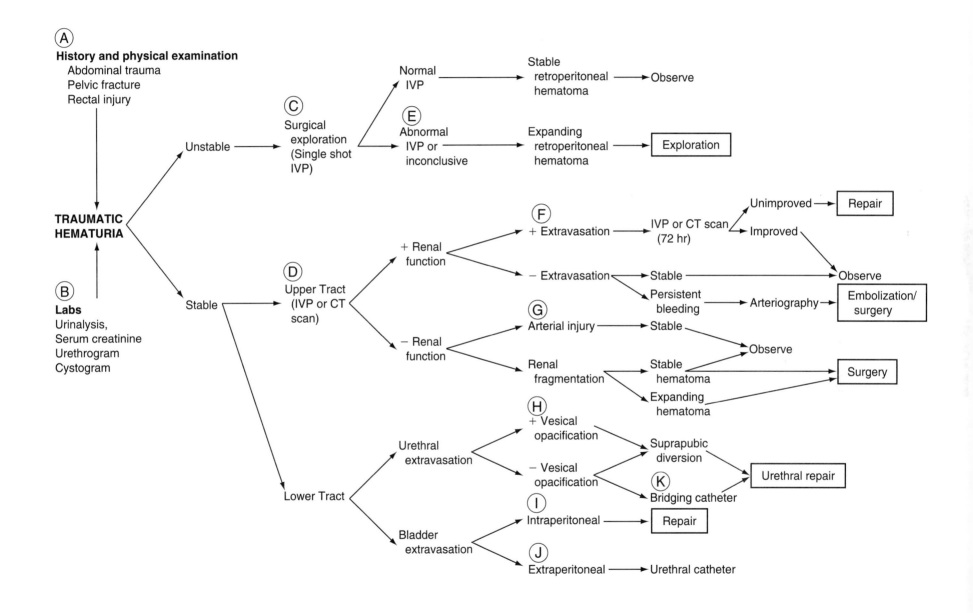

Ⓐ
History and physical examination
   Abdominal trauma
   Pelvic fracture
   Rectal injury

TRAUMATIC HEMATURIA

Ⓑ
Labs
Urinalysis,
Serum creatinine
Urethrogram
Cystogram

Unstable

Ⓒ Surgical exploration (Single shot IVP)

Normal IVP → Stable retroperitoneal hematoma → Observe

Ⓔ Abnormal IVP or inconclusive → Expanding retroperitoneal hematoma → Exploration

Stable

Ⓓ Upper Tract (IVP or CT scan)

+ Renal function

Ⓕ + Extravasation → IVP or CT scan (72 hr) → Unimproved → Repair
                                 → Improved

– Extravasation → Stable → Observe
              → Persistent bleeding → Arteriography → Embolization/surgery

– Renal function

Ⓖ Arterial injury → Stable → Observe

Renal fragmentation → Stable hematoma → Observe / Surgery
                       → Expanding hematoma → Surgery

Lower Tract

Urethral extravasation

Ⓗ + Vesical opacification → Suprapubic diversion

– Vesical opacification → Suprapubic diversion / Urethral repair

Ⓚ Bridging catheter → Urethral repair

Bladder extravasation

Ⓘ Intraperitoneal → Repair

Ⓙ Extraperitoneal → Urethral catheter

Chapter 152 *Pelvic Fractures*

WADE R. SMITH, MD • STEVEN J. MORGAN, MD

(A) Pelvic fractures are high-energy injuries with significant risk of death. The kinetic energy required to disrupt the pelvis also injures vital organs, particularly in the retroperitoneum, abdomen, and thorax. Mortality may result from exsanguination, the acute impact of associated injuries, or the combined sequalae of injury and massive resuscitation. Multidisciplinary protocols for acute pelvic injury management have been recognized as reducing morbidity and mortality, especially in the hemodynamically unstable patient. The goal of pelvic fracture algorithms is to quickly identify potential sources of shock and to prioritize management in a logical and efficacious sequence. By design, protocols overtriage in order to avoid missing a significant injury. Effective protocols will have a relatively low overtriage rate and will allow the trauma team to focus on key decision-making. Time is often critical, and standardization of basic pathways is essential. The key for the trauma team is to view pelvic algorithms as resuscitation strategies, not as definitive treatment guidelines.

The criteria for entering the algorithm should be well defined. Definitions of hemodynamic instability continue to be controversial. Accepted criteria are systolic blood pressure less than 90 mm Hg and transfusion of at least one unit of red blood cells (RBC) with evidence of a pelvic ring injury.

(B) Portable chest and a single AP pelvis x-ray are used to search for potential causes of shock. There is no role for special views of the pelvis and acetabulum during resuscitation. Thoracic aortic injuries cannot be ruled out by chest x-ray alone; however, a widened mediastinum indicates need for further diagnostic investigation.

(C) Resuscitation begins with 2 liters of crystalloid, establishment of central venous access, and initiation of blood transfusion. RBCs are transfused 1:1 with fresh frozen plasma (FFP). For *every* 5 units of packed RBCs, 5 units of platelets are administered to prevent coagulopathy.

Massive transfusion over a brief period is not uncommon, and without aggressive factor replacement pelvic injury patients can quickly decompensate because of coagulopathy despite adequate volume resuscitation.

(D) Initiation of the protocol requires immediate notification of all personnel whose interventional skills have been predetermined to be potentially necessary for the unstable pelvic injury patient. In cases of massive injury, unusual resuscitation maneuvers (e.g., hemipelvectomy or iliac artery ligation) may be urgently required. Experienced surgeons need to be available in these cases.

(E) In specific injury patterns, mechanical stabilization may be helpful in reducing and stabilizing the pelvis. However, stabilization should be viewed as a resuscitation maneuver and performed quickly within the flow of evaluation and treatment. Simple pelvic binders, wrapping of the pelvis with a sheet, or placement of an anterior C-clamp for anterior-posterior compression injuries should take less than 10 minutes and are sufficient during the hemodynamically unstable phase. More sophisticated techniques that require significant time should be deferred until the patient is stable.

(F) Focused abdominal sonography for trauma (FAST) is a critical screening tool for intra-abdominal injury. The key in the unstable patient is to determine and prioritize sources of bleeding. Ignoring an intra-abdominal injury in favor of a dramatic-appearing AP pelvis x-ray can lead the patient to the incorrect treatment pathway and potential disaster. A positive ultrasound in the face of hemodynamic instability requires urgent laparotomy. Further injury definition in the CT scanner may delay inevitable surgery and control of bleeding. Local associated injuries impact treatment decisions. Open fractures, including perineal or vaginal lacerations, increase mortality to 50% and require urgent operative exploration. Diverting colostomy should be considered in all open pelvis fractures.

Urogential injuries occur in 15% of cases but are often missed. The negative ultrasound patient with continued instability and no evidence of thoracic injury may merit diagnostic peritoneal lavage and/or pelvic angiography. The stable patient can continue resuscitation in the surgical intensive care unit (SICU). Diagnostic Peroneal Lavage (DPL) is reserved for patients with refractory shock and a high degree of suspicion of intra-abdominal bleeding.

(G) At the time of urgent laparotomy, all potential sources of bleeding should be addressed. If the retroperitoneum is exposed, consideration should be given to deep pelvic packing. Arterial bleeds in the pelvis, particularly from large vessels, can be addressed at laparotomy.

(H) In the stable patient, more definitive fixation (e.g., symphyseal plating, iliosacral screw, or external fixation placement) can be considered. The patient with continued instability mandates a reconsideration of missed injuries and/or pelvic angiography.

(I) Less than 10% of pelvic fractures have significant arterial bleeding. Though arteriography can often demonstrate some type of bleeding, in many cases the blood loss is not significant. The majority of injuries result in venous bleeding and bleeding from fracture surfaces, both of which are not amenable to angiographic embolization. Therefore angiography should not be a primary intervention in the algorithm. Over-enthusiastic use of angiography can lead to delay in the diagnosis and treatment of more common sources of blood loss. However, angiography can offer dramatic hemorrhage control in selected cases.

(J) Pelvic fixation can be temporary or definitive. Splinting of the pelvis by external binders, C-clamps, or fixators may stabilize pelvic volume, protect clot formation, and prevent ongoing soft tissue damage, although the extent of these effects is controversial. Early mechanical stabilization should be considered to help control venous and bone bleeding.

More definitive fixation at the time of laparotomy should be considered because this simplifies management and may provide better pelvic stability. In the acute period, however, the role of fixation is to assist in limiting ongoing hemorrhage. Time-consuming maneuvers can impede resuscitation and should be avoided.

Ⓚ When shock control is achieved, aggressive resuscitation and monitoring should continue

in the SICU. Follow-up CT scan will be required to fully document intra-abdominal pathology and to better characterize the pelvic injury.

REFERENCES

Biffl WL, Smith WR, Moore EE et al: Evolution of a multidisciplinary clinical pathway for the management of unstable patients with pelvic fractures. Ann Surg 233:843–850, 2001.

Eastridge BJ, Starr A, Minei JP et al; The importance of fracture pattern in guiding therapeutic decision-making in patients with hemorrhagic shock and pelvic ring disruptions. J Trauma 53:446–451, 2002.

Grisoni N, Connor S, Marsh E et al: Pelvic fractures in pediatric level I trauma center. J Orthop Trauma 16:458–463, 2002.

Gruen G, Leit M, Peitzman A et al: The acute management of hemodynamically unstable multiple trauma patients with pelvic ring fractures. J Trauma 36:706–713, 1994.

McIntyre RC Jr., Bensard DD, Moore EE et al: Pelvic fracture geometry predicts risk of life-threatening hemorrhage in children. J Trauma 35L:423–429, 1993.

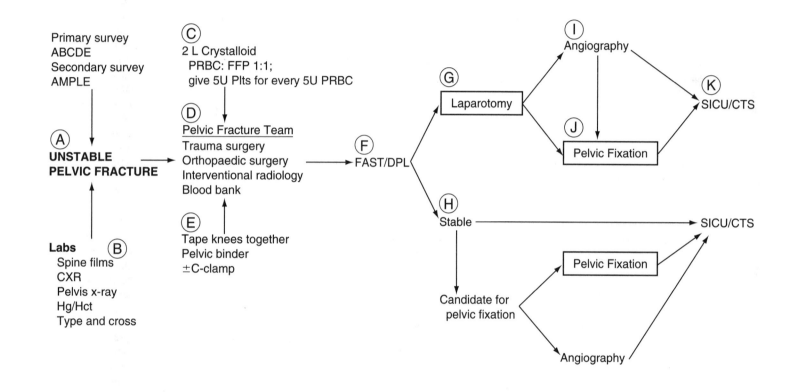

Chapter 153 *Closed Head Injury*

MARJORIE C. WANG, MD • ROBERT E. BREEZE, MD

(A) The neurologic examination is a critical part of the primary survey recommended by the American College of Surgeons Advanced Trauma Life Support protocols. Maintenance of airway, breathing, and circulation are of utmost importance.

(B) Brain injury is thought to occur in two phases. The first phase occurs at the time of impact and is irreversible. The second phase occurs from that moment on and is caused by effects ultimately related to poor cerebral perfusion or oxygenation of the penumbra. Injury occurring during the latter phase may be ameliorated by intervention.

(C) Data suggest that maintaining a cerebral perfusion pressure (cerebral perfusion pressure equals mean arterial pressure minus intracranial pressure) greater than 70 mm Hg, an intracranial pressure less than 20 mm Hg, pCO_2 of 30 to 35 mm Hg, and a pO_2 of greater than 60 mm Hg may help lessen secondary brain injury.

(D) Injury to the central nervous system is often assessed by the Glasgow Coma Scale (GCS). The GCS measures motor response, verbal response, and eye opening. Motor response is graded as follows: follows commands (6 points), localizes (5 points), withdraws to pain (4 points), decorticate or flexor posturing (3 points), decerebrate or extensor posturing (2 points), and no response (1 point). Verbal response is graded as follows: oriented (5 points), confused (4 points), inappropriate (3 points), incomprehensible sounds (2 points), no response (1 point). Eye opening is graded as follows: spontaneous (4 points), open to voice (3 points), open to pain (2 points), no response (1 point). The best score is 15 and the worst score is 3. Although this scale measures global function and consciousness, it is not sensitive to focal neurologic deficits or pupillary reactivity that may alter treatment. Repeat neurologic examinations are crucial to clinical decision making. Deteriorating examinations may indicate the need for urgent neurosurgical intervention.

(E) Confounding factors such as chemical paralysis or alcohol intoxication will often obscure a single neurologic assessment.

(F) Decreased mental status or level of consciousness may indicate the need for intracranial pressure monitoring. If serial neurologic examinations are not possible (e.g., because of sedation), intracranial pressure should be monitored by a fiberoptic pressure transducer or ventriculostomy. A GCS score of 8 or less is an indication for intracranial pressure monitoring. Certainly any patient with a significant head injury and the need for an operative procedure should be monitored for intracranial hypertension throughout that operation.

(G) Patients who are fully alert and who have a normal examination may be observed. Patients who have had a seizure should be monitored closely. In the setting of intracranial hemorrhage, prevention of early post-traumatic seizures may be managed by phenytoin given for 1 week; however, this does not appear to alter the incidence of late onset (more than 7 days) seizures.

(H) Intubation and hyperventilation to a pCO_2 of 30 to 35 mm Hg decreases intracranial pressure; however, a pCO_2 below this level is thought by some to be harmful because it might exacerbate cerebral ischemia. Osmotic diuretics such as mannitol also aid in decreasing intracranial pressure with intermittent doses. Glucocorticoids such as dexamethasone are not recommended in severe head injury. Elevation of the patient's head in reverse Trendelenburg is a simple maneuver to decrease intracranial pressure while maintaining spine precautions. Care should be taken to ensure that the cervical collar is not so overly snug that jugular venous outflow is impaired. Computed tomography (CT) is sensitive for most traumatic intracranial pathology. Repeat CT should be performed if there is obvious intracranial pathology on the initial scan or if the neurologic examination changes.

Scans performed within a few hours of injury may not accurately reflect intracranial pathology. Diffuse axonal injury may not show any manifestations on CT scans.

(I) If a focal neurologic deficit cannot be explained by CT, carotid injury should be suspected and radiographic evaluation (e.g., angiography, CT angiography, or magnetic resonance angiography) should be performed.

(J) Patients with normal CT scans and normal neurologic examinations who are not under the influence of drugs or alcohol may be observed or sent home under the direct supervision of a responsible individual. A post-traumatic seizure warrants observation in the hospital. Concussion can be graded by several scales; these generally take into account confusion, loss of consciousness, amnesia, and duration of symptoms. Estimates of the duration of unconsciousness before arrival to the ER are often unreliable; however, post-traumatic amnesia correlates with the severity of concussion and with prognosis. Patients with a loss of consciousness should undergo a CT scan. Postconcussive syndrome may ensue after trauma and may last days to months. Headache, nausea, dizziness, vertigo, short-term memory loss, difficulty with concentration, irritability, and fatigue are manifestations of this syndrome. These symptoms gradually resolve; however, if they are associated with focal neurologic deficits or if they persist, a repeat CT scan is indicated. In addition, severe headache during the days following trauma is another indication for a repeat CT scan. Return to sports after concussion should await complete resolution of any and all symptoms related to the injury. Resuming activity before resolution of symptoms may result in severe damage even if the second head injury is mild.

(K) Intracranial hemorrhages are evacuated via craniotomy depending on the extent of the mass effect and the neurologic examination. Posterior fossa pathology often requires urgent neurosurgical intervention. Closed depressed skull fractures may be repaired electively depending on the cosmetic deficit.

REFERENCES

Ali J, AC, Bell RM et al: Advanced Trauma Life Support for Doctors, 6th ed. Chicago: American College of Surgeons, 1997.

Biffl WL et al: Optimizing screening for blunt cerebrovascular injuries. Am J Surg 178:517–522, 1999.

The Brain Trauma Foundation: The American Association of Neurological Surgeons. The Joint Section on Neurotrauma and Critical Care. J Neurotrauma 17:457–462, 2000.

Bulger EM, Nathens AB, Rivara FP et al: Management of severe head injury: Institutional variations in care and effect on outcome. Crit Care Med 30:1870–1876, 2002.

Bullock M, Chesnut RM, Clifton GL: Management and Prognosis of Severe Traumatic Brain Injury: Part I: Guidelines for the Management of Severe Traumatic Brain Injury: Part II: Early Indicators of Prognosis in Severe Traumatic Brain Injury. New York: Brain Trauma Foundation, 2000.

Chesnut RM et al: The role of secondary brain injury in determining outcome from severe head injury. J Trauma 34:216–222, 1993.

McAllister TW, Arciniegas D: Evaluation and treatment of postconcussive symptoms. NeuroRehabilitation 17:265–283, 2002.

Teasdale G, Jennett B: Assessment of coma and impaired consciousness: A practical scale. Lancet 2:81–84, 1974.

Temkin NR et al: Valproate therapy for prevention of posttraumatic seizures: A randomized trial. J Neurosurg 91:593–600, 1999.

Young B et al: Failure of prophylactically administered phenytoin to prevent late posttraumatic seizures. J Neurosurg 58:236–241, 1983.

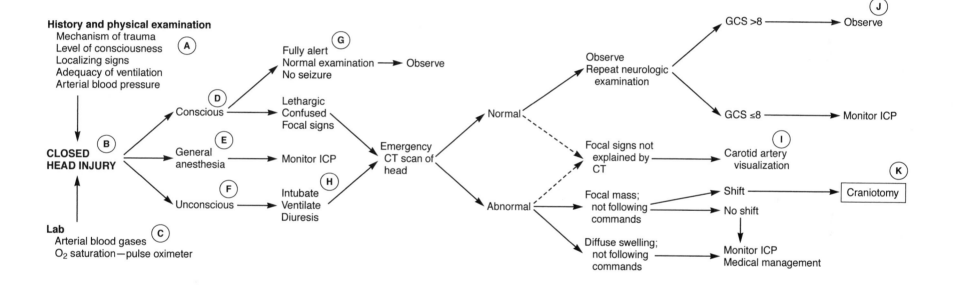

Chapter 154 *Cervical Spine Fractures*

MARJORIE C. WANG, MD • ROBERT E. BREEZE, MD

(A) Recognition of a cervical fracture is of paramount importance. Neck or midscapular pain, muscle spasm, or neurologic deficit in the setting of trauma should raise suspicion for a cervical fracture. Change in level of consciousness or drug use can sometimes obscure these clues, but mechanism of injury should also alert the physician to the possibility. Motor vehicle accidents, falls, and diving accidents are common causes of cervical spine fractures. Gunshot wound victims do not usually sustain spine fractures unless the trajectory of the bullet nears the spine. Some studies have also found an association between head injury and cervical spine fractures, most commonly in the upper cervical spine.

(B) Neurologic deficit will alter treatment options. Motor or sensory deficit, absence of rectal tone, loss of bulbocavernosus reflex, priapism, paradoxical respirations (use of accessory muscles), or bradycardia and hypotension (neurogenic shock) are indicators of cervical spine injury. Monoplegia or a Horner's sign are more suggestive of a brachial plexus injury. Progressive neurologic deficit demands emergent imaging (e.g., x-ray, CT, or MRI) followed by intervention.

The role of methylprednisolone in spinal cord injury was studied in the NASCIS I, II, and III trials. Although still controversial, there is evidence to suggest that high-dose methylprednisolone sodium succinate given within 8 hours of injury may facilitate neurologic improvement, more so in incomplete spinal injury. Benefit was seen after an intravenous loading dose of 30 mg/kg over 15 minutes followed by 5.4 mg/kg/hour infusion for 24 hours if given up to 3 hours after injury, or 48 hours if given from 3 to 8 hours after injury. Decreased neurologic recovery was noted if methylprednisolone was administered more than 8 hours after injury. Although some studies have shown a higher incidence of adverse events after use of high-dose methylprednisolone, a systematic review did not reveal any significant increase in complications; however, those patients receiving treatment for 48 hours may be at higher risk for pulmonary complications (reported in NASCIS III). There is also some evidence to suggest that maintenance of a mean arterial pressure greater than 85 mm Hg for 7 days postinjury may improve neurologic outcome.

(C) The presence of neck or midscapular pain should prompt a thorough radiographic work-up. Plain films are often used first for screening. Abnormalities on plain film lead to more detailed investigation with thin-cut CT scans and reconstructions. Helical CT may be more efficacious and cost effective for screening in trauma patients. MRIs or angiograms are sometimes indicated to rule out ligamentous or vascular injury. If no fracture is elucidated but pain persists, patients should be maintained in a cervical collar until pain resolves and flexion/extension x-rays can be obtained. Care should be taken to ensure that all radiographs are of adequate quality and that all segments of the cervical spine including the cervicothoracic junction are well visualized.

(D) Marked subluxation generally requires reduction. Most clinicians will proceed with CT evaluation of the fracture site first, but in the presence of a neurologic deficit, early reduction may be attempted. Traction is applied through a halo ring or Gardner-Wells tongs. After reduction is achieved, traction should be removed in order to prevent overdistraction or further neurologic injury. Generally, 5 to 19 pounds of weight per cervical level are utilized. Neurologic recovery has not been clearly proven to be related to early decompression or surgical intervention.

(E) Patients who are cooperative and awake, and who are neurologically intact without pain, can usually be evaluated with plain films. Radiographic abnormalities in this scenario should be assessed for age of defect as well as for stability. Thin-cut CT scans with reconstructions and flexion/extension x-rays often assist with the diagnosis.

(F) Patients with neurologic deficits but no bony abnormalities should be evaluated with MRI or CT myelogram. Acutely herniated disks, epidural hematomas, or spinal cord injury without radiographic (x-ray) abnormality (SCIWORA) may be diagnosed by these studies. CT myelograms should be performed both above and below any complete block in order to fully assess any pathologic process.

(G) The decision to treat a patient with external fixation or surgical fusion is generally based on the degrees of bony and ligamentous disruption.

(H) If the fracture is markedly unstable or displaced, or there is extensive ligamentous injury, surgical fusion is usually necessary. Anterior or posterior approaches depend on the nature of the injury itself.

(I) Compressive lesions generally require surgical intervention. Patients with canal compromise and no neurologic deficit or an incomplete neurologic injury may be considered for surgical treatment for decompression. Anterior decompressions usually take the form of diskectomy or vertebrectomy/corpectomy. Posterior decompressions are achieved by laminectomy. Decompressions may be followed by open reduction or fusion depending on the injury.

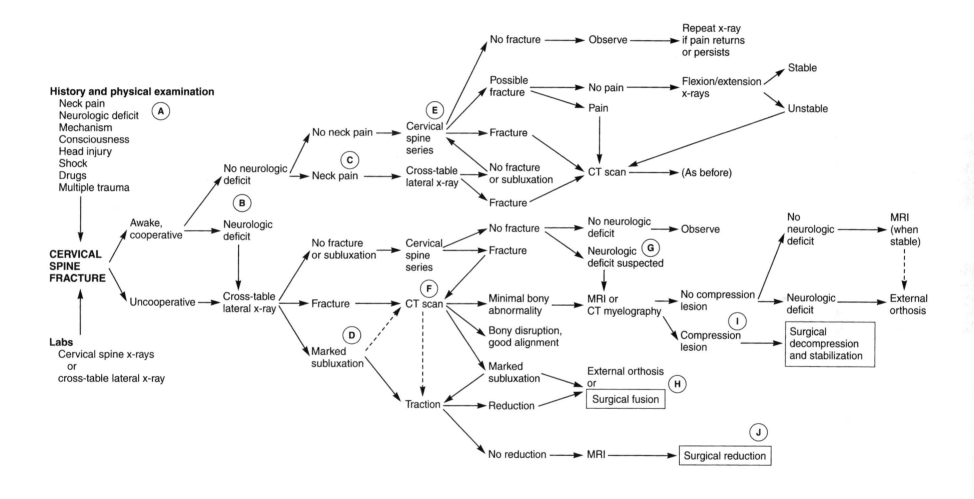

History and physical examination
Neck pain
Neurologic deficit (A)
Mechanism
Consciousness
Head injury
Shock
Drugs
Multiple trauma

CERVICAL
SPINE
FRACTURE

Labs
Cervical spine x-rays
or
cross-table lateral x-ray

Awake,
cooperative

Uncooperative

No neurologic
deficit

(B) Neurologic
deficit

Cross-table
lateral x-ray

No neck pain

(C) Neck pain

Cervical
spine
series (E)

Cross-table
lateral x-ray

No fracture
or subluxation

(D) Fracture

Marked
subluxation

Cervical
spine
series

CT scan (F)

Traction

No fracture

Possible
fracture

Fracture

No fracture
or subluxation

Fracture

No fracture

Fracture

Minimal bony
abnormality

Bony disruption,
good alignment

Marked
subluxation

Reduction

No reduction

Observe

No pain

Pain

CT scan

No neurologic
deficit

Neurologic
deficit suspected (G)

MRI or
CT myelography

External orthosis
or
Surgical fusion (H)

MRI

Repeat x-ray
if pain returns
or persists

Flexion/extension
x-rays

(As before)

Observe

No compression
lesion

Compression
lesion (I)

Surgical reduction (J)

Stable

Unstable

No
neurologic
deficit

Neurologic
deficit

Surgical
decompression
and stabilization

MRI
(when
stable)

External
orthosis

(J) Surgical or open reduction is performed if alignment cannot be achieved by traction. Locked facets represent one type of injury often reduced in the operating room. Other injuries such as fracture dislocations may require multiple interventions (e.g., anterior decompression, anterior fusion, and posterior fusion). A full radiographic evaluation better defines fracture patterns that, in turn, dictate treatment options.

REFERENCES

Blackmore CC, Mann FA, Wilson AJ: Helical CT in the primary trauma evaluation of the cervical spine: An evidence-based approach. Skeletal Radiol 29:632–639, 2000.

Bracken MB: Methylprednisolone and acute spinal cord injury: An update of the randomized evidence. Spine 26:S47–S54, 2001.

Bracken MB: Steroids for acute spinal cord injury (Cochrane Review). The Cochrane Library, 2003(1).

Bracken MB, Shepard MJ, Holford TR et al: Administration of methylprednisolone for 24-48 hours or tirilazad mesylate for 48 hours in the treatment of acute spinal cord injury: Results of the third national acute spinal cord injury randomized controlled trial. JAMA 277(20):1597–1604, 1997.

Chen TY, Dickman CA, Eleraky M et al: The role of decompression for acute incomplete cervical spine injury in cervical spondylosis. Spine 23(22):2398–2403, 1998.

Hadley MN: Blood pressure management after acute spinal cord injury. Neurosurgery (Suppl) 50:S58-S62, 2003.

Holly LT, Kelly DF, Counelis GJ et al: Cervical spine trauma associated with moderate and severe head injury: Incidence, risk factors, and injury characteristics. J Neurosurg 96(3 Suppl):285–291, 2002.

Marshall LF, Knowlton S, Garfin SR et al: Deterioration following spinal cord injury: A multicenter study. J Neurosurg 66:400–404, 1987.

Sauerland S, Nagelschmidt M, Mallmann P et al: Risks and benefits of preoperative high dose methylprednisolone in surgical patients: A systematic review. Drug Saf 23:449–461, 2000.

Terzis JK, Papakonstantinou KC: The surgical treatment of brachial plexus injuries in adults. Plast Reconstr Surg 106:1097–1122; quiz 1123–1124, 2000.

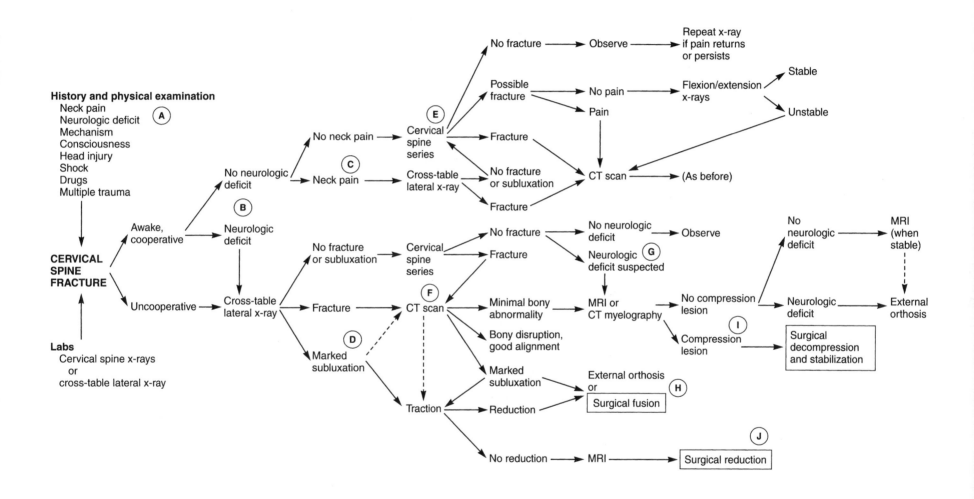

History and physical examination
Neck pain
Neurologic deficit (A)
Mechanism
Consciousness
Head injury
Shock
Drugs
Multiple trauma

CERVICAL SPINE FRACTURE

Labs
Cervical spine x-rays
or
cross-table lateral x-ray

Awake, cooperative

Uncooperative

No neurologic deficit

Neurologic deficit (B)

Cross-table lateral x-ray

No neck pain

Neck pain (C)

Cervical spine series

Cross-table lateral x-ray

No fracture or subluxation

Fracture

Marked subluxation (D)

Cervical spine series

CT scan (F)

Traction

No fracture → Observe → Repeat x-ray if pain returns or persists

Possible fracture → No pain → Flexion/extension x-rays → Stable / Unstable

Pain → CT scan

Fracture → CT scan

No fracture or subluxation → CT scan

Fracture → CT scan

CT scan → (As before)

No fracture → No neurologic deficit → Observe

Fracture → Neurologic deficit suspected (G)

Minimal bony abnormality → MRI or CT myelography

Bony disruption, good alignment

Marked subluxation → External orthosis or Surgical fusion (H)

Reduction → External orthosis or Surgical fusion (H)

No reduction → MRI → Surgical reduction (J)

MRI or CT myelography → No compression lesion → No neurologic deficit → MRI (when stable) → External orthosis

No compression lesion → Neurologic deficit → External orthosis

Compression lesion (I) → Surgical decompression and stabilization

Chapter 155 *Maxillary Fractures*

MICHAEL LEO LEPORE, MD

(A) Maxillary fractures are associated with high-speed motor vehicle accidents in approximately 8.7% of cases. Most injured victims may have associated injures to the cervical spine, the airway (larynx), and intracranial injuries manifested by CSF leak.

(B) The maxilla is constructed to absorb and dissipate forces in an inferosuperior direction through a series of buttresses (i.e., nasomaxillary, zygomatic maxillary, and pterygoids). An arc formed by the inferior and superior orbital rims and the zygomatic arches supports superiorly the nasomaxillary and zygomatic maxillary buttresses. In fractures of the maxilla, the internal and external pterygoid muscles pull the maxilla postero-inferiorly, creating the classic open bite deformity because of premature contact of the molars. Emergency care consists of establishing an airway, either by intubation, cricothyroidotomy, or by tracheotomy according to the severity of the injury. Cervical spine stabilization is of utmost importance until cleared clinically and radiographically. Bleeding must be controlled as a part of the resuscitative efforts. Once the patient is hemodynamically stabilized, a complete facial examination is carried out. This examination consists of the following:

1. Look for lacerations
2. Nose and ear drainage (CSF)
3. The skull is examined for depressions
4. Bimanual palpation is important to denote bony discontinuity particularly involving the orbit and zygomatic arches
5. Check for crepitance
6. Occlusion is evaluated (open bite deformity)
7. Check for palatal ecchymosis indicating palatal fractures
8. Check for mobility of the maxilla (often this may be absent because of impaction of the maxilla)
9. Check for sensory changes in the distribution of the infraorbital nerve (e.g., cheek and lateral aspect of the nose)
10. Perform an ocular examination checking the following:
    a. Visual acuity
    b. Extraocular muscle mobility
    c. Fundoscopy is done to determine existence of intraocular hemorrhage
    d. Intercanthal distance (33 to 34 mm in men and 32 to 34 mm in women).

(C) Midfacial fractures traditionally are classified into LeFort I (Guerin), II (pyramidal), and III (naso-orbital-ethmoidal) based on the level of injury. LeFort I is horizontal above the nasal spine. LeFort II is at the level of the fronto-nasal suture line. LeFort III is at the level of the fronto-orbital–nasal region, giving rise to the classic elongated faces look. Because various combinations can occur in one patient, most surgeons will give an anatomic description of the fractures instead of using the traditional classification.

(D) Radiologic evaluation is complementary to your clinical examination. Computed tomography is the preferred radiologic modality. If a cervical spine injury is suspected, high-resolution 1-mm axial films with coronal reconstructions may be obtained to determine the extent of bony involvement.

(E) Isolated fractures of the alveolar ridge normally involve a segment of bone with teeth present. This type of fracture may be managed in a variety of ways including monomaxillary fixation alone, use of a single arch bar, or by the application of palatal splints.

(F) Treatment may be delayed up to 2 weeks according to the overall condition of the patient.

Nondisplaced maxillary fractures without malocclusion are treated with observation only.

(G) Isolated fractures of the zygomatic maxillary complex without cosmetic or orbital involvement are managed by observation. If a cosmetic defect is present, or if there is involvement of the orbit, then open reduction and fixation of the fractures are performed with orbital floor exploration (particularly if the inferior rectus muscle is entrapped, causing diplopia on upward gaze).

(H) Fractures of the nasoethmoidal complex may be isolated or a component of the LeFort II or III type injury. Nasoethmoidal fractures are managed by open reduction and internal fixation, paying close attention to the position of the medial canthal ligaments.

(I) In general, treatment of the classic LeFort type I, II, and III fractures depends on the patient's occlusion and severity of the displaced fractured segments. The goal of surgical intervention is the reestablishment of normal occlusion (preaccident occlusion), vertical height, and anterior posterior projection of the maxilla as it relates to the mandible. Classically, LeFort I, II, and III fractures are treated with intermaxillary-mandibular fixation to restore dental occlusion, followed by plating of the fracture sites through a gingivobuccal approach. Associated orbital and nasal injuries are addressed individually through various surgical approaches according to the displaced segments.

(J) Mixed and complex fractures of the maxilla are individualized according to the complexity of the injury. Some of the fractures may be managed in the traditional ways if there is no loss of bone. If bone loss is present, early bone grafting may be necessary to stabilize the maxilla to achieve normal occlusion, vertical height, and anterior-posterior projection.

REFERENCES

Adamo AK, Pollick SA, Lauer SA et al: Zygomatico-orbital fractures: Historical perspective and current surgical management. J Cranio-Maxillofacial Trauma 1:26–31, 1995.

Dingman R, Natvig P: Surgery of Facial Fractures. Philadelphia: WB Saunders, 1964.

Foresca RJ, Walker RV (eds): Oral and Maxillofacial Trauma, 2nd edition: Philadelphia, WB Saunders, 1997.

Lauer SA, Snyder B, Rodriguez E et al: Classification of orbital floor fractures. J Cranio-Maxillofacial Trauma 2:6–11, 1996.

Manson PN: Facial Injuries. In McCarthy JG (ed): Plastic Surgery. Philadelphia: WB Saunders, 1990.

Manson PN, Crowley WA, Yaremchuk MJ et al: Midface fractures: Advantages of immediate extended open reduction and bone grafting. J Plast Reconstr Surg 76:1–10, 1985.

Padilla RR et al: Treatment and prevention of alveolar fractures and related injuries. J Cranio-Maxillofacial Trauma 3:22–27, 1997.

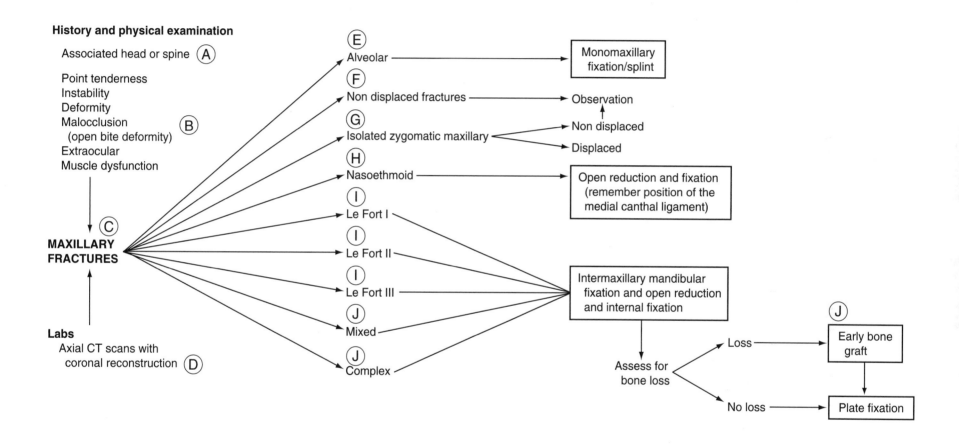

Chapter 156 *Mandibular Fractures*

MICHAEL LEO LEPORE, MD

Ⓐ Signs and symptoms of mandibular fractures include the following: malocclusion (i.e., change in the patient's bite), pain and swelling in the region of the fracture, anesthesia of the lower lip caused by involvement of the inferior alveolar nerve, loose teeth, trismus, hematomas, ecchymosis, and intraoral lacerations at the fracture site. On bimanual palpation one may feel movement of the fractured segments.

Ⓑ The major causes of mandibular fractures worldwide are motor vehicle accidents and assaults. Any force capable of causing a mandibular fracture may cause other injuries, particularly to the cervical spine, abdominal and thoracic regions. In severe fractures of the mandible, do not forget to study the carotid system.

Mandibular fractures may be classified in a variety of ways. Fractures may be open or closed; simple (i.e., no communication with the oral cavity) or compound (i.e., communication with the oral mucosa is present); favorable (fractured segments are drawn together) or unfavorable (fractured segments are distracted or displaced); greenstick (one cortex involved) or comminuted (bone is splintered or crushed). Most surgeons classify mandibular fractures according to their location: body (29%), condyle (26%), angle (25%), symphysis (17%), ramus (4%), or coronoid process (1%).

Ⓒ The most common radiologic studies ordered include CT scans, which are particularly useful for condylar or coronoid fractures; or plain films consisting of a mandibular series (e.g., anterioposterior, left and right, lateral oblique, and Towne's projections). Occasionally, 3D CT coronal reconstructions are helpful. However, the most useful plain film is the panoramic view (Panorex). The advantages of the Panorex include simplicity of the technique, the ability to visualize the entire mandible in one radiograph, and the generally good detail. One disadvantage is that the patient needs to be erect, something that is difficult in the trauma victim.

Ⓓ The following may be treated by closed techniques: nondisplaced, favorable fracture; grossly comminuted fractures; fractures exposed to significant loss of overlying soft tissue; edentulous mandibular fractures; and ramus, unilateral condylar, and coronoid process fractures.

Ⓔ Bilateral symphyseal-parasymphyseal fractures cause a flail mandible. The mandible is displaced inferiorly and posteriorly by the pull of the digastric, geniohyoid, and genioglossus muscles. These patients are usually in respiratory distress requiring the establishment of an airway either by intubation, cricothyroidotomy, or tracheotomy. After the airway is secured, this fracture is normally treated with maxillomandibular fixation and open reduction and internal fixation.

Ⓕ In the case of multiple mandibular fracture sites, patients are normally treated with maxillomandibular fixation and open reduction and internal fixation. The maxillomandibular fixation is accomplished by the use of arch bars spanning the maxillary arch and mandibular arch. These bars are then circumferentially wired together in order to reduce the fractures and obtain preaccident occlusion. The patient is left in occlusion for 3 to 6 weeks, depending on the sites fractured.

Ⓖ If malocclusion is present, the fracture may be treated with closed techniques (maxillomandibular fixation) or open techniques, depending on the type of fractures involved. Symphyseal, body, and angle fractures are normally associated with malocclusion because of the pull of muscular attachments. Angle fractures may be unfavorable because of the action of the masseter, temporalis, and medial pterygoid muscles. Most vertically unfavorable fractures tend to occur in the body and symphysis-parasymphysis region. The anterior segment of vertically unfavorable body and symphysis-parasymphyseal fractures is displaced posteromedially by the pull of the mylohyoid and other suprahyoid muscles.

Ⓗ The primary goal in the treatment of mandibular fractures is the re-establishment of preaccident occlusion. Patients with compound mandibular fractures should be placed on antibiotics.

Ⓘ The treatment of condylar fractures with open reduction and internal fixation (ORIF) remains controversial. Each case must be individualized. Absolute indications for opening reduction include the following:

1. Displacement of the condyle in the middle cranial fossa
2. Lateral extracapsular displacement of the condyle
3. Good occlusion cannot be obtained by closed techniques
4. Bilateral condylar fractures with an associated comminuted, unstable, midfacial fracture
5. Unilateral or bilateral fractures when closed reductions are not indicated for medical reasons

Ⓙ Because of the possible injury to tooth buds in children, fractures are treated conservatively with the application of splints with circumferential wiring.

REFERENCES

Dingman R, Natvig P: Surgery of Facial Fractures. Philadelphia: WB Saunders, 1964.

Fonseca RJ: Oral and Maxillofacial Trauma. Philadelphia, WB Saunders, 1991.

Lazow SK: The mandible fracture: A treatment protocol. J Craniomaxillofacial Trauma 2:24–30, 1996.

Rodriquez ED, Adams AK, Anastassov GE: Open reduction of subcondylar fractures via an anterior parotid approach. J Craniomaxillofacial Trauma 3:28–34, 1997.

Spiessl B: Internal Fixation of the Mandible: A Manual of AO/ASFI Principles. Berlin, Germany: Springer-Verlag, 1989.

Zide MF, Kent JN: Indications for open reduction of mandibular condyle fractures. J Oral Maxillofac Surg 41:89–98, 1983.

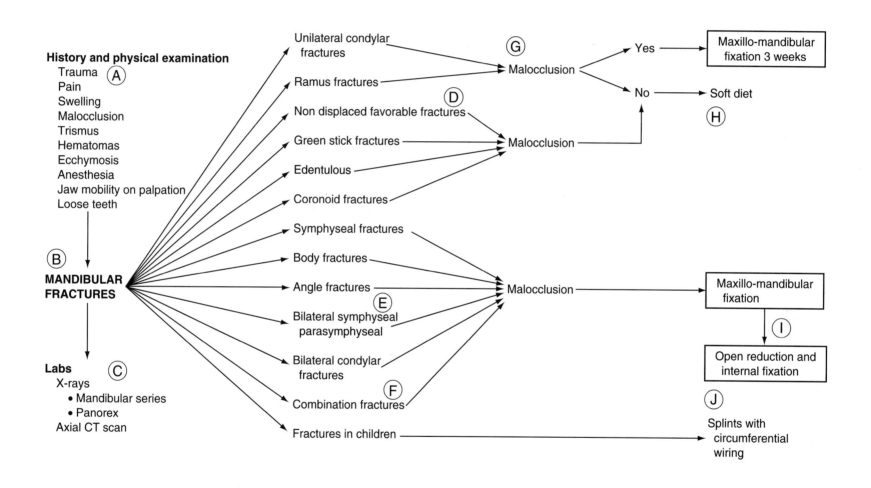

History and physical examination
Trauma (A)
Pain
Swelling
Malocclusion
Trismus
Hematomas
Ecchymosis
Anesthesia
Jaw mobility on palpation
Loose teeth

(B)

**MANDIBULAR
FRACTURES**

Labs (C)
X-rays
• Mandibular series
• Panorex
Axial CT scan

Unilateral condylar
fractures

Ramus fractures

(G)

Malocclusion

Yes → Maxillo-mandibular
fixation 3 weeks

No → Soft diet

(H)

Non displaced favorable fractures (D)

Green stick fractures

Edentulous

Coronoid fractures

Malocclusion

Symphyseal fractures

Body fractures

Angle fractures

(E)

Bilateral symphyseal
parasymphyseal

Bilateral condylar
fractures

Combination fractures (F)

Malocclusion → Maxillo-mandibular
fixation

(I)

Open reduction and
internal fixation

(J)

Fractures in children → Splints with
circumferential
wiring

Chapter 157 *Hand and Wrist Fractures*

MICHAEL J.V. GORDON, MD

(A) The most important aspect of care for those with fractures of the upper extremity is a thorough understanding of the patient. Different treatment protocols will be devised for the same injury depending on the patient's age, sex, occupation, avocations, health status, mechanism of injury, and associated injuries. A seemingly minor issue such as a patient's desire to do needlework or an upcoming once-in-a-lifetime vacation may dictate treatment considerations far more than obvious considerations such as occupation.

(B) It can be said that fractures are universally caused by trauma; it is the magnitude of that trauma that can be questioned. Pathologic weakening of a bone can occur with systemic disease (e.g., osteoporosis) or local disease (commonly, a nonmalignant enchondroma). Treatment of the underlying disease is then mandatory in addition to the resultant fracture.

(C) Fractures of the distal upper extremity are one of the most common injuries sustained in all age groups. Although most commonly caused by blunt trauma, the mechanisms can vary from gunshot wounds to pathologic fracture. The intricate mechanical nature of the hand makes the importance of fracture treatment vary dramatically depending on which bone and at what level the fracture occurs. Some fractures are merely a nuisance to daily life while the bone heals, whereas others have severe long-term impacts on the function of the hand.

(D) Evaluation of the injury is begun with a careful visual inspection to identify any open wounds and to ascertain likely areas of bony injury. Most open wounds do not immediately identify an open fracture; instead, these are usually concomitant soft tissue lacerations unrelated to the bony injury. Nonetheless, it is the physician's responsibility to differentiate between coincidental soft tissue injury with minimal risk of infection and direct bony contamination with high risk of infection. The former requires suturing of a wound, whereas the latter necessitates operative irrigation.

Functional evaluation (movement by the patient) is limited in value secondary to pain issues but is often helpful. Palpation is likewise of limited value in the zone of obvious injury, but it is clearly important to confirm the absence of injury in other areas (e.g., making sure that an obvious digital fracture does not also have a less apparent associated wrist fracture). Radiographic evaluation is mandatory in all cases of hand trauma. More elaborate testing (e.g., CT scan or MRI) is rarely indicated in the evaluation of the acute injury.

The general principles of fracture management (i.e., reduction and stabilization) are applicable to these fractures; however, there are specific modifications that must be considered. The loss of motion associated with an intra-articular fracture can be acceptably tolerated, but the potential for traumatic arthritis and the pain associated with it can be devastating. Thus intra-articular fractures typically require exacting reduction. Fractures involving displacements of 2 mm are considered unacceptable. If at all possible, alignment should be anatomic.

The other critical issue is stiffness. Stiffness can occur as a result of scar tissue formation from the trauma itself; however, it can also occur as the result of lack of mobility (during a period of immobilization) leading to contracture of uninjured ligamentous structures. Although hand function can be adapted to compensate for this loss, the goal in the delivery of care is to avoid this complication. The easiest way to prevent stiffness is early range of motion, but this has to be balanced against the potential loss of reduction, particularly in small bones that heal quite slowly.

There are several different techniques available for holding fracture segments still until healing occurs. These include external fixation (e.g., casting/splinting or placement of an external fixator) and internal fixation (e.g., Kirschner wires, screws, or plates and screws). External fixation usually sacrifices some degree of anatomic reduction for decreased

trauma to the already injured area, thus preserving local circulation as well as decreasing scar formation. Early range of motion is also not allowed with this technique. Internal fixation typically allows better anatomic alignment and rigid fixation, which permits early range of motion; however, the cost is disruption of marginal blood supply to bones and scar tissue that can cause decreased range of motion. Pins or wires that transit the skin increase the risk of infection, which has to be weighed against other alternatives.

(E) Fractures of the distal phalanx are quite common because the fingertip is readily exposed to crush injuries. The result is a fracture of the distal tuft. For the most part these are nuisance fractures, causing limited use during the healing process secondary to pain but rarely causing long-term disability. Because the fracture occurs distal to the insertion of the flexor or extensor tendons, there are no forces leading to the displacement of the fracture, excepting direct trauma. Usually a cap-type splint that straps to the middle phalanx (or proximal phalanx in the case of the thumb) is adequate to prevent trauma to the fracture site.

Fractures less commonly occur in the shaft of the distal phalanx. Because the nail bed is adherent to this area, secondary deformity of the nail might result if left untreated. Closed reduction, frequently with K-wire fixation, is adequate for treatment. If the nail bed has been disrupted, it is imperative that the nail bed be repaired (usually with 6-0 or 7-0 absorbing suture and splinting of the eponycheal fold).

Another common fracture that might occur is a mallet fracture; this is a result of a forceful flexion of the distal phalanx at the same time that there is tension in the extensor tendon. The result can be a rupture of the extensor tendon itself; an avulsion of the insertion of the extensor tendon with a minimal fragment of bone; or, rarely, a moderately sized intra-articular fragment of bone avulsed with the extensor tendon. The first two situations are treated

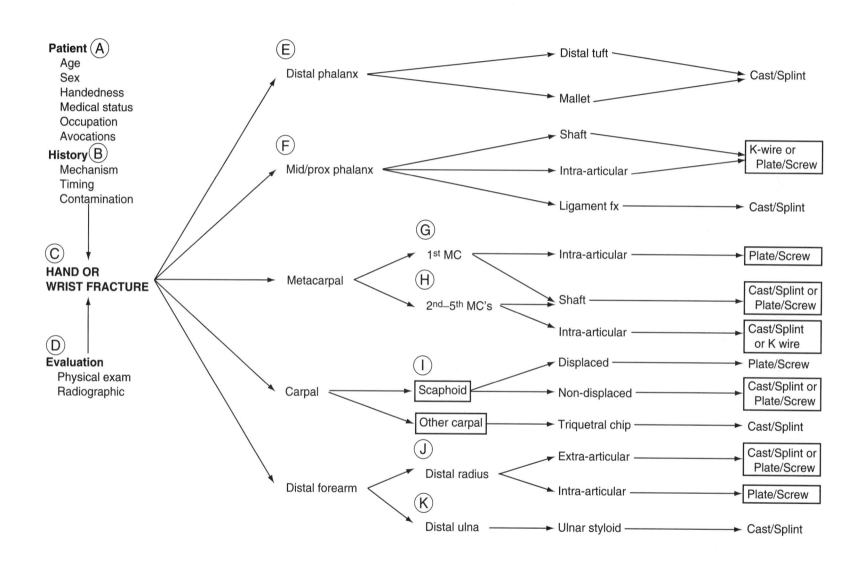

Patient Ⓐ
Age
Sex
Handedness
Medical status
Occupation
Avocations

History Ⓑ
Mechanism
Timing
Contamination

Ⓒ
**HAND OR
WRIST FRACTURE**

Ⓓ
Evaluation
Physical exam
Radiographic

Ⓔ Distal phalanx → Distal tuft → Cast/Splint
Distal phalanx → Mallet → Cast/Splint

Ⓕ Mid/prox phalanx → Shaft → K-wire or Plate/Screw
Mid/prox phalanx → Intra-articular → K-wire or Plate/Screw
Mid/prox phalanx → Ligament fx → Cast/Splint

Metacarpal → Ⓖ 1st MC → Intra-articular → Plate/Screw
Metacarpal → Ⓗ 2nd–5th MC's → Shaft → Cast/Splint or Plate/Screw
Metacarpal → Ⓗ 2nd–5th MC's → Intra-articular → Cast/Splint or K wire

Carpal → Ⓘ Scaphoid → Displaced → Plate/Screw
Carpal → Scaphoid → Non-displaced → Cast/Splint or Plate/Screw
Carpal → Other carpal → Triquetral chip → Cast/Splint

Distal forearm → Ⓙ Distal radius → Extra-articular → Cast/Splint or Plate/Screw
Distal forearm → Distal radius → Intra-articular → Plate/Screw
Distal forearm → Ⓚ Distal ulna → Ulnar styloid → Cast/Splint

as soft-tissue injuries (even though there is a small fragment of bone in the second case) with hyperextension splinting of the DIP joint. Because the extensor tendon does not retract significantly, just placing the joint in hyperextension is enough to reapproximate the ends of the tendon (or the bone). If, however, there is a significant intra-articular fragment of bone (usually greater than 30%), then reduction by either closed or open technique with fixation is warranted.

(F) Middle and proximal phalangeal fractures are fraught with a high complication rate. Both flexor and extensor tendons lie extremely close to the bone and can easily become involved either in the primary fracture or caught up in the healing process. If the fracture is non–intra-articular and relatively transverse, simple closed reduction and splint immobilization may be all that is necessary. Intra-articular fractures will typically require open reduction. Unfortunately, the prolonged healing associated with these fractures (6 to 8 weeks) often results in marked stiffness, particularly at the PIP joint. This is a significant morbidity, and alternative methods of stabilization have been attempted. K-wire fixation is convenient, but it is not uncommon for the K-wires to limit motion by piercing the tendons themselves or by causing pain and irritation to the skin. External K-wires have the additional disadvantage of potentially leading to infection. Plate or lag screw fixation produces significant scar, which causes adhesions to the adjacent tendons and resultant long-term limitation of motion. Many times a compromise between these factors is sought by attempting rigid internal fixation (plate or lag screw) with early range of motion to prevent tendon adhesions. Although conceptually sound, the practice still does not universally result in good motion. In general, these are some of the most morbid fractures in the hand.

Ligamentous injuries, particularly of the PIP joint, are commonly associated with small avulsion fractures of the insertions of the ligaments (collateral ligaments or volar plate). For the most part the fractures may be ignored and the injuries treated essentially as soft-tissue injuries. As with the mallet fracture of the DIP joint, on occasion there might be a large fragment that requires reduction and fixation. Without question, intra-articular fractures of the PIP joint are the most common cause of morbidity, with decreased range of motion and the eventual development of arthritis. Preservation of motion at the PIP joint contributes most to the functional use of the hand, followed by preservation of motion at the MP joint. Motion at the DIP joint is useful and desirable but not nearly as critical as the other two joints.

(G) Metacarpal fractures typically cause less morbidity than phalangeal fractures, mostly because there is more soft tissue separating the bones from the tendons. As a result, open reduction is less likely to cause adhesions. Similarly, internal fixation is also not as likely to create secondary problems. The size of the metacarpals is also greater than the phalanges and so stabilization is easier. This results in less need to cross joints (and therefore less stiffness) to achieve stable fixation. Finally, the larger bones and better blood supply translate into more rapid healing (e.g., around 4 to 6 weeks).

As the dominant digit with a different type of articulation at its base, the thumb has some relatively unique fracture patterns. Transverse fractures occur as they do with the other metacarpals; but for early range of motion, stable internal fixation is preferred to splint/cast immobilization. There are also two specific fractures at the base of the first metacarpal that typically require intervention. The Bennett's fracture is an intra-articular fracture at the base of the first metacarpal that usually has the main body of the fracture dorsal, radial, and distal. The smaller fragment is attached volarly to the ligament and is technically hard to visualize (operatively). The fracture is inherently unstable because the APL is attached to the larger fragment at the radial base of the bone and constantly pulls the fracture apart. Because this joint is one of the most critical to daily use of the hand, anatomic reduction is warranted, though not particularly easy. The Rolando fracture is a three-piece, intra-articular fracture at the base of the first metacarpal. As with the Bennett's fracture, anatomic alignment is the desired goal, using open reduction and internal fixation.

(H) Fractures occur more commonly in the ulnar metacarpals as opposed to the second or third. The most famous fracture has been dubbed the "boxer's fracture." The original use of this term was to apply to a fracture at the head/neck area of the fifth metacarpal. Common (inaccurate) usage has come to mean just about any fracture pattern involving the metacarpal. Interestingly, the true boxer's fracture does not typically occur with real boxers; rather it is extremely frequent in amateur bar fighters or in those with self-control problems who strike a wall out of anger. Fortunately these fractures usually can be readily reduced by closed reduction techniques and splint/cast immobilized. Occasionally, lack of stability or inability to reduce the fracture adequately necessitates a closed reduction in the operating room using imaging equipment and K-wire fixation. Treatment of these fractures is both for cosmetic reasons (i.e., the loss of the fifth metacarpal head when a fist is made) as well as functional reasons (i.e., displacement of the metacarpal head volarly results in pressure and pain on the metacarpal head when power grasp is needed). The literature refers to the critical angulation of the fracture at 30 degrees to 40 degrees. This should be used as a guide because it can be quite difficult to make an accurate measurement of the angle of the fracture. Lesser angulation can usually be compensated for by motion at the CMC joint. Because there is less and less motion available at the CMC joint moving towards the radial metacarpals, less and less angulation should be tolerated in those fractures.

Oblique, non–intra-articular fractures of the metacarpals are also commonly seen. As opposed to transverse fractures, these are inherently unstable. There is almost always shortening involved in these fractures. A small amount of shortening (less than 5 mm) is not likely to functionally impact the use of the hand; however, many times the fracture includes a spiral element, which will cause rotation of the bone as it shortens. This will result in significant morbidity because the digit will cross over its neighbor digit when flexed. This crossing over may not be apparent with the digits in an extended position; many times it can only be observed when a fist is made—something almost impossible to do in the acute setting.

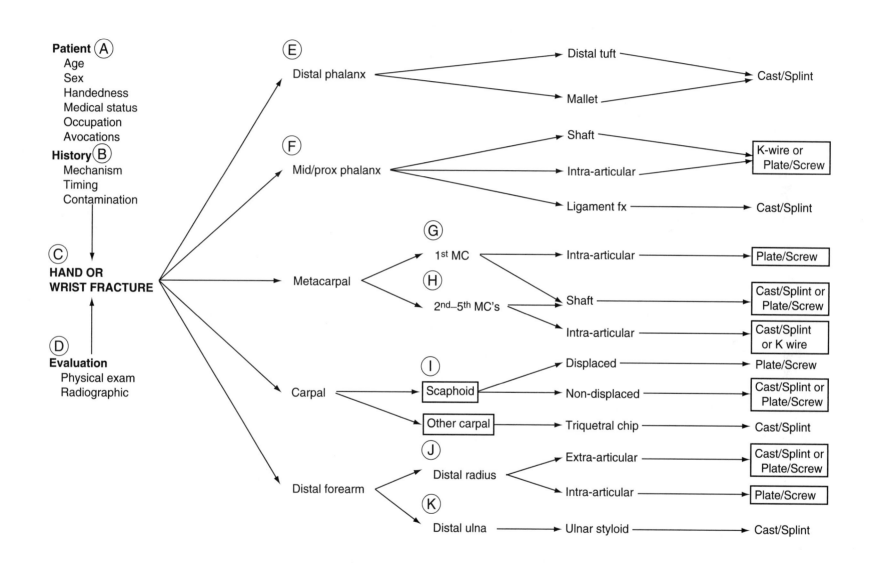

Patient (A)
Age
Sex
Handedness
Medical status
Occupation
Avocations

History (B)
Mechanism
Timing
Contamination

(C)
**HAND OR
WRIST FRACTURE**

(D)
Evaluation
Physical exam
Radiographic

(E) Distal phalanx
Distal tuft
Mallet
Cast/Splint

(F) Mid/prox phalanx
Shaft
Intra-articular
K-wire or Plate/Screw
Ligament fx
Cast/Splint

Metacarpal
(G) 1st MC
Intra-articular
Plate/Screw
(H) 2nd–5th MC's
Shaft
Cast/Splint or Plate/Screw
Intra-articular
Cast/Splint or K wire

Carpal
(I) Scaphoid
Displaced
Plate/Screw
Non-displaced
Cast/Splint or Plate/Screw
Other carpal
Triquetral chip
Cast/Splint

Distal forearm
(J) Distal radius
Extra-articular
Cast/Splint or Plate/Screw
Intra-articular
Plate/Screw
(K) Distal ulna
Ulnar styloid
Cast/Splint

Intra-articular fractures at the bases of the metacarpals deserve special consideration. As opposed to the first metacarpal, intra-articular fractures at the bases of the second, third, and fourth metacarpals are usually not treated to the same level of exacting reduction because these joints do not have a great deal of motion associated with them. As a result the long-term risk for arthritic complications is smaller. The fifth metacarpal, however, still has a moderate amount of motion at the carpal metacarpal joint and so it may be considered for reduction. This fracture is analogous to the first metacarpal fracture, with the extensor carpi ulnaris creating an imbalance and distracting the fracture much the same way that the abductor pollicus longus does in a Bennett's fracture. The fracture is typically quite comminuted, and anatomic reduction is extremely difficult. Fixation is a challenge because of the thinness of the cortex at the base of the metacarpal. Many times gross alignment of the bones with fixation to the fourth metacarpal and hamate with K-wires is the best that can be achieved.

(I) The scaphoid is the most commonly fractured bone of the wrist because it spans the distance between the proximal and distal carpal rows. Hyperextension of the wrist causes significant forces to be exerted across the scaphoid, leading to fracture. The dominant circulation enters the bone dorsally and through the distal half of the bone. As a result, the proximal pole receives its blood supply through branches coming from the distal pole. If a fracture occurs proximal to the entry of the feeding vessel, the circulation to the proximal pole may be compromised by disruption of the interosseus vessels. The final effect is that such fractures might lead to avascular necrosis of the proximal pole and

long-term traumatic arthritis. Fear of arthritis has led to more exacting standards of anatomic reduction. Because the healing can be quite delayed (presumably secondary to issues of circulation), it has become popular to perform rigid internal fixation with either percutaneous or open-screw placement to allow earlier range of motion and avoid the long-term stiffness from prolonged immobilization. It is clear that the late treatment of scaphoid fractures is associated with very high rates of morbidity secondary to the traumatic arthritis.

(J) In general, other carpal bone fractures are less common than scaphoid fractures. The principle of anatomic reduction is adhered to, with exceptions for non–intra-articular fractures or severe injuries. Ligamentous injuries are quite common. The scapholunate ligament is the most commonly damaged, followed by the TFCC (triangular fibrocartilage complex, a stabilizer of the ulnar styloid process to the ulnar edge of the radius) and the lunotriquetral ligament. A relatively common injury resulting from a hyperextended wrist is a dorsal triquetral chip fracture. Such an injury probably occurs from a direct blow to the triquetrum on the distal ulna rather than a torque across the bone or avulsion of a ligamentous attachment. Because there are no static or dynamic forces at the fracture site, treatment is mostly symptomatic with a short period of immobilization followed by range of motion and a prolonged period of dorsal tenderness.

(K) Options for distal radius fractures continue to evolve as newer techniques are introduced and compared with the latest standards. Critical factors remain the amount of shortening of the radius compared with the ulna, the angle of the distal radial articular surface (normally slightly volarly

inclined), and the displacement (if any) of the intra-articular fracture segments. Closed reduction with cast immobilization, closed reduction with external fixation, closed reduction with internal fixation, open reduction with internal fixation, arthroscopically assisted reduction with fixation, and minimally invasive open reduction with fixation with allograft- or cement-assisted support are all viable alternatives for the treatment of distal radius fractures, depending on the specifics of the patient and the nature of the injury.

(L) The most common distal ulna fracture is that of the ulnar styloid process (attachment of the TFCC). Most fractures occur in combination with a distal radius fracture. In most cases there is minimal displacement of this structure, and therefore treatment is generally immobilization. If a significant displacement is noted, reduction and fixation is performed in combination with the treatment for the distal radius fracture. More extensive fractures are uncommon, and treatment is based on the specifics of the injury.

REFERENCES

Chung K, Spilson S: The frequency and epidemiology of hand and forearm fractures in the United States. J Hand Surg 26: 908–915, 2001.

Freeland AE, Sud V: Unicondylar and bicondylar proximal phalangeal fractures. J Hand Surg 1:14–24, 2001.

Hofmeister E P, Mazurek MT, Shin AY et al: Extension block pinning for large mallet fractures. J Hand Surg 28:453–459, 2003.

Stern P: Management of fractures of the hand over the last 25 years. J Hand Surg 25:817–823, 2002.

Trumble TE, Vo D: Proximal pole scaphoid fractures and nonunion. J Hand Surg 1:155–171, 2001.

Weinstein LP, Hanel DP: Metacarpal fractures. J Hand Surg 2:168–180, 2002.

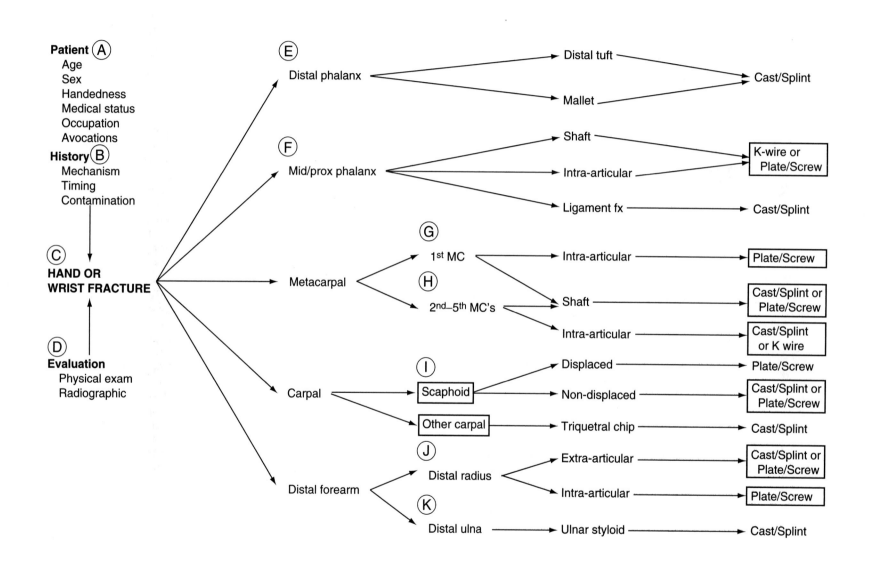

Chapter 158 *Flexor Tendon Injuries of the Hand*

DAVID P. SCHNUR, MD • LAWRENCE L. KETCH, MD

(A) Severed flexor tendons in the hand must be treated as major injuries despite their often benign appearance. The potential for disability can be out of proportion to the immediate appearance of the injury. Important management factors include repair in the operating room using proper anesthesia, tourniquet control, meticulous wound care, and atraumatic technique. The repair should be performed with a core suture using 3-0 or 4-0 braided synthetic nonabsorbable suture on a taper needle and a small-caliber (5-0 or 6-0) monofiliment peripheral epitenon suture.

(B) Treatment and prognosis depend on location of the injury, which is classified by zones (illustration). Primary repairs in Zone II or "no man's land" are the most challenging. Tendon adhesion and rupture occur in this zone more often than in any other as a result of limited space and close anatomic association between the superficial and deep flexor tendons. Although still a point of debate, most authors feel that both tendons should be repaired in this zone whenever possible.

(C) Only contaminated wounds require culture before irrigation and debridement. Tetanus prophylaxis and broad-spectrum antibiotics are routine in this situation.

(D) Delayed primary repair of contaminated injuries is performed 72 hours or more after the trauma when a decrease in the bacterial count has been documented by quantitative cultures.

In cases of prolonged contamination, secondary reconstruction of the tendon should be considered.

(E) Any suture placed within the tendon weakens it. Studies have shown that tendons in Zone II with a laceration of less than 60% treated without repair have better outcomes than those treated with repair. If a partial laceration is not repaired, rough edges of the tendon can be trimmed to prevent triggering.

(F) Injuries of the nerves, arteries, and soft tissue seriously compromise prognosis and must be managed before or concurrent with tendon repair. Pulley destruction requires Silastic rod implantation and staged repair.

(G) Inflammatory or fibroblastic response within the fibrosseous canal (Zone II) results in scarring of both the superficial and deep flexors and, subsequently, compromised function. Definitive treatment of this injury is difficult and should be referred immediately to an experienced hand surgeon for repair.

(H) Primary tendon repair is used when there is less than a 1.5- to 2-cm gap in tendon substance; otherwise, a free tendon graft should be used. A graft is contraindicated when there is gross contamination, skin loss, extensive pulley destruction, comminuted raw bone, or a severe crush injury.

(I) Return of sensation and motor function to an injured digit is the criterion for determining

success, regardless of the quality of the tenorrhaphy. Arthrodesis is the salvage after a severe injury or failed reconstruction.

(J) If a tendon is severed less than 1 cm proximal to its insertion, it may be advanced and reinserted into the bone. If it is severed more than 1 cm from its insertion, intratendinous repair is suitable.

(K) Immobilization significantly decreases tendon tensile strength. Guarded, passive range of motion exercise increases healing, minimizes contracture and joint stiffness, and decreases adhesions. This results in improved function with fewer ruptures. Rehabilitation should be started in the first few days after tendon repair. This is an essential part of treatment and should be carried out by a certified hand therapist.

(L) Repair after 4 weeks results in muscle shortening. This necessitates tendon grafting, which decreases excursion and may limit range of motion of the digit.

REFERENCES

Hunter JM, Schneider LH, Mackin EJ et al: Tendon Surgery in the Hand. St. Louis: CV Mosby, 1987.

Ingari JV, Pederson WC: Update on tendon repair. Clinics Plastic Surg 24:161–173, 1997.

Strickland JW: Flexor Tendons—Acute Injury. In Green DP, Hotchkiss RN, Pederson WC (eds): Operative Hand Surgery, 4th ed. New York: Churchill Livingstone, 1993.

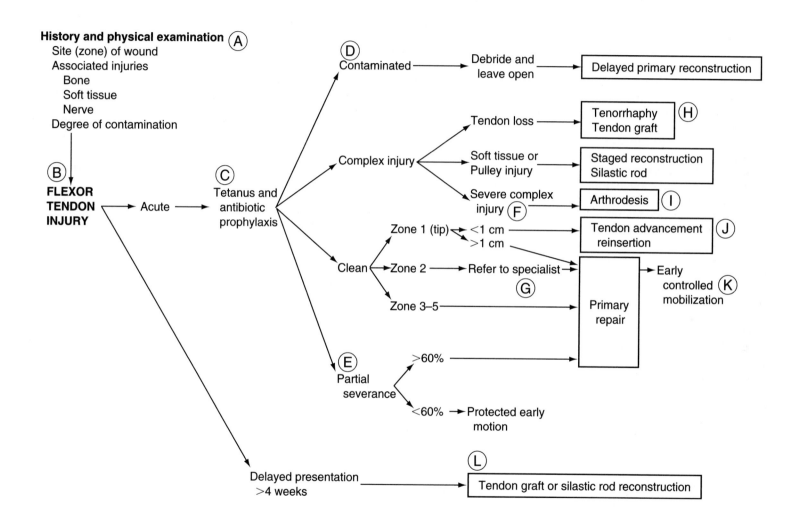

History and physical examination (A)
    Site (zone) of wound
    Associated injuries
        Bone
        Soft tissue
        Nerve
    Degree of contamination

(B)
FLEXOR TENDON INJURY

Acute → (C) Tetanus and antibiotic prophylaxis

(D) Contaminated → Debride and leave open → Delayed primary reconstruction

Complex injury
    Tendon loss → Tenorrhaphy / Tendon graft (H)
    Soft tissue or Pulley injury → Staged reconstruction / Silastic rod
    Severe complex injury (F) → Arthrodesis (I)

Clean
    Zone 1 (tip)
        <1 cm → Tendon advancement reinsertion (J)
        >1 cm
    Zone 2 → Refer to specialist (G)
    Zone 3–5 → Primary repair → Early controlled mobilization (K)

(E) Partial severance
    >60% → Primary repair
    <60% → Protected early motion

Delayed presentation >4 weeks → (L) Tendon graft or silastic rod reconstruction

Chapter 159 *Mangled Extremity*

STEVEN J. MORGAN, MD • WADE R. SMITH, MD

Ⓐ   A mangled extremity is a severe injury that often includes damage to the bone, muscle or tendons, vascular structures, and nervous tissue. Although isolated in some settings, the injury is often associated with multisystem trauma, the result of a high-energy mechanism. Mangled extremities, which include amputations, are dramatic and often distracting to the care team. It is imperative that attention not be diverted from resuscitation efforts and continued evaluation of the ABCs.

Ⓑ   If the mangled extremity consists of an amputated limb or digit, appropriate care of the part will maximize its potential benefit in the reconstructive phase of limb salvage. Although not every amputated extremity can be replanted, viable tissue can be salvaged from the amputated portion of the limb and used in the reconstruction of the remaining residual limb. Appropriate care for the amputated extremity includes removal of gross debris, wrapping the amputated part in a moist gauze bandage, and placement of the part into a sealed bag. The part should then be placed on a bed of ice to maintain tissue viability.

Ⓒ   Regardless of retention or amputation of the mangled extremity, care of the victim with a mangled extremity focuses on hemorrhage control and minimization of further damage to the injured extremity. In most cases, hemorrhage control can be obtained with direct pressure in the area of active bleeding, in combination with splinting of the extremity. Splinting limits motion, allowing for clot formation and decreasing the likelihood of clot disruption in the areas of active bleeding. Arterial ligation and tourniquet application should be avoided in the emergency department. If these procedures are undertaken as a life-saving maneuver, the decision to perform amputation of the mangled extremity has essentially been made. Open injuries should be covered with a dilute Betadine dressing. Cultures of open wounds in the emergency department are to be avoided. Systemic antibiotics, consisting of a first-generation cephalosporin, are generally

sufficient for the initial prevention of infection, in combination with routine tetanus prophylaxis. A medical history is important because some medical conditions resulting in immune suppression (e.g., diabetes or AIDS) may be a contraindication to limb salvage.

Ⓓ   The decision to proceed with limb salvage is not always based on the status of the injured extremity; rather, the decision is driven by the status of the patient. In a patient with continued hemodynamic (HD) instability following initial resuscitation, limb salvage may not be an option.

Ⓔ   In the presence of ongoing HD instability, it is important to differentiate the source of hemorrhage. The ability to perform limb salvage will largely be based on this decision, as well as on the rapidity of control and the systemic effects of ongoing blood loss.

1. When a correctable associated injury is the cause of continued HD instability, and minimal procedures to the limb do not pose a substantial risk to life, then limb salvage should be attempted by stabilizing the extremity with rapid application of external fixation and debridement of devitalized tissue. If the associated injury is not rapidly correctable, and a substantial threat to life exists (e.g., with issues such as coagulopathy and hypotension), then prolonged attempts at limb salvage should be avoided and amputation should be viewed as a potential life-saving procedure.

2. If the mangled extremity is the source of HD instability and is an imminent threat to life, then amputation should be performed. This situation is evident in large injuries to muscle surfaces in the face of coagulopathy. If the source of bleeding is easily controlled, and the imminent threat to life is minimized, then continued efforts at limb salvage are warranted. This is often the case in arterial injuries.

Ⓕ   The identification of a vascular injury that requires repair is key to successful limb salvage.

Careful physical examination for pulse asymmetry is critical. In cases with pulse asymmetry or diminished pulse on examination, an ankle brachial index (ABI) measurement should be performed when possible. An ABI of less than 0.9 is suggestive of arterial injury, and formal arteriography is warranted. In some instances, the severity of the soft tissue injury will prohibit ABI measurements, and progression directly to angiography is necessary. In the HD unstable patient, formal angiography may be prohibited and either direct exploration of the vascular structures or on-the-table angiogram should be performed. A formal angiogram may also be useful in later soft-tissue reconstructive procedures, specifically free tissue transfer.

Ⓖ   In the event of a vascular injury that requires repair, a decision regarding the timing of skeletal stabilization is necessary. When ischemia time is minimal and the skeletal stabilization procedure is brief, initial skeletal stabilization should be performed. This will restore limb length and stabilize the soft tissue envelope in which to perform the vascular repair. When ischemia time is prolonged, or in instances when prolonged skeletal stabilization procedures must be undertaken, temporary vascular shunting is an excellent procedure for restoration of flow before definitive vascular repair. In rare cases, vascular repair can be attempted first, with the understanding that subsequent orthopedic procedures may disrupt the repair. If restoration of flow is not possible, then the limb should be amputated.

Ⓗ   Successful limb salvage is predicated on achieving a stable soft tissue environment. This goal is achieved by stabilizing the bone. External fixation is rapidly applied and allows access to the soft tissues for continued assessment and debridement removal of nonviable tissue. The high-energy nature of these injuries, in conjunction with vascular disruption, increases the risk of compartment syndrome. Fasciotomies should be employed liberally to prevent or limit the deleterious effects of compartment syndrome. Achieving a stable soft

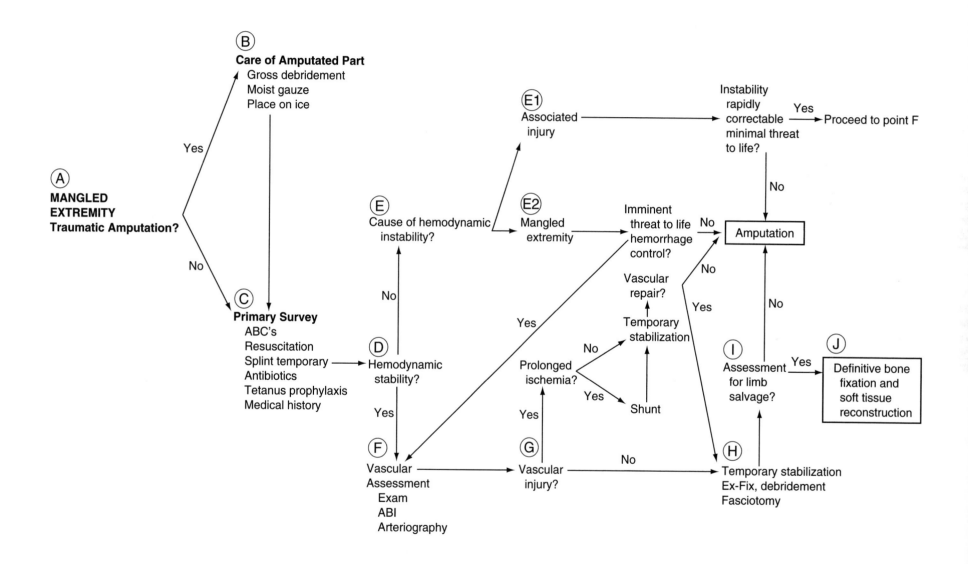

tissue envelope may require multiple debridements over time.

(I)   The ultimate goal of limb salvage is to achieve the best functional outcome possible with the goal of returning to the patient to pre-injury status. This goal may or may not be achieved with limb salvage, and in some cases amputation may provide the same or superior results. Determining when limb salvage or limb amputation is preferred has been the subject of debate and study over the last two decades. As a general rule, complete amputations of the lower extremity are not considered for replantation, whereas the upper extremity is considered on an individual basis. In limbs without traumatic amputation, the most widely used scoring system to help determine the appropriateness of limb salvage is known as the Mangled Extremity Severity Score (MESS). The MESS assigns points for the following areas: skeletal/soft-tissue injury, limb ischemia, shock, and patient age. Combined points greater than 7 are considered predictive for

failed limb salvage and amputation is recommended. Unfortunately, validation of this scoring system has not been achieved in other studies. The Lower Extremity Assessment Project (LEAP), a NIH multi-institutional study to evaluate the mangled lower extremity, was unable to validate the MESS and has demonstrated great difficulty in predicting functional outcome based on injury evaluation alone. The decision to move ahead with limb salvage at this point should be made by the patient and the surgical team (orthopaedic, plastic, trauma surgeons) with experience in limb salvage. A complete understanding of potential functional limitations, associated complications, and potential for amputation at any time during the reconstructive phase should be discussed. Involving the patient in the discussion may improve psychologic outcome. The reconstructive period in some instances may last as long as 2 years.

(J)   Definitive fixation with internal fixation, or modification of the initial external fixation, is undertaken at this point in reconstruction.

Stabilization of the soft tissue envelope may require the use of free tissue transfer or local transfer to achieve a durable soft tissue envelope. Definitive soft tissue reconstruction and skeletal stabilization within 7 days of injury or sooner is associated with decreased complications.

REFERENCES

Bosse MJ, MacKenzie EJ, Kellam JF et al: A prospective evaluation of the clinical utility of the lower-extremity injury-severity scores. J Bone Joint Surg Am 83A:3–14, 2001.

Dirschl DR, Dahners LE: The mangled extremity: When should it be amputated? J Am Acad Orthop Surg 4:182–190, 1996.

Helfet DL, Howey T, Sanders R et al: Limb salvage versus amputation: Preliminary results of the Mangled Extremity Severity Score. Clin Orthop 256:80–86, 1990.

Johansen K, Daines M, Howey T et al: Objective criteria accurately predict amputation following lower extremity trauma. J Trauma 30:568–572, 1990.

McNamara MG, Heckman JD, Corley FG: Severe open fractures of the lower extremity: A retrospective evaluation of the Mangled Extremity Severity Score (MESS). J Orthop Trauma 8:81–87, 1994.

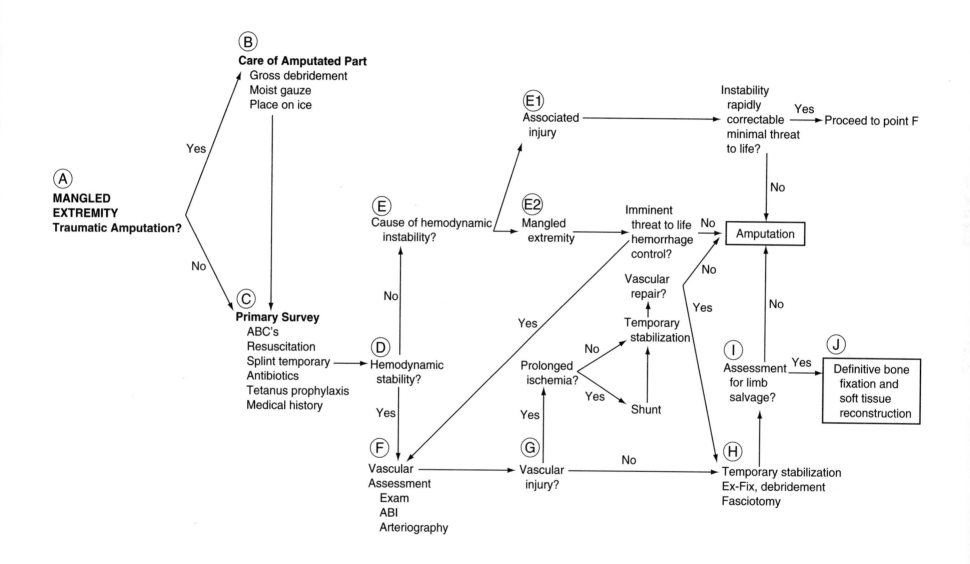

Chapter 160 *Popliteal Artery Injury*

KRISTIN MEKEEL, MD • JON M. BURCH, MD

(A) Popliteal artery injury is caused by penetrating trauma in 56% of cases. Blunt trauma follows, causing 28% of popliteal injuries but with a higher amputation rate. Popliteal artery injuries are associated with crush injuries, distal femur fractures, proximal tibia fractures, and posterior knee dislocations. Iatrogenic injury is a rare cause of popliteal artery injury and is usually associated with total knee replacement.

(B) The physical examination for popliteal vascular injury should include monitoring for the hard signs of vascular trauma:
1. Active hemorrhage
2. Pulsatile or expanding hematoma
3. Bruit or thrill
4. Absent pulses
5. Distal ischemia (pain, pallor, pulseless, parasthesias, coolness)

(C) The physical examination may be unreliable if the patient has pre-existing vascular disease, a large amount of soft tissue or bone loss, multiple sites of injury, or a delayed presentation 12 to 24 hours after injury. These patients need angiography.

(D) Even if the hard signs of vascular injury are absent, 10% to 24% of patients may still have injury. If there is a concern injury, the ankle brachial index (ABI) should be completed. The ABI is the systolic pressure of the injured limb compared with systolic pressure of the uninjured limb and arm. An ABI of less than 0.9 has a sensitivity of 95% and a specificity of 97% in predicting arterial injury. A patient with an ABI of less than 0.9 needs angiography.

(E) Options for operative intervention include revascularization, amputation, and possible fasciotomies. Revascularization should be done before orthopedic fixation. Revascularization is completed either through the standard trauma incision (i.e., a medial longitudinal incision 1 cm posterior to the distal femur and proximal tibia) or through a posterior S-shaped incision. The optimal repair would be an end-to-end anastomosis; however, if more than 2 cm of the artery is injured, an interposition vein graft should be used. Prosthetic grafts should only be used as a last resort because they are problematic across the knee joint. All concomitant venous injuries should be repaired primarily if possible, using ligation as a last resort. Ligation of the popliteal vein results in a higher incidence of compartment syndrome and amputation.

(F) Immediate amputation should be considered in patients with the following injuries that have a high rate of limb loss when associated with arterial injury:
1. Open, comminuted tibia/fibula fracture
2. Severe crush injuries or injuries with extensive soft tissue loss
3. Multiple comminuted skeletal fractures with bone loss
4. Sciatic or tibial nerve transection
5. Other life-threatening injuries that preclude long operative times

(G) Popliteal artery injuries place patients at a high risk (33%) of compartment syndrome. Patients who have concomitant venous injury, prolonged ischemia of longer than 4 hours, and complex injury with crush and multiple fractures should have prophylactic fasciotomies. The signs and symptoms of compartment syndrome include pain out of proportion to examination, neurologic deficits, and tenseness of his lower extremity. Definitive treatment is 4-compartment fasciotomies.

(H) Although most arterial injuries require operative intervention, minor nonocclusive injuries including vessel narrowing of less than 25%, small intimal flap, small AV fistula, or small false aneurysm can be watched nonoperatively with anticoagulation. Some 10% of these injuries will eventually require operative intervention.

REFERENCES

Frykberg et al: Popliteal vascular injuries. Surg Clin North Am 82:67–89, 2002.

Hafez HM et al: Lower extremity arterial injury: Results of 550 cases and review of the risk factors associated with limb loss. J Vasc Surg 33:1212–1219, 2001.

Johansen J et al: Noninvasive vascular reliably exclude occult arterial trauma in injured extremities. J Trauma 31:515, 1991.

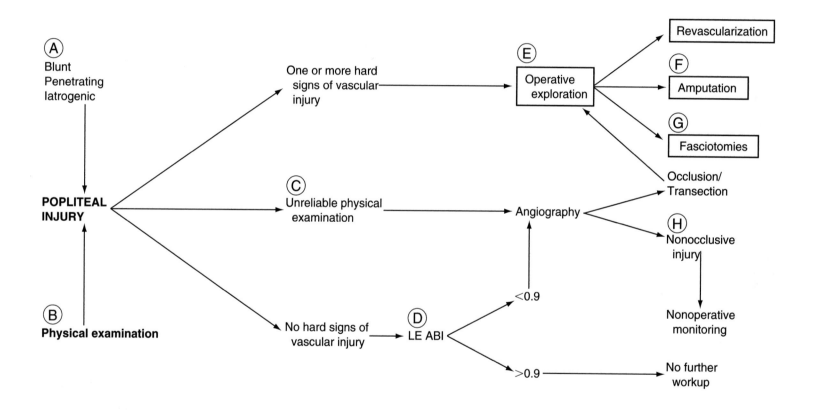

(A)
Blunt
Penetrating
Iatrogenic

**POPLITEAL
INJURY**

(B)
Physical examination

One or more hard
signs of vascular
injury

(C)
Unreliable physical
examination

No hard signs of
vascular injury

(D)
LE ABI

<0.9

>0.9

(E)
Operative
exploration

Revascularization

(F)
Amputation

(G)
Fasciotomies

Occlusion/
Transection

Angiography

(H)
Nonocclusive
injury

Nonoperative
monitoring

No further
workup

Chapter 161 *Burns*

DAVID T. HARRINGTON, MD ● WILLIAM G. CIOFFI, Jr., MD

(A) The skin provides a barrier function for fluid and heat loss, an antimicrobial border for prevention of infection, and has a cosmetic and aesthetic function. Because depth of burn is dependent on temperature, duration of contact, and heat content of the offending agent, minimizing continued exposure should be one of the first priorities of management. For thermal injury, immediate application of cool fluids may reduce temperature of the skin and reduce depth of burn; however, large burned areas should not be treated in this manner because hypothermia may result. Chemical injuries should be treated by brushing off excess liquid or powder and then diluting the agent with copious water irrigation. Adherent, hot materials (e.g., tar or melted plastics) should be cooled and removed as expediently as possible. Tar can be removed with a petroleum-based product. Once completed, the burn patient should be covered in a dry, clean sheet for temperature regulation and to prevent bacterial contamination.

(B) Airway injury following thermal trauma can occur in the upper or lower airway. Upper airway injury, injury above the glottis, (predominantly a heat injury) is often not apparent at presentation but develops in the first 8 hours, creating airway obstruction. If an upper airway injury is suspected, early assessment by bronchoscopy in the first 2 to 3 hours postinjury is warranted. Waiting for stridor can be dangerous because stridor occurs only after 70% of the cross-sectional diameter and 90% of the cross-sectional area of the glottis has been compromised. Lower airway injury, defined as injury below the level of the glottis, is predominantly a chemical injury and is most commonly referred to as smoke inhalation injury. The injury is produced from incomplete products of combustion transmitted to the lower airway as fumes, mists, and liquids precipitated on soot. Bronchoscopy shows soot in the lower airway. Smoke inhalation injury rarely has clinical sequela in patients with minor body surface area burns. In patients with significant body surface area burns, the injury's effects of poisoning the mucociliary apparatus, hypersecretion of the respiratory goblet cells, and sloughing of the tracheal mucosa can result in distal airway occlusion. This occlusion and the host's inflammatory response independently increase mortality following thermal injury.

(C) Edema occurs both in the burned and nonburned tissues. Edema formation is greatest in the first 8 hours but continues for 24 to 48 hours. Resuscitation with lactated Ringer's is meant to partially replace this volume loss and maintain adequate plasma volume. Various formulas estimate expected resuscitation needs in the first 24 hours after burn. The Brooke formula is 2 cc per kilogram body weight per body surface area burned. The Parkland formula is 4 cc per kilogram body weight per percent body surface area burned. Patients with less than 20% TBSA burned can often resuscitate themselves orally, but larger burns need intravenous resuscitation. Half of the calculated volumes are given in the first 8 hours, and the second half in the next 16 hours.

Smoke inhalation injury or delay for treatment following thermal trauma can increase resuscitation requirements. Both formulas are only starting points of resuscitation. Volumes should be titrated to a urine output of 0.5 to 1.0 cc/kg/hour. Colloid resuscitation is generally avoided in the first 24 hours after injury and is initiated once the endothelial leak of the burn injury has been reduced. Some burn centers utilize hypertonic saline and colloid combinations in the first 24 hours to reduce resuscitation volume. Children are resuscitated based on a formula of 3 cc per kilogram body weight per percent body surface area burned using lactated Ringers, but these patients also require maintenance fluid of $D_5\frac{1}{2}$ NS.

(D) In addition to confounding nonburn-related problems (e.g., hypoglycemia and electrolyte imbalances), hypoxia, carbon monoxide poisoning, cyanide poisoning, and central nervous system trauma can all result in a depressed mental status. Patients should have nonburn causes of change in mental status evaluated and should all be placed on 100% oxygen. Blood gas analysis with a co-oximeter to measure directly the percent of hemoglobin saturated with carbon monoxide is necessary. Standard blood gas oximeters and cutaneous oxygen saturation monitors do not accurately measure carbon monoxide. Treatment of carbon monoxide poisoning with hyperbaric oxygen is controversial because the half-life of carbon monoxide is reduced by only 20 minutes. Cyanide poisoning is an uncommon but potentially fatal event and should be suspected in a patient who appears to be tolerating resuscitation with reasonable urine output, good oxygen saturation and no carbon monoxide poisoning, yet is deteriorating in terms of unexplained mental status depression or progressive metabolic acidosis. Blood cyanide levels should be obtained, but therapy can be started before the levels return if the clinical situation warrants it.

(E) Exposure relates to three issues. Exposure means complete disrobing of the thermally injured patient to assess extent and depth of burn and examine for other potential injuries. Exposure also implies concern for the patient's body temperature. Once the patient is fully exposed and assessed, he or she should be covered with a dry clean sheet. The patient should only be exposed in an environment that allows for protection of temperature. Lastly, exposure means that the health care practitioner should wear a cap, mask, gown, and gloves that are not only protective of the practitioner but also protects the burn patient from potential contamination of the skin with hospital-acquired pathogens.

(F) During the exposure of the patient, associated injuries should be sought by a careful head-to-toe examination for external trauma. Up to 5% of burn patients have associated injuries such as solid organ or head injury. Injuries should be suspected in patients who were involved in falls or motor vehicle crashes.

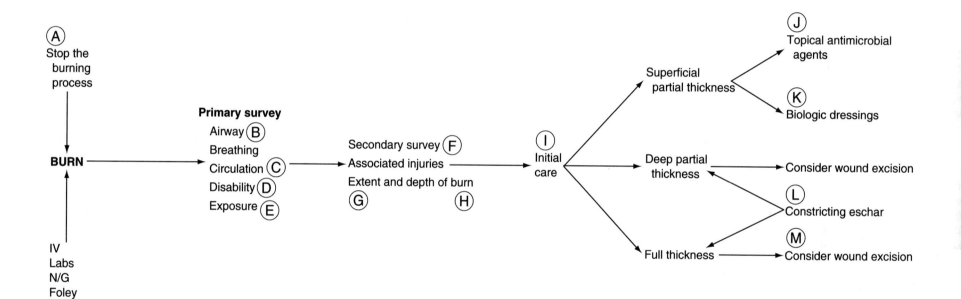

G During the exposure phase of treatment, extent of burns should be assessed. This evaluation is important, not only to predict resuscitation needs but to assess need for operative intervention, calculate estimated length of stay (1 to 1.5 days per percent body surface area burned), and estimate predicted mortality. Extent of burn can be roughly evaluated by the rule of 9s, whereby the head is 9%, the anterior torso is 18%, the posterior torso is 18%, the upper extremities are 9% each, and the lower extremities are 18% each, leaving 1% for the perineum. This rule is reasonably accurate in adults; however, children have a greater proportion of their body surface area in their heads. An infant under the age of 6 months may have up to 18% of the body surface area accounted for by his or her head and only 14% for each lower extremity. Another way to estimate body surface area burn is to use the palmar surface of the patient's hand. The palmar surface includes both the palm and fingers and represents roughly 1% of the body surface. These two methods are only rough estimates of true extent of burn. The use of a Lund-Browder diagram or other device is more accurate.

H The assessment of burn depth is most accurate in the first 48 hours after burn. By 2 or 3 days later, burn wounds often are covered with a pseudoeschar, which can mimic the appearance of a true eschar and make assessment of burn depth unreliable. Dermal burns, also called second-degree or partial thickness burns, are commonly categorized as superficial, mid- or deep dermal burns. Superficial dermal burns are pink, moist, and very tender. Even brief exposure to air causes pain. These burns will generally heal in 5 to 7 days, primarily by re-epithelization, with little functional or cosmetic defects. Mid-dermal burns are similar in appearance to superficial burns in that they are also pink, moist, and tender; however, parts of the dermis often are white and opaque secondary to a true eschar. These burns take up to 2 to 3 weeks to heal and will occasionally cause scar or require grafting. Deep dermal burns share characteristics of full-thickness burns. They are opaque, not moist, and are significantly less tender than superficial and mid-dermal burns. These burns take several weeks to heal, heal with a significant component of contraction, and heal less by primary re-epithelization. They often heal with hypertrophic scar. Large confluent areas of deep dermal burn should be considered for excision and grafting, especially in functional areas. Full-thickness burns are white, dry, and insensate. These will heal only by contraction and, unless they are small burns in nonfunctional locations, require surgery.

I Patients with greater than 20% burn often have a gastric ileus, which should be decompressed with a nasogastric tube for patient comfort. The urine should be assessed for pigment and the presence of myoglobin. Myoglobin occurs in the presence of deep burn or a limb compartment syndrome. Patients with over 30% burn often require enteral nutritional supplementation to meet the stress response to their injury. Patients often cannot consume appropriate calories orally to meet their needs; therefore enteral supplementation with a nasoduodenal tube is recommended. The hypermetabolic response to burn overwhelms the ability to deliver adequate calories to protect lean body mass, even with early enteral feeding and measuring of metabolic rates to estimate metabolic demands. Loss of significant lean body mass affects rehabilitation and, in large burns, survival. Adjunctive treatments to modulate the stress response in order to preserve lean body mass and improve outcomes have focused on subcutaneous growth hormone and the oral synthetic androgen oxandrolone.

J Silver sulfadiazine and mafenide acetate are the most commonly used topical antimicrobial agents. Silver sulfadiazine has broad antimicrobial activity and can be applied once or twice a day, generally with gauze dressing. The silver sulfadiazine does not penetrate eschar well and, when used as the only agent on large body surface area burns, will allow for colonization with resistant bacteria. For these reasons some burn centers use mafenide acetate to augment silver sulfadiazine. Because mafenide acetate can penetrate eschar, this agent can help control bacteria colonization. In situations where burns involve thin skin overlying cartilaginous structures (e.g., the ears), mafenide acetate may prevent severe infection. Lastly, in very large burns where there is some concern over development of wound infection, alternating silver sulfadiazine and sulfamylon can be employed. Although mafenide acetate penetrates burn eschar and provides a wide range of activity against bacteria, it is painful when applied. Further, it can create renal tubular acidosis when used twice a day because it is a carbonic anhydrase inhibitor.

K Multiple wound dressings are available that can substitute for topical antimicrobials. Many of these wound covers can be left on for 7 or more days until the wounds have healed, thereby avoiding the pain and cost of daily dressing changes. However, infection may develop under the dressing. Common wound covers are Biobrane, which is a bilaminate membrane recommended for superficial partial thickness burns. Trancyte is also a bilaminate membrane with an inner layer composed of a mixture of human glucosaminoglycans and collagen. This product should be placed within 72 hours of burn injury and can be left until the wound has healed. Porcine xenograft is also a good wound cover. Acticoat and Acticoat 7, which are silver-based dressings, have a strong antimicrobial activity lacking in Biobrane and Transcyte. The Acticoat dressings need to be moistened two or three times a day to release the silver from the dressing.

L A full-thickness burn wound on a limb can act as a constricting tourniquet. Because the burned skin is denatured, it will not expand as edema is formed in the subcutaneous and muscle compartments. This can result in a limb "compartment syndrome," with the level of constriction not at the level of the muscle fascia but at the level of the skin. Monitoring is accomplished with a Doppler flow probe. Alternatively, compartment pressures can be directly measured with a needle. Releasing the skin with appropriately placed escharotomy incisions prevents development of tissue ischemia as the pressure underneath the unyielding eschar increases and allows the tissue to swell during resuscitation. To prevent limb compartment syndrome, judicious fluid resuscitation is warranted, elevation of burn extremity is mandatory, and gentle active and passive range of motion of the limbs to augment the venous pump of the muscle compartment is helpful. A similar phenomenon can occur with

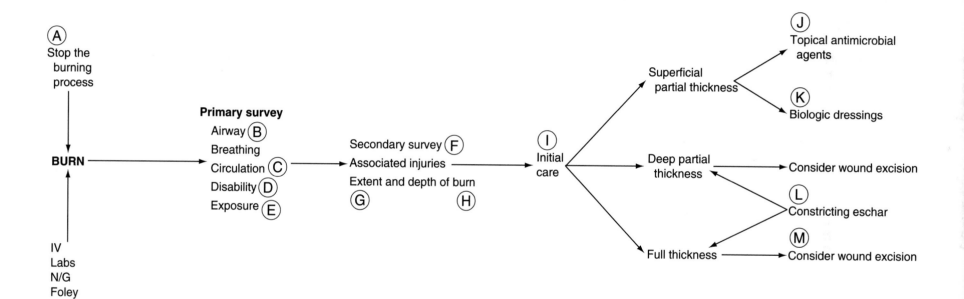

circumferential chest wounds because underlying chest wall edema limits chest wall excursion and pulmonary compliance. Chest wall escharotomies should be considered in patients with full-thickness circumferential chest wall burns and rising airway pressures (volume-cycled ventilation) or decreasing tidal volumes (pressure-cycled ventilation).

(M) Superficial or mid-dermal burns, which should heal in 7 to 14 days, should not be excised and grafted. Although these burns may occasionally result in scarring, spontaneous healing generally results in a better outcome than surgery. Deep dermal and full-thickness burns generally should be excised. Spontaneous healing results in prolonged epithelial instability and significant hypertrophic scar. Areas of deep partial and full-thickness burn that are small and sited in nonfunctional or not cosmetically important areas can be allowed to heal spontaneously. Excision and grafting of burn wounds should be initiated as soon as burn depth can be accurately assessed. Some centers employ immediate excision with the goal of removing all full-thickness burns and covering the excised beds with autograft, allograft, or skin substitute within the first 48 hours of injury. Most centers employ an early excision approach with all full-thickness burns excised within the first 2 to 3 weeks of burn. During burn excision of the limbs, adjunctive measures to prevent blood loss (e.g., tourniquets)

are warranted. Grafting should employ nonmeshed skin when burn size and available donor sites allow; however, when burn size exceeds 20% of body surface area, meshing of the donor skin allows coverage of larger areas. In patients with burns of 40% or greater, other adjuncts for wound coverage may be necessary. Temporary skin substitutes (e.g., cryopreserved allograft and new commercially available substitutes such as Integra) can be employed to biologically seal the wound after removal of the burn eschar. These products allow for early or immediate excision of all full-thickness burn even in the absence of available donor skin for autografting. Once the donor sites have healed, the cryopreserved allograft or the top silicon layer of the Integra is removed and the donor sites are recropped for autografting. In these massively burned patients, sheet autograft is rarely employed except over highly functional or cosmetically important areas such as the face and hands. Mesh autografts, even up 4:1 and 6:1, may be necessary.

REFERENCES

Grube BJ, Marvin JA, Heimbach DM: Therapeutic hyperbaric oxygen: Help or hindrance in burn patients with carbon monoxide poisoning? J Burn Care Rehabil 9:249–252, 1988.

Hart DW, Wolf SE, Ramzy PI et al: Anabolic effects of oxandrolone after severe burn. Ann Surg 233:556–564, 2001.

Heimbach DM, Warden GD, Luterman A et al: Multicenter postapproval clinical trial of Integra dermal regeneration template for burn treatment. J Burn Care Rehabil 24:42–48, 2003.

Horton JW, White DJ, Hunt JL: Delayed hypertonic saline dextran administration after burn injury. J Trauma 38:281–286, 1995.

Purdue GF, Hunt JL: Multiple trauma and the burn patient. Am J Surg 158:536–539, 1989.

Ryan CM, Schoenfeld DA, Malloy M et al: Use of Integra artificial skin is associated with decreased length of stay for severely injured adult burn survivors. J Burn Care Rehabil 23:311–317, 2002.

Suman OE, Thomas SJ, Wilkins JP et al: Effect of exogenous growth hormone and exercise on lean mass and muscle function in children with burns. J Appl Physiol 94:2273–2281, 2003.

Tredget EE, Shankowsky HA, Groeneveld A et al: A matched-pair, randomized study evaluating the efficacy and safety of Acticoat silver-coated dressing for the treatment of burn wounds. J Burn Care Rehabil 19:531–537, 1998.

Wolf SE, Thomas SJ, Dasu MR et al: Improved net protein balance, lean mass, and gene expression changes with oxandrolone treatment in the severely burned. Ann Surg 237:801–810, 2003.

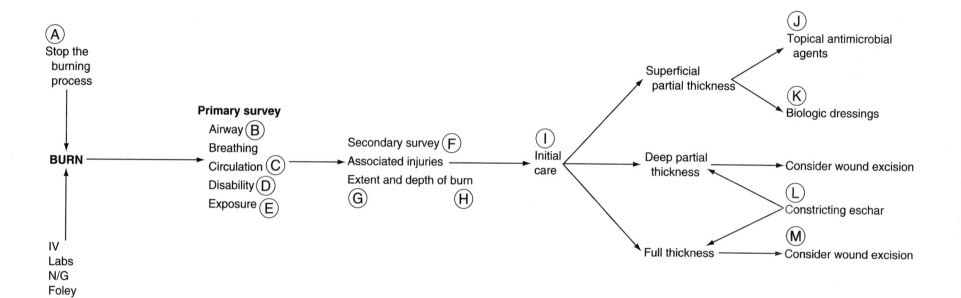

INDEX

Note: Page numbers followed by f indicate figures; those followed by t indicate tables.